WT
100
DHA

KU-148-313

MCARDLE LIBRARY

0151 604 7223

John Aitken Library

T7217

CLINICAL
GERIATRICS

JOHN A... ...RARY
WIRRAL POSTGR.
CLATT... ...DICAL
BEBING
TE...

C

CLINICAL GERIATRICS

Edited by

T.S. DHARMARAJAN, MD, FACP, AGSF

Chief, Division of Geriatrics, and Director, Geriatric Medicine Fellowship Program
Our Lady of Mercy Medical Center, University Hospital of New York Medical College, Bronx, New York; and
Associate Professor of Medicine, New York Medical College, Valhalla, New York

and

ROBERT A. NORMAN, DO, MPH

President and CEO, Dermatology Healthcare, Tampa; and
Nova Southeastern University, Fort Lauderdale, Florida

The Parthenon Publishing Group
International Publishers in Medicine, Science & Technology

A CRC PRESS COMPANY
BOCA RATON   LONDON   NEW YORK   WASHINGTON, D.C.

Library of Congress Cataloging-in-Publication Data
Data available on request

Published in the USA by
The Parthenon Publishing Group
345 Park Avenue South 10th Floor
New York, NY 10010, USA

Published in the UK and Europe by
The Parthenon Publishing Group
23–25 Blades Court, Deodar Road
London SW15 2NU, UK

Copyright © 2003 The Parthenon Publishing Group

British Library Cataloguing in Publication Data

Clinical geriatrics
  1. Geriatrics
  I. Dharmarajan, T.S. II. Norman, Robert A., 1955-
618.9′7

ISBN 1842141120

*No part of this publication may be reproduced in any
form without permission from the publishers, except for
the quotation of brief passages for the purpose of review.*

Typeset by Siva Math Setters, Chennai, India

Printed and bound by CPI Bath, UK

Notice: Our knowledge in clinical sciences is constantly changing as a result of new
developments in diagnosis and management. The editors, authors and publishers
have made every effort to provide updated information compatible with standards
at time of publication, but cannot be held responsible for any omissions or inadvertent errors, nor can they warrant that the work is accurate in every respect. This is
particularly true in the area of pharmacology, where the reader is encouraged to
review the package insert for each drug.

Contents

Geriatric syndromes

List of contributors

Srinivasa R. Adapa, MD
Senior Fellow, Geriatric Medicine
Our Lady of Mercy Medical Center
Bronx, NY

G.U. Adiga, MD
Fellow, Geriatric Medicine
Our Lady of Mercy Medical Center
Bronx, NY

Nanakram Agarwal, MD, MPH, FRCS, FACS
Chief, Surgical Intensive Care Unit
Our Lady of Mercy Medical Center, Bronx;
Professor of Surgery
New York Medical College
Valhalla, NY

Shamim Ahmed, MD
Senior Fellow, Geriatric Medicine
Our Lady of Mercy Medical Center
Bronx, NY

Mehmet K. Albulak, MD, FCCP
Attending, Pulmonary and Critical Care
   Medicine
Our Lady of Mercy Medical Center
Bronx, NY

Ravinder K. Annamaneni, MD, FRCS
Senior Resident, Department of Surgery
Our Lady of Mercy Medical Center
Bronx, NY

Maria de Araujo, MD
Associate Clinical Professor, Department of
   Physical Medicine and Rehabilitation
New York Medical College, Valhalla;
Director, Department of Physical Medicine
   and Rehabilitation
Our Lady of Mercy Medical Center
Bronx, NY

Shahrad Aynehchi, MD
Clinical Instructor, Department of Urology
New York Medical College
Valhalla, NY

Alan S. Berkower, MD, PhD
Assistant Professor of Otolaryngology
New York Medical College, Valhalla;
Chief, Department of Otolaryngology
Our Lady of Mercy Medical Center
Bronx, NY

Niyati Bhagwati, MD
Assistant Professor of Medicine
New York Medical College, Valhalla;
Department of Hematology and Oncology
Our Lady of Mercy Medical Center
Bronx, NY

Megan Bock, PA
Physician Assistant
Dermatology Healthcare
Tampa, FL

May Luz F. Bullecer, MD
Senior Fellow, Geriatric Medicine
Our Lady of Mercy Medical Center
Bronx, NY

Daisy G. Ciocon, PhD, ARNP
Associate Professor, Florida International
    University, Miami;
Nurse Researcher, VA Medical Center
Miami, FL

Jerry O. Ciocon, MD, FACP, AGSF, FACA
Chairman, Department of Geriatric
    Medicine
Cleveland Clinic Florida, Weston;
Assistant Professor, University of Miami
    Medical Center–Veterans Adminstration
    Medical Center
Miami, FL

Marilou O. Corpuz, MD, FACP
Chief, Infectious Disease
Our Lady of Mercy Medical Center, Bronx;
Associate Professor of Clinical Medicine
New York Medical College
Valhalla, NY

Christina M. Davitt, MSN, GNP
Geriatric Nurse Practitioner
Section of Geriatric Medicine
Saint Vincent Catholic Medical Centers
St. Vincent's Hospital Manhattan, NY

Lekshmi Dharmarajan, MD, FACP, FACC
Clinical Associate Professor of Medicine
Weill Medical College of Cornell University;
Chief, Division of Cardiology
Lincoln Medical and Mental Health Center
Bronx, NY

T.S. Dharmarajan, MD, FACP, AGSF
Associate Professor of Medicine
New York Medical College, Valhalla;
Chief, Division of Geriatrics
Director, Geriatric Medicine Fellowship
    Program
Our Lady of Mercy Medical Center
Bronx, NY

Seshagiri Rao Doddi, MD
Clinical Associate Professor of Psychiatry
New York Medical College, Valhalla;
Director of Psychiatry
Our Lady of Mercy Medical Center
Bronx, NY

Janice P. Dutcher, MD
Professor of Medicine, New York Medical
    College, Valhalla;
Associate Director for Clinical Affairs
Comprehensive Cancer Center
Our Lady of Mercy Medical Center
Bronx, NY

Majid Eshghi, MD, FACS
Professor and Chief, Section of
    Endourology
Department of Urology
New York Medical College
Valhalla, NY

Etta M. Eskridge, MD, PhD
Attending, Internal Medicine
Saint Joseph Medical Center
Yonkers, NY

Suzanne D. Fields, MD
Chief, Geriatrics and General
    Internal Medicine
Associate Professor of Clinical Medicine
SUNY Stony Brook School of Medicine
Stony Brook, NY

Barry Fomberstein, MD, FACP, FACR
Associate Professor of Clinical Medicine
New York Medical College, Valhalla;
Chief, Division of Rheumatology
Program Director, Internal Medicine
    Residency Program
Our Lady of Mercy Medical Center
Bronx, NY

Abdolreza Ghazinouri, MD
Fellow, Geriatric Medicine
Our Lady of Mercy Medical Center
Bronx, NY

J. Neil Henderson, PhD
Vice Chair, Department of Health
  Promotion Sciences
College of Public Health
University of Oklahoma Health
  Sciences Center
Oklahoma City, OK

John T. Hughes, MD
Assistant Professor of Neurology
New York Medical College, Valhalla;
Chief, Department of Neurology
Our Lady of Mercy Medical Center
Bronx, NY

Lisa C. Hutchison, PharmD, MPH, BCPS
Associate Professor, College of Pharmacy;
Clinical Pharmacist, Donald W. Reynolds
  Center of Aging
University of Arkansas for Medical Sciences
Little Rock, AR

Kenneth B. Juechter, MD
Chief, Department of Ophthalmology
Our Lady of Mercy Medical Center, Bronx;
University Hospital of New York
  Medical College
Valhalla, NY

M. Kanagala, MD
Assistant Professor of Medicine
New York Medical College, Valhalla;
Attending Physician, Geriatric Medicine
Our Lady of Mercy Medical Center
Bronx, NY

Ajit J. Kokkat, MD
Senior Fellow, Geriatric Medicine,
Our Lady of Mercy Medical Center
Bronx, NY

Kenneth J. Koval, MD
Chief, Orthopaedic Trauma Service
Associate Professor, Department of
  Orthopaedic Surgery
New York University/Hospital for Joint
  Diseases, NY

Susan D. LaMonica RN, C, MSN, MBA, CNA
Assistant Vice-President of Nursing
Peninsula Hospital Center
Far Rockaway, NY

Anna Skokowska-Lebelt, MD
Fellow, Geriatric Medicine
Our Lady of Mercy Medical Center, Bronx;
University Hospital of New York
  Medical College
Valhalla, NY

William Lewis, MSW, CSW
Clinical Social Worker
Saint Vincent Catholic Medical Centers
Mary Immaculate Hospital
Jamaica, NY

Rosemarie Lifrieri, RN, C, MSN, MBA, CNA
Vice-President, Geriatric Services
Our Lady of Mercy Medical Center
Bronx, NY

Frank A. Liporace, MD
Department of Orthopaedic Surgery
New York University/Hospital for
  Joint Diseases, NY

Vincent Marchello, MD, CMD
Medical Director
Kings Harbor Multicare Center, Bronx;
Assistant Professor of Medicine
Albert Einstein College of Medicine of
  Yeshiva University
Bronx, NY

Merville C. Marshall Jr, MD, FACP, FACE
Director
The Endocrine Institute
White Plains, NY

Monisha Medhi, MD
Clinical Instructor in Medicine
Fellow, Geriatric Medicine
New York Medical College
Valhalla, NY

Michelle L. Moehl, MD
Staff Physician
LifePath Hospice and Palliative Care, Inc.
Tampa, FL

Mario Nelson, MD
Associate Clinical Professor
Department of Physical Medicine
 and Rehabilitation
New York Medical College
Valhalla, NY

Edward P. Norkus, PhD, FACN, ABNS
Director, Medical Research
Our Lady of Mercy Medical Center, Bronx;
Associate Professor of Community and
 Preventive Medicine
New York Medical College
Valhalla, NY

Robert A. Norman, DO, MPH
President and CEO
Dermatology Healthcare, Tampa;
Department of Dermatology
Nova Southeastern University
Fort Lauderdale, FL

Wilson P. Pais, MD
Fellow, Geriatric Medicine
Our Lady of Mercy Medical Center
Bronx, NY

Bhavesh S. Patel, MD
Assistant Professor of Medicine
New York Medical College, Valhalla;
Attending Physician
Saint Vincent Catholic Medical Centers
Mary Immaculate Hospital
Jamaica, NY

C.S. Pitchumoni, MD, FACP, FRCP(C), MACG, MPH
Professor of Medicine, New York Medical
 College, Valhalla;
Chief, Division of Gastroenterology and
 Clinical Nutrition
Our Lady of Mercy Medical Center
Bronx, NY

Suresh Pitchumoni, MD
Resident, Department of Medicine
Thomas Jefferson University Hospital
Philadelphia, PA

Areta D. Podhorodecki, MD
Clinical Assistant Professor, Rehabilitation
 Medicine
New York Medical College, Valhalla;
Attending, Rehabilitation Medicine
Saint Vincent Catholic Medical Centers
St. Vincent's Hospital Manhattan, NY

Kevin D. Reilly, MD
Assistant Professor, Obstetrics
 and Gynecology
New York Medical College, Valhalla;
Director, Department of Obstetrics
 and Gynecology
Our Lady of Mercy Medical Center
Bronx, NY

Seema Sami Rizvi, MD
Fellow, Geriatric Medicine
Our Lady of Mercy Medical Center
Bronx, NY

Robin O. Russell, MD
Assistant Professor of Medicine
New York Medical College, Valhalla;
Attending, Geriatric Medicine
 and Nephrology
Our Lady of Mercy Medical Center
Bronx, NY

Albert A. Samadi, MD
Assistant Professor, Laparoscopy and
 Endourology
Department of Urology
New York Medical College
Valhalla, NY

Noah S. Scheinfeld, MD
Department of Dermatology
St. Lukes-Roosevelt Hospital Center;
Beth-Israel Medical Center, NY

Ronald S. Schonwetter, MD
Professor and Director
Division of Geriatric Medicine
University of South Florida College
  of Medicine;
Chief Medical Officer, LifePath Hospice
  and Palliative Care, Inc.
Tampa, FL

Jonathan A. Ship, DMD
Professor, Department of
  Oral Medicine
Director, Bluestone Center for Clinical
  Research
New York University College of
  Dentistry, NY

Robert M. Simon, MD
Associate Chairman, Graduate
  Medical Education
Department of Physical Medicine
  and Rehabilitation
Saint Vincent Catholic
  Medical Centers
St. Vincent's Hospital Manhattan, NY

Upinder Singh, MD
Clinical Director
Independent Living Services
N. Syracuse, NY

William D. Spielfogel, DPM, FACFAS
Clinical Instructor
Department of Orthopaedics
Mount Sinai School of Medicine, NY

Margaret M. Squillace, MD, MPH
Clinical Assistant Professor
  of Medicine
Clinical Assistant Professor of Community
  and Preventive Medicine
New York Medical College, Valhalla;
Associate Program Director,
  Internal Medicine
Our Lady of Mercy Medical Center
Bronx, NY

Harvey Strauss, DPM, FACFAS
Chief, Division of Podiatric Medicine
  and Surgery
Director, Podiatric Residency
  Training Program
Our Lady of Mercy Medical Center
University Hospital of New York
  Medical College
Valhalla, NY

Mary-Letitia Timiras, MD, FACP
Chief, Geriatrics
Associate Director, Internal Medicine
Overlook Hospital
Atlantic Health System
Summit, NJ

Joey T. Ugalino, MD
Assistant Professor of Medicine
New York Medical College, Valhalla;
Attending Physician, Geriatric Medicine
Our Lady of Mercy Medical Center
Bronx, NY

Dilip Unnikrishnan, MD
Fellow, Geriatric Medicine
Our Lady of Mercy Medical Center
Bronx, NY

Durairaj Venkatasamy, MD
Fellow, Geriatric Medicine
Our Lady of Mercy Medical Center
Bronx, NY

Jeffrey M. Weinberg, MD
Attending, Department of Dermatology
St. Luke's-Roosevelt Hospital Center;
Beth-Israel Medical Center
Philips Ambulatory Care Center, NY

J. Elizabeth Whiteman, MD
Assistant Professor of Medicine
UCLA Department of
  Geriatric Medicine
UCLA Medical Center
Los Angeles, CA

Peter H. Wiernik, MD
Professor of Medicine and
    Radiation Oncology
New York Medical College, Valhalla;
Director, Comprehensive Cancer Center
Our Lady of Mercy Medical Center
Bronx, NY

Joseph D. Zuckerman, MD
Chairman and Professor
Department of Orthopaedic Surgery
New York University/Hospital for Joint
    Diseases, NY

Preface

Trends in global aging necessitate that our health community make changes in the way in which it provides care to older adults. The geriatric segment of the population is presently large and will grow rapidly to occupy an even larger segment of an aging society. Many of these older individuals lead active and independent lives. However, others are burdened and made dependent by crippling illness with impaired quality of life. Are we really prepared to meet the explosive growth and demands of this population? Readiness requires planning in several domains including the hospital, community, sub-acute and long-term care settings, public health and education. Both primary and specialty care providers in practice today must make adjustments in their delivery of health care. In addition, we must train future generations of health providers to handle the daunting task of caring for older adults in this century.

Until the world is ready to provide trained geriatricians for the global needs of the elderly, most primary health-care providers and some specialists will have no choice but to provide 'geriatric care'. The primary care provider in particular has the challenging task of dealing with the range of complex problems of the geriatric individual. Thus, to serve the needs of the elderly, one must enrich the fund of knowledge of both primary care and specialist providers in geriatric and gerontological areas of their practice. The quality of care provided to our elderly will depend considerably on continuing education of both the provider in practice today as well as the students and trainees who will provide care in the years to come. Textbooks and journals in geriatric medicine are valuable tools for providing the foundation for appropriate and effective care practices. The objective of this textbook of *Clinical Geriatrics* is to contribute to the soaring educational needs in geriatrics the world over.

The first edition of *Clinical Geriatrics* is broadly divided into five sections, each of which comprises several chapters. The first section describes the basic principles of geriatrics; the second discusses typical geriatric syndromes; the third focuses on commonly encountered neuropsychiatric problems in older adults; the fourth is a compilation of chapters on systems involvement; and the final section depicts miscellaneous problems of growing importance in the elderly. The range of subjects provided is by no means vast, but appears reasonable. We have attempted to organize chapters in a practical manner and simplify the material for easy reading. Most chapters are illustrated with tables and figures to provide concise data. Efforts have been made to provide up-to-date references.

This textbook seeks to provide satisfying reading for primary care physicians in internal medicine and family practice, nurse practitioners, nurses and physician assistants who provide care for the elderly. The work also offers ample material for medical, nursing and physician assistant students. Fellows training in geriatric medicine have access to several excellent texts; while this book is certainly not all-inclusive, it is likely to be a helpful grounding in geriatric medicine.

We are grateful to the many individuals who helped convert this idea into a textbook. We are indebted to our mentors, trainees and contributors who have freely donated time from their busy teaching and practice schedules to impart ideas and experiences to help complete this project. In addition, we give our sincere thanks to the staff members of CRC Press/Parthenon Publishing for their co-operation and assistance in the creation of this text. Finally, we would like to dedicate this work to our wives and children who have been sources of great joy, patience, understanding and support during a difficult year that has been demanding on our time.

While geriatric medicine has been a mainstay in Europe for over half a century, the maturing of this discipline has been noted only in the past few decades in the USA. Our older patients have taught us much and have been instrumental in this development. The editors as well have enhanced their knowledge through both their practice of clinical geriatrics and this undertaking. It is our hope that this book proves timely and contributes in a small way to improving the knowledge and skills of those who wish to provide their time and lives for the elderly.

T.S. Dharmarajan, MD, FACP, AGSF
Robert A. Norman, DO, MPH

Foreword

As the aging population increases in numbers worldwide, healthcare professionals from all adult medical disciplines need to become aware of geriatric issues as important components of their clinical practices. The major features of geriatric medicine are not just the aging process itself, but the preservation and restoration of function. Geriatric practice does not mean caring for older individuals, but implies a mindset that is incorporated into all medical specialties, which is to improve the health and well-being of patients with chronic disease and/or disability throughout life.

Geriatrics is a relatively new specialty in the United States, and to date, most of the textbooks on the subject are directed at individuals who plan to work in this discipline as their major career path. There is a need for a geriatrics book that critically and succinctly encompasses all the available information on this subject for the primary care physician, nurse and medical trainee. *Clinical Geriatrics* fills this important void, and its editors, Drs. Dharmarajan and Norman, accomplish this task in a masterful fashion. Both are distinguished geriatric clinicians, teachers, and researchers. Remarkably, almost half of the chapters in this book are co-authored by these same individuals, which provides for great consistency in style and content. The other contributors are noted experts in their fields. The book is well-organized, easy to read, and inclusive of basic geriatric principles, geriatric syndromes, and organ-specific clinical problems seen in older patients. Moreover, each chapter provides updated references for the reader who wishes to pursue a topic in greater detail.

Clearly, *Clinical Geriatrics* is a 'labor of love', and the editors and their collaborators should be congratulated for their fine effort. The book provides an excellent foundation for geriatricians and non-geriatricians to learn the principles and practice of geriatric medicine as they continue their self-education and apply modern up-to-date information for the well-being of their patients.

William H. Frishman MD, MACP
Barbara & William Rosenthal Professor of Medicine; Chair of Medicine
New York Medical College, Valhalla, NY;
Director of Medicine
Westchester Medical Center, Valhalla, NY;
Co-Principal Investigator,
The Bronx Longitudinal Aging Study

August 2002

1 Aging and public health

J. Neil Henderson, PhD

INTRODUCTION

Never before have so many people lived so long. Although today's unprecedented longevity began in the early 20th century, the link of public health with aging is one of the newest constructs of the public health paradigm. Today, the demographics of the American and international populations create an imperative for the inclusion of aging as an integral part of the public health mission. In fact, in 1978, a few American Public Health Association members initiated a special interest group titled 'Gerontological Health'. Now, there is a rapidly growing interest in the development of this topic as reflected in new and specific curricular and text offerings in public health and aging in colleges of public health across the nation. Still, overall, public health response trails far behind the constantly advancing surge of aging citizens.

The corrective for the problems of public health and aging is as multifaceted as the phenomenon itself. While there are apparently fixed biologic parameters regarding a person's longevity and disease risks, there are also known behavioral 'interventions' that can be employed in early and midlife to provide some protection in late life. For example, early optimal nutrition and brain development are clearly linked[1,2]. Also, risk for skin cancer in late life is a function of early life experiences of sunburn[3,4]. Lifetime attention to cardiovascular health, such as hypertension, may also contribute to protection from strokes[3,5]. Last, Alzheimer's disease may be symptomatically moderated in those with large brain reserve capacities due to inheritance and lifetime cognitive stimulation[6]. Research has also indicated that estrogen replacement therapy may delay the clinical manifestations of dementia in women[7,8].

In terms of medical advances, the cures for chronic disease will probably remain elusive, but their symptomatic management will probably increase in effectiveness. For example, diabetes management is currently being improved with nasal inhalants so that behavioral obstacles are significantly reduced[9]. Even Alzheimer's disease continues to have more advances in drugs to improve the cognitive capacities of victims so that better years will be a reality.

Educationally, those in health sciences training and practice have increased amounts of scientific literature and continuing education available. The US Public Health Service has developed a division of geriatric initiatives in its Bureau of Health Professions branch. One result is the development of several geriatric education centers across the nation. These also have a strong responsibility toward attention to aging in a culturally diverse world[10].

Policy issues for improving the health of elders in communities include new methods of financing and delivering long-term care.

A primary part of such a scenario is the development of support for in-home care as a means of reducing the use of institutional care, which is the most costly of all long-term care types[11]. Also, less obvious matters must be considered. For example, the National Institute on Aging is now conducting experiments to determine the most effective means by which to train at-home caregivers for Alzheimer's disease victims[12]. Most people know the name of the disease, but little else, and certainly not the specifics of providing care to confused and forgetful adults.

The most obvious connection of public health and aging is not age segmentation. It is most productive to examine public health and aging from the perspective of life span[13]. Gerontology, while seemingly defined as specific to old age, is actually an examination of the *process* of aging. The process of aging is a life-long phenomenon. This life span conceptual base leads to the concept of 'preventive gerontology'[14]. Preventive gerontology accounts for the health-relevant events of pre-senescent life in terms of risk identification and avoidance. The product of such behavior should be the reduction of certain deleterious outcomes in senescence.

DEMOGRAPHICS

Old is new. This means that while there have always been some people who have lived well into their sixties and seventies or even beyond, the magnitude of this longevity today is a very recent development among the human species. If age at death is plotted for the human evolutionary line beginning about 3–5 million years ago, most hominids were dying in their teens and twenties. By the time the first *Homo sapiens* of the Neanderthal subspecies were around, human life averaged about 30–38 years. The date was 100 000 years ago. By 50 000 years ago, the first *Homo sapiens* were present and lived into their late thirties and early forties as a group. It is true that some lived into their sixties, but only a few. By 10 000 years ago, humans had discovered how to grow plants and tend herd animals for an improved food supply. Yet, longevity stayed basically the same as it had been for the past 40 000 years. The probable cause for the ceiling effect on longevity was the lack of control over infectious disease[15,16].

It was not until the 20th century that human longevity began commonly to climb to its current extent of 75+ years for most people in technologically developed societies. In AD 1900 in the USA, the average age of death was 49 years, due primarily to problems of high infant mortality. However, by the mid-century mark, the rapid ascent of human longevity was well on its way. It has not yet stopped climbing. Today, public health is practiced in the face of an unprecedented demographic event marked by common and extreme longevity.

Global aging is happening at a record-breaking rate of 800 000 new members entering the 65+ cohort per month according to *An Aging World: 2001*[17]. Also from Kinsella and Velkoff[17], the geographic distribution of this growth is surprisingly uneven. More than three-quarters of this burgeoning global growth is in still-developing countries. The USA is 32nd in worldwide ranking of 65+ populations while Italy has the highest national percentage of 65+ citizens: 18%. However, for the oldest cohort (80+ population), more than 33% live in three nations: China (11.5 million), the USA (9.2 million) and India (6.2 million).

Data reported by Kinsella and Velkoff[17] show that Western Europe is now nearly dominated by nations whose 65+ population is over 13%, whereas Canada and the USA have fewer elders, representing 8–12.9%. However, in less than 30 years, Canada and the USA will join Western Europe in the 13% bracket of elders aged 65+ in the total population. In Europe, the 2000 census showed a shift from Sweden as the nation with the highest percentage of 65+ (17.3%) to Italy, with 18.1% of its population aged 65 and older. Also, Greece (17.3%) now shares second place with Sweden.

It is obvious from the preceding text that the USA is a major player in global aging. In 2000, there were 35 million people over age 65 in the USA, comprising a little under 13% of the US population[18]. By the year 2030, this number will double to 70 million and constitute 23% of the total population[18]. For those surviving to age 65, men will live another 15.2 years and women another 19.1 years[19]. The fastest growing age segment is the 85 and over group[20,21]. Today, the 85+ cohort is 4.2 million people which is 34 times larger than the same cohort in 1900[18]. On November 1st, 2000, the 68 000 American centenarians represented a doubling since 1990, but even more stunning is that, in little more than 45 years, this 100-year-old group will reach 1.1 million members[22]. It is exactly these oldest groups that have the highest risk for becoming symptomatic for several chronic diseases, many of which produce incapacitating dependencies.

Across the USA, the geographic distribution of the older adult population is uneven. By population numbers, California ranks first (3.6 million), Florida second (2.8 million) and New York third (2.4 million)[18]. However, by percentage, Florida ranks first with 17.6% of its population over age 65 compared to the nation's 12.9% over the age of 65[18]. Within states there can be great variation, too. In Florida, for example, the west coast counties average 34% of elders over age 65 while the inland adjacent counties are at about the national average[23].

Among older adults in the USA, the Hispanic population is the fastest growing of the so-called ethnic minority groups with a projected increase of 91% by 2030[19]. African-American elders will increase by 159% and Native Americans by 294%[19]. In 2000, about 16% of persons aged 65+ were considered a minority, and these will increase to 25% in 2030[18].

EXPOSURE TO TIME

There are several conditions for which increased risk occurs as a function of advancing years of life. These include the major diseases of mortality such as cardiovascular diseases, cancers, brain injuries such as strokes, metabolic disorders such as diabetes mellitus type II, osteoporosis and dementing diseases such as Alzheimer's disease and vascular dementias. There are no illusions that health science will eliminate death, nor would this be desirable. However, there are good chances of moderating the direct effects of these chronic diseases at the population scale, as well as pushing their onset into the future. The result is that, while the disease is not eradicated, its effects are postponed. Consequently, the elusive couplet of longevity and quality of life moves from fantasy to viable experiential reality.

The upper limit of human longevity is about 110–115 years[24]. This is determined by studies of various animals' metabolic rates related to their body mass. The index figure generated by this calculation is plotted against the species-specific life span of several animals including humans. For example, dogs' species-specific life span years correspond to about 12–15 chronological years, whereas those of horses correspond to about 40–45 chronological years. At an extreme, some tortoises map onto the chronological year line at about 175 years. In this mix is the human group that maps onto the line at about 110–115 years. The biological lesson is that longevity is predetermined at the species level[3]. The question then becomes how much of the biological upper limit of years of life will be attained in the context of running the gauntlet of life?

Extending the upper biologic limit of human lifespan is probably not possible. Enthusiasm for telomere length as a human longevity indicator and changeable factor has waned[25–29]. Although much fervor for 'anti-aging medicine' has arisen over the last decade, no claims to reverse or stop aging are credible[28,29]. However, reducing the disease burden associated with aging and increasing the years of high functioning healthy life, is a meritorious and feasible goal. Such a goal is attainable by attention to the basics currently known, such as nutrition, exercise, and risk reduction practices[29].

THE GERIATRIC PATIENT PROFILE

Older adults as patients have several characteristics that collectively produce the need for a unique knowledge base and set of skills in order to provide optimal care for them. First, the older adult is more likely than other age groups to express symptoms 'atypically'[4,30]. A propensity for atypical presentation of symptoms introduces the risk for misdiagnosis or misinterpretation[4]. For example, older adults may not always have high temperatures in the presence of significant infectious disease. Also, myocardial infarction may be 'silent'. The medical texts may describe the patient's complaint as a 'crushing substernal chest pain with possible radiation into the left arm', Yet the older adult may show none of these typical signs. They may present without pain, some nausea or gastrointestinal distress, or may walk in to the hospital, and generally not seem to be in a medical crisis.

Mental health conditions such as depression can also be expressed atypically. The 'masked depression' is more common among older adults and challenges clinicians to detect the altered signs[20]. For example, typical signs of significant depression can include sadness of affect, expression of despair, changes in appetite, changes in sleep and a general slowing of motion, reflexes and movement. Older depressed persons may not clearly show any of these signs. There may be loss of appetite, sleep disturbance, a cognitive awareness of sadness, loss, or despair, and inadequate energy to feel comfortable in conducting ordinary activities of daily living. However, some of these signs of masked depression may be considered a normal part of aging. The older adult may not eat as much as in the past, may change the sleep pattern, may be observed to move more slowly and have less energy than in earlier life. Still, the clinician alert to the increased probabilities of masked depression in older adults will have to distinguish between normal age-related change and those associated with underlying depression.

The older adult population will have increased instances of 'multiple pathologies'[3,4]. This means that older adults often have several co-morbidities at any one time. Many of these will be chronic diseases for which there is no cure but only symptom management.

The older adult population is more at risk of 'polypharmacy' than their younger counterparts[3–5]. This is related to the phenomenon of multiple pathologies. Clinicians treating multiple diseases and conditions will prescribe medications to ameliorate the older adult's symptoms or improve function. However, some of the prescribing may occur among several different clinicians who may not be aware of each other's actions. Even so, when one clinician treats one older adult patient there is increased risk of noxious interactive effects and several predictable side-effects.

'Impaired homeostasis' is another characteristic of older adult life that effects health-care interventions[4]. This means, in general physiological terms, that the ability of the older adult to maintain normal functioning and/or to recover from alterations to normal functioning is reduced. Also, bed rest can produce loss of muscle tone very rapidly compared to younger adults. Some have suggested that 1 day of bed rest for elders is equivalent to 3 days of bed rest for younger adults in terms of muscle tone and possible atrophy. Even the occurrence of acute disease such as the flu can take the older adult much longer to recover to baseline function and wellness than younger adults.

Iatrogenic disease is a type of malfunction resulting from application of medical care. *Iatros* is Greek for physician. The current use of 'iatrogenic disease' does not always, however, mean specifically the physician, but, rather, exposure to the health-care system as a whole or individual practitioners resulting in compromised health[4,5]. All people are at some unavoidable risk, such as post-surgical infections or other nosocomial infections during hospital care. However, older adults are at heightened risk. To ignore the unique attributes of older adult health commits the 'one size fits all' fallacy and, worse, heightens the vulnerability index already applicable to the elderly.

PUBLIC HEALTH AND AGING: THE ROLE FOR PREVENTION

The National Health Interview Survey reports that most older persons have at least one chronic condition and many have multiple chronic conditions. In 1995, those 70+ reported the following conditions (ranked by frequency of occurrence): 58% with arthritis, 45% hypertension, 21% heart disease, 19% cancer, 12% diabetes and 9% stroke[22]. It is clear that considerable attention must be given to preventive aspects of aging over the life span.

Prevention, moderation and treatment of disease in older adults can be seen from at least two viewpoints. One is the 'prevention in remaining years' view and another is the 'preventive gerontology' or life span view. First, it is simply wrongheaded to ignore the current elderly population in terms of prevention during their remaining years. While many effects of long unhealthy lifestyles cannot be obliterated, they can be modified[4].

It is necessary to remember that longevity today and in the future means that older adults can expect decades of life after reaching 65 years of age. In fact, it may be all the more important to attend to prevention at this time of life, due to the increased health vulnerability common to longevity. For example, primary prevention in the form of vaccinations against influenza for older adults is critical in older age compared to its importance in their earlier years, because their risk of death from the flu is now higher. While in youth, flu vaccines were highly recommended with the main risk for not getting vaccinated was getting the flu and experiencing much discomfort. Whereas the 'discomfort index' was very high, the 'mortality index' was comparatively low. In old age, both indices are high for influenza.

Smoking and physical activity have also been found sensitive to modification in old age. For example, in a study of 70–79-year-olds who had no cognitive dysfunction, no functional limitations and one or no chronic disease, those who currently smoked had a doubling of risk of death within 3 years compared to those who never smoked[31]. It is also clear that smoking is related to reduction in physical activity and functioning over the course of the lifetime. Moreover, reduction in physical activity has numerous and rapid effects on exaggerating the functional status of a person negatively, simply due to disuse of the body. For example, immobility or disuse of the body can have compounding effects which can introduce the risk for and actual occurrence of serious morbidity and even mortality. The cascade of smoking, physical inactivity and increased immobility can lead to a linked scenario such as gait unsteadiness, fear of falling, more immobility, actual falls, skeletal fractures, surgical repairs, hospital stays, infection, pneumonia and death. The human and fiscal costs of such a cascade are huge and, largely, preventable.

Functional status generally decreases with aging. While this may be universally true, the extent to which decline in function is related to inherent changes of aging and/or to lifestyles is difficult to determine[32]. Ethnic minority status also has been associated with drastically lowered health and function within older age cohorts. African-Americans report their functional status on activities of daily living as fair or poor much more often than do Whites[18]. These functional losses are the pathways to dependency, requiring assistance in the form of specialized long-term care and/or personal surveillance in one's own home.

PUBLIC HEALTH AND AGING: THE FUTURE

The future of public health and aging is driven by a demographic and political engine[33]. Components of this engine include the effects of the aging baby boomers and an epidemiologic transition of increased chronic disease. However, future older adults will be better-educated and wealthier, they will work longer prior to retirement and be more politically assertive. Yet they will experience highly diverse family support systems due to family composition change related to divorce, remarriage or remaining single.

Kodner[33] has pointed out that, today and in the future, there is a national tendency to value a restrained governmental role in public welfare issues. This includes social security, Medicare and Medicaid, which continue to be threatened targets for tax cuts. In spite of this, the need for expensive long-term care increases. In-home long-term care does not mean 'free' long-term care, but, rather, it shifts the expenditures of dollars for caring for dependent elders. The future of long-term care will involve new ways of financing and possibly more interest in preventing the need for it during the earlier years of a person's life.

What is unknown is the effect of technological breakthroughs on diseases of old age that today are seemingly resistant to medical cure. For example, osteoporosis was long considered a near normal part of aging for many women. As it became more appropriately conceptualized and biologically understood, the 'cure' was the long-term pathway of early life nutrition and physical activity to ward off the risk of bone fracture by building a reserve capacity of high bone density[34].

Another example is the near frenzy of research on Alzheimer's disease to treat or prevent its effects of killing brain cells and leaving people confused and in need of supervised help. It is quite correct that more cases of Alzheimer's disease will be present simply because more people are living into the ages of greatest risk. However, recent genetic studies are helping to understand its causation and to create potential predictive formulae for determining probabilities of occurrence. Also, new medications are available to improve thinking ability during the early stages of the disease. New medications are in experimental trials that will postpone the symptoms by several years. Actual prevention is a wish, but is not considered to be an imminent reality. A future scenario, which was unimaginable just a few years ago, includes a person in their twenties getting a genetic test, providing a family history relative to dementing disease and, if considered a high-risk case, beginning to take protective medications in midlife. The intent is to protect the brain for as long as possible so that the person will die from some other condition before brain function is severely compromised. This compresses the amount of life experienced with severe brain impairment into a shorter capsule of time and eliminates much of the patient's and family's burden of long-term care.

The concept of compressing morbidities into a relatively small increment of time in late life has been discussed as a desirable future in which long-term care becomes short-term care. More specifically, the notion is to compare the ages at which chronic disease becomes apparent and limits function relative to age at death. The current curve shows that, after age 65, the number and seriousness of functional limitation increases significantly while the life expectancy is still high, hence the need for long-term care. However, if there is some success in the efforts of health promotion and disease prevention, the effects may be manifest in late life by compressing the time of chronic disease and functional limitations to many fewer years prior to death. Overall, people live longer and healthier, at least as measured by physical health and functional status[24,35].

The future for public health and aging has numerous imperatives. Kodner[33] has enumerated several implications for preparing for the predictable 'baby boom' demographic peak. First, there is a need to prevent disability. This is consistent with the notion that the prevention of death or all disease is absurd, but the effects of one's inevitable demise can be much better managed than the experience of today's cohort of older adults. There is also the need to strengthen informal care of older adults. This means that the most expensive long-term care will be drastically reduced by rewarding the use of in-home, non-professional long-term care. Also required would be better systems of

delivering preventive care and final long-term care. The need for properly trained professionals and paraprofessionals is clear. Related to this need is the need for the ordinary citizen to have access to learning how best to manage the needs of a dependent elder. Many middle-aged people today are experiencing 'parent care' without benefit of familial models or professional models for such tasks.

In summary, the health of communities in which one in four is over the age of 65 is a function of how a nexus of participants manage the life experience. The participants include the older adults themselves, whose behavior influences their health over the entire life span. Other participants include their social support environment. The community resource network of in-home and assisted care will determine much of elders' quality of community life. Also, medical professionals will impact functional status and quality of life more by 'caring' for chronic disease than by cure. Last, doctors who value a multidisciplinary approach, and have taken the time to explore the elder patient's community resource 'bank', will be most able to optimize quality of life.

References

1. Greenspan S. *The Growth of the Mind and the Engendered Origins of Intelligence.* New York: Addison-Wesley, 1997
2. Huttenlocher PR. Synaptogenesis: synapse elimination and neural plasticity in human cerebral cortex. In Nelson CA, ed. *Threats to Optimal Development: Integrating Biological, Psychological, and Social Risk Factors.* Minnesota: The Minnesota Symposia in Child Psychology, 1994:35–54
3. Brookbank J. *The Biology of Aging.* New York: Harper and Row, 1990
4. Ham R, Sloane P, Warshaw G. *Primary Care Geriatrics, 4th edn.* Syracuse, NY: State University of New York, 2001
5. Kane RL, Ouslander, JG, Abrass IB. *Essentials of Clinical Geriatrics.* New York: McGraw-Hill, 1984
6. Mortimer JA. The continuum hypothesis of Alzheimer's disease and normal aging: the role of brain reserve. In *Alzheimer's Disease and Normal Aging: the Role of Brain Reserve* 1995;1:67–70
7. Barrett-Conner E, Kritz-Silverstein D. Estrogen replacement therapy and cognitive function in older women. *J Am Med Assoc* 1993;269:2637–41
8. Rowe J, Kahn R. *Successful Aging.* New York: Pantheon Books, 1998
9. Marks JB. Diabetes management in the future: a whiff and a long shot? *Clin Diabetes* 1998;16:140–5
10. Henderson JN. Ethnogeriatrics. In Klein S, ed. *A National Agenda for Geriatric Education.* Rockville, MD: US Bureau of Health Professions, 1995:119–42

11. Binstock RH, Cluff LE, von Mering O. Issues affecting the future of long-term care. In Binstock RH, Cluff LE, v. Mering O, eds. *The Future of Long-term Care*. Baltimore: Johns Hopkins University Press, 1996:8–12

12. Ory M, Schulz R. Resources for enhancing Alzheimer's care-giving in health (REACH). *Gerontologist* 1996;36:100–1

13. Morgan L, Kunkel S. *Aging: The Social Context*. Thousand Oaks: Pine Forge Press, 1998

14. Balsam AL, Bottum CL. Understanding the aging and public health networks. In Speers MA, Prohaska TR, eds. *Public Health and Aging*. Baltimore: Johns Hopkins University Press, 1997:19–21

15. Harrison GA, Weiner JS, Tanner JM, Barnicot NA. *Human Biology*, 2nd edn. Oxford: Oxford University Press, 1997

16. Moore MJ. The human life span. In Silverman P, ed. *The Elderly as Modern Pioneers*. Bloomington: Indiana University Press, 1987:54–72

17. Kinsella K, Velkoff V. *An Aging World: 2001*. Washington, DC: US Census Bureau. Series P95/01-1. US Government Printing Office, 2001

18. Fowles D, Greenberg S. *A Profile of Older Americans: 2000*. Washington, DC: Administration on Aging, 2001

19. Haley WE, Han B, Henderson JN. Aging and ethnicity: issues for clinical practice. *J Clin Psychol Med Settings* 1998;5: 393–409

20. Kausler DH, Kausler BC. *The Graying of America*. Chicago: University of Illinois Press, 1996

21. Williams FT, Temkin-Greener H. Older people, dependency, and trends in supportive care. In Binstock RH, Cluff LE, Mering OV, eds. *The Future of Long-Term Care*. Baltimore: Johns Hopkins University Press, 1996:51–7

22. Administration on Aging. *Fact Sheet for Features from the Census Bureau*. Washington, DC: Administration on Aging, 2001

23. West Central Florida Area Agency on Aging. *Florida: Highest Proportion of Elders in the Nation*. Tampa, FL: West Central Florida Area Agency on Aging, 1990

24. Sidell M. *Health in Old Age*. Philadelphia: Open University Press, 1995

25. Campesi J, Dimri G, Hara E. Control of replicative senescence. In Schneider E, Rowe J, eds. *Handbook of the Biology of Aging*, 4th edn. San Francisco: Academic Press, 1996:134–5

26. Chang, E, Harley CB. Telomere length and replicative aging in human vascular tissues. *Proc Natl Acad Sci USA* 1995;92:11190–4

27. Hoffman SM, Hromas R, Amemiya C, Mohrenweiser HW. The location of MZF-1 at the telomere of human chromosome 19q makes it vulnerable to degeneration in aging cells. *Leukemia Res* 1996;20:281–3

28. Olshansky SJ, Hayflick L, Carnes B. Position statement on human aging. *J Gerontol: Biol Sci* 2002;57A(no.8): B292–B297

29. Butler RN, Fossel M, Harman SM, et al. Is there an antiaging medicine? *J Gerontol: Biol Sci* 2002;57A(no.9):B333–B338

30. Wallace R. Variability in disease manifestations in older adults: implications for public and community health programs. In Hickey T, Speers M, Prohaska T, eds. *Public Health and Aging*. Baltimore: Johns Hopkins University Press, 1997:75–86

31. Schoenfeld D, Malmrose L, Blazer D, et al. Self-rated health and mortality in the high functioning elderly. A closer look at healthy individuals. MacArthur Field Study of Successful Aging. *J Gerontol* 1994;49: M109–15

32. Kosorok MR, Omenn GS, Diehr P, et al. Conditions associated with restricted activity days among older adults. *Am J Public Health* 1992; 82:1263–7

33. Kodner DL. Foreseeing the future of long-term care: the highlights and implications of the Delphi Study. In Binstock RH, Cluff LE, v. Mering O, eds. *The Future of Long-Term Care*. Baltimore: Johns Hopkins University Press, 1996:275–91

34. Prince R. Diet and the prevention of osteoporotic fractures. *N Engl J Med* 1997; 337:701

35. Fries JF. Aging, natural death and the compression of morbidity. *N Engl J Med* 1980;303:130–5

2 The physiology of aging

T.S. Dharmarajan, MD, FACP, AGSF, and Joey T. Ugalino, MD

INTRODUCTION

The world population of older adults is increasing significantly; by the year 2050, adults older than 65 years will comprise one-fifth of the global population. In the US there are about 35 million individuals (or 13% of the population) aged 65 years and older[2] and by 2020 these will comprise a fourth of the US population. Interestingly, the age group 85 and older is the fastest growing segment of the population and, at present rates of growth, there will be more than 380 000 centenarians by the year 2030. A basic understanding of the aging process will enable health-care providers to distinguish age-related physiological changes from disease-related pathological processes[1-3].

DEFINITIONS

While *aging* is an ongoing process, *senescence* involves the post-maturational processes that lead to diminished homeostasis and increased vulnerability of the organism. *Normal aging* involves inevitable changes related to physiological processes occurring at certain stages in life, e.g. menopause. *Usual aging* refers to age-related diseases that typically occur in older individuals, e.g. coronary artery disease and hypertension. *Life expectancy* is the age reached by half a given population and varies with race, gender and geographical influences. The *maximum life span potential* is the age attained by the longest-lived member of

a given population[4]. The oldest properly documented human (Jeanne Calment) died at age 122 in 1997[5]. In 1997, life expectancy at birth in the USA was 79.4 years for women and 73.6 years for men; at age 85, it was 6.6 and 5.5 years, respectively[2]. In general, the female outlives the male with reference to the human and most species.

THEORIES OF AGING

The search for a satisfactory explanation of the aging process continues, with several theories proposed. *Stochastic theories* explain that random damage to vital molecules (e.g. DNA, proteins) results in progressive decline in cellular function and eventual death. Included are the somatic mutation/DNA repair theory, the error catastrophe theory, the protein modification theory and the free radical/mitochondrial DNA theory[4]. Free radicals are highly reactive by-products of cellular metabolism that can affect cell components and result in accumulation of dysfunctional molecules[6].

The belief that genes program an individual's growth from birth to death is the basis for the *genetic theory*. Longevity appears to be associated with the apo E ε-2 allele or possibly the lack of the ε-4 allele[5]. Genetics play a significant role in accelerated aging syndromes such as Werner's syndrome (adult progeria), Hutchinson–Gilford syndrome (childhood progeria) and Down's syndrome. The genetics of aging differ substantially from the genetics of longevity[5].

The *immunological theory* states that alterations in the immune system increase susceptibility to disease and affect longevity. The *neuroendocrine theory* suggests that the hypothalamus–pituitary–adrenal axis may function as a time keeper and play a central role at different stages of growth, e.g. menopause[4].

Based on some of these theories, therapies are being explored with the hope of slowing down the aging process. Two of these are caloric restriction and hormonal therapy. Restricting caloric intake by about 30% has been shown to prolong life in animals. Hormonal therapy with estrogen benefits the bone and lipid profile in women, preventing complications such as osteoporotic fractures that can increase morbidity and mortality. However, the Women's Health Initiative Study recently also revealed the adverse effects (increase in coronary and cerebrovascular disease, cancer and thromboembolism) resulting from the use of estrogen and progestin over a 5-year period[7].

Another theory is that aging causes changes in the vascular system, resulting in functional alterations and co-morbid processes; this in turn is the explanation for age-related changes in the coronaries, vascular stiffening, abnormal vasomotor regulation and disabilities involving the heart, brain, and skeletal muscle performance. This is the rationale to efforts in improving vascular health[8]. Genetic manipulation and transplantation of cells or cellular extracts (e.g. pancreatic cells in diabetes mellitus) are being explored[9].

BODY COMPOSITION, HEIGHT AND WEIGHT

Height increases until the third decade. Thereafter, it may decrease 5 cm by the seventh decade of life; the basis is a decrease in height of the vertebral body, thinning of the intervertebral discs, flexion of the hips and knees, and flattening of the arch of the foot[10]. Arm span remains constant.

An individual's weight is affected by multiple factors including dietary habits, activity level, culture and economic status. In Western society, weight increase occurs in men and women until the age of 50 and 60, respectively, with a decline thereafter[10].

Total body water decreases with age. While lean body mass decreases by 1% per year from age 55[11], the fat compartment doubles to 30% of the body weight by the seventh decade in men; in women, the lipid compartment is even larger at all ages. Thus, while total body weight may not necessarily be altered, relative increase in fat and decrease in water compartments occur, with the pattern more pronounced in females. Fat becomes centrally distributed, deposited in the abdomen and muscle tissues[12]. These alterations profoundly affect the pharmacokinetics and pharmacodynamics of medications. Smaller doses of water-soluble drugs (e.g. aminoglycosides) achieve therapeutic levels while lipid-soluble drugs (e.g. benzodiazepines) remain stored in fat depots, exerting their effect long after withdrawal of the drug.

MUSCULOSKELETAL SYSTEM

Lean body mass decreases by as much as 40% from the third to the eighth decade of life. Although handgrip strength decreases substantially, overall loss of strength is more in the lower than in the upper extremities. Sarcopenia is the result of alterations in neuronal, muscular and neuromuscular transmission. Muscle loss mainly involves type 2 fibers, where a decrease in size or number of myofibrils and altered innervation are observed. An exception is the diaphragm. Lipofuscin accumulation is a notable feature[10].

Joints become stiffer with age as water content in tendons, ligaments, cartilage and synovial compartments decreases. The keratin sulfate and hyaluronic acid content of cartilage increases[10].

With age, net bone formation takes place until the thirties; thereafter, bone resorption of 1% and 0.7% per annum occurs in females and males, respectively. As a result of estrogen loss during menopause, bone loss accelerates in females up to 5% annually for several years, eventually decelerating to its previous rate[13].

GAIT AND BALANCE

Gait velocities, both usual and maximal, are maintained until the seventh decade. The gait of older adults is slower; they have shorter stride length and spend longer time in stance with both feet on the ground. Arm swing and plantar flexion are diminished. Due to hip flexion, an anterior flexed posture is adopted. The older individual has a greater propensity to fall under trying conditions due to greater body sway when standing, impaired ability to stand longer on one leg and lesser capacity to lean anteriorly with aging[14,15]. Disease processes and medications influence balance and may predispose the elderly to falls.

INTEGUMENT

Skin changes may be intrinsic or extrinsic (photoaging). The epidermal turnover time (the period keratinocytes take to migrate outward from the basal cell layer) is longer. The epidermal–dermal junction flattens, lessening surface contact between these two layers. Decreases in blood supply and the number of Langerhans cells (immune) and melanocytes occur. Xerosis (dry skin) is common as a result of decreased activity of sweat and sebaceous glands. These changes predispose the aging skin to injury with mild trauma or infection with a prolongation of healing time.

Wrinkling of the skin is the result of fewer dermal fibers (e.g. collagen, elastin) and loss of subcutaneous fat. The dermal thickness is reduced by 20%. Usual hair loss is between 50 and 100 strands per day; hair thinning is due to decreasing number of follicles, slower growth rate and lesser diameter of hair. Graying of the hair is from progressive loss of melanocytes[16]. The rate of nail growth is reduced by 50%.

Vitamin D production by the skin is reduced due to lesser concentration of epidermal provitamin D_3. Further, inadequate sunlight compounds the risk of hypovitaminosis D and osteoporosis.

Changes from photoaging are due to sun exposure, accounting for much of the visible skin changes and are cosmetically undesirable. The use of a transretinoic acid preparation may reverse some of the intrinsic and photoaging changes.

SENSORY CHANGES WITH AGING

Eyes

The tissues around the orbital areas show atrophy with aging. The eyelids may lose tone and, along with fibrous changes, may manifest as ptosis, ectropion or entropion. Tear production by the lacrimal glands and goblet cells is decreased. The outward displacement of the lacrimal punctum results in abnormal tear drainage and causes 'teary eyes'. The conjunctiva becomes atrophied and yellow. The aging iris responds sluggishly to light stimulation due to increasing rigidity. Yellowing of the lens results from photo-oxidation of tryptophan in lens protein, affecting blue color perception. Glare occurs when light is scattered by changes in the lens. Presbyopia begins in the earlier decades of life as a result of decreasing lens elasticity and ciliary muscle atrophy, but manifests many years later[10].

Production of aqueous humor decreases with age. Floaters are condensations in the vitreous gel resulting from a collapsing collagen framework. The retina becomes thinner with loss of rods in the center; the number of cones in the fovea is maintained.

Both light and dark adaptation are impaired with aging. Contrast sensitivity is diminished. The use of night lamps and glare-free lights lessen the risk of injury.

Ears

Changes occur in the external, middle and inner ears that impact on hearing. Anatomical changes render the external auditory canal narrower, predisposing the older individual to cerumen impaction. The cerumen becomes drier and the hair in the canal gets coarser, more so in men, predisposing to conductive hearing loss from impaction. This alone can result in substantial diminished hearing acuity[17]. The ossicles in the middle ear may ossify with aging. Changes in the inner ear are degenerative, with vascular changes from atherosclerosis contributing to hair cell loss (in the organ of Corti) and cochlear neuronal loss. These changes are compounded by other factors such as diet, dyslipidemia, medication, noise, and genetics[18,19]. The result is a bilateral symmetric hearing loss involving higher frequencies referred to as presbycusis. Unilateral hearing loss is not a result of the aging process alone.

Taste and smell

The olfactory threshold increases consistently with age, with a 50% decline in the capacity to perceive smell by the age of 80. Alteration in taste is less consistent[20,21]. Taste perception deteriorates with decreased ability to detect salt, bitter, sweet and sour tastes[11]; preferences vary and the ability for fine discrimination is affected. The number of taste buds is constant but the amount of lingual papillae decreases[20,21]. Alterations in taste and smell result in diminished enjoyment of food. However, profound anorexia in the elderly is mostly a result of disease and/or medications. When possible, dietary restrictions should be minimized in older individuals with anorexia.

While avoiding excessive addition of sugar and salt to make food tastier, flavor enhancement of food may help. Examples are pepper, cinnamon, vinegar, vanilla and ginger, among others[20].

GASTROINTESTINAL SYSTEM

Common physiological changes with aging are enumerated in Table 1. The oral mucosal epithelium thins with aging. The gum recedes fairly consistently, exposing the tooth to plaques, inflammation and infection. Years of tobacco and beverage (e.g. tea, coffee) consumption results in yellow discoloration of teeth. Attrition (wearing out of tooth surface) is the result of lifelong chewing. The edentulous state is commonly the result of disease. Preventive dental hygiene should be encouraged early in life[22].

The parotid and submandibular glands may lose up to 30% of the parenchyma; in spite of replacement by fat and fibrous tissue, stimulated salivation is unchanged[11]. Salivary production, necessary for oropharyngeal health, is intact with healthy aging. Reduction is a result of disease, medications and radiotherapy to the neck. Drug-induced basis appears the most common etiology as older individuals typically are on numerous medications[23]. Medications with strong anticholinergic effect may cause a dry mouth. Chewing of food is likewise affected; older adults tend to chew longer but less efficiently and swallow larger portions of food[24].

Swallowing is unaffected by aging, *per se*. The onset and duration of primary esophageal contractions are preserved. Despite a 20% decrease in the number of myenteric ganglion cells[11] and decreased amplitude of contraction[25], food movement through the esophagus is unaffected. The presence of dysphagia warrants evaluation for disease. Presbyesophagus, a condition arising from disease rather than a part of normal aging, encompasses a group of findings that includes decreased amplitude of

Table 1 Age-related changes in the gastrointestinal system. Reprinted with permission from reference 22

Gastrointestinal system component	Characteristic changes
Oral cavity	quantity of taste buds is not significantly affected; quantity of papillae decreases
	taste perception is altered
	dentition is not significantly affected
Esophagus	swallowing and motility functions are not significantly affected
Stomach	distensibility is decreased; early satiety occurs
	acid production is not significantly affected;
	gastric emptying time is not significantly affected
Small intestine	transit time is not significantly affected
	absorption of some micronutrients is impaired (e.g. calcium, vitamin D)
Large intestine	tendency to diverticulosis
	motility is decreased
Liver	hepatic size, mass and blood flow are decreased
	liver function parameters are not significantly affected
Pancreas	displaced inferiorly
	exocrine and endocrine function are not significantly affected

peristaltic contractions, incomplete sphincter relaxation, delayed esophageal emptying, frequent tertiary contractions and esophageal dilatation[11,26].

Gastric acid production, both basal and stimulated, does not decline appreciably with aging. Decreased acidity, however, may be seen in disease processes (e.g. chronic atrophic gastritis) or with the use of medications. Gastric chief cell mass and function decline, resulting in decreased basal and stimulated pepsin secretion. Early satiety in older individuals may be due to decreased distensibility of the stomach. Gastric motility and gastric emptying time are minimally affected and effects may be due to dysfunction of the autonomic nervous system[11].

Small intestinal changes include moderate villous atrophy and loss of myenteric neurons. However, transit time remains constant. Absorption of calcium declines, due to impaired active transport of calcium and fewer vitamin D receptors[11]. Among fat-soluble vitamins, absorption of vitamins A and K is unaffected, while that of vitamin D is decreased[10]. Decreasing lactase levels may cause intolerance to dairy products.

In the large intestine, hypertrophy of the muscularis mucosa, atrophy of the muscularis externa and mucosa, and increased collagen deposition in the wall with aging compromise mechanical integrity. An increase in opioid receptors and slower transit time (inconsistently demonstrated) predispose to constipation and colonic diverticulosis[11,24]. Fecal incontinence is a result of disease, not normal aging.

The number of hepatocytes in the liver decreases from the sixth decade, accelerating in the eighties, and accounts for a reduced liver mass[27]. As a result of decreasing cardiac output and splanchnic blood flow, hepatic blood flow diminishes by 10% every decade, affecting the hepatic metabolism of drugs with high first-pass metabolism such as labetalol and nitrates[27]. Some decline in the production of vitamin K-dependent coagulation factors occurs. Liver function tests are generally normal.

The proximal common bile duct dilates with aging while the preampullary common bile duct becomes narrower. Although there is no change in the function and morphology of the gallbladder, the older adult is predisposed to gallstone formation due to lithogenic bile. The pancreas is displaced inferiorly and its weight decreases after the seventies; exocrine and endocrine functions are preserved[24,27].

CARDIOVASCULAR SYSTEM

An increase in left ventricular wall mass occurs with aging (Table 2). Hypertrophy involves both cellular and non-cellular components (e.g. collagen, fibrous tissue). The left atrium enlarges and the circumference of the cardiac valves, especially that of the aortic valve, increases. Although valvular cusps become thicker and calcified, valvular dysfunction is not expected with normal aging.

The cardiac conduction system is affected. About 90% of pacemaker cells in the sinus node disappear by age 75[28]. Heart rate is unaffected at rest. With exercise, there is a decrease in the inotropic, chronotropic and maximum heart rate (Max HR) response. Unlike in younger individuals, cardiac output is maintained by increasing the stroke volume instead of the heart rate during physical activity. The diminished response to catecholamine stimulation or a subnormal β-adrenergic response remains unclear, but it has been theorized to be the result of altered adenylate cyclase or G protein activity[10]. Max HR in both genders can be estimated using the following formulae[10]:

$$\text{Max HR (males)} = 220 - \text{age}$$
$$\text{Max HR (females)} = 190 - (\text{age} \times 0.8)$$

Large vessels undergo an increase in diameter and loss of compliance resulting from collagen deposition, fragmentation of elastin and calcification of the vessel walls. As a result, elevated systolic blood pressure is common in older adults, while diastolic blood pressure appears to plateau by the sixties.

RESPIRATORY SYSTEM

The anterior–posterior diameter of the chest wall increases (Table 3). Calcification of the costochondral cartilage and greater intercostal

Table 2 Age-related changes in the cardiovascular system. Reprinted with permission from reference 22

Morphologic changes
Increased atrium size
Increased left ventricular wall mass and thickness
Increased proportion of collagen and fibrous tissue
Increased deposition of lipofuscin
Increased valve circumference
Thickening and calcification of valve cusps
Decreased number of sinoatrial nodal cells
Loss of compliance of large vessels

Functional changes
Diastolic dysfunction
Increased systolic blood pressure
Cardiac output stable at rest
Submaximal increase in heart rate with activity

muscle contraction lead to a stiffer, less compliant chest wall. The cough reflex is less efficient, causing poorer mucociliary clearance. Alveolar washings demonstrate a decrease in macrophages and an increase in IgA, IgG, albumin and neutrophils[10]. Lung compliance increases, counteracted by a stiffer chest wall, with a decline in total compliance.

Loss of elastic tissues leads to enlargement of alveolar ducts. The dependent airways close at a higher 'closing volume' with less area available for gas exchange. The residual volume and functional residual capacity increase, with the total lung capacity remaining constant with aging. An increase in ventilation–perfusion (V/Q) mismatch is observed in older adults, especially in the supine position[10]. These changes account for the decreased partial pressure of oxygen (Pa_{O_2}) and arterial oxygen saturation (Sa_{O_2}) observed with aging. Expected Pa_{O_2} in older adults is calculated by the following formula:

$$Pa_{O_2} = 100 - (\text{age}/3)$$

Arterial Pco_2 and pH are not affected with aging. Pulmonary diffusing capacity for carbon dioxide declines by 5% per decade[29]. In non-smoking men, forced expiratory volume in 1 s (FEV_1) and forced vital capacity decrease by 0.15–0.30 1/decade[10].

Table 3 Age-related changes in the respiratory system. Reprinted with permission from reference 22

Respiratory system component	Characteristic changes
Chest wall	increased anteroposterior diameter
	costochondral cartilage calcification
	decreased compliance of rib cage
Lungs	increased lung compliance
	poor mucociliary clearance
	decreased efficiency of cough
Capacities and volumes	total lung capacity not significantly affected
	increased residual volume, functional residual capacity
	Decreased vital capacity, FEV_1, forced vital capacity
	increased closing volume
	increased $\dot{V}/\dot{Q}$ mismatch
Arterial blood gas values	Decreased Pao_2, Sao_2
	$Paco_2$, pH not significantly affected

FEV_1, forced expiratory volume in 1 s; Pao_2, arterial partial pressure of oxygen; $Paco_2$, arterial partial pressure of carbon dioxide; Sao_2, arterial oxygen saturation; $\dot{V}/\dot{Q}$, ventilation–perfusion ratio

KIDNEYS AND BLADDER

Kidney size decreases with aging (Table 4). The decline in weight is 10–43% by the eighth decade, mainly affecting the renal cortex; the number of glomeruli and proximal tubules decreases[30]. By age 75, fewer glomeruli remain functional due to diffuse sclerosis. Each glomerulus will have fewer capillary loops and epithelial cells, with an increase in mesangial cells. Tubules become shorter. Small diverticuli of unknown significance are noticeable in distal convoluted tubules[30].

Renal blood flow decreases 10% per decade beyond the age of 30. The glomerular filtration rate (GFR) usually declines with aging; creatinine clearance decreases by 8.0 ml/min per 1.73 m²/decade from the third decade. However, the decline in renal function may be less pronounced in a third or may not occur at all in another third of the population[10,30].

Serum creatinine values in older adults reflect a lower creatinine clearance compared to younger individuals with the same creatinine value. This is the result of a decline in muscle mass that occurs with aging. The 24-h creatinine clearance remains the most accurate clinical estimate of the GFR[30]. However, when renal function is stable, the Cockcroft and Gault formula (given below) may be used to estimate the creatinine clearance[31].

Table 4 Age-related changes in the kidneys. Reprinted with permission from reference 22

Morphologic changes
Decreased size (mainly cortex)
Sclerosis of glomeruli
Loss of nephrons with long tubules

Functional changes
Decline in creatinine clearance (from third decade of life)
Decline in tubular secretion
Impaired capacity to concentrate or dilute urine
Decreased ability to handle sodium and potassium load
Decreased ability to excrete an acid load

Hormonal changes
Decreased secretion of renin
Decreased synthesis of 1,25-dihydroxyvitamin D_3
Decreased metabolism of parathyroid hormone, glucagon, calcitonin
Erythropoietin synthesis not significantly affected

$$\text{Creatinine clearance} = \frac{(140 - \text{age in years}) \times (\text{weight in kg})}{72 \times \text{serum creatinine in mg/dl}} \times 85\% \text{ (in females)}$$

Table 5   Age-related changes in the endocrine system. Reprinted with permission from reference 22

Endocrine system component	Characteristic changes
Thyroid	decreased size
	increased fibrosis and nodularity
	levels of T_4, thyroid-stimulating hormone not significantly affected
	decreased peripheral conversion of T_4 to T_3
Insulin	increased insulin level due to decreased clearance
	increased peripheral insulin resistance
	increased fasting glucose level (1% increase per decade)
Glucagon	glucagon level not significantly affected
Growth hormone	decreased growth hormone secretion
	decreased insulin-like growth factor I level
Antidiuretic hormone (ADH)	increased ADH levels due to tubular resistance
Atrial natriuretic peptide (ANP)	increased ANP level
Prolactin	loss of pulsatile secretions
Parathyroid hormone (PTH)	increased PTH levels; decreased metabolism
Vitamin D	decreased synthesis of 25-hydroxyvitamin D_3 and 1,25-dihydroxyvitamin D_3
Calcitonin	biologically active calcitonin level not significantly affected
Adrenocorticotropic hormone (ACTH), cortisol	secretion of ACTH or cortisol not significantly affected
Renin, aldosterone	decreased renin, aldosterone levels
Catecholamines	increased norepinephrine level
	catecholamine secretion not significantly affected

T_3, tri-iodothyronine; T_4, thyroxine

Tubular secretion diminishes at a rate of 0.7–1% annually. The renal threshold for glucose is lowered, with urine testing less reliable than the glucometer for the monitoring of diabetes mellitus in older people. Maximal urine concentration and dilution by the kidneys become impaired. The aging kidneys also have decreased ability to conserve and excrete sodium. Likewise, the capacity to handle a potassium load is impaired. Last, the kidneys are unable to excrete an acid load or maximally acidify the urine. These functional changes predispose the older adult to fluid and electrolyte disturbances such as dehydration, fluid overload, hyponatremia, hypernatremia and hyperkalemia[32].

Erythropoietin synthesis is preserved with aging. There is a decrease in renin synthesis, vitamin D hydroxylation to the active form and metabolism of parathyroid hormone, glucagon and calcitonin[33].

Urinary bladder capacity and contractility, and the ability to postpone voiding decline with age. Postvoid residual urine volume increases, with up to 100 ml considered normal. Fluid excretion patterns are altered, with most fluid excreted at night. Nocturia may be a consequence[34].

ENDOCRINE SYSTEM

Endocrine changes occur with aging, affecting the levels of several hormones (Table 5).

Adrenocorticotropic hormone and cortisol

Adrenocorticotropic hormone (ACTH) and cortisol levels are largely unchanged with age. The cortisol response to stress is preserved in the elderly unless adrenal function is suppressed by use of steroids or by disease[35–37].

Antidiuretic hormone

The antidiuretic hormone (ADH) response to hypovolemia and hypotension is attenuated but remains sensitive to changes in serum osmolarity. With aging, water conservation is impaired as the collecting tubules develop resistance to ADH[38]. These changes, along with a blunted response to the thirst sensation, predispose the older adult to dehydration.

Atrial natriuretic peptide

Similar to ADH, renal resistance to atrial natriuretic peptide (ANP) with aging results in elevated serum levels, both basal and stimulated, in response to volume expansion[33].

Catecholamines

The catecholamine production by the adrenal medulla in response to stress is unaffected by aging. Epinephrine and norepinephrine levels are increased[35]. The α-receptor responsiveness is unchanged, while that of the β-receptor is diminished[37].

Growth hormone

The pituitary response to growth hormone releasing hormone (GHRH) attenuates with aging, with a decrease in secretion of growth hormone. The level of integrated growth factor 1, a mediator of growth hormone action in peripheral tissues, declines with age[36].

Insulin and glucagon

Insulin release from the aging pancreas is impaired under hyperglycemic situations. However, plasma insulin levels are elevated due to increased peripheral tissue resistance and decreased clearance of the hormone. The enlarging fat compartment and decreasing muscle mass in older adults account for the insulin resistance (as lipid tissues contain fewer insulin receptors). Glucagon levels remain constant despite impaired renal metabolism. Fasting glucose level increases by 1% per decade from age 20 while postprandial glucose level increases by 10 mg/dl and

5 mg/dl per decade at 1 and 2 h, respectively[10]. The effect of these changes on glycosylated hemoglobin level is minimal[39]. Acceptable normal ranges for fasting glucose level and glycosylated hemoglobin are the same irrespective of age.

Parathyroid hormone, vitamin D and calcitonin

Parathyroid levels increase with age in an effort to maintain serum calcium concentration. Vitamin D synthesis in the skin is diminished, along with levels of 25-hydroxyvitamin D and 1,25-dihydroxyvitamin D. The fact that there are fewer intestinal receptors for this vitamin results in impaired intestinal calcium absorption. Although total calcitonin levels decrease with aging, the active component levels are intact. Metabolism of parathyroid hormone and calcitonin in the kidneys is impaired[33,35].

Prolactin

Prolactin levels are variable. Nocturnal pulsatile secretion of prolactin is lost[10].

Renin and aldosterone

Serum levels of renin and aldosterone decline with age. The response of both hormones to postural changes and sodium restriction is blunted, causing a decreased ability to conserve sodium and excrete potassium[37]. A predisposition to hyperkalemia is noted in the elderly.

Thyroid

The size of the thyroid gland decreases, with more fibrosis and nodularity. Thyrotropin (TSH) and thyroxine (T_4) levels do not change with age. There is less peripheral conversion of T_4 to tri-iodothyronine (T_3). Nevertheless, normal ranges of T_3 are maintained. Alteration in the TSH level suggests abnormal thyroid function[36,40].

REPRODUCTIVE AND SEXUAL FUNCTION

The aging ovary is barely visible on radioimaging as it becomes fibrotic and involutes; its weight decreases to 2.5 g from 20 g at menopause. The ovary becomes less responsive to follicle stimulating hormone (FSH) and luteinizing hormone (LH), with resultant decreased production of estrogen, progesterone, testosterone and androstenedione. The uterus atrophies with age. Vaginal secretions decrease in amount and acidity, resulting in alteration of normal flora. The postmenopausal breast undergoes atrophy of glands, narrowing of ductal lumina with cystic changes and increase in fat tissue. The breast contour is altered as a result of relaxation of ligamentous support and loss of muscle tone. As the aging breast may give a nodular feel on examination, additional tests such as mammography may be required[10].

The ability to procreate is maintained in males, since germ cells are produced continuously. Sperms may manifest chromosomal abnormalities. The seminiferous tubules degenerate while Leydig cells decrease in number. After age 50, total and free testosterone levels decrease along with an increase in FSH and LH levels. The prostate gland increases in size; benign prostatic hyperplasia is seen in 90% of men by age 85. However, the amount of prostate secretion in ejaculate and urine is decreased[10].

The aging female experiences a slow decline in libido mainly from a decrease in testosterone. Due to less vaginal lubrication, vaginal bleeding and dyspareunia may be presentations. Orgasmic contractions are fewer and weaker but the ability to experience multiple orgasms remains. Local or systemic estrogen use and vaginal lubricants may resolve some of the aforementioned problems. In men,

decreasing testosterone level also affects libido. More direct and prolonged stimulation is required to achieve an erection adequate for intercourse. A decrease in seminal vesicle secretions accounts for a lesser amount of seminal fluid[41].

HEMATOPOIESIS

Although bone marrow mass decreases with an increase in the marrow fat with aging, red blood cell, white blood cell and platelet counts remain in the normal range. Aging is associated with a slight increase in red cell size and membrane viscosity with a minimal decline of the red cell lifespan, perhaps brought about by alterations in enzyme content and metabolic activity. More recently, alterations in the levels of interleukins 2 and 6 are said to influence hematopoiesis[42,43].

IMMUNE SYSTEM

The skin's efficacy as a barrier against infection is compromised due to lower acidity and moisture (from decreased glandular activity) and fewer immune cells (Langerhans cells)[44]. Skin injury takes longer to heal due to intrinsic changes with aging (see 'Integument'). Altered mucus secretion in the genitourinary and respiratory tracts facilitates bacterial adherence. Urine is less acidic; a decrease in Tamm–Horsfall urinary protein and lesser antibacterial activity of prostatic fluid increase susceptibility to infection. Decreased clearance of the airway due to less effective coughing may predispose to respiratory infection.

The number and function of neutrophils including chemotaxis, adherence and phagocytic activity are preserved. Some macrophage functions are altered; secretion of transforming growth factor (TGF)-β, tumor necrosis factor (TNF)-α and interleukin (IL)-6 increases while IL-1 may decrease. Complement activity is maintained[10].

Involution of the thymus along with a decline in thymic hormones begins after puberty; by age 50, the thymus weighs only 5–10% of its original mass[11]. As a result, T cells are affected with aging. Memory cells increase while naive cells decrease in number. Antibody response to vaccines is attenuated due to defects in B-cell and possibly helper T-cell function. This is the basis for the two-step tuberculin test including the booster dose[45]. As a result of impaired thermal regulation, the older adult with septicemia may be afebrile.

CENTRAL AND PERIPHERAL NERVOUS SYSTEM

The mass of the brain decreases in parallel with the decrease in cerebral blood flow by 20%. Cerebral autoregulation is progressively lost. Neuronal loss mainly involves the large neurons of the cerebellum, superior temporal gyrus and subcortical regions (locus ceruleus, substantia nigra). Modest losses are seen in the brainstem, hypothalamus and nucleus basalis of Meynert[10]. Accumulation of lipofuscin is observed.

In the spinal cord, loss of motor neurons occurs with age and mainly affects the anterior horn cells. Diminished ankle vibratory sensation occurs with aging; when involving the knee, the cause may be pathological. While deep tendon reflexes tend to become hypoactive with ankle reflex often absent, the knee jerk can still be elicited[46].

Changes in neurotransmitters, receptors and non-neurotransmitters occur but do not imply abnormal behavior or thinking. Examples include a decrease in carbonic anhydrase and acetylcholinesterase, a decreased number of receptors (dopaminergic, muscarinic and serotonin), and alterations in substance P and vasoactive intestinal polypeptide[47].

Vocabulary is generally preserved. Older adults complain of memory loss and difficulty in recalling names. Recall is affected more than recognition. The use of adaptive techniques (e.g. reminders, lists) can compensate for impairment of short-term memory. Studies of general intelligence test performance show a decline in the sixties but this remains modest until the eighties. However, more time is required to accomplish complex tasks, while simple tasks are often performed satisfactorily[47].

Table 6 Examples of disorders *not* attributable to normal aging

Anemia
Anorexia
Cataract
Constipation
Dementia
Dry mouth
Dysphagia
Edentulous state
Erectile dysfunction
Falls
Fecal incontinence
Glaucoma
Hearing loss (unilateral)
Hypoalbuminemia
Malnutrition
Syncope
Tinnitus
Urinary incontinence

SLEEP

Normal sleep comprises rapid eye movement (REM) sleep and non-REM sleep, the latter with four stages. Stages 3 and 4, the deepest and most restorative, are decreased in older adults. Likewise, the number of awakenings and arousal after sleep onset is increased. Therefore, inadequate or restless sleep is a common perception on the part of older adults. In addition, sleep efficiency (actual sleep time divided by time spent in bed) is diminished while sleep latency (time needed to fall asleep) is prolonged, with a tendency to awaken during the early morning hours[48,49].

THERMOREGULATION

Physiologic alterations render the elderly susceptible to hypothermia and hyperthermia. The lowered basal metabolic rate from a decline in lean body mass predisposes to hypothermia. Other contributing factors include inability to appropriately perceive alterations in environmental temperature, a decreased dermal insulation role from loss of subcutaneous fat and an increased latency for shivering.

In spite of fever or hyperthermia, the sweat response is diminished, due to decreased activity and number of sweat glands; a higher core temperature threshold is needed to induce sweating. Decreased thirst perception predisposes to dehydration[50,51].

THE PSYCHOSOCIAL FACTOR

As one ages, the geriatric individual is subject to substantial stress and demands upon the body, which necessitates adjustment to the environment. Society may be demanding or impose restrictions. Living alone can result in depression and health problems. Retirement is associated with fear and lack of adjustment. Co-morbid problems result in further burden. And finally, family and community support may be wanting. Aging, therefore, presents a challenge to the older person to develop strategies to cope with these difficulties[52].

HEALTHY AGING AND THE FUTURE

The gradual increase in life expectancy has led to a growth in the elderly population. Advances in health care including preventive measures, better sanitation and the availability of antibiotics have contributed to a healthier older population[53]. Perhaps in the future, life expectancy may approach the current maximum life span. However, it is equally likely that the older adult will have age-related disorders that may diminish the quality of life. Table 6 enumerates examples that should not be attributed to healthy aging and, on the contrary, need evaluation.

Quality of life is enhanced when disabilities are minimized and function maintained. Many age-related disorders are preventable. While average genes allow the human to attain the eighties in generally good health, several years are lost by failure to observe 'healthy' life-style measures[5]. Counseling for appropriate nutrition, regular exercise and avoidance of smoking and excessive alcohol consumption can be offered early in life and these help increase life expectancy[54,55]. Screening for and treatment of diseases with periodic review of medication regimens (prescribed and over-the-counter) and avoidance of polypharmacy are useful measures. Gene therapy is unlikely to dramatically change the aging process in the foreseeable future. Stem cell research might help modify the course of diseases. Estrogen has been widely used but its benefit with regards to cardiovascular and cognitive functions remains questionable. Of all the measures, caloric restriction with provision of essential nutrients has shown promise in animal experiments, although this has been difficult to demonstrate in humans[9]. Nevertheless, the ultimate goal of prolonging healthy life and maintaining function continues to be challenged.

References

1. Jackson SA. The epidemiology of aging. In Hazzard WR, Blass JP, Ettinger WH Jr, et al., eds. *Principles of Geriatric Medicine and Gerontology*, 4th edn. New York: McGraw-Hill, 1999:203–25

2. Federal Interagency Forum on Aging-Related Statistics. *Older Americans 2000: Key Indicators of Well-Being*. Washington, DC: US Government Printing Office, 2000

3. Furner SE, Brody JA, Jankowski LM. Epidemiology and aging. In Cassel CK, Cohen HJ, Larson EB, *et al.*, eds. *Geriatric Medicine*, 3rd edn. New York: Springer, 1997:37–43

4. Troen BR, Cristofalo VJ. The biology of aging. In Cobbs EL, Duthie EH Jr, Murphy JB, eds. *Geriatrics Review Syllabus*, 4th edn. Dubuque, IA: Kendall/Hunt Publishing, 1999:5–10

5. Perls T, Kunkel LM, Puca A. The genetics of exceptional human longevity. *J Am Geriatr Soc* 2002;50:359–68

6. Miller RA. The biology of aging and longevity. In Hazzard WR, Blass JP, Ettinger WH Jr, *et al.*, eds. *Principles of Geriatric Medicine and Gerontology*, 4th edn. New York: McGraw-Hill, 1999:3–19

7. Rossouw JE, Anderson GL, Prentice RL, *et al.* Risks and benefits of estrogen plus progestin in healthy postmenopausal women: principal results from the Women's Health Initiative randomized controlled trial. *JAMA* 2002;288:321–33

8. Forman DE. Paradigm of vascular aging: conceptual strides slowed by technical limitations. *J Am Geriatr Soc* 2002;50:1159–60

9. Vojta CL, Fraga PD, Forciea MA, Lavizzo-Mourey R. Anti-aging therapy: an overview. *Hosp Pract* 2001;36:43–9

10. Taffet GE. Age-related physiological changes. In Cobbs EL, Duthie EH Jr, Murphy JB, eds. *Geriatrics Review Syllabus*, 4th edn. Dubuque, IA: Kendall/Hunt Publishing, 1999:10–23

11. Blechman MB, Gelb AM. Aging and gastrointestinal physiology. *Clin Geriatr Med* 1999;15:429–38

12. Harris T. Weight and age: paradoxes and conundrums. In Hazzard WR, Blass JP, Ettinger WH Jr, *et al.*, eds. *Principles of Geriatric Medicine and Gerontology*, 4th edn. New York: McGraw-Hill, 1999:967–72

13. Dharmarajan TS, Ugalino JT. Current trends in the prevention and treament of osteoporosis. *Family Practice Recertification, 2000: Special Geriatric Issue*: 17–26

14. Judge JO, Ounpuu S, Davis RB III. Effects of age on the biomechanics and physiology of gait. *Clin Geriatr Med* 1996;12:659–78

15. Baddour RJ, Wolfson L. Nervous system disease. In: Duthie EH Jr, Katz PR. eds. *Practice of Geriatrics*. 3rd edn. Philadelphia: WB Saunders, 1998:317–27

16. Berger R, Gilchrest BA. Skin disorders. In Duthie EH Jr, Katz PR, eds. *Practice of Geriatrics*, 3rd edn. Philadelphia: WB Saunders, 1998:467–80

17. Moore AM, Voytas J, Kowalski D, Maddens M. Cerumen, hearing and cognition in the elderly. *J Am Med Dir Assoc* 2002;3:136–9

18. Marcincuk MC, Roland PS. Geriatric hearing loss: understanding the causes and providing appropriate treatment. *Geriatrics* 2002;57:44–59

19. Meyerhoff W. Age-related disorders of the ear, nose and throat. *Geriatrics* 2002;57:43

20. Schiffman SS. Taste and smell losses in normal aging and disease. *J Am Med Assoc* 1997;278:1357–62

21. Shao W, Ondrey F. Smell and taste. In Lunenfeld B, Gooren L, eds. *Textbook of Men's Health*. New York: Parthenon Publishing, 2002:513–26

22. Dharmarajan TS, Ugalino JT. The aging process. In Dreger D, Krumm B, Yoder D, eds. *Hospital Physician Geriatric Medicine Board Review Manual*. Wayne, PA: Turner White Communications, 2000;1:1–12

23. Ship JA, Pillemer SR, Baum BJ. Xerostomia and the geriatric patient. *J Am Geriatr Soc* 2002;50:535–43

24. Dharmarajan TS, Pitchumoni CS, Kokkat A. The aging gut. *Pract Gastroenterol* 2001; 25:15–27

25. Dharmarajan TS, Kathpalia RK. A review of geriatric nutrition. In Dreger D, Krumm B, Garrison L, eds. *Hospital Physician Geriatric Medicine Board Review Manual*. Wayne, PA: Turner White Communications, 2000;1:1–12

26. Sallout H, Mayoral W, Benjamin SB. The aging esophagus. *Clin Geriatr Med* 1999;15: 439–56

27. Dharmarajan TS, Pitchumoni CS, Kumar KS. Drug-induced liver disease in older adults. *Pract Gastroenterol* 2001;25: 43–60

28. Lakatta EG. Circulatory function in younger and older humans in health. In

Hazzard WR, Blass JP, Ettinger WH Jr, et al., eds. *Principles of Geriatric Medicine and Gerontology*, 4th edn. New York: McGraw-Hill, 1999:645–60

29. Enright PL. Aging of the respiratory system. In Hazzard WR, Blass JP, Ettinger WH Jr, et al., eds. *Principles of Geriatric Medicine and Gerontology*, 4th edn. New York: McGraw-Hill, 1999:721–8

30. Jassal SV, Oreopoulos DG. The aging kidney. In Oreopoulos DG, Hazzard WR, Luke R, eds. *Nephrology and Geriatrics Integrated*. Boston: Kluwer Academic Publishers, 2000:27–36

31. Cockcroft DW, Gault MH. Prediction of creatinine clearance from serum creatinine. *Nephron* 1976;16:31–41

32. Beck LH. Changes in renal function with aging. *Clin Geriatr Med* 1998;14:199–209

33. Beck LH. Changes in renal function with aging. Genitourinary problems. *Clin Geriatr Med* 1998;14:199–209

34. Brandeis GH, Resnick NM. Urinary incontinence. In Duthie EH Jr, Katz PR, eds. *Practice of Geriatrics*, 3rd edn. Philadelphia: WB Saunders, 1998:189–98

35. Perry HM. The endocrinology of aging. *Clin Chem* 1999;45:1369–76

36. Lamberts SWJ, van den Beld AW, van der Lely AJ. The endocrinology of aging. *Science* 1997;278:419–24

37. Davis PJ, Davis FB. Endocrine disorders. In Duthie EH Jr, Katz PR, eds. *Practice of Geriatrics*, 3rd edn. Philadelphia: WB Saunders, 1998:563–78

38. Gruenewald DA. Aging of the endocrine system. In Hazzard WR, Blass JP, Ettinger WH Jr, et al., eds. *Principles of Geriatric Medicine and Gerontology*, 4th edn. New York: McGraw-Hill, 1999:949–65

39. Halter JB. Diabetes mellitus. In Hazzard WR, Blass JP, Ettinger WH Jr, et al., eds. *Principles of Geriatric Medicine and Gerontology*, 4th edn. New York: McGraw-Hill, 1999:991–1011

40. Mooradian AD. Normal age-related changes in thyroid hormone economy. *Clin Geriatr Med* 1995;11:159–69

41. Gentili A, Mulligan T. Sexual dysfunction in older adults. *Clin Geriatr Med* 1998;14: 383–93

42. Walsh JR. Hematological problems. In Cassel CK, Cohen HJ, Larson EB, et al., eds. *Geriatric Medicine*, 3rd edn. New York: Springer Verlag, 1997:627–36

43. Carmel R. Anemia and aging: an overview of clinical diagnostic and biological issues. *Blood Rev* 2001;15:9–18

44. Gilcrest BA. Aging of the skin. In Hazzard WR, Blass JP, Ettinger WH Jr, et al., eds. *Principles of Geriatric Medicine and Gerontology*, 4th edn. New York: McGraw-Hill, 1999:573–90

45. Cantrell M, Norman DC. Infections. In Duthie EH Jr, Katz PR, eds. *Practice of Geriatrics*, 3rd edn. Philadelphia: WB Saunders, 1998:563–78

46. Jordan B, Cumming JL. Mental status and neurological exam in the elderly. In Hazzard WR, Blass JP, Ettinger WH Jr, et al., eds. *Principles of Geriatric Medicine and Gerontology*, 4th edn. New York: McGraw-Hill, 1999:1209–17

47. Aldwin CM, Levenson MR, Ober BA. Psychology of aging. In Reuben DB, Yoshikawa TT, Besdine RW, eds. *Geriatric Review Syllabus*, 3rd edn. Iowa: Kendall/ Hunt Publishing, 1996:24–9

48. Pressman MR, Fry JM. What is normal sleep in the elderly? *Clin Geriatr Med* 1988;4: 71–81

49. Bundlie SR. Sleep in aging. *Geriatrics* 1998;53(suppl 1):S41–3

50. Hirsh CH. Hypothermia and hyperthermia. In Duthie EH Jr, Katz PR, eds. *Practice of Geriatrics*, 3rd edn. Philadelphia: WB Saunders, 1998:244–55

51. Ballester JM, Harchelroad FP. Hyperthermia: how to recognize and prevent heat-related illnesses. *Geriatrics* 1999;54:20–4

52. Gall JS, Szwabo PA. Psychosocial aspects of aging. *Clin Geriatr* 2002;10:48–52

53. Cassell CK. Successful aging. *Geriatrics* 2001;56:35–9

54. Lunenfeld B, Gooren L. Aging men – challenges ahead. In Lunenfeld B, Gooren L, eds. *Textbook of Men's Health*. New York: Parthenon Publishing, 2002:3–14

55. Fillit HM, Butler RN, O'Connell AW, et al. Achieving and maintaining cognitive vitality with aging. *Mayo Clin Proc* 2002;77:681–96

3 Comprehensive geriatric assessment

T.S. Dharmarajan, MD, FACP, AGSF, Shamim Ahmed, MD, and Srinivasa R. Adapa, MD

INTRODUCTION

Aging, with longer life expectancy, has characterized the world human population in the past century. Although most older people enjoy reasonable health, the number of elderly with multiple illnesses and disabilities appears to be increasing worldwide[1]. Older adults tend to have obscured illnesses, atypical presentation of common disease and a vulnerability to iatrogenic medical problems, posing challenges to the physician in management[2]. In the 1970s, when geriatrics entered its renaissance, health providers began to analyze the specific problems and needs of older adults, noticed differences between age-related physiologic alterations and diseases, between caring and curing, and realized the need to focus on improving the functional status of the older individual[3]. The benefit of interdisciplinary team effort in managing co-morbidity has become apparent[3]. Evaluation of the elderly with such an approach is different and much more than the standard medical evaluation; broadly termed 'geriatric assessment', the theme evolved from efforts of geriatricians in the UK and the USA[4,5]. When geriatric assessment involves an intensive interdisciplinary process of organizing the extensive database to manage complex, interacting problems of the elderly, it is termed 'comprehensive geriatric assessment' (CGA). From the demographic standpoint, non-geriatricians are currently managing most patients older than 65 years; the concept of CGA has become an established part of medical practice for all healthcare providers, to be utilized when indicated and appropriate[6].

CONCEPT AND DEFINITION OF COMPREHENSIVE GERIATRIC ASSESSMENT

Since the early 1970s and up to 1987, various approaches had been tried to explore the effectiveness of CGA[3]. The data from these studies and presentations by experts were used to develop a consensus for geriatric assessment methods for clinical decision-making by the National Institutes of Health (NIH) in the USA in 1987[3]. CGA was defined, the goals were determined and different settings, processes and elements of geriatric assessment were discussed. Studies have since demonstrated significant benefits, including improvement in diagnosis and functional status, reduced rates of institutionalization and hospital admissions, and increased survival (Table 1). Other benefits included reduction in medication use, improved affect and cognition and overall reduction in medical care costs[3]. Effectiveness of CGA varied with the assessment process, settings, target population and personnel involved in the team

23

Table 1 Benefits of comprehensive geriatric assessment

Unmasks underlying illness
Reduces medication-related adverse effects
Improves affect and cognition
Improves independent function
Improves quality of life
Decreases hospital stay and admissions
Decreases nursing home admissions
Decreases health-care cost
Decreases mortality and improves survival

Table 2 The process of comprehensive geriatric assessment (CGA)

Identify population at risk
Involve appropriate team members or consultant
Assess CGA elements
   physical health
   mental health
   functional status
   social and economic status
   environmental characteristics
Co-ordinate data and develop a plan
Implement plan and monitor progress

effort. Comprehensive geriatric assessment in practice includes evaluation, management and monitoring of progress. Data are gathered by team members, a comprehensive management plan is developed and implemented, and the progress is monitored (Table 2).

The NIH consensus conference on CGA defined CGA as: 'A multidisciplinary evaluation in which multiple problems of older persons are uncovered, described, and explained, if possible, and in which the resources and strengths of the person are catalogued, need for services assessed, and a coordinated care plan developed to focus interventions on the person's problems'[3]. Simply stated, CGA is a clinical approach to screening and diagnosis designed to achieve the best possible health outcome and highest level of functional status in the geriatric patient.

GOALS

The well-being of older adults depends on their physical and psychological health, social and economic support, environmental factors and functional status. The functional status influences and is influenced by the above domains of geriatric health; improvement in function is often the most appropriate goal of CGA. The goals are to assist in accurate diagnosis, unmask illness that may have been otherwise undetected, plan and provide appropriate management and treatment to restore or maintain health, improve or maintain function, suggest and refer as indicated for optimum environmental and social support, predict outcome and monitor progress[3,7].

THE TEAM MEMBERS

The terms 'multidisciplinary' and 'interdisciplinary' are often used interchangeably to describe the involved team effort; in reality, a subtle difference exists[8]. A multidisciplinary team is a group of health-care providers who assess the patient 'independently', with the information shared amongst team members. The interdisciplinary team members assess the patient in a co-ordinated manner, interacting together and working 'interdependently'[8]. The interdisciplinary team includes a core group consisting of a physician, nurse and social worker, each with special expertise in caring for older people. When appropriate, the interdisciplinary team may also include physical and occupational therapists, a nutritionist, pharmacist, audiologist, optician, dentist and psychiatrist. Support from other medical specialties, such as neurology, ophthalmology, physiatry and urology is often required. Although, in the early phases of evolution of geriatrics, the concept of CGA included mostly multidisciplinary effort, with increased interest in cost effectiveness, the composition of the assessment team has changed to include in many instances only one health professional, with provision of expert consultant involvement as needed[4]. Also, depending on the setting, the composition of team members can vary. The concept of a virtual interdisciplinary team has been gaining interest recently; here, members are included as needed, and communicate electronically[4].

THE SETTINGS FOR COMPREHENSIVE GERIATRIC ASSESSMENT

CGA may be performed in many settings, including acute care, ambulatory care, long-term care and home care. In the UK, Canada and Australia, CGA is performed in out-patient facilities termed 'geriatric day hospitals'[9]. The elements of assessment, as well as team composition, differ with the setting. While the most effective CGA programs initially were institution based, in this era of cost cutting with hospitalizations, more CGA programs rely on post-discharge and community-based settings[5,9]. With this change, the focus has also changed. While the earlier programs stressed tertiary prevention by rehabilitation, the newer programs focus on primary and secondary prevention.

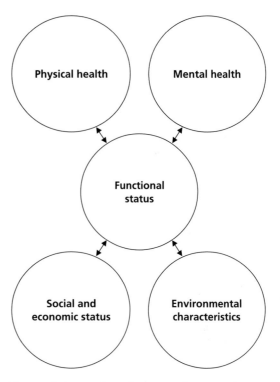

Figure 1 Interacting domains of comprehensive geriatric assessments

TARGET POPULATION

Selection of the appropriate candidates for comprehensive assessment is important, as some older but vigorous adults will not benefit from the same program meant for frail elderly; the latter group, at risk for functional compromise and nursing home placement, will benefit most from CGA[10,11]. Several criteria have been suggested to identify the frail elderly. The frail older individual has very limited reserves and the potential to decline rapidly into dysfunction and dependency[12]. The number of co-morbid problems, prescription medications and presence of functional limitations predict increased hospital use[11]. Frail geriatric patients, who are at high risk for repeated hospitalizations, longer length of hospital stay and nursing home placement, appear appropriate candidates for CGA[11]. The prevalence of functional limitations increases with age; hence, those aged 75 or over are more likely to benefit from periodic functional assessment[7,11].

THE ELEMENTS OF COMPREHENSIVE ASSESSMENT

Elements of geriatric assessment include different domains of health (Figure 1). These domains interact in the sense that a decline in any one element may eventually affect general well-being, other domains and functional status. Thus, to achieve optimum health in older subjects, all domains should be assessed and managed simultaneously (Table 3). The domains of health include physical health, mental health, social and economic status, functional status and the environmental states[3]. Counseling, emphasizing factors that affect lifestyle, such as nutrition, exercise, smoking, alcohol and injury prevention, is relevant in this regard[6,13]. Also important are discussions on patient preferences regarding

Table 3 Elements of comprehensive geriatric assessment

Physical health
Chronic illnesses
Vision and hearing
Falls, gait and balance
Weight changes; nutritional assessment
Incontinence, sexual function
Prescription and over-the-counter medications
Screening: cholesterol, thyroid function tests,
  colonoscopy, mammogram, Pap smear,
  prostate-specific antigen
Immunization: influenza, pneumonia, tetanus,
  diphtheria
Counseling: diet, supplements (calcium, vitamin D),
  exercise, smoking, alcohol, injury prevention
Advance directives

Mental health
Assessment for recent memory changes
Assessment of cognition
Screen for depression

Functional status
Ability to maintain advanced activities of daily living:
  maintaining occupational, social, community and
  recreational activities
Instrumental activities of daily living: use of telephone
  and public transportation, shopping, housekeeping,
  meal preparation, intake of medications,
  management of finances
Assessment of basic activities of daily living: bathing,
  dressing, toileting, transferring, eating, maintaining
  continence

advance directives[14]. The appointment of a responsible other person helps to make decisions on treatment options in the setting where the ability to communicate is impaired for any reason.

Physical health

Older adults are vulnerable to disease. Often, the presentation of common diseases is atypical and can be missed. An adequate history is crucial; this is often obtained from the caregiver, as the patient may be incapable of giving a reasonable history. A history of smoking, alcohol use, exercises, immunization status and review of medications need emphasis. Sexual function, often overlooked, should be ascertained, as it may relate to well-being;

older individuals maintain sufficient interest in sexual activities[3,6]. Screening for treatable diseases should be individualized depending on the presenting condition and prognosis. Depending on the setting for comprehensive assessment and patient status, specific preventive processes (primary, secondary and tertiary) receive emphasis[15]. The physical examination should focus on areas relevant to the presenting complaint and other common conditions. The latter include vision, hearing, gait and balance, nutrition and continence. Iatrogenic problems are common in the elderly, with polypharmacy often the clue to diagnosis of many complaints. Medical evaluation in CGA extends beyond the standard examination to include possible geriatric syndromes[4]. The overall goal is to achieve the best possible health and improve the quality of life[8].

Vision

Changes in vision occur with aging; visual impairment is a common problem in the elderly resulting in disability, falls and functional impairment[6]. Impairment of visual functions such as acuity of vision, contrast sensitivity, effects from glare and level of illumination, and ability for dark adaptation increase exponentially with age[16]. Over 90% of older people require eyeglasses, and a fifth of the over-85 age group have difficulty seeing even with eyeglasses[17]. The most common causes include presbyopia, cataract, glaucoma, diabetic retinopathy and macular degeneration[6]. The US Preventive Services Task Force (USPSTF) recommends regular vision screening for patients 65 years or older[6,18].

The visual acuity test with the Snellen eye chart is an easy screening process. If patients are unable to read satisfactorily, referral to an ophthalmologist is indicated. Risk factors include diabetes mellitus, family history of glaucoma, hypertension, myopia, African-American race and steroid therapy; periodic tonometry, fundoscopy and visual field examination is recommended in this group[5,6].

Hearing

Hearing impairment is extremely common, particularly in the very old, the prevalence rate ranging from 23 to 48% in the over-65 age group[17,19]. The most common cause of hearing impairment is presbycusis, a progressive, high-frequency, bilateral hearing loss. Those with presbycusis usually do not complain of a hearing disorder, rather report difficulty in understanding speech[19]. Hearing impairment is associated with poor self-esteem, emotional vulnerability, irritability, social isolation, depression and cognitive impairment. Screening for hearing impairment appears to be underutilized; only one-fifth of primary care providers routinely screen older individuals for hearing disorders[6]. Sadly, patients do not appear to seek help either.

Several screening methods are available; the whisper voice test is the simplest, where the examiner whispers a series of words, standing out of sight and 12 inches away from the testing ear; the patient is expected to repeat at least 50% of the words[17,19]. Another screening tool is a ten-item questionnaire called the Hearing Handicap Inventory for the Elderly – Screening version (HHIE-S)[6,19]. The gold standard for screening is the Welch Allyn Audioscope, with built-in audiometer[19]. When unable to hear either the 1000- or the 2000-Hz frequency in both ears or both frequencies in one ear, an audiology referral is appropriate[17]. The Clinical Glidepath recommends yearly screening for the elderly[18]. Cautious use or avoidance of ototoxic drugs and use of hearing aids improve functional status and quality of life.

Gait, balance and falls

Gait and balance problems increase with aging, affecting a fifth of community elderly, and predispose to falls[5,17]. A multifactorial

basis is usual; consequences of falls include soft tissue injuries, fractures, fear of recurrent falls, restricted mobility and decline in functional status[20]. Musculoskeletal disorders including arthritis, vascular and/or neurodegenerative disorders are common in the elderly and contribute to gait and balance problems.

Screening and detailed assessment are effective in identifying those at risk for falls; intervention may reduce the risk. It is a good practice to observe the gait while the patient is entering the office[4]. Often, the presence of specific gait disturbances (such as a Parkinsonian gait) may provide diagnostic clues[21]. Several gait and balance tests are available and easy to perform. Asking the patients to fold their hands across the chest and rise from an armless chair provides clues about quadriceps strength[20]. Tandem walking may reveal difficulties with balance. Impaired proprioception may be assessed by Romberg's test[21]. The ability to stretch and reach an object, a measure of functional reach, can be a predictor. In the timed 'Up & Go' test, the patient is asked to rise from an arm chair, walk 10 feet, turn, walk back and sit again; it permits evaluation of postural stability, steppage, stride length and sway[5,20]. A duration over 20 s to perform the maneuver suggests the need for further evaluation[4].

Nutrition

Malnutrition encompasses a broad range of conditions ranging from undernutrition to overnutrition. The prevalence of malnutrition in the geriatric population varies considerably, ranging from 1 to 60% with higher numbers in institutions[22]. Obesity is not uncommon, particularly among community-dwelling-elderly. Malnutrition is associated with poor immune function, susceptibility to infection, poor wound healing, osteoporosis and additional co-morbidity[22]. Data from the National Health and Nutrition Examination Survey III suggest that median energy intake is often lower than recommended in the elderly, leading to protein–energy malnutrition[5,22]. Certain vitamin deficiencies (vitamin B_{12}, folate and vitamin D) are common; calcium intake is inadequate in most, compounded by the presence of lactose intolerance[22]. The US diet contains far less than the recommended amount of fiber (20–35 g/day) in the diet. A modified dietary pyramid for older adults emphasizes the above measures and suggests an adequate water intake of approximately 2 litres daily[23]. A flag at the apex of the pyramid stresses the importance of calcium, vitamin D and B_{12} supplements[22,23].

The health-care provider should inquire about unintentional weight loss (or gain) of 10% or more in 6 months and compare weights periodically[5,21]. A history of unexplained weight change warrants further evaluation. The Mini Nutritional Assessment (MNA) is a screening tool for nutritional evaluation inclusive of anthropometric, general, dietary and self assessments[24]. Out of a maximum possible score of 30, a score range of 17–23.5 suggests risk of malnutrition and a score below 17 indicates frank malnutrition. Assessment includes a complete blood cell count, total lymphocyte count, and total serum protein, albumin and cholesterol levels[22]. Serum albumin levels do not change with normal aging. A cholesterol level below 130 mg/dl is associated with a poor prognosis[22]. While albumin has a half-life of 2–3 weeks, another marker, prealbumin, has a shorter half-life (2–3 days), which is helpful in monitoring acute changes in nutritional status[22].

Continence

Older adults typically underreport urinary incontinence, as they are embarrassed, and often consider it as an uncorrectable consequence of aging. A third of community-dwelling older women have some degree of urinary incontinence[25]. Men have a lower prevalence until age 80, after which they are equally affected from an increase in prevalence of benign prostatic hyperplasia

(BPH) with age[25]. Urinary incontinence is associated with urinary tract infection, falls, sleep deprivation, social withdrawal and depression, all of which impact on the quality of life. It may even be the basis for nursing home placement[25]. Fecal incontinence, on the other hand, is far less common than urinary loss but not rare[21]. The evaluation of urinary incontinence should include assessment of cognition, fluid intake, mobility, medications, prior urologic or gynecologic surgery and a focused physical examination. All older adults should be screened for urinary incontinence; a cure or significant improvement is often achievable. Evaluation and specialty consultation should be individualized.

Review of medications

The increase in co-morbidity with age is associated with an increase in use of medications, both prescribed and over-the-counter[26]. Most elders, on average, use three or more medications at any given time[26]. Many visit multiple physicians; often the primary care physician may be unaware of the total number and actual medications consumed[4]. 'Polypharmacy' is associated with increased risk of drug–drug, drug–disease, and drug–nutrient interactions, contributed to by age-related changes in pharmacokinetics and pharmacodynamics. Thus, older adults are predisposed to adverse drug events (ADEs)[26]. Falls, incontinence, delirium and cognitive impairment are only a few of the several ADEs in the elderly. A careful periodic review and revision of the drug regimen minimizes ADEs. This is accomplished by instructing the patient to bring in all medications at every visit, including prescribed and over-the-counter medications; vitamins, herbal products and ophthalmic preparations tend to be overlooked[4,26,27]. The need to continue each medication should be justified.

Preventive geriatrics

Screening Depending on the health status and life expectancy, the focus of preventive services should vary from extending life for appropriate candidates to preserving or improving quality of life for others[13]. Thus, decisions on screening should be individualized and discussed with the patient and/or caregiver. Recommendations vary based on the sources or guidelines. Hypertension is extremely common among men and women above 60 years of age. Detection and treatment of hypertension has demonstrated benefit in this age group. Screening for hypertension is appropriate every 1–2 years in all candidates for treatment[13]. The Adult Treatment Panel III (ATP III) favors screening for dyslipidemia and considers treatment beneficial in the elderly as much as or more than the younger age group[28]. Hypothyroidism is common in older women and often goes undetected. The Clinical Glidepath recommends thyroid stimulating hormone (TSH) assay every 2 years[18]. Vitamin B_{12} deficiency is common in the elderly with a prevalence of 3–40%, warranting screening for B_{12} deficiency in geriatric patients[29]. Cancer screening is quite complex in the elderly, with benefits of screening less well defined in those older than 65 years, whereas 60% of cancers occur in this age group[30]. Screening for breast, colon and cervical cancer is recommended for appropriate older candidates, and is discussed elsewhere in the text[13,30]. The USPSTF strongly recommends screening adults over 50 years for colorectal cancer, and mentions that benefits from screening outweigh potential harm; it stated that there is insufficient data as to the best screening procedure in terms of cost, benefits and potential risk[31]. As there is no agreement regarding prostate cancer screening among the American Cancer Society, USPSTF and American College of Physicians, the Clinical Glidepath recommends an individualized approach after discussing the pros and cons of prostate cancer screening with patient and/or caregiver[13,18,30].

The USPSTF recently recommended screening women over 65 years routinely for osteoporosis and that screening should begin at age 60 for those at risk for osteoporotic fractures[32]. The evidence was good that risk for osteoporosis and fractures increased with age; bone mineral density predicted risk for fractures and treatment in asymptomatic women reduced the risk for fractures[32].

Immunizations Assessment of the immunization status of geriatric patients is important. Older adults should receive annual influenza vaccine, as influenza is a major preventable cause of morbidity and mortality[13,15,18]. The vaccine is moderately effective and serious adverse reactions are rare. Pneumococcal pneumonia is common and associated with significant mortality and morbidity. The USPSTF recommends the current 23-valent polysaccharide pneumococcal vaccine for all aged 65 years and over[13,15,18]. Revaccination is suggested for those who received vaccine before age 65 and 5 or more years have elapsed, and for those immunocompromised. Tetanus still occurs in older individuals and is associated with high mortality. Fewer than half the elderly are immunized against tetanus and diphtheria. Tetanus–diphtheria (Td) toxoid is recommended every 10 years after the initial administration of a three-injection series; vaccination is 100% effective[6,13].

Counseling Health-care providers should counsel older people to exercise regularly, using an activity that is generally liked by the individual[3,33]. The benefits of exercise have been shown consistently with hypertension, cardiovascular disease, osteoporosis and other disorders[33]. The USPSTF recommends counseling on dietary measures, namely to increase intake of fruits, vegetables and grains and decrease fat consumption. An adequate calcium (1200–1500 mg/day) and vitamin D (400–800 IU/day) intake is recommended unless contraindicated[13,22]. Counseling for smoking cessation is always worthwhile, with benefits noted even if one quits smoking after age 70[13]. Provision of nicotine patch or gum is helpful. Brief counseling about the effects of alcohol and limits on consumption of alcohol is appropriate[34]. The USPSTF recommends counseling the elderly on injury prevention. Burns and scald injuries may be avoided by using smoke detectors, avoidance of smoking in bed and setting tap water (heater) temperature to 120–130°F (49–54°C)[13]. The elderly driver is at risk for injury from physical and cognitive impairments; the involved health-care provider should suggest using seat belts, curtailing alcohol use and determining the capacity to drive when appropriate.

Advance directives

Advance care planning by an individual with intact cognition provides help in medical decision-making for the period when the individual becomes decisionally incapacitated[14]. Advance directives are the expressions and/or documentations of such an individual's advanced care planning. Advance directives should be discussed with all geriatric patients, preferably in the out-patient setting while they are stable and receptive, and reviewed at the time of admission to a hospital or nursing home. The health-care provider must discuss life-sustaining care options and document individual preferences on resuscitation, mechanical ventilation and options on nutrition. Advance directives can be instructional (e.g. Living Wills, other written directives) or appointment of a health-care proxy, who acts as a spokesperson for decision-making[14]. Patients may change their preferences at any time as long as cognition is intact.

Mental health

Assessment of cognition, behavioral and emotional status of the older adult is an essential part of CGA. In particular, detection of dementia, delirium and depression are important, as their prevalences increase with age.

Assessment of cognition

The prevalence of dementia increases above the age of 65; up to 50% of those 85 and over have Alzheimer's disease, the most common basis. Screening instruments used for assessing cognition include the Clock Drawing Test, Short Portable Mental Status Questionnaire (SPMSQ), the Information–Memory–Concentration Mental Status Test (IMCT) and, the most commonly used, the Mini-Mental State Examination (MMSE) of Folstein and Folstein[4,5,35]. The MMSE is brief, easy to administer, and a recognized tool for quantifying the degree of cognitive impairment. The MMSE assesses orientation, registration, attention and calculation ability, recall, language and ability to follow simple commands[35]. Age, education, language and sensory impairments (of the patient) influence performance and score in the MMSE; these factors need to be considered prior to interpretation of the score. Out of a maximum score of 30, less than 24 is consistent with cognitive impairment but not necessarily diagnostic of dementia. Likewise, a score above 24 does not exclude dementia; thus, a near normal score may fail to detect early dementia, sometimes entailing a detailed psychiatric interview, neurobehavioral consultation and/or comprehensive neuropsychologic testing[5,35].

Assessment of affect

Depression is common in the elderly, with a prevalence of more than 10% in the community[5,17]. Risk factors include chronic illness, functional or cognitive decline, recent loss of a close one and socioeconomic factors, amongst others[17]. Often overlooked, the assessment for depression is essential as a component of CGA. Several screening instruments are available to aid in identifying the person at risk. The Geriatric Depression Scale (GDS) has three different versions (five-, 15- and 30-item versions), is easy to administer, and a well validated screening test[17,36]. Another instrument, the Hamilton Depression Scale, measures the severity of depression[37]. Positive screening warrants a more detailed evaluation. When a diagnosis of depression is made, it is important to verify in a non-threatening manner the risk for suicide.

Functional health

Assessment of functional status is an essential component of geriatric assessment. Functional status depends on physical health, cognition and adequate social and environmental support. Impairment of functions frequently goes unrecognized and undertreated by the health-care provider. Chronic conditions such as musculoskeletal disorders, diabetes, strokes, incontinence and sensory impairments are significant predictors of onset of functional limitation[38]. Early detection and specific interventions for risk factors for functional impairment may help reduce functional decline. Information on functional status may be gathered by direct observation of the patient by family or health-care provider. Function is measured by the ability to perform different levels of daily activities (Table 4). These include activities of daily living (ADL), instrumental activities of daily living (IADL) and advanced activities of daily living (AADL)[17,39].

Basics ADL are physical functions and include bathing, dressing, toileting, transferring, continence and feeding, often the one eventually lost[39]. When patients are unable to perform the basic ADL, they are unlikely to be able to live alone safely in the community and may require assistance at home or will need to live in a supervised environment[7]. IADL are behavioral and social activities that require a higher level of cognition and judgement; IADL include activities such as use of the telephone or public transportation, shopping for groceries, preparing meals, doing

Table 4 Activities of daily living (ADL), instrumental activities of daily living (IADL) and advanced activities of daily living (AADL)

ADL
Bathing
Dressing
Toileting
Continence
Transferring
Feeding

IADL
Use of telephone
Use of public transportation
Shopping
Preparation of meals
Housekeeping
Washing personal clothing
Taking medication properly
Managing personal finance

AADL
Occupation related
Traveling
Volunteer activities
Recreational activities
Community tasks
Organizing events

housework and laundry, taking medication and finally managing financial tasks, often the first noticeable decline[40]. Independent living in the community requires capacity for ADL and many IADL. AADL are more complex tasks to fulfil responsibilities to the family, society and community including recreational and occupational activities[16]. Several standardized questionnaires or self-report tools are available for assessing functional status[39,40]. The need for and the level of supportive assistance required can be determined by using these instruments.

Social and economic status

Assessment of social support network is an important component of CGA, as social isolation is common in patients aged 75 years and older. Any impairment or dependency in ADL or IADL prompts the need for

Name:			Date of Birth:		Gender:		

Physical Health
Chronic disorder:

Vision:	Adequate	Inadequate	Eye glasses:	Y	N	Needs evaluation
Hearing:	Adequate	Inadequate	Hearing Aids:	Y	N	Needs evaluation
Mobility:	Ambulatory:	Y	N	Assistive device:		
	Falls:	Y	N			Needs evaluation
Nutrition:	Albumin:		TLC:	HCT:		
	Weight:		Wt. Loss or gain:	Y	N	Needs evaluation
Incontinence:	Y	N	Treatment:	Y	N	Needs evaluation
Medications:	Total number:		Reviewed & revised: Y	N		
	Adverse effects/Allergy:					
Screening:	Cholesterol:	TSH:		B_{12}:		Folate:
	Colonoscopy:	Date:		N/A		
	Mammogram:	Date:		N/A		
	Osteoporosis	Date:		N/A		
	Pap smear:	Date:		N/A		
	PSA:	Date:		N/A		
Immunization:	Influenza:	Date:				
	Pneumonia:	Date:				
	Tetanus:	Date:		Booster:		
Counseling:	Diet	Exercise	Calcium	Vitamin D		
	Smoking	Alcohol	Driving	Injury Prevention		

Mental Health

Dementia:	Y	N	MMSE Score:	Date:	Cause (if known):	
Depression:	Y	N	GDS Score:	Date:	Treatment: Y	N

Functional Status

ADL:	Bathing:	I	D	Dressing:	I	D	Toileting:	I	D
	Transferring: I	D		Feeding:	I	D	Continence: Y	N	
IADL:	I	D	Partially dependent						

Home Health Services:		Not required	Required		Needs evaluation

Advance Directive

	Living Will:	Y	N		Health Care Proxy: Y	N
	DNR:	Y	N		Comments:	

(Y: Yes;   N: No;   N/A: Not applicable;   I: Independent;   D: Dependent)

Health Care Provider:		Date:

Figure 2   Comprehensive geriatric assessment

caregivers while still in the community. The health provider should inquire about the present and potential caregivers, who would be able to take care of patients, when incapacitated. Occasionally, the caregiver, most often a female, either family member or paid attendant, suffers a high level of stress from the physical and emotional burdens of providing care. Caregiver stress should be identified to avoid potential 'burn out'[5-7]. Referral to support groups is often helpful.

Economic concerns should be discussed with the patient and/or caregiver after establishing rapport to avoid misunderstanding. The elderly are often unaware of agencies that can provide help and unnecessarily may suffer a drain on their resources. By exploring the financial status, the health provider may assist in determining eligibility and need for state or other benefits for services. Personal values, such as cultural, ethnic and spiritual, should be given importance.

Possible outcome and options in management (such as placement in a nursing home) should be part of the discussions.

Environmental characteristics

For the frail elderly at risk for falls, the home environment should be assessed for potential hazards by a health professional, through a home visit, to determine adequacy and safety[21]. Adaptive devices such as shower bars and raised toilet seats should be recommended for those with impaired mobility and balance. Also, loose floor coverings, insufficient lighting and widened doors for wheelchair access deserve consideration to facilitate a safe environment, and to promote the ability to live independently. The means to access personal and health services from their current living situation should be assessed, to assure an adequate quality of life.

COORDINATE DATA AND DEVELOP A PLAN

Following comprehensive assessment by the team members or individual consultant, data are gathered and co-ordinated by the team leader or a health professional, to identify problems, determine goals and develop treatment plans. There is often a tendency to postpone evaluation of chronic conditions and geriatric syndromes (dementia, incontinence, falls, etc.) because of time constraints[41]. Evaluation of common geriatric problems with the aid of prescreening questionnaires and guided geriatric care protocols may lead to the identification and treatment of more problems than usual care[41,42]. A sample of a comprehensive assessment data sheet is illustrated in Figure 2. Recommendations are made to address the physical, mental, functional, social and environmental problems to improve overall outcome and quality of life. As there can be a large number of problems, recommendations should be prioritized to focus on the major or urgent issue. While some interventions are immediately necessary, many recommendations are best implemented after the patient is stabilized[4].

IMPLEMENT PLAN AND MONITOR PROGRESS

It is critical to implement recommendations; the success of CGA depends on compliance with the recommendations and periodic monitoring of outcome. Non-adherence to the treatment plans leads to failure of CGA programs[43]. The primary care physician or health providers should assume the responsibilities to implement recommendations and monitor progress; if needed, the treatment plan should be revised and modified[44].

SUMMARY

Accumulated evidence indicates that comprehensive geriatric assessment is effective when implemented and monitored, although effectiveness has varied in different settings. Concordance between the patient and healthcare provider is a powerful predictor of implementation and patient adherence to CGA recommendations[45]. Careful selection of patients and adherence to the plan by participants and providers will maximize the benefit from the comprehensive assessment program. The most consistent benefits of CGA have been reduced use of hospital and nursing home, reduced medical care costs and prolonged survival. Improvement in mental health and reduction in functional decline can be achieved by geriatric evaluation and management in both inpatient and outpatient settings[46]. Likewise, reduced mortality has been shown in the management of the acutely ill, frail elderly when cared for in a geriatric evaluation and management unit, compared to care in the general medical ward[47]. The goal is to preserve function and provide a better quality of life with maximum attainable health to our elders.

References

1. Lubitz JD, Eggers PW, Gornick ME, Villafranca NP. Demography of aging. In Cobbs EL, Duthie EH, Murphy JB, eds. *Geriatrics Review Syllabus*, 4th edn. Dubuque, IA: Kendall/Hunt Publishing, 1999:1–5

2. Williams ME. Approach to managing the elderly patient. In Hazzard WR, Blass JP, Ettinger WH Jr, Halter JB, Ouslander JG, eds. *Principles of Geriatric Medicine and Gerontology*, 4th edn. New York: McGraw Hill, 1999:249–53

3. Solomon D, Chairman, Consensus Development Panel. National Institutes of Health Consensus Development Conference Statement: Geriatric Assessment Methods for Clinical Decision-making. *J Am Geriatr Soc* 1988;36:342–7

4. Reuben DB. Principles of geriatric assessment. In Hazzard WR, Blass JP, Ettinger WH Jr, Halter JB, Ouslander JG, eds. *Principles of Geriatric Medicine and Gerontology*, 4th edn. New York: McGraw Hill, 1999:467–81

5. Palmer RM. Geriatric assessment. *Med Clin North Am* 1999;83:1503–23

6. Miller KE, Zylstra RG, Standridge JB. The geriatric patient: a systematic approach to maintaining health. *Am Fam Physician* 2000;61:1089–104

7. Gudmundsson A, Carnes M. Geriatric assessment: making it work in primary care practice. *Geriatrics* 1996;51:55–65

8. Elon R, Phillips C, Loome JF, *et al.* General issues and comprehensive approach to assessment of elders. In Osterweil D, Brummel-Smith K, Beck JC, eds. *Comprehensive Geriatric Assessment*. New York: McGraw Hill, 2000:1–39

9. McGann PE. Geriatric assessment for the rheumatologist. *Rheum Dis Clin North Am* 2000;26:415–32

10. Williams TF. Comprehensive geriatric assessment. In Duthie EH Jr, Katz PR, eds. *Practice of Geriatrics*, 3rd edn. Philadelphia, PA: WB Saunders, 1998:15–22

11. Laird RD, Studenski SA. Assessment. In Cobbs EL, Duthie EH Jr, Murphy JB, eds. *Geriatrics Review Syllabus*, 4th edn.

Dubuque, IA: Kendall/Hunt Publishing, 1999:75–9

12. Rockwood K, Silvius JL, Fox RA. Comprehensive geriatric assessment, helping your elderly patients maintain functional well-being. *Postgrad Med* 1998;103:247–64

13. Mehr DR. Preventive geriatrics. In Cobbs EL, Duthie EH Jr, Murphy JB, eds. *Geriatrics Review Syllabus*, 4th edn. Dubuque, IA: Kendall/Hunt Publishing, 1999:69–75

14. Pearlman RA. Advance directives. In Osterweil D, Brummel-Smith K, Beck JC, eds. *Comprehensive Geriatric Assessment*. New York: McGraw Hill, 2000:611–37

15. Bloom HG. Preventive medicine, when to screen for disease in older patients. *Geriatrics* 2001;56:41–5

16. West CG, Gildengorin G, Haegerstrom-Portnoy G, *et al.* Is vision function related to physical functional ability in older adults? *J Am Geriatr Soc* 2002;50:136–45

17. Koretz BK, Moore AA. Assessment of the geriatric patient: a practical approach. *J Clin Outcome Manage* 2001;8:35–40

18. Health maintenance in the elderly. *Home Health Care Consult* 2001;8:28–35

19. Bess FH. Hearing impairment. In Cobbs EL, Duthie EH Jr, Murphy JB, eds. *Geriatrics Review Syllabus*, 4th edn. Dubuque, IA: Kendall/Hunt Publishing, 1999:123–7

20. Rubenstein LZ. Falls and gait disorders. In Osterweil D, Brummel-Smith K, Beck JC, eds. *Comprehensive Geriatric Assessment*. New York: McGraw Hill, 2000:573–87

21. Paist SS III, Jafri A. Functional assessment in older patients, key to improving quality of life. *Postgrad Med* 1996;99:101–8

22. Dharmarajan TS, Kathpalia RK. A review of geriatric nutrition. In Dreger D, Krumm B, eds. *Hospital Physician Geriatric Medicine Board Review Manual*, vol 1. Wayne, PA: Turner White Communications, 2000:2–12

23. Russell RM, Rasmussen H, Lichtenstein A. Modified food guide pyramid for people over seventy years of age. *J Nutr* 1999;129:752

24. Vellas B, Guigoz Y, Garry PJ. *Nutrition* 1999;15:116–22
25. DuBeau CE. Urinary incontinence. In Cobbs EL, Duthie EH Jr, Murphy JB, eds. *Geriatrics Review Syllabus*, 4th edn. Dubuque, IA: Kendall/Hunt Publishing, 1999:115–23
26. Dharmarajan TS, Ugalino JT. Understanding the pharmacology of aging. In Dreger D, Krumm B, eds. *Hospital Physician Geriatric Medicine Board Review Manual*, vol 1. Wayne, PA: Turner White Communications, 2000:2–12
27. Dharmarajan TS, Tota R. Appropriate use of medications in older adults. *Fam Pract Recert* 2000;22:29–38
28. Sherman FT. New guidelines on high cholesterol. *Geriatrics* 2001;56:3–4
29. Dharmarajan TS, Norkus EP. Approaches to vitamin B12 deficiency. *Postgrad Med* 2001;110:99–106
30. Heflin MT, Cohen HJ. Cancer screening in the elderly. *Hosp Pract* 2001;36:61–9
31. Berg AO, Allan JD, Frame PS, *et al.* Screening for colorectal cancer: recommendation and rationale. US Preventive Services Task Force. *Ann Intern Med* 2002;137:129–31
32. Berg AO, Allan JD, Frame PS, *et al.* Screening for osteoporosis in postmenopausal women: recommendations and rationale. *Ann Intern Med* 2002;137:526–8
33. Schwartz RS, Buchner DM. Exercise in the elderly: physiologic and functional effects. In Hazzard WR, Blass JP, Ettinger WH Jr, Halter JB, Ouslander JG, eds. *Principles of Geriatric Medicine and Gerontology*, 4th edn. New York: McGraw Hill, 1999:143–58
34. Jones TV, Adams WL. Alcohol, tobacco, and drug abuse. In Cobbs EL, Duthie EH, Jr, Murphy JB, eds. *Geriatrics Review Syllabus*, 4th edn. Dubuque, IA: Kendall/Hunt Publishing, 1999:190–5
35. Folstein MF, Folstein SE, McHugh PR. 'Mini-mental state.' A practical method for grading the cognitive state of patients for the clinician. *J Psychiatr Res* 1975;12:189–98
36. Yesavage JA. Depression in the elderly: how to recognize masked symptoms and choose appropriate therapy. *Postgrad Med* 1992;91:255–61
37. Hays JC, Steffens DC, Flint EP, *et al.* Does social support buffer functional decline in elderly patients with unipolar depression? *Am J Psychiatry* 2001;158:1850–5
38. Dunlop DD, Manheim LM, Sohn MW, *et al.* Incidence of functional limitation in older adults: the impact of gender, race, and chronic conditions. *Arch Phys Med Rehabil* 2002;83:964–71
39. Katz S. Assessing self-maintenance: activities of daily living, mobility, and instrumental activities of daily living. *J Am Geriatr Soc* 1983;31:721–7
40. Lawton MP, Brody EM. Assessment of older people: self maintaining and instrumental activities of daily living. *Gerontologist* 1969;9:279–85
41. Philpot CD, Cefalu CA, Thomas DR. Comprehensive geriatric assessment. *Res Staff Phys* 2002;48:17–24
42. Bogardus ST, Richardson E, Maciejewski PK, *et al.* Evaluation of a guided protocol for quality improvement in identifying common geriatric problems. *J Am Geriatr Soc* 2002;50:328-35
43. Aminzadeh F. Adherence to recommendations of community-based comprehensive geriatric assessment programmes. *Age Ageing* 2000;29:401–7
44. Reuben DB, Frank JC, Hirsch SH, *et al.* A randomized clinical trial of outpatient comprehensive geriatric assessment coupled with an intervention to increase adherence to recommendations. *J Am Geriatr Soc* 1999;47: 269–76
45. Maly RC, Leake B, Frank JC, *et al.* Implementation of consultative geriatric recommendations: the role of patient-primary care physician concordance. *J Am Geriatr Soc* 2002;50:1372–80
46. Cohen HJ, Feussner JR, Weinberger M, *et al.* A controlled trial of inpatient and outpatient geriatric evaluation and management. *N Engl J Med* 2002;346:905–12
47. Saltvedt I, Mo EO, Fayers P, *et al.* Reduced mortality in treating acutely sick, frail older patients in a geriatric evaluation and management unit. A prospective randomized trial. *J Am Geriatr Soc* 2002;50:792–8

4 Hospital care

T.S. Dharmarajan, MD, FACP, AGSF, *and Abdolreza Ghazinouri*, MD

Although hospitalization usually deals with the diagnosis and treatment of specific disorders, functional outcomes are often overlooked. This chapter focuses on risks associated with functional decline from hospitalization, means to avoid them and ways to maintain independence and quality of life. Furthermore, in-patient interventions represent only the initial step to avoid functional decline, with the need to extend the process into the post-discharge period. Patients aged 65 years and older have the highest rates of hospitalization, the longest length of stay and the greatest risks of functional decline and nursing home placement. The use of hospital care by the geriatric age group is anticipated to grow by 250%, with a significant increase in hospital days of care[1].

ACUTE CARE GERIATRIC UNITS

Acute care of elders (ACE) units, also referred to as geriatric evaluation and management (GEM) units, are different from other general medical units in their environmental design, patient population and organization. Besides administering medical treatment, the emphasis is on maintaining functional independence and self-care through multidisciplinary collaboration and comprehensive discharge planning. Randomized clinical trials have demonstrated that ACE units can improve functional outcomes, with lower length of hospital stay, fewer nursing home placements and higher satisfaction with care[2]. Suggestions have been made

to create geriatric hospitals for common medical and surgical problems, with provision for rehabilitation[3].

Units are ideally designed to suit the needs of older individuals. 'Gerodesign' includes glare-free lighting, use of appropriate furniture (chairs and beds) to suit elder needs, clocks that are easy to read, calendars with minimum data (date, day, month, in large font), easy to use telephones and appropriately designed bathrooms (hand-held showers, non-skid surfaces). Wheelchair and stretcher access should be easy, with clutter avoided. Most of these features have been in use in our 75-bed in-hospital acute care geriatric unit (in the Bronx) and have contributed substantially to better overall patient satisfaction and perhaps outcome. Nursing staff in this unit should be ideally those interested in caring for the older individual and preferably with additional training in this area[4].

In-patient geriatric units should provide for rendering primary care and the availability of geriatric consultations when requested. A recent controlled trial suggested that in-patient geriatric units had no effects on survival, but significantly impacted on function in a favorable manner without increase in costs[5]. Further, studies suggest that patients and caregivers value benefits from these programs[6].

FUNCTIONAL STATUS

Although hospitalization usually focuses on treatment of acute illness, functional outcomes are the critical determinants of the quality of life, independence, cost of care and prognosis[7]. These functional issues are often not considered by physicians who are preoccupied with the diagnostic evaluation and treatment of acute illness. The causes of functional decline are 'multifactorial, cumulative and interactive', and include the effects of the acute illness itself, and adverse effects of medical and surgical treatments[8].

Studies of patients hospitalized for a variety of illnesses have demonstrated that acute medical diagnosis alone is a poor predictor of functional decline[7,9–11]. In the Harvard Medical Practice Study, the rate of adverse events occurring in hospitalized patients aged 65 and older was higher than that for any age group and more than twice the rate of adverse events recorded for the age group of 16–44[12,13]. Hospitalized elderly had the highest rate of diagnostic and therapeutic mishaps, falls and fractures[8]. The consequence is loss of independence and self-esteem resulting from the need to rely on others for basic needs[8]. A decline in function is also associated with a longer length of stay[7,10].

Patients at risk for functional decline in the hospital should be identified early. Such decline occurs more often in those aged 75 years and older, with cognitive impairment and dependence on two or more instrumental activities of daily living (IADL) prior to admission[11]. There is also a correlation with pressure ulcers, baseline functional dependency and/or a history of low social activity[14]. Depression and delirium are consistent associations.

Identification of functional impairment is obtained via self-reports of activities of daily living (ADL) and bedside observations during rounds. Balance and gait can be assessed by observing the patient move around. Those with ADL dependence and gait and balance impairment may benefit from physical and occupational therapy. Increased physical activity, avoidance of restraints and the use of assistive devices help improve self-dependence.

Attention to maintaining functional status should begin on the day of hospitalization and is the responsibility of all staff, not just the physical and occupational therapists[15].

IATROGENICITY

The rate of iatrogenic illness is higher in the elderly, partly due to the higher rates of co-morbidity and subsequent longer lengths of hospitalization[16]. Examples of iatrogenic illnesses include nosocomial infections, complications of diagnostic or therapeutic procedures (e.g. contrast-associated nephropathy), pressure ulcers resulting from prolonged and sometimes enforced bedrest, trauma (e.g. falls), fluid and electrolyte disturbances and hematomas from venipuncture[2].

Iatrogenic illnesses can also arise from use of broad-spectrum antibiotics that eliminate normal body flora and lead to infections with resistant micro-organisms such as methicillin-resistant *Staphylococcus aureus* (MRSA) and vancomycin-resistant enterococcus (VRE). These infections are increasingly recognized in the hospitalized elderly. VRE infections are associated with prolonged hospitalization, intra-hospital spread between floors and prior use of broad-spectrum antimicrobials[2]. Another example is infection due to *Clostridium difficile*, a common cause of nosocomial diarrhea[15]. C. *difficile* infection follows antibiotic therapy; nearly every antibiotic has been implicated. C. *difficile* diarrhea is noticed in both community and nursing home residents who need hospitalization; outcome is determined by the co-morbidity rather than age[17,18].

Nosocomial infections can be transmitted by caregivers and/or hardware (e.g. unclean stethoscopes)[16]. Overwhelming evidence supports a causal relationship between indwelling urinary catheters and urinary tract infections[15]. Suggestions that help reduce nosocomial infections and iatrogenic illnesses are listed in Table 1[15,16].

Table 1 Measures to reduce nosocomial infections and Iatrogenic illnesses

Follow universal precautions
Use hygienic hand washing techniques between patient visits
Limit use of urinary catheters and intravenous lines
Narrow the spectrum of empirically selected antibiotics when cultures available
Limit the length of hospitalization
Use appropriate posture for feeding and institute aspiration precautions
Practice rational drug prescribing, understand the pharmacology of aging
Be knowledgeable of drug interactions
Avoid psychoactive drugs if alternatives are available
Be aware of adverse drug events
Minimize diagnostic procedures (e.g. contrast media associated)
Maintain adequate hydration and nutrition
Prevent development of pressure ulcers

POLYPHARMACY

Older adults tend to be on numerous medications, both prescribed and over-the-counter drugs, in addition to eye drops and topical agents. The use of multiple drugs (polypharmacy) predisposes the individual to drug–drug, drug–nutrient and drug–disease interactions. Adverse drug events, such as falls, appear to be linked to the number of medications taken. It is the role of the health provider to review medications periodically, and dose based on altered pharmacokinetics related to aging or disease (e.g. renal function). On discharge from the hospital, regimens may need further alteration in the out-patient setting with changes in physical status, activity and diet[6,19,20].

SURGERY

Preoperative assessment may be performed in the out-patient setting for elective surgery or in the hospital (see Chapter 11, on perioperative management). It may be reasonable to schedule older individuals earlier in the day to reduce the anxiety and duration of 'nothing by mouth' (NPO).

SKIN INTEGRITY

Patients at risk for development of pressure ulcers should be identified early. Predisposing factors such as pressure, immobility, shearing, friction, moisture and malnutrition should be recognized and attended to. Periodic examination is indicated of potential sites for skin breakdown[21].

BOWEL FUNCTION

Prolonged immobilization, dehydration, certain medications and electrolyte imbalance may result in constipation and fecal impaction. This in turn may lead to poor appetite, malnutrition, depression and prolonged hospitalization[15]. Furthermore, as stated earlier, excessive use of antibiotics places the patient at risk for development of diarrhea.

NUTRITION

Undernutrition is a significant problem in the hospitalized elderly, and is associated with higher morbidity and mortality. Dramatic weight loss and hypoalbuminema quickly follow acute hospitalization, often in days[22]. Undernutrition increases the risk of nosocomial infections and pressure ulcers, and delays healing after surgery[15].

Malnutrition can be diagnosed on a clinical basis, by a history of unintentional weight loss, anthropometric measurements and by biochemical measures of nutrition. Biochemical parameters suggestive of protein–calorie malnutrition include serum albumin levels of less than 3.5 g/dl, low serum cholesterol and a low total lymphocyte count. Other serum markers, such as prealbumin, with a shorter half-life, reflect more recent nutritional changes[23].

Malnourished individuals or those at risk of undernutrition may benefit from consultation with a nutrition support team. These nutritionally deficient hospitalized elderly are not the best candidates for dietary restrictions for long-term benefits to lower cholesterol or blood pressure[15]. Furthermore, in order to encourage intake, the food should be palatable, calorie-dense and nutritious. Studies indicate that nutritional supplements containing balanced mixtures of amino acids, carbohydrates, fat, minerals and vitamins may improve the prognosis of older adults with lung infections and hip fractures[2]. The old saying 'if the gut works, use it' holds true for oral feeding, which is preferred to peripheral alimentation. When enteral feeding is contraindicated for an indefinite period of time, for example in inflammatory bowel disease or bowel obstruction, total parenteral nutrition is indicated. Older patients, whether on tube feeds or capable of oral intake, are often at risk for aspiration pneumonia. In such situations, evaluation with the help of a nutritionist to determine the dietary prescription, including consistency, is warranted.

COGNITION

Cognitive dysfunction in the geriatric population is usually secondary to delirium, dementia or depression. A missed diagnosis is not unusual. Delirium or acute confusional state commonly occurs in elderly individuals at admission or during hospitalization, and often goes unrecognized[24]. Dementia is an important risk factor for the development of delirium. Other contributing factors are medications, dehydration, iatrogenic events, medical illnesses, infection, metabolic derangement, alcohol or drug withdrawal, environmental influences, psychosocial factors, advanced age and vision or hearing impairment, particularly superimposed on those with restricted immobility[24].

Delirium is potentially a medical emergency and should be suspected in individuals with recent changes in mental status. It might be the only sign of underlying life-threatening illness such as myocardial infarction, pneumonia or urosepsis in the geriatric population.

The cardinal signs of delirium are its acute onset (hours to days), inattention and its fluctuating course. It remains a clinical diagnosis[24], based on careful bedside observations, including tests of attention and cognition. The diagnosis of delirium should prompt the clinician to look for an etiology.

On the other hand, while dementia is often recognized, a greater awareness for the diagnosis of depression in older subjects is warranted. Sometimes, it is difficult to distinguish between the two, and a trial of antidepressants is warranted. Medications should always be considered in the etiology.

MOBILITY AND FALLS

Impaired mobility is common in the hospitalized elderly and predisposes to adverse physiological effects. Deconditioning brought on by inactivity or prolonged bedrest results in diminished functional capacity and increases complications such as hypoxemia, bone demineralization, muscle atrophy, contractures, constipation, pressure ulcers, urinary incontinence, deep vein thrombosis, postural hypotension and falls[2,25]. Further exacerbation results from use of physical or chemical restraints, and restrictions imposed by intravenous lines and catheters. Prevention of deconditioning requires a multifaceted approach, from medical, nutritional, rehabilitational and psychosocial services. Falls occur during hospitalization and may be multifactorial; factors include co-morbidity, decreased sensory input, medications, restraints and an unfamiliar environment. It is essential for the staff to familiarize hospitalized adults about the surroundings and leave a night light when indicated. Falls need to be evaluated, as they tend to recur.

RESTRAINTS

Restraints are any physical, chemical (i.e. drugs) and mechanical devices or equipment attached to or near the patient's body that would restrict one's movement or access. Examples of physical restraints include hand mittens, wrist or leg restraints, Posey jackets, lap belts or sheets, full side rails and restraining chairs[26]. The subject of physical restraints is a paradox. On the one hand, they are used in hospitalized patients primarily to prevent disruption of medical therapies for confused patients and to prevent falls. On the other hand, they are perceived as a form of physical and psychological abuse. The use of physical restraints has undesirable sequelae, such as limb ischemia, pressure ulcers, deconditioning and mortality[2]. The most commonly reported danger is strangulation from vest restraints[27]. Health professionals also believe that they may be subject to legal liability if an unrestrained patient suffers an injury[28]. Although hospitals have a clear duty to protect patients from harm, they 'do not have a duty to restrain'[26,29]. Guidelines for the use of physical restraints define the parameters of liability and have become the standard for customary practice to establish policies and procedures. A reasonable approach to restraint use is to avoid them until all alternative approaches have been implemented or determined not feasible[2]. Alternatives require use of targeted approaches with environmental, social and pharmological interventions.

Medications are considered to be chemical restraints when applied to modify behavior that is normally not thought by the patient to require drug treatment[27]. The medications most often used are the benzodiazapines or the antipsychotics. The pharmacology and side-effects of these medications are well recognized. Oversedation can add to the risk of falls, aspiration, confusion and respiratory arrest.

THE INTERDISCIPLINARY TEAM

Changes in the health system have led to shorter hospital stays, resulting in earlier discharge of older patients with complex care needs. The criteria for discharge remain contingent on trajectory of illness, baseline physical and cognitive function, social support and, most importantly, the patient preferences. Function, the ability to manage day-to-day activities, is the best predictor of the patient's health and post-hospital care needs[30].

An interdisciplinary (ID) team assumes the responsibility of addressing the complex medical, physical and psychological needs in order to decrease the functional decline in hospitalized, medically ill, older patients. A geriatric ID team often includes a core group of individuals such as a geriatrician (or primary physician), a clinical nurse specialist or nurse practitioner, staff nurses, a social worker, a dietitian and a physical or occupational therapist. Other team members such as a pharmacist, speech and swallow therapist, psychologist or psychiatric clinical nurse, and a spiritual leader may be involved, depending on the patient's needs. The strength of the ID team lies in communication and trust in each other's competency and expertise, and the ability to work together toward common goals[30]. The goals are to help with placement after discharge, identify post-hospital care needs and services, educate the patient and family about diagnosis, prognosis and choices for discharge location, review medications, home situation and safety, and estimate/reduce the length of stay. If possible, tentative plans for discharge are made at the time of admission.

The ID team should focus on complex, high-risk patients, and those at risk for functional decline. Suggestions may be written on the interdisciplinary communication sheet placed in the patient's chart. This will serve as a communication tool between the team and primary care physician[30]. The process is efficacious, and evidence suggests that the approach helps prevent functional decline, restores function and provides continuity of care and the best disposition following discharge.

The majority of hospitalized patients are discharged home, while others require short-term or long-term care facilities post-hospitalization. Patients able to perform daily activities independently may return home with or without the need for home care services. On the other hand, patients with chronic disease who lack sufficient support may be transferred to long-term care facilities. Recruiting skilled nursing care and home physical therapy are other options that enable completion of medical treatment restorative services at home. Rehabilitation hospitals may be a reasonable option for patients with good rehabilitation potential after a stroke or hip fracture. Frail elderly patients may benefit from short-term rehabilitation in a subacute care unit until they regain functional independence. Hospice care at home or in a facility is an option for a terminally ill patient with life expectancy less than 6 months.

References

1. Rice DP. Beneficiary profile: yesterday, today and tomorrow. *Health Care Financing Rev* 1996;18:23–45

2. Palmer RM. Acute care. In Hazzard WR, Blass JP, Ettinger WH, Jr, Halter JB, Ouslander JG, eds. *Principles of Geriatric Medicine and Gerontology*, 4th edn. New York: McGraw-Hill, 1999:483–92

3. Gillick MR. Do we need to create geriatric hospitals? *J Am Geriatr Soc* 2002;50:174–77

4. Dharmarajan TS, Lifrieri R, Gerstner LS. Launching a geriatric unit. *Health Prog* 1998;79:46,47,51

5. Cohen HJ, Feussner JR, Weinberger M, et al. A controlled trial of inpatient and outpatient geriatric evaluation and management. *N Engl J Med* 2002;346:905–12

6. Campion EW. Specialized care for elderly patients. *N Engl J Med* 2002;346:874

7. Landefeld CS, Palmer RM, Kresevic D, et al. A randomized trial of care in a hospital medical unit especially designed to improve the functional outcomes of acutely ill older patients. *N Engl J Med* 1995;332:1338

8. Sager MA, Rudberg MA. Function decline associated with hospitalization for acute illness. *Clin Geriatr Med* 1998;14:669–79

9. Inouye SK, Wagner DR, Acampora D, et al. A controlled trial of a nursing-centered intervention in hospitalized elderly medical patients: the Yale Geriatric Care Program. *J Am Geriatric Soc* 1993;41:1353–60

10. Sager MA, Franke T, Inouye SK, et al. Functional outcomes of acute medical illness in hospitalized older persons. *Arch Intern Med* 1996;156:645–52

11. Sager MA, Rudberg MA, Jalaluddin M, et al. Hospital Admission Risk Profile (HARP): identifying older patients at risk for functional decline following acute medical illness and hospitalization. *J Am Geriatr Soc* 1996;44:251–7

12. Brennan TA, Leape LL, Laird NM, et al. Incidence of adverse events and negligence in hospitalized patients: results of the Harvard Medical Practice Study I. *N Engl J Med* 1991;324:370–6

13. Brennan TA, Leape LL, Laird NM, et al. The nature of adverse events in hospitalized patients: results of the Harvard Medical Practice Study II. *N Engl J Med* 1991;324:377–84

14. Inouye SK, Wagner DR, Acampora D, et al. A predictive index for functional decline in hospitalized elderly medical patients. *J Gen Intern Med* 1993;8:645–52

15. Riedinger JL, Robbins LJ. Prevention of iatrogenic illness. *Clin Geriatr Med* 1998; 14:681–98

16. Palmer RM. Acute care. In Duthie EH Jr, Katz PR, eds. *Practice of Geriatrics*, 3rd edn. Philadelphia: Saunders, 1998:65–72

17. Dharmarajan TS, Sipalay M, Shyamsunder R, et al. Comorbidity not age predicts

outcome in older adults with *Clostridium difficile* colitis. *World J Gastroenterol* 2000;6:198–201

18. Dharmarajan TS, Patel B, Sipalay M, Norkus EP. *Clostridium difficile* colitis in older adults from long term care facilities and the community: do their outcome differ? *J Am Med Dir Assoc* 2000;1:58–61

19. Dharmarajan TS, Ugalino JT. Understanding the pharmacology of aging. In Dreger D, Krumm B, eds. *Hospital Physician Geriatric Medicine Board Review Manual*. Wayne, PA: Turner White Communication, 2001;1:1–12

20. Dharmarajan TS, Tota R. Appropriate use of medications in older adults. *Fam Pract Recertific* 2000;22:29–38

21. Dharmarajan TS, Ugalino JT. Pressure ulcers: clinical features and management. *Hosp Physician* 2002;38:64–71

22. Thomas DR, Zdrowski CD, Wilson MM, *et al*. Malnutrition in subacute care. *Am J Clin Matr* 2002;75:308–13

23. Dharmarajan TS, Kathpalia RK. A review of geriatric nutrition. In Dreger D, Krumm B, eds. *Hospital Physician Geriatric Medicine Board Review Manual*. Wayne, PA: Turner White Communication, 2000;1:1–12

24. Inouye SK. Delirium in hospitalized older patients. *Clin Geriatr Med* 1998;4:745–64

25. Mahoney JE. Immobility and falls. *Clin Geriatr Med* 1998;14:699–726

26. Frengley JD, Lorraine CM. Physical restraints in the acute care setting. *Clin Geriatr Med* 1998;4:727–43

27. Marks W. Physical restraints in the practice of medicine. *Arch Intern Med* 1992;152:2203–6

28. Francis J. Using restraints in the elderly because of fear of litigation. *N Engl J Med* 1989;320:870–1

29. Kapp MB. Legal issues of physical restraints in hospital. Reducing physical restraints in hospitals: issues and approaches. Presented at *50th Annual Meeting of the Gerontological Society of America*, Cincinnati, 1997

30. Kresevic D, Holden C. Interdisciplinary care. *Clin Geriatr Med* 1998;14:787–98

5 Community care

T.S. Dharmarajan, MD, FACP, AGSF, and Abdolreza Ghazinouri, MD

The aim of geriatric care, besides diagnosis and management of specific disease entities, is to maintain function and self-care. Minute changes in functional and cognitive status often lead to significant improvement in the patients' quality of life. While hospitalization provides acute care, community care deals with prevention of disease and functional decline, and with maintenance of health. This chapter reviews the different community settings in which geriatric care is rendered. Each locale has its advantages and disadvantages and may or may not require change of residence of the patient. Services provided in certain settings may vary depending on the location, state laws and licensing regulations.

OFFICE VISIT

The office visit provides the physician with an opportunity to perform a comprehensive geriatric assessment and to provide preventive services. The physician must have an organized and systematic approach. Standardized forms for geriatric assessment that are easy to follow will facilitate this process and save time. This comprehensive assessment involves the evaluation of the physical, psychosocial and environmental factors that impact on the well-being of the elderly. Evaluation for activities of daily living (ADL), instrumental activities of daily living (IADL), advance activities of daily living (AADL), cognition, mood, gait, falls, nutrition, incontinence,

sensory impairments, polypharmacy, social support, elder abuse, provision of primary, secondary and tertiary prevention, and implementing advance directives are all possible in the office[1].

Older individuals require more time for a complete evaluation. The initial examination may be spread over two (or more) visits, based on the extent of evaluation needed. Prolonged office visits may fatigue the patient. Sometimes the help of a physician's assistant (or suitable other) to obtain basic information from the caregiver using standardized questionnaires may be of considerable benefit. Much of the history can be gathered by someone other than the physician. A long time spent by the doctor does not always translate into greater patient satisfaction[2]. Caregiver help is often necessary to obtain a complete history.

Proper documentation with standard or electronic charts is essential. Our educational background teaches us that, if it is not on paper, it never took place. It is important that communications with the patient, examination findings and revision of regimens be appropriately documented in the patient's chart.

Patients should be instructed to bring all their medications for review at each office visit. It is imperative that all medications including prescribed, over-the-counter, herbal, topical, ocular and nutritional supplements be reviewed. Older adults often visit multiple health providers; they should be encouraged to use only one pharmacy if possible. The primary physician should co-ordinate these visits and review the regimen carefully, attempting to discontinue unnecessary drugs. Every symptom does not need to be treated with a medication.

Often times, the physician is faced with the task of preparing an older individual for elective surgery in the out-patient setting. With the present trends toward shorter hospitalizations, the individual is frequently hospitalized on the morning of surgery or not hospitalized at all, with a discharge within hours following surgery. Perioperative management involves obtaining a history, including relevant past medical history and present co-morbidities, focused physical examination, basic laboratory tests, electrocardiogram and radiological tests (the last two often indicated in older adults, as the likelihood of abnormalities in asymptomatic individuals exists) to assess risks. An assessment, and if indicated, a revision of the medication regimen should take place. A postoperative follow-up evaluation is recommended by the physician, at the time of discharge, following surgery[3,4] (see Chapter 11).

The office environment itself should suit the needs of the older individual. Approach should be provided for wheelchair access. Cluttering is to be avoided. Glare-free lighting, with avoidance of slippery floors and scatter rugs, should be the norm. The examination room must be appropriately furnished, keeping in mind the functional limitations of the older adult.

HOME CARE

As a result of earlier hospital discharge, home health care has grown considerably. Studies have shown that home care can reduce hospital days, readmission and nursing home placement. The Outcome and Assessment Information Set (OASIS) enables the home-health-care agency to assess the patient's needs for services and therapy. By law, the physician who is part of the interdisciplinary team is responsible for the patient's care plan and health-care needs[5]. The physician with the aid of other team members develops the plan of care, and is in charge of certification or recertification. An interdisciplinary team approach in Sweden demonstrated that implementation of education and exercise programs, with modification of environment and review of drug regimens, resulted in fewer falls and injuries, particularly femoral fractures. Fewer hospitalizations may also be a result[6]. An in-home multidimensional geriatric assessment found a modest but non-significant effect on the prevention of nursing home admissions, functional decline and all-cause mortality[7]. Models for delivery of primary care to older adults have been designed and suggest that an enhanced inter-disciplinary collaboration holds the greatest promise for improving management and outcomes in geriatric care[8]. Furthermore, a recent study comparing multidisciplinary restorative care models (based on principles from geriatric medicine, nursing, rehabilitation and goal attainment) with usual care suggested that the former could enhance health outcomes of older patients without increasing health-care utilization[9].

Home care helps to evaluate the environment at home for safety and risks. This includes assessment for safety issues in the bathroom such as the need for a hand-held shower, proper fitted handrails, anti-skid flooring in the shower area, adequate but glare-free lighting, appropriate water-heater temperature (to be kept below 120°F (49°C)), smoke-detectors, avoidance of scatter rugs and loose cords, etc. Assessment for determining the need for canes, walkers or a wheelchair may be made. Environmental modification may prevent unforeseeable falls, and improve one's ease of moving around the home. The ability to access health care in emergency situations must be readily available and provided for. A list of emergency numbers should be easily accessible[10].

HOUSE CALLS

House calls by physicians are back and on the increase. While most physicians make home visits, many do so only rarely. The physician visit to a patient's home helps recognize the support system, environment, psychological and medical status, and scope for abuse, amongst other aspects. Patients suitable for such visits are those who are terminally ill, individuals known to have repeated 'missed appointments', when elder abuse is likely or suspected, and when transportation becomes problematic for any reason.

Home visits provide an excellent opportunity to verify the medications that the patient is on, both prescribed and non-prescribed. Bottles should be inspected for duplication, expired items and clues suggesting a compliance issue. Sometimes, containers which are child-proof are also adult-proof! Pill boxes can be useful; these come in various forms[1].

While it is easy for a health provider to verify the patient's blood pressure, monitor glucose control or verify the status of a wound including change of dressing, more importantly home visits provide the opportunities in the post-hospitalization period for monitoring progress. Examples include follow-up for newly diagnosed heart failure, myocardial infarction or strokes, decision on antibiotic therapy for pneumonia, ambulatory status following orthopedic surgery, newly initiated tube feeding, intravenous therapy and care of urinary catheters[10].

The health provider who provides home visits should be properly equipped to render the visits meaningful. The list of equipment may be compiled based on one's practice patterns and neatly carried in a bag(s). Prescribing can be rendered easier by carrying either a pocket-sized reference pharmacopeia or a hand-held device. Record keeping can also be facilitated by a hand-held device. Table 1 provides a useful list that may be considered for this purpose.

While house call programs have the potential for financial rewards, the non-economic satisfaction derived is high, for both the patient and the health provider. Billing codes for reimbursement to the health provider are available for both new and established patients. Home visits can be a single visit, annual or as needed. Follow-up can also be achieved via a telephone conversation. In any case, proper documentation in the patient's record is essential.

OTHER COMMUNITY-BASED SERVICES

Adult day care

Day care centers may be located in community centers or religious institutions. They offer a variety of social and support services ranging from non-skilled custodial care to

Table 1 A list of supplies and tools for house calls[5]

Medical supplies
Audioscope
Bandages and wound dressing materials
Cerumen curette
Cotton tip applicators
Emergency drugs
Foley catheter
Gloves
Glucometer, lancets and strips
Intravenous and phlebotomy kits
Intravenous fluids
Lubricating jelly
Oto-ophthalmoscope
Portable electrocardiograph machine
Portable sphygmomanometer
Reflex hammer
Specimen containers
Stethoscope
Stool guaiac cards with developer
Thermometer
Tongue depressors
Tuning fork
Urine dipsticks
Weighing scale

Tools and stationery
Advance directive forms
Appointment cards
Instruments for assessing cognition and depression
Pocket-sized reference book or a hand-held device for medications, dosing and drug interactions
Prescription pads
Stationery

advanced skilled services. Primary medical care may be provided. Demented individuals benefit from such settings where supervision and help with ADL are provided while the primary caregiver is at work. These may also serve as a form of respite for caregivers. Relief is provided for part of a day or week, and includes meals, and variable degrees of nursing support. The opportunity to socialize with fellow residents exists. Medicare does not pay for adult day care, whereas Medicaid may reimburse partially. Overall, the cost entailed is far less in day care programs than that for similar services in the hospital or nursing home settings[11].

Assisted living

Services provided in this setting vary from state to state based on differing licensing requirements. The common features entail living services such as meals, housekeeping, laundry, transportation and limited provision for health care. Residents may have a variety of choices depending on their financial capabilities. Payment is mainly by the client, while there is a provision in some locales for reimbursement through Medicaid. Due to fewer services provided in this setting, assisted living facilities are less expensive than nursing homes[5]. They may be located close to a hospital or have the means to provide medical care through a health-care provider on a limited basis (e.g. weekly); individuals ought to be capable of ADL and some IADL and assessed for suitability for assisted living by a physician.

Group homes

This setting provides homes or apartments where several unrelated people cohabit. Group homes often house individuals with dementia or chronic mental illnesses. The living arrangement reduces the cost of living and at the same time promotes socialization with fellow residents. Most are funded privately and are for profit.

Housing shelters

These settings are sheltered homes that provide food, housekeeping and help for personal care. They are funded through the Older American Act and are subsidized for senior citizens and disabled residents. Charges are determined and proportionate to one's income and ability to pay[5].

Home hospital

The home hospital renders hospital-level care in the home for acutely ill patients who would otherwise be hospitalized. Hospital-at-home originated in France in 1961, and has since become an area of increasing interest worldwide[12]. The complexity of care varies broadly. Many diagnostic and therapeutic modalities are carried out in the home setting. Studies performed outside the USA indicate that the care is comparable and provides a high degree of satisfaction. One retrospective study performed in the USA illustrated that, under conditions of equal outcome, preference for home versus hospital were equal[13]. The profile of those who preferred home hospital care included the educated, Caucasians, married individuals and those dependent for ADL[13]. There is accumulating evidence that hospital-at-home effectively complements other forms of health care; the cost-effectiveness of this form of home care is unclear[12]. A pilot study has substantiated the usefulness of the home hospital concept for certain acutely ill patients[14].

TRANSPORTATION

Transporting the older patient often poses a challenge. The use of an ambulette or an ambulance adds substantially to cost. Transportation services and entitlements vary widely. Some community settings offer their own services for patients. Patients with cognitive impairment require more attention, since these individuals tend to wander off and may get lost; such individuals need to be escorted between locations and appropriately monitored to avoid accident or undesired consequences.

ADVANCE DIRECTIVES

Ideally advance directives (which include Living Wills and durable power of attorney that are not mutually exclusive) should be discussed when the patient is not acutely ill, is of sound mind and capable of expressing his or her wishes. The durable power of attorney for health care entails choosing a surrogate (the agent) to help decision-making when the patient loses capacity in the future. The agent may (but need not) be a family member. Patients may retain capacity to make decisions even in early dementia. When the patient is not acutely ill, office visits provide the physician with an opportunity to discuss this issue. Often times, written advance directives are unavailable in an acute situation[15]. It is essential that advance directives be properly transferred to the hospital, long-term care facilities or site of care, so that the patient does not suffer unwanted consequences. A 'do not' decision may be revoked or changed at any time. It is the physician's responsibility to provide the patient with relevant new information necessary for re-evaluation of a previously placed 'do not' order[16].

CAREGIVER BURDEN

Family members, commonly women, render most of the care received by older individuals in the community. Caregiving is time consuming and stressful, and may take a toll on the caregiver's physical and emotional health. Caregivers of patients with Alzheimer's dementia are known to suffer from a higher prevalence of hypertension, depression and musculoskeletal disorders. Often they also look to the same physician for their health-care needs. Furthermore, caregiver burden is associated with increased risk of nursing home placement of patients with dementia[17]. Caregiver burnout must be suspected when there is a decline in patient status or there are signs of frequent calls for help or impatience on the part of the caregiver. Attention should be given to the caregiver's own needs; the help from support groups in such circumstances may be crucial[10].

SUMMARY

As our elderly increase in numbers and tend to live longer, a variety of community setting options are available for medical care and/or residence. These are in addition to the well accepted and time tested home visits by the health provider and the visit to the doctor's office. Considerable support is provided by the family member, and only a small number of the elderly live in nursing homes, a more expensive option. Goals are targeted to maintain function and improve quality of life, with simple measures making a difference. Difficulties in financing these avenues for care are an issue and unlikely to be resolved in the foreseeable future.

References

1. Tangalos EG. Office practice. In Duthie EH Jr, Katz PR, eds. *Practice of Geriatrics*, 3rd edn. Philadelphia: Saunders, 1998: 89–97
2. Robbins JA, Bertakis KD, Helms LJ, *et al.* The influence of physician practice behaviors on patient satisfaction. *Fam Med* 1993;25: 17–20
3. Francis J. Perioperative management of the older patient. In Hazzard WR, Blass JP, Ettinger WH Jr, Halter JB, Ouslander JG, eds. *Principles of Geriatric Medicine and*

Gerontology, 4th edn. New York: McGraw-Hill, 1999:365–76

4. Keating HJ III, Lubin MF. Perioperative responsibilities of the physician/geriatrician. *Clin Geriatr Med* 1990;4:459–67

5. Eleazer GP. Community-based care. In Cobbs EL, Duthie EH Jr, Murphy JB, eds. *Geriatrics Review Syllabus: A Core Curriculum in Geriatric Medicine*, 5th edn. Malden, MA: Blackwell Publishing for the American Geriatric Society, 2002:93–100

6. Jensen J, Lundin-Olsson L, Nyberg L, Gustafson Y. Fall and injury prevention in older people living in residential care facilities. *Ann Intern Med* 2002;136:733–41

7. Stuck AE, Egger M, Hammer A, *et al.* Home visits to prevent nursing home admission and functional decline in elderly people: systematic review and meta-regression analysis. *J Am Med Assoc* 2002; 287:1022–8

8. Coleman EA. Innovative approaches to improving delivery of primary care to older adults. *J Clin Outcomes Man* 2002;9:33–9

9. Tinetti ME, Baker D, Gallo WT, *et al.* Evaluation of restorative care vs usual care for older adults receiving an acute episode of home care. *J Am Med Assoc* 2002;287: 2098–105

10. Boling PA, Abbey LJ. In-home assessment. In Osterweil D, Brummel-Smith K, Beck JC, eds. *Comprehensive Geriatric Assessment*. New York: McGraw-Hill, 2000:203–23

11. Finucane TE, Burton JR. Home care and community-based long-term care. In Hazzard WR, Blass JP, Ettinger WH Jr, Halter JB, Ouslander JG, eds. *Principles of Geriatric Medicine and Gerontology*, 4th edn. New York: McGraw-Hill, 1999: 529–36

12. Corrado OJ. Caring for older hospital-at-home patients. *Age Ageing* 2000;29:97–8

13. Fried TR, van Doorn C, O'Leary JR, *et al.* Older persons' preferences for home vs hospital care in the treatment of acute illness. *Arch Intern Med* 2000;160:1501–6

14. Leff B, Burton L, Guido S, *et al.* Home hospital program: a pilot study. *J Am Geriatr Soc* 1999;47:697–702

15. Danis M, Southerland LI, Garrett JM, *et al.* A prospective study of advance directives for life-sustaining care. *N Engl J Med* 1991; 324:882–8

16. Kapp MB. Legal perspective on ethical issues. *Clin Geriatr* 2002;10:52–62

17. Yaffe K, Fox P, Newcomer R, *et al.* Patient and caregiver characteristic and nursing home placement in patients with dementia. *J Am Med Assoc* 2002;287:2090–7

6 Long-term care

Vincent Marchello, MD, CMD

Institutional care has made significant changes over the past 10 years. Both young and old disabled individuals can spend time in a long-term care facility. The goals and expectations may be different today than in the past. The services provided by these institutions are no longer limited to custodial care, but have expanded. This chapter addresses the care of individuals in long-term care facilities.

TYPES OF CARE

While there are no standardized definitions of the different types of care seen in long-term care facilities, three distinct areas are identifiable: sub-acute care, long-term care and specialized care.

Patients who stay in a long-term care facility for a short time, usually with a discharge plan to home, are considered sub-acute. These include individuals admitted for rehabilitative care, complex medical care and/or wound care. Most of these individuals were previously hospitalized, requiring skilled nursing care, and continue their care plan in the long-term care facility.

Those individuals who suffer from multiple chronic diseases and are no longer able to live in the community reside in a long-term care facility receiving custodial care. This type of institutional care can be considered the traditional nursing home.

Patients receiving specialized care are those individuals who may not necessarily have a discharge plan to the community and most likely will spend the rest of their lives in a long-term care facility, but also require a specialized service. Examples of this population include those in specific programs in dementia care, dialysis and hospice care. These individuals usually require a specially trained staff and programs to address their unique needs.

DEMOGRAPHICS

It has been estimated that approximately 43% of people who turned 65 in 1990 will be admitted into a long-term care facility at some time in their life[1]. As the elderly segment of the population ages and as the prevalence of those with chronic diseases increases, there will continue to be an increase in the utilization and expansion of long-term care facility beds. In 1964, in the USA, approximately half a million people were in long-term care facilities. In 1987, that number increased to nearly 2 million people.

Another important factor contributing to these numbers is the interaction of long-term care with acute care. In many instances the acute care hospital is the portal of entry into long-term care. The number of patients admitted to long-term care facilities has increased with a reduction in the length of hospital stay. In the USA, the proportion of individuals over the age of 65 rose from 4% of the total population in 1900 to 11% in 1980, and it is projected to reach 20% by the year 2030. The over-85 age group, which has the highest institutionalization rate, is also the fastest growing group[2]. The continued expansion of the older population and the increased prevalence of chronic disease and disability in the elderly has led to a dramatic increase in institutional care. In 1993, nursing home expenditures reached $70 billion and accounted for 8% of health-care spending in the USA; this number is likely to increase. Approximately 40% of institutional care expenditures was paid from out of pocket by residents and their families, and the rest by public funds.

Although private long-term care insurance is available, this option has not proved to be popular in the USA. In 1995 only 2.9 million policies had been sold for an over-65 population of more than 31 million[3]. Modification in long-term care policies (such as increasing the number of direct admissions from home, the physician's office and the emergency department in acute hospitals to institutions, or providing on-site treatment of acute decompensations within the nursing home) can have a significant impact on both acute and long-term care costs.

ADMISSION EVALUATION

Admissions to a long-term care facility can be of two types: the short-term admission and the long-term admission. The short-term admission usually comes with specific instructions and a focused care plan. The long-term admission is usually the result of marked functional or cognitive impairment and the absence of adequate social support in the community. Nursing home residents represent a very heterogeneous population. Clearly, the evaluation and management of an individual with a hip fracture admitted for rehabilitation and one with a severe cognitive impairment and behavioral disorders have little in common. The goals of care must be individualized; it is impossible to recommend a common approach to all nursing home residents. Some general guidelines can nevertheless be proposed. These are discussed below.

Table 1 Admission assessment of nursing home residents

Medical history
  description of acute medical conditions and
    identification of co-morbidities
  results of laboratory tests done to monitor active
    medical problems
  list current medications
Review of systems
  review symptoms common in nursing home residents
Physical examination
Functional status
  current status with ADL assessment
  assess rehabilitation potential (if relevant)
Social status and supports
Health maintenance
  screening evaluations
    audiologic
    ophthalmologic/optometric
    dental
    immunizations such as tetanus, influenza
      and pneumococcal vaccines
    tuberculosis testing
Advanced directives
Care plans

ADL, activities of daily living

The admission evaluation should go beyond the traditional history and physical examination, and requires a team approach. It should include a comprehensive assessment, using validated tools (Table 1), and should lead to the establishment of an appropriate plan of care. The goals of care for each resident need to be well defined upon admission and reviewed on a regular basis.

Goals of care in an institutional setting may differ from those of the acute hospital. The emphasis is placed on maximizing function, maintaining quality of life, and comfort care, rather than on curing disease. It is important to communicate with the resident's family, to address their fears and concerns, when present, and to ensure their participation in the development of the care plan. Follow-up care includes interventions to handle acute events, periodic reassessments of the patient's status, and implementation of preventive programs to meet the specific goals of the resident. Scheduled evaluations and sick visits provide an opportunity to review the resident's and staff concerns, monitor vital signs (including weight), identify changes in the physical examination, re-examine the medication list and review the care plan.

ADVANCED DIRECTIVES

The importance of evaluating nursing home residents for medical decision-making capacity and the securing of advanced directives is essential to quality care. Advanced directives such as the DNR (do not resuscitate), Living Will and health-care proxy appointment should be secured as part of the admission assessment. Residents' fears regarding illness and dying should be explored and their wishes regarding resuscitation, hospitalization and medical interventions should be discussed.

The geriatric long-term care population often suffers from dementia, resulting in a progressive cognitive impairment that makes this vulnerable group unable to express their wishes or participate fully in their own care. Advanced directives can facilitate the decision-making process that respects a resident's values and wishes.

A DNR gives specific instruction to the health-care staff pertaining to resuscitation, chest compressions and mechanical ventilation. A Living Will enables an adult with capacity to leave written instructions regarding future care, in the event that the individual becomes incapable of decision making. A health-care proxy appointment enables an adult with capacity to appoint an agent and an alternative agent to make health-care decisions in case of future incapacity. Individuals entering nursing homes have frequently already lost the capacity to participate in many, but not necessarily all, medical decisions. In the ideal world, individuals dwelling in the community should be encouraged by their physicians, usually in the office practice setting, to designate a health-care proxy or write a Living Will at the time when they are capable of such documentation[4].

Table 2 Requirements for the use of physical restraints (Omnibus Budget Reconciliation Act of 1987)

Consultation with physical and/or occupational therapy
Documentation that less restrictive measures were considered
Physician's order
Consent of the resident or family
Documentation that the restraint enables the resident to maintain maximum functional and psychosocial well-being

RESTRAINTS

Physical and chemical restraints have long been a controversial yet frequently employed modality in the care of nursing home residents. They are used in an effort to promote safety, prevent falls and control violent behavior. Unfortunately, restraints may increase the risk of injury-producing falls[5]. Physical restraints have been associated not only with increased injury, but also with increased mental impairment, decubitus ulcers, nosocomial infections and increased agitation. Surveys performed in the 1970s and 1980s in the USA revealed a physical restraint prevalence as high as 75% in some facilities, and psychotropic use as high as 90%[6]. Many factors, such as a better understanding of the risks related to restraints, an increase in public awareness and dignity issues, led towards a concern regarding the appropriateness of physical and chemical restraints.

This culminated in the USA in a detailed regulatory framework governing the use of such restraints, as contained in the Nursing Home Reform Amendments of the Omnibus Budget Reconciliation Act of 1987[7] (OBRA'87). OBRA'87, which was fully implemented in all states by 1991, placed freedom from restraint within the broader context of residents' rights and quality of life. According to these regulations, when a physical restraint is employed, the long-term care facility must demonstrate evidence that less restrictive measures were considered earlier. These and other requirements are listed in Table 2.

The challenges put forth by this new legislation entailed reformulation of policy, re-education of staff, exploration of alternatives to restraint use and, most importantly, adoption of new attitudes. Restraints should be avoided. They represent a last resort, to be used only after thorough nursing and medical assessment and evaluation for less restrictive measures. Most long-term care facilities have responded with dramatic reductions in physical restraint use[8].

Chemical restraints also need to be identified and addressed. Psychoactive medications should be given only to treat specific conditions such as psychotic symptoms and specific behaviors that cause residents to endanger themselves or others. They should not be prescribed to control resident behavior for the convenience of the facility staff. Appropriate monitoring guidelines need to be implemented and many of these medications should undergo weaning trials. This is best accomplished with an interdisciplinary team and a geropsychiatrist.

PREVENTION IN THE NURSING HOME

Preventive care in long-term care should continue what began in youth and middle age. Some interventions have been shown to remain quite effective even in the very old. These include the treatment of isolated systolic hypertension, for example[9], and continued efficacy of the influenza and pneumococcal vaccines. Most clinical and laboratory screening performed annually and upon admissions to nursing homes may be of limited value[10]. The most appropriate preventive interventions in the nursing home are those directed at preservation of function and quality of life. Tertiary prevention, which is aimed at preventing the complications of disease, should be emphasized. Screening for hearing problems, cognitive disorders, mobility impairment, malnutrition and incontinence, as well as optometry, podiatry and dental needs is recommended[11,12].

Prevention of contagious diseases is also important. Tuberculosis can be endemic and epidemic in nursing homes and remains a major concern[13]. Purified protein derivative (PPD) skin testing should be performed on all entering residents who are not known to have had tuberculosis or a positive PPD test in the past. When the initial test is negative, a two-step testing procedure should be performed (second skin test 1–3 weeks after a negative first test) to check for a booster phenomenon. This occurs when waning skin reactivity is boosted by the initial PPD injection, resulting in a positive response to the second PPD skin test[14]. A vaccination program should be in place with policies and procedures for each individual vaccine. These include influenza vaccine annually and pneumococcal vaccine upon admission (if not already vaccinated within the past 6 years).

Tetanus and diphtheria immunization are recommended in the absence of a clear vaccination history[15]. Influenza is a major cause of death in institutions. Influenza vaccine is highly effective in preventing complications, hospitalization and death from both influenza A and influenza B. Amantadine and rimantadine are effective in the early treatment and prevention of influenza A, but not influenza B. Their use has been advocated for the control of influenza outbreaks in the nursing home[16]. Vaccine remains the most effective and best tolerated prophylaxis against influenza[17].

INFECTION CONTROL

The institutionalized elderly are at particular high risk for infection, because their immunity may be impaired by age and co-morbidities, and at the same time they live in a closed environment. New arrivals from the acute hospital setting may bring with them virulent and resistant organisms such as vancomycin-resistant enterococcus, methicillin-resistant *Staphylococcus aureus* and *Clostridium difficile*, which are difficult to treat. The average incidence rate in US long-term care facilities is 1–2 infections per resident per year[18]. These infections are responsible for a significant portion of acute hospital transfers and mortality[19].

The major elements of a successful infection control program include a rational approach to prevention and screening (including a vaccination program), a procedure for identifying and investigating infections, treatment of infections and supervision of epidemics.

The facility must educate its staff on proper preventive measures including the use of universal precautions, the importance of simple hand washing, aseptic technique and proper disposal of contaminated materials and solutions. A procedure for reporting infections should be developed. Awareness of these infections and appropriate precautions are important in minimizing spread to other nursing home patients. Most facilities have specific policies and procedures for identifying and investigating infections and an infection control co-ordinator responsible for evaluating and monitoring infections. Infections are classified according to location, such as urinary tract, upper and lower respiratory tract, skin and soft tissue. The infection control co-ordinator, usually a registered nurse, works closely with the medical director, tracking by way of line-listing and following infections in the facility, ensuring proper treatment protocols and responses. Most state Department of Health agencies have highly specific reporting requirements for a variety of infections. Infection control committee meetings are scheduled to review statistics and rates of infection. Quality assurance reports are generated and discussed. The information from these meetings is used to educate staff and improve the quality of care rendered in these facilities. Epidemics in nursing homes are a serious matter with potentially devastating results. Fortunately outbreaks are infrequent. An interdisciplinary team effort is critical in containing the outbreaks when they occur.

QUALITY ASSURANCE

Quality assurance programs which began in the 1970s comprised the first attempts to measure health-care quality. The conceptual framework for quality assurance was first described by Donabedian in 1978[20].

Quality improvement (also known as continuous quality improvement or total quality management) represents an advancement on quality assurance, because it incorporates specific principles of system change that had originally been devised and tested for industry. These principles, originally described by W. Edwards Deming[21] include both philosophical and statistical methodologies.

The focus on quality assurance and quality improvement in long-term care is relatively recent. Implementation of these principles is possible with the identification of valid quality indicators. Most authorities agree that these can include structural indicators such as staffing ratios, process indicators such as restraints prevalence, and outcome indicators such as decubitus ulcers. Successful approaches to quality assurance necessitate facility-wide participation involving the administrative staff and the direct primary care providers, usually in a committee model. The concept of quality improvement evaluates, monitors and addresses all areas, not only those where a problem exists, thereby continually improving the overall system of care.

ACADEMICS IN LONG-TERM CARE

Medical education is traditionally oriented toward hospital-based acute care. This provides little exposure to the natural course of chronic illness. With today's trend toward progressively shorter hospital stays, students and house staff in classic programs are rarely exposed to follow-up care.

Training programs have just begun to extend beyond the medical center's walls. Settings such as physicians' offices, home care, hospices and nursing homes can provide a unique understanding of the natural course of medical illness[22]. In 1983 the Association of American Medical Colleges (AAMC) departed from its traditional reticence in addressing categorical subjects in medical school curricula and published a guideline for geriatrics curriculum assessment, outlining ways in which courses in basic science and clinical medicine could be strengthened in the areas of geriatrics and gerontology[23]. The AAMC indicated that medical schools should accept responsibility for offering a variety of clinical settings (including ambulatory, long-term institution and home care experiences) through which students can learn special arrangements for the care, diagnosis and treatment of the elderly.

Most medical students, residents, and fellows are trained in the hospital environment. Challenges arise from design and implementation of community-based training. This fact is magnified in the teaching of geriatrics. Geriatrics training in medical schools has not advanced to meet the need in educating the future physician in providing high-quality medical care to older people. Possible reasons for this are manifold. First, and probably of paramount importance, is the obvious shortage of skilled teachers in geriatrics. Second is the lack of utilization of ancillary locations as part of the rotations. Sites such as long-term care facilities, sub-acute units and physician offices need to be used as the center or site of the rotation, rather than 'visits' or 'tours' of the rotation.

Although efforts at implementing geriatric training in nursing homes have been hampered by a lack of qualified teachers, many medical schools now offer training in geriatrics and long-term care[24]. These programs allow students to further develop their fund of geriatric knowledge, learn specific geriatric skills and develop into comprehensive practitioners who can apply the team approach to address all the medical, functional, psychosocial and ethical aspects of caring for the elderly[25].

Table 3   Role of the medical director

Organizing the medical staff
  credentialing and privileging physicians and physician extenders
  ensuring adequate medical coverage and availability
Overseeing policies and procedures
Establishing and using committees effectively
Infection control responsibilities
  influenza and pneumococcal vaccination programs
  methicillin-resistant *Staphylococcus aureus*
  Clostridium difficile
  infection tracking
Employee health programs
  post-offer physical examination
  annual evaluation

Research is another mandate of the academic nursing home. The chronically ill elderly, particularly the very old, have often been excluded from scientific studies[26]. Long-term care institutions offer significant advantages for the study of this population, and also represent the most appropriate site for research into costs and quality of nursing home care. Nursing home-based studies have increased in quantity and quality over the past decade[27].

ROLE OF THE MEDICAL DIRECTOR

The role of the medical director presently encompasses not only clinical oversight of the medical care rendered, but also administrative functions such as policy development and quality assurance (Table 3). The role of the medical director can be described in several different areas. The American Medical Directors Association (AMDA) has a specific program to certify medical directors for long-term care facilities and be designated as a certified medical director (CMD).

Organizing the medical staff

There are many different models of primary physician coverage in nursing homes. The two most common can be described as the closed and open system models. The closed system model involves full- or part-time employment of the medical staff by the nursing facility. In an open system, physicians practicing in the community carry a panel of patients in the nursing home. Physicians and physician extenders, such as physician assistants and nurse practitioners, are employed to deliver medical care to nursing home residents. The medical director is responsible for appointing, credentialing and privileging all physicians and physician extenders and ensuring that the medical staff are qualified and meet the needs of the residents. He or she must serve as an opinion leader and a role model. The individual must educate caregivers and provide specific feedback to all physicians. This is usually done during regularly scheduled medical board meetings.

Overseeing policies and procedures

The medical director is responsible for actively participating in the co-ordination and development of policies and procedures relating to patient care in the nursing home. The medical director must ensure that they accurately reflect laws and regulations, but also must understand the purpose of policies in order to educate physicians and other staff about the value of following them. The medical director must help implement procedures and evaluate their effectiveness.

Establishing and using committees effectively

Most nursing homes now include many committees addressing such issues as infection control, ethics, pharmacy, safety, emergency procedures and quality assurance. Involvement in committees and using them effectively is an important role for the medical director. Participation in committees represents an opportunity to interact with other institutional staff, to help direct care, and to effect change.

Overseeing employee health program

The medical department in nursing facilities is responsible for developing and implementing an employee health program within the institution. Components of employee health include:

(1) Ensuring that employees are physically and mentally capable of performing their duty;
(2) ensuring appropriate handling of occupational injuries;
(3) ensuring the safety of the workplace;
(4) encouraging personal health by utilizing periodic assessments such as medical questionnaires.

Direct patient care

Many medical directors are the primary physician for a panel of residents in their facility. They may also be called upon in emergency situations. This provides the opportunity to function as a role model and to become fully familiar with the system of care. In one study, 19% of medical directors indicated that direct patient care and acting as a physician of last resort were the most important tasks they performed[28].

Leadership

The role of the medical director, today and in the future, is constantly being redefined. The medical director is a key player in improving the quality of care in the facility, disseminating information, educating staff, teaching medical students and residents, and promoting research. The frail institutionalized elderly deserve to be cared for by dedicated and knowledgeable professionals. It is the responsibility of the medical director to ensure that this occurs.

CONCLUSION

Residents in long-term care institutions should receive the best possible care available, should be treated with dignity, and should be allowed to benefit from continued advances in the body of knowledge of geriatrics. It should also be recognized that admission to a long-term care facility does not necessarily imply custodial care. The care plan must meet the social needs of patients, respect their privacy and autonomy, and maintain their dignity. An interdisciplinary team of dedicated and knowledgeable professionals is essential to address the multiple medical co-morbidities, psychiatric, rehabilitative, and social aspects of caring for the residents in a long-term care facility.

References

1. Kemper P, Murtaugh CM. Lifetime use of nursing home care. *N Engl J Med* 1991; 324:595–600
2. Brody JA. Aging: where have we been and where are we going? *Prognosis Clin Biol Res* 1989;287:7–25
3. Mellor JM. Private long term care insurance and the asset protection motive. *Gerontologist* 2000;40:596–604
4. Meier DE, Gold G, Mertz K, *et al.* Enhancement of proxy appointment for older persons: physician counselling in the ambulatory setting. *J Am Geriatr Soc* 1996; 44:37–43
5. Tinetti ME, Liu WL, Ginter SF. Mechanical restraint use and fall-related injuries among residents of skilled nursing facilities. *Ann Intern Med* 1992;116:369–74
6. Tinetti ME, Liu, WL, Marottoli RA, Ginter SF. Mechanical restraint use among residents of skilled nursing facilities: prevalence, patterns and predictors. *J Am Med Assoc* 1991;265:468–71
7. *The OBRA'87 Enforcement Rule: Implications for Attending Physicians and Medical Directors.* Columbia, MD: American Medical Directors Association, 1995
8. Levine JM, Marchello V. Progress toward a restraint-free environment in a large academic nursing facility. *J Am Geriatr Soc* 1995; 43:914–18
9. SHEP Cooperative Research Group. Prevention of stroke by antihypertensive drug treatment in older persons with isolated systolic hypertension: final results of the Systolic Hypertension in the Elderly Program (SHEP). *J Am Med Assoc* 1991;265:3255–64
10. Wolf-Klein GP, Holt T, Silverstone FA. Foley C, Spatz M. Efficacy of routine annual studies in the care of elderly patients. *J Am Geriatr Soc* 1985;33:325–9
11. Ouslander JG, Osterweil D. Physician evaluation and management of nursing home residents. *Ann Intern Med* 1994;120: 584–92
12. Heath I. Longterm care for older people. *Br Med J* 2002;324:1534–5
13. McCray E. The epidemiology of tuberculosis in the United States. *Clin Chest Med* 1997;18:99–113
14. Vega Torres RA. Prevalence of tuberculin reactivity and risk factors for the development of active tuberculosis upon admission to a nursing home. *P R Health Sci J* 1996; 15:275–7
15. *Report of the U.S. Preventive Services Task Force. Guide to Clinical Prevention Services – an Assessment of the Effectiveness*, 2nd edn. Baltimore: Williams and Wilkins, 1986
16. Gomolin IH, Leib HB, Arden NH, Sherman FT. Control of influenza outbreaks in the nursing home: guidelines for diagnosis and management. *J Am Geriatr Soc* 1995;43: 71–4
17. Nicholson KG. Use of antivirals in the elderly: prophylaxis and therapy. *Gerontology* 1996;42:280–9
18. Yoshikawa, TT, Normal DC. Infection control in long-term care. *Clini Geriatr Med* 1995;11:467–80
19. McNeil SA. Methicillin-resistant *Staphylococcus aureus*: management of asymptomatic colonization and outbreaks of infection in long-term care. *Geriatrics* 2002;57:16–27

20. Donabedian A. The quality of medical care. *Science* 1978;200:856–64

21. Deming E. *Out of Crisis*. Cambridge, MA 1986

22. Butler RN. Education and research: key components of healthcare reform. *Geriatrics* 1992;47:11–12

23. Executive council of the Association of American Medical Colleges. Preparation in undergratudate medical education for improved geriatric care – a guideline for curriculum assessment. *J Med Ed* 1983;58:501–26

24. Writing Group of the American Geriatrics Society. *Core Competencies for the Care of Older Patients: Recommendations of the American Geriatrics Society. Acad Med* 2000;75:252–5

25. Gold G. Education in geriatrics: a required curriculum for medical students. *Mt Sinai J Med* 1993;60:461–4

26. Bene J, Liston R. The special problems of conducting clinical trials in elderly patients. *Rev Clin Gerontol* 1977;7:1–3

27. Katz P, Karuza J, Counsell SR. Academics and the nursing home. *Clin Geriatr Med* 1995;1:503–13

28. Katz PR. Medical practice with nursing home residents: results from the National Physician Professional Activities Census. *J Am Geriatr Soc* 1997;45:911–17

7 Preventive health assessment in the older adult

Margaret M. Squillace, MD, MPH

INTRODUCTION AND SCOPE OF THE PROBLEM

Increased average life expectancy will have a significant impact on the future state of medical management. It is estimated that within three decades, persons 65 years of age and above will represent nearly 25% of the United States population and consume nearly half of the expenditure on health care[1]. The possibility of restricted use of medical treatment and therapeutic measures in the future makes the use of preventive care more compelling. The comprehensive health evaluation of a geriatric patient may reduce overall morbidity suffered by the patient and hence the patient's utilization of health resources.

Screening for the early detection of disease has been associated with reduced morbidity and mortality of certain illnesses. The goal of prevention in medical care is not only to decrease morbidity, but also to prolong and improve the quality of life. Classically, there are three tiers of preventive care. Primary prevention is intended to minimize risk factors and prevent disease. This level of prevention includes immunizations as well as programs that educate and promote healthy behaviors. Primary prevention is an important part of medical care for those who will one day become older, but provides limited benefit to those already of an advanced age.

Secondary prevention consists of screening for diseases in order to detect an illness in its early stages. Tertiary prevention, on the other hand, applies to the treatment and management of an established disease to prevent further morbidity and complications secondary to the illness. Secondary and tertiary prevention play an important role in the health care of older adults.

Two major preventive medicine tasks forces, the Canadian Task Force on the Periodic Health Examination and the US Preventive Services Task Force, have reviewed the literature to determine methods by which the periodic health examination should be enhanced to incorporate all levels of prevention. The quality of an intervention was based on the strength of the evidence in the literature that supported its effectiveness. Evidence obtained from randomized controlled trials or well designed studies received more weight than expert opinions. Through these means a classification of preventive service recommendations was constructed. The list of recommendations for screening of older adults (Table 1) is based on the findings and recommendations of the US Preventive Services Task Force[2].

Proper medical treatment and frequent behavioral counseling can impact positively

Table 1 General evaluation for preventive medical care of the older adult. From reference 2

Height
Weight
Blood pressure
Assess visual acuity
Assess for glaucoma
Assess for skin lesions
Assess for hearing problems
Assess for problem drinking
Assess risk of cardiovascular disease
Assess for changes in cognitive function
Assess for signs and symptoms of depression
Assess for subtle signs of thyroid dysfunction
Assess for signs of peripheral vascular disease
Assess beliefs regarding end-of-life issues
Assess social support systems
Assess risk for elder abuse
Counsel smoking cessation
Counsel use of smoke detectors
Counsel safe storage of firearms
Counsel use of seat belts and helmets
Advise adequate calcium and vitamin D intake
Advise regular weight-bearing exercise
Advise regular dental care
Advise on the use of multivitamins
Administer appropriate immunizations
Assess need for referral for cancer screening: Pap smear, mammogram, colorectal screening
Advise outdoor activity such as walking to improve musculoskeletal strength and sun exposure
Review list of medications and avoid polypharmacy/ stop all unnecessary medications

on the overall health of a geriatric patient. Health risk appraisals, frequent health assessments and physical examinations, as well as proper referrals to specialists, may reduce co-morbidity and complications of disease, and prevent future hospitalizations.

Targeted questionnaires (see Table 2) to help assess the patient's current state of health should be completed by the caregiver and, when appropriate, by the patient. The evaluation of the elderly person's ability to perform the normal activities of daily life and instrumental activities of daily living should be an integral part of any comprehensive health assessment. Inquiries into whether the patient continues to operate a motorized vehicle offers insight into the patient's overall physical function, independence and cognitive ability. Local licensure requirements vary.

Firm counseling regarding the suitability of an elderly patient's operation of a motorized vehicle may be warranted in persons taking certain medications or in whom some functional impairment has been demonstrated. Both the patient and the caregiver should be counseled regarding the appropriate use of seat belts and protective helmets when required.

In addition to information regarding past medical illnesses, use of prescribed medications, surgical history and prior hospitalizations, the medical history of the geriatric patient must also include dietary patterns, nutrition, presence of incontinence, history of trauma or falls, and over-the-counter medications including herbal supplements and teas. The patient's sexual function, risk of sexually transmitted diseases or other infectious diseases, including HIV, should be assessed.

The patient's social history should include an inquiry into the patient's participation in community affairs or religious activities as well as an evaluation of the older adult's social support system including neighbors, family and friends. A discussion of those opinions and values that might impact upon end-of-life decisions should be clearly documented in the medical record and witnessed if possible. If an advanced directive or Living Will exists, a copy should be kept in the patient's medical record and updated as needed.

Preventing falls and accidental injury begin with a thorough assessment of the patient's musculoskeletal strength. Risk factors for falls include gait and balance disturbances, polypharmacy, postural hypotension, use of sedative–hypnotic medications and environmental hazards[3]. Increased risk may warrant a complete multidisciplinary fall-risk evaluation. A focused physical examination should include assessment of muscle strength, mobility, flexibility and the 'Get Up & Go' test[4-6]. In addition to evaluating gait and balance, fall prevention may necessitate an evaluation of living quarters. Removing environmental hazards from the home, such as

Table 2 Model of a comprehensive preventative medicine examination form that should be applied every 1–3 years in patient 65 years and older

MEDICAL EXAMINATION	Current complaints	
	Comorbid conditions	
	Significant medical/surgical history	
	Family history	
	Social history including end of life beliefs if appropriate	
	Current prescription medications	
	Use of over-the-counter medications	
	Use of alternative medical treatments	
SCREENING	Weight	
	Height	
	Blood pressure	
	Vision screening	
	Depression	
	Cognitive impairment	
	Domestic violence	
	Assess for hearing impairment	
	Annual fecal occult blood test and/or sigmoidoscopy every 3–5 years and/or colonoscopy or double-contrast barium enema	
	Annual clinical breast exam and/or mammogram every 1–2 years	
	Pap test in sexually active females if cervix present or if no history of three documented tests in prior 3 years or if not offered in prior 10 years	
	Assess for skin lesions	
IMMUNIZATIONS	Current tetanus and diptheria	
	Pneumococcal vaccine one 23 polyvalent vaccine or repeat every 5 years if high risk	
	Annual influenza vaccine	
COUNSELING	Injury prevention	Seat belts
		Motorcycle and bicycle helmets
		Fall prevention
		Smoke detector
		CPR training for household members
		Safe storage/removal of firearms
		Set hot water heater < 130°F (54°C)
	Sexual behavior	STD prevention
		Avoid high risk behavior
	Substance abuse	Avoid tobacco use
		Avoid alcohol
		Avoid intoxication especially when driving, boating, swimming, etc.
	Diet & exercise	Adequate caloric intake
		Limit fat and cholesterol
		Consume fruit, vegetable, grains
		Adequate calcium intake
		Regular physical exercise
	Dental health	Regular dental care
		Daily floss
		Daily brushing with fluoride toothpaste

Continued

Table 2 Continued

CHEMOPROPHYLAXIS	Discuss use of HRT or SERM		
HIGH RISK	Institutionalized persons	PPD	
		Hepatitis A vaccine	
		Amantidine/rimantadine	
	Persons at risk for falls	Fall prevention intervention	
	Age > 75 years, or		
	Age > 70 years and:		
	using > 4 medications		
	impaired cognition		
	use of psychoactive medication		
	use of cardiac medication		
	impaired strength, balance, gait		
	Intravenous drug use or	HIV screen	
	exchange of sex for drugs	RPR/VDRL screen	
		Hepatits A vaccine	
		Hepatitis B vaccine	
		PPD	
		Advice to reduce infection risk	
	High risk sexual behavior	HIV screen	
	Exchanges sex for drugs/money	RPR/VDRL screen	
	Partner who exchanges sex for drugs/money	Hepatitis A vaccine Hepatitis B vaccine	
	More than two sexual partners within one year	Advice to reduce infection risk	
	STD in past		
	Partner with STD history		
	Recurrent gonorrhea		
	Male having sex with men		
	Partner of male having sex with men		
	Blood product recipient	HIV screen	
	Hemodialysis patient	Hepatitis B screen	
	Blood transfusion during 1978–1985	Hepatitis C screen	
	Cardiovascular risk	Consider lipid screening	
	Diabetes, smoking, coronary artery disease, hypertension		
	Immigrant, low income, medically underserved, alcoholics, homeless persons, close contacts of persons with TB, HIV positive persons, chronic medical conditions	PPD	
	Travellers to developing nations	Hepatitis A vaccine Hepatitis B vaccine	
	Health care/laboratory workers Persons with occupational exposure to blood or blood products	PPD Influenza vaccine Hepatitis A vaccine Hepatitis B vaccine	
	Persons susceptible to varicella	Varicella vaccine	
SUMMARY OF HEALTH RISK APPRAISAL AND REFERRAL PLAN:			

loose rugs or obstructing furniture, and lowering the height of the bed can help reduce the risk of falls. Similar prevention can be accomplished by installing hand-rails in the bathrooms and shower stalls.

The older adult person's daily diet should be evaluated for adequacy of calories and nutrition. The elderly should be instructed to consume a sufficient amount of daily fluid, pro-teins, fruits and vegetables, as well as 1500 mg of calcium, 400–800 IU of vitamin D and a daily multivitamin. Overnutrition and obesity should be avoided. The condition of being overweight may lead to physical inactivity and add unnecessary stress and strain on joints.

Virtually every adult would benefit from increased physical activity. Even small increases in physical activity may be beneficial in the elderly. Exercise should match the needs and lifestyle of the individual. Recom-mended programs should include walking, for endurance, as well as flexibility and strength-building exercises[7]. Physical activity will not only improve physical conditioning but also help foster a more positive emotional outlook. Avoidance of alcohol and tobacco should be counseled. Efforts at smoking cessation should be encouraged.

The elderly are more vulnerable to envi-ronmental changes. Even small changes often yield dramatic impact. The senior adult should be advised to maintain an adequate level of heat in their home environment, to dress in layers if necessary and to reduce the hot water temperature to < 130°F (54°C). The importance of the installation and main-tenance of smoke detectors in homes should be stressed. Firearm safety and proper stor-age of guns should be shared with both the patient and the caregiver.

IMMUNIZATION

Immunization is the best example of success-ful primary prevention. The recommendations for immunization in the geriatric population include the administration of vaccines against influenza, pneumococcal disease and tetanus. Vaccination against infection with influenza and pneumococcal pneumonia in this target population is clinically beneficial and cost-effective[8].

Antiviral drugs such as amantadine and rimantadine block an early step in replication of the influenza A virus and are an effective prophylaxis in the elderly when influenza A has been documented in the community. Antiviral drugs are usually administered to those senior residents exposed to influenza A but who are unimmunized, recently immunized or otherwise expected to have a suboptimal response to immunization. The medication is administered daily for approxi-mately 2 weeks, or until 1 week after the out-break has ended. Although oseltamivir, a neuraminidase inhibitor, initially marketed as treatment for influenza, won recent approval for the prophylactic management of both influenza A and B in adults, its use as a pro-phylactic agent in the institutionalized geri-atric population has yet to be demonstrated.

Influenza vaccine should be administered annually to all persons aged 65 years or older. Two strains of influenza A and one strain of influenza B viruses are chosen annually based on the latest worldwide surveillance data to formulate the yearly vaccine. Influenza A viruses are highly mutagenic and demonstrate strong antigenic drift. The virus has its most significant impact on a population when new strains emerge against which most of the pop-ulation lacks immunity. Influenza A viruses are classified into subtypes on the basis of two antigens: hemagglutinin (three subtypes, H_1, H_2, H_3) and neuraminidase (two subtypes, N_1, N_2). It is the immunity to these antigens that reduces the likelihood of infection and ameliorates the severity of disease in vacci-nated persons.

Pneumococcal vaccine is recommended for all immunocompetent persons who are aged 65 years and older. Routine revaccination is not recommended, but may be considered in persons vaccinated more than 5 years previously, and those who received other than the 23-valent vaccine or are at significant risk for morbidity and mortality from pneumococcal illness. There are no contraindications to pneumococcal vaccine. Side-effects are virtually absent.

The tetanus and diphtheria toxoids adsorbed (Td) series should be completed for all patients who have not received the primary series. If there is an uncertain history of vaccination, reinitiating the primary series may be considered. Adults should receive periodic Td boosters every 10 years. A universal administration of the Td booster at the age of 65 years is generally recommended. The Td booster should be given again after 5 years if the patient suffers a dirty wound. Older adults may sustain injuries from minor falls while residents in long-term care facilities have a high prevalence of pressure ulcers; hence, the benefits of tetanus toxoid are clear.

It is important to immunize high-risk seniors against infection with hepatitis B virus and hepatitis A virus. Seniors may be at risk because of social, occupational or environmental conditions that increase the likelihood of exposure. Rabies vaccine is considered for seniors who hunt, trap, explore caves or travel to endemic areas.

VISION AND HEARING

The elderly require screening for visual and hearing impairment[9,10]. Diminished vision and hearing in the elderly can lead to motor vehicle accidents, improper use of medications, falls, other forms of accidental injury and a feeling of isolation. Although decreased visual acuity and hearing loss are common in the geriatric population, patients do not complain for fear of loss of independence. The most common causes of visual impairment in the geriatric population include cataract, glaucoma, age-related macular degeneration and presbyopia. Loss of visual acuity can be easily detected by the use of a Snellen chart. The optimal frequency for screening is left to clinical discretion. Referral

to an ophthalmologist should be recommended if visual acuity scores are worse than 20/40 vision while using corrective lenses, or if impairment interferes with normal functions of daily life. Diabetics should undergo annual ophthalmologic evaluations. Persons over 65 years of age remain at risk for glaucoma and should be screened periodically for the disorder.

Hearing loss in the elderly can adversely affect physical safety and emotional health by increasing isolation. Impaired hearing may interfere with cognitive assessment. The optimal frequency of screening for hearing impairment is left to clinical discretion. Screening older adults for hearing impairment can be achieved by questioning them, asking them to repeat instructions regarding medication or to follow commands. It has been recommended that clinicians counsel patients regarding the availability of hearing aid devices and make referrals when appropriate.

COGNITIVE ASSESSMENT

Testing an older person's cognitive ability remains an essential part of every patient encounter, even if it involves merely checking different components of the patient's history for accuracy and consistency. The clinician should engage the senior in conversations regarding past encounters, current events or family matters. Persons suffering from early dementia usually retain their social graces and offer agreeable and co-operative conversation. The information gathered during these sessions should be verified for accuracy by questioning the caregiver. Orientation to person, place and time should be easy to ascertain during the initial few minutes with the patient. Further comfortable conversation regarding items of mutual interest to both patient and the clinician should verify the orientation of the patient as well as determine the person's current mood and affect.

Depression should not be overlooked in an elderly patient[11]. Screening for depression can be performed with any variety of tools and should be coordinated with the appropriate intervention and follow-up[12,13]. The depressive episode may be due to a feeling of isolation from familiar friends or activities. The change in affect may be associated with the onset of decreased visual acuity or hearing loss. Simple changes such as acquiring a hearing aid or adjustment of lenses, as well as engagement in new activities, may alleviate the depressed mood. Any senior developing cardiovascular illness, malignancy, substance abuse or chronic pain, or presenting with insomnia, apathy or weight change should be screened for depression[14]. The use of medications to counteract the depression should be considered.

Dementia may coexist with depression and delirium in an elderly patient. Formal assessment of cognitive function should help discriminate one from the other. The appropriate frequency for performing a mini-mental test on elderly patients should be individualized and left to the discretion of the clinician. Evaluation of cognitive function and screening for depression is discussed elsewhere in this text.

The patient's caregiver should be questioned regarding episodes of wandering and getting lost, and accidental dangers such as leaving the stove on after cooking. Any noticeable deterioration in the older person's cognitive abilities should prompt a search for the cause, which may be a yet unidentified systemic illness and/or medications. Even small changes in medication can have a dramatic impact on an older adult. The evaluation of the patient's medications, especially those recently prescribed, and an effort to eliminate polypharmacy should be undertaken.

The patient and family should be encouraged to consider future plans, including the need for chronic care. The discussion of personal preferences surrounding continued mechanical ventilation, permanent nutritional support, advanced directives, Living Wills, health-care proxies and timely planning should be encouraged and documented whenever possible.

ELDER ABUSE

Family violence, also known as domestic violence, crosses all socioeconomic and cultural barriers[15–17]. There appears to be no age limit placed on the victims of sexual abuse, physical abuse, financial abuse or emotional abuse. All indications suggest that elder abuse is grossly underreported. Clinicians should screen every geriatric individual for potential abuse in their daily life[18].

Abuse can take various forms. Most abuse falls into one of the following categories: physical abuse, neglect, exploitation, psychological abuse and violation of rights. Physical abuse is an act of violence causing bodily harm or mental anguish. Neglect is the withholding of assistance vital to daily living. Neglect may include, but is not limited to, deprivation of meals, grooming, housework or medical care. Emotional trauma results from psychological abuse often inflicted by repeated verbal threats or cruel words. Improper use by another of an older adult's financial resources or property for self-benefit is labeled exploitation. Depriving a person of an inalienable or legal right such as voting, privacy or liberty is viewed as a violation of that person's rights.

Detection of abuse is dependent on the clinician's awareness of the problem and ability to detect the possibility of abuse. Obvious indications of abuse include unexplained bruises, injuries or burns. The presence of extremely poor hygiene, pain or misuse of medication may suggest the possibility of abuse. A pattern of missed appointments or frequent changing of health-care providers should sound an alarm. Finally, the interaction between the patient and the caregiver may hint at the problem. Relieving the caregiver burden for a few hours per week by arranging for substitute companions or nurses, or placing the older individual in a senior day care center for some hours per week may prevent the onset of the elder abuse paradigm.

OSTEOPOROSIS

Bone mineral density may decrease with age, placing the elderly at increased risk for osteoporosis or osteopenia. Osteoporosis leads to vertebral collapse or the threat of fracture from even minor trauma. Age-related osteoporosis may be associated with a smoking history, the presence of a hypogonadal state, lack of weight-bearing exercise, low calcium intake, significant family history and use of certain medications.

Primary preventive strategies to avoid osteoporosis in old age must be initiated early in life. A diet adequate in calcium and an active lifestyle will help prevent osteopenic complications. The daily consumption of 1000–1500 mg of calcium through either calcium supplements or several servings of milk, yogurt or cheese, daily exposure to sunlight for vitamin D synthesis, and regular mild to moderate exercise in the form of walking most days a week or weight training are recommended to maintain strong bones. Secondary prevention may include the use of hormone replacement therapy, calcium intake, exercise, calcitonin, biphosphonates or selective estrogen receptor modulators (SERMs)[19]. Asymptomatic women at risk for osteoporosis, with osteopenia, or osteopenic bone densitometry can be managed medically. The treatment of osteoporosis with medications may not succeed in preventing injury after minor trauma or during disease states, so the prevention of falls is still of paramount importance in avoiding fractures.

CARDIOVASCULAR HEALTH

Cardiovascular disease is the number one cause of mortality in the older adult. A baseline electrocardiogram (ECG) should be obtained in all geriatric patients. There is no evidence to suggest routine or repeated ECG evaluation in asymptomatic elderly patients as a screening for cardiovascular illness. The cardiovascular examination includes documentation of heart rhythm, pulse, heart sounds, murmurs and vascular bruits. Any significant change from prior examinations, even in an asymptomatic patient, should warrant further evaluation.

Screening for hypertension is indicated at every physician/patient encounter[20]. The initial measurement of blood pressure should include readings in lying and standing positions. The patient should be questioned regarding sensations of light-headedness, and orthostatic changes should be documented. Control of hypertension in the elderly has been shown to reduce the incidence of new cardiovascular events. Ideally, blood pressure should be maintained below 140/90 mmHg. Non-pharmacologic therapy includes salt restriction, diet low in saturated fat, weight reduction, regular exercise, adequate nutrients and avoidance of smoking and excessive alcohol intake[21,22].

There has been insufficient evidence to recommend regular screening of cholesterol levels among persons aged 65 year of age or older, because most trials do not include adequate numbers of older individuals[23,24]. Growing evidence supports the aggressive management of dyslipidemia in the elderly especially in the 65–75 year age group[25,26]. The National Cholesterol Education Panel suggests screening for hyperlipidemia every 5 years beyond age 65 of the high-risk patient who would benefit from long-term lipid management. The most recent recommendations of the National Cholesterol Education Panel advocate a fasting lipoprotein profile as initial screening in adults, especially in those never before screened and with a life expectancy sufficient to allow benefits of therapy. These Adult Treatment Panel (ATP III) guidelines suggest that high low-density lipoprotein (LDL) cholesterol, low high-density lipoprotein (HDL) cholesterol and high triglyceride levels have predictive value for coronary heart disease. A 10-year coronary artery disease risk is estimated based on several items: gender, age, smoking history, lipid profile and blood pressure, and is used to determine management. The first-line therapy in older adults remains therapeutic lifestyle changes including dietary management and exercise. LDL-cholesterol-lowering drugs should be considered for older persons at higher risk, since secondary prevention trials have shown significant risk reduction in older adults treated with statin lipid-lowering medications.

Currently, there is no recommendation for the use of hormone replacement therapy in the prevention of cardiovascular disease[27]. The most recent studies support an increased risk for venous thromboembolism with the use of postmenopausal estrogen replacement[28]. Use of hormone replacement therapy or SERMs must be determined on an individual basis[29].

The management of the older patient after myocardial infarction may require the use of a lipid-lowering drug to decrease serum cholesterol, along with β-blockers and aspirin given indefinitely. Persons with a left ventricular thrombus or persistent and paroxysmal atrial fibrillation should be maintained on long-term anticoagulant therapy. Angiotensin converting enzyme inhibitors should be given to persons with congestive heart failure, anterior myocardial infarction and left ventricular ejection fraction of < 40%[30]. Although the benefits of cardiac rehabilitation have not been clearly demonstrated, cardiac rehabilitation offers an opportunity to improve the quality of life in the older adult[31].

While aspirin has a clear role in secondary prevention of cardiovascular disease, its use in primary prevention in the older adult requires assessment of risks and benefits. The US Preventive Services Task Force found that, while aspirin decreases the incidence of coronary heart disease in adults at risk, including postmenopausal women and men over 40 years of age, it increases the risk of gastrointestinal bleeding and possibly hemorrhagic stroke. Calculation of individual 5-year coronary artery disease risk is recommended for making decisions regarding the use of aspirin for primary prevention; the recommended daily dose is 75 mg[32,33].

Recommendations regarding the use of anti-platelet medications in the prevention of stroke among the elderly population have not been firmly established. It may be prudent to use platelet antiaggregant therapy in the patient with asymptomatic carotid artery stenosis. In patients aged < 70 years with atrial fibrillation without additional risk factors, aspirin may be an effective prophylactic agent, while anticoagulants may be considered if the patient is older than 70 years[34]. Clinicians should individualize use of these agents in geriatric patients, taking into account contraindications and life expectancy.

CANCER SCREENING

The burden of cancer-related morbidity and mortality has fallen disproportionately on geriatric patients. Cancer is the second most important cause of death after cardiovascular disease. Approximately one-half of cancer deaths occur in this population. The early identification and treatment of cancer may allow for improved survival, comfort or quality of life. The eventual decision to screen for cancer belongs to the patient and/or caregiver. Co-morbidity, life expectancy, frailty, the stress associated with early diagnosis or threatened disability may alter the risk/benefit ratio of screening the elderly. Clearly, the early detection of a potentially treatable malignancy in an individual with many years of productive and active life ahead of them would prove an important part of their health maintenance. When cancer screening is offered, it should be done in a positive manner to facilitate the screening process[35,36].

The current recommendations for colorectal cancer screening suggest initiating screening at 50 years of age in asymptomatic persons at average risk. Screening options include an annual home fecal occult blood test, flexible sigmoidoscopy, the combination of fecal occult blood test and flexible sigmoidoscopy, colonoscopy and double-contrast barium enema[37,38]. The fecal occult blood test should follow the guidelines for sampling collection.

In addition, a flexible sigmoidoscopy should be performed every 5 years, or a colonoscopy or air-contrast barium enema every 10 years[39,40]. Although there is no upper age limit specified by either the American College of Physicians, the American Gastroenterology Association or the United States Preventive Services Task Force (USPSTF), screening for colorectal cancer beyond 85 years of age, in a healthy low-risk individual in whom prior flexible sigmoidoscopic screenings have proved negative for colorectal cancer, may not be required. An abnormal finding on any screening test would necessitate an examination of the entire colon and rectum by colonoscopy or contrast barium enema. Cost analysis may recommend colonoscopy as a first-line screening test in the future[41].

Evaluation of the prostate gland should be performed during the annual digital rectal examination. The use of prostate-specific antigen (PSA) level as a screening test for prostate disease has remained controversial. Screening with PSA after age 50 in males with at least a 10 year life expectancy is recommended by the American Cancer Society and the American Urological Society, but not endorsed by the American College of Physicians or the USPSTF[42–45]. At the present time the use of PSA as a screening tool for prostate cancer should be at the discretion of the clinician. Prior to screening, the patient should be counseled on the interpretations of abnormal results and possible need for further evaluation.

Recent recommendations from the USPSTF are for screening mammography with or without clinical breast examination every 1 or 2 years for women aged 40 or older. Women aged 70 or older face a higher absolute risk of breast cancer. Since the probability of benefits of regular mammography increase with age, as the likelihood of harms from screening diminish, annual or biennial mammography in women aged 70 and older is recommended[46]. Annual mammography should be considered in women with a family history of breast cancer and on current hormone replacement therapy. A mammogram and Pap smear should be performed in all women prior to initiating hormone replacement therapy[47,48]. The routine use of SERMs for the primary prevention of breast cancer is not recommended. The use of SERMs as chemoprevention in women with high risk of breast cancer may be considered after frank discussion of the potential benefits and risks[49,50].

Periodic Pap smears are not necessary for women who have undergone complete hysterectomies including the removal of the cervix. Elderly women do not benefit from Pap testing if repeated cervical smears have consistently been normal in the past. In such cases no further screening is needed after age 65. A Pap smear should be offered to women who have not been screened in the previous 10 years[51].

There are no serious risks from total-body skin examination, but screening may detect large numbers of benign skin conditions in the elderly which may lead to unnecessary biopsies. Clinicians should remain alert, however, for skin lesions in seniors which demonstrate malignant features or resemble atypical moles[52].

References

1. Rice DP, Feldman JJ. Living longer in the United States: demographic changes and health needs of the elderly. *Milbank Mem Fund Q* 1983;61:362–96

2. *Guide to Clinical Preventive Services: Report of the US Preventive Services Task Force*, 2nd edn. Alexandria, VA: International Medical Publishing, 1996.

3. Tinetti ME. Prevention of falls and fall injuries in elderly persons: a research agenda. *Prevent Med* 1994;23:756–2

4. Okimiya K, Matsubayashi K, Nakamura T, *et al.* The time 'up and go' test is a useful predictor of falls in community-dwelling older people [letter]. *J Am Geriatr Soc* 1998;46:928–9

5. Mathias S, Nayak US, Isaacs B. Balance in elderly patients: the 'get up and go' test. *Arch Phys Med Rehabil* 1986;67:387–9

6. Ostchega Y, Harris TB, Hirsch R, *et al.* Reliability and prevalence of physical performance examination assessing mobility and balance in older persons in the US: data from the Third National Health and Nutrition Examination Survey. *J Am Geriatr Soc* 2000;48:1136–41

7. Christmas C, Andersen RA. Exercise and older patients: guidelines for the clinician. *J Am Geriatr Soc* 2000;48:318–24

8. Stein BE. Adult vaccinations: protecting your patients from avoidable illness. *Geriatrics* 1993;48:46–55

9. Miller KE, Zylstra RG, Standbridge JB. The geriatric patient: a systematic approach to maintaining health. *Am Fam Physician* 2000;61:1089–104

10. Rosenthal BP. Screening and treatment of age-related and pathologic vision changes. *Geriatrics* 2001;56:27–31

11. Irwin MI, Artin KH, Oxman MN. Screening for depression in the older adult. *Arch Intern Med* 1999;159:1701–4

12. US Preventive Services Task Force. Screening for depression: recommendations and rationale. *Ann Intern Med* 2002;136:760–4

13. Pignone M, Gaynes BN, Rushton JL, *et al.* Screening for depression in adults: a summary of the evidence for the US Preventive Services Task Force. *Ann Intern Med* 2002; 136:765–76

14. Wenger NS, Shekelle P, Davidoff F, *et al.* Quality indicators for assessing care of vulnerable elders. *Ann Intern Med* 2001;135: 653–68

15. Kleinschmidt KC. Elder abuse: a review. *Ann Emerg Med* 1997;30:463–72

16. Tatara T. *Elder Abuse: Questions and Answers. An Information Guide for Professional and Concerned Citizens,* 6th edn. Washington DC: National Center for Elder Abuse, 1996

17. Bourland MD. Elder abuse: from definition to prevention. *Postgrad Med* 1990;87: 139–44

18. Bloom JS, Ansell P, Bloom MN. Detecting elder abuse: a guide for physicians. *Geriatrics* 1989;44:40–56

19. Ettinger B, Black D, Mitlak B, *et al.* Reduction of vertebral fracture risk in post-menopausal women with osteoporosis treated with raloxifene. *J Am Med Assoc* 1999;282:637–45

20. Laird RD, Studenski SS. Management of hypertension for stroke prevention in older people. *Clin Geriatr Med* 1999;15:663–84

21. Prisant LM, Moser M. Hypertension in the elderly. *Arch Intern Med* 2000;160:283–9

22. Goldberg TH, Chavin SI. Preventive medicine and screening in older adults. *J Am Geriatr Soc* 1997;45:344–54

23. US Preventive Services Task Force. Screening for lipid disorders: recommendations and rationale. *Am J Prev Med* 2001; 20(3S):73–6

24. Mormando RM. Lipid levels: applying the Second National Cholesterol Education Program Report to geriatric medicine. *Geriatrics* 2000;55:48–53

25. Grundy SM, Cleeman JI, Rifkind BM, *et al.* Cholesterol lowering in the elderly population. *Arch Intern Med* 1999;159:1670–8

26. Executive Summary of the Third Report of the National Cholesterol Education Program (NCEP) Expert Panel on Detection, Evaluation, and Treatment of High Blood Cholesterol in Adults (ATP III). *J Am Med Assoc* 2001;285:2486–97

27. Writing Group for the Women's Health Initiative Investigations. Risks and benefits of estrogen plus progestin in healthy post-menopausal women: principal results from the Women's Health Initiative Randomized Controlled Trial. *JAMA* 2002:288:321–33

28. Miller J, Chan BKS, Nelson HD. Post-menopausal estrogen replacement and risk for venous thromboembolism: a systemic review and meta-analysis for the US Preventive Services Task Force. *Ann Intern Med* 2002;136:680–90

29. American Heart Association. Hormone replacement therapy and cardiovascular disease. *Circulation* 2001;104:499

30. Aronow WS. Management of older persons after myocardial infarction. *J Am Geriatr Soc* 1998;46:1459–68

31. Forman DE, Farquhar W. Cardiac rehabilitation and secondary prevention programs for elderly cardiac patients. *Clin Geriatr Med* 2000;16:619–29

32. US Preventive Services Task Force. Aspirin for the primary prevention of cardiovascular events: recommendations and rationale. *Ann Intern Med* 2002;136:157–60

33. Hayden M, Pignone M, Phillips C, *et al.* Aspirin for the primary prevention of cardiovascular events: a summary of the evidence for the US Preventive Services Task Force. *Ann Intern Med* 2002;136:161–72

34. Weinberger J. Prevention and management of cerebrovascular events in primary care. *Geriatrics* 2002;57:38–43

35. Robinson B, Beghe C. Cancer screening in the older patient. *Clin Geriatr Med* 1997; 13: 97–118

36. Zoorob R, Anderson R, Cefalu C, *et al.* Cancer screening guidelines. *Am Fam Physician* 2001;63:1101–12

37. US Preventive Services Task Force. Screening for colorectal cancer: recommendations and rationale. *Ann Intern Med* 2002;137:129–31

38. Pignone M, Rich M, Teutsch SM, *et al.* Screening for colorectal cancer in adults at average risk: a summary of the evidence for the US Preventive Services Task Force. *Ann Intern Med* 2002;137:132–41

39. USPSTF Recommendation. Colon cancer screening. *J Am Geriatr Soc* 2000;48:333–5

40. American Cancer Socity guidelines on screening and surveillance for the early detection of adenomatous polyps and cancer – update 2001. In American Cancer Society guidelines for the early detection of cancer. *CA Cancer J Clin* 2001;51:44–54

41. Sonnenberg A, Delco F, Inadomi JM. Cost-effectiveness of colonoscopy in screening for colorectal caner. *Ann Intern Med* 2000; 133:573–84

42. Barry MJ. Prostate-specific-antigen testing for early diagnosis of prostate cancer. *N Engl J Med* 2001;344:1373–7

43. Gambert SR. Prostate cancer: when to offer screening in the primary care setting. *Geriatrics* 2001;56:22–31

44. American Urological Society. Prostate specific antigen (PSA): best practice policy. *Oncology* 2000;14:267–86

45. Recommendations from the American Cancer Society Workshop on Early Prostate Cancer Detection, May 4–6, 2000 and American Cancer Society guideline on testing for early prostate cancer detection: update 2001. In American Cancer Society guideline for the early detection of cancer. *Cancer J Clin* 2001;51:39–44

46. US Preventive Services Task Force. *Screening for Breast Cancer: Recommendations and Rationale*, 3rd edn. http:// www.ahrq.gov/clinic/3rduspstf/breastcancer/ brcanrr.htm.

47. American Geriatrics Society Clinical Practice Committee. Breast cancer screening in older women. *J Am Geriatr Soc* 2000;48: 842–4

48. Tishler J, McCarthy EP, Rind DM, *et al.* Breast cancer screening for older women in a primary care practice. *J Am Geriatr Soc* 2000;48:961–6

49. Cummings SR, Eckert S, Krueger KA, *et al.* The effect of raloxifene on risk of breast cancer in postmenopausal women. Results for the MORE randomized trial. *J Am Med Assoc* 1999;281:2189–97

50. *Chemoprevention of Breast Cancer. Recommendations and Rationale, July 2002.* Agency for Healthcare Research and Quality, Rockville MD. http://www.ahrq. gov/clinic/3rduspstf/breastchemo/breastch emorr.htm

51. Mehr DR. Preventive geriatrics. *Clin Geriatr* 2001;9:1931

52. US Preventive Services Task Force. Screening for skin cancer: recommendations and rationale. *Am J Prev Med* 2001;20:44–6

8 Exercise in the elderly

Areta D. Podhorodecki, MD, and Robert M. Simon, MD

INTRODUCTION

The human body was originally designed for much shorter wear and tear. Prior to the 20th century, average life expectancy was about 45 years. Although the dawning of the new millennium has not seen 'the pursuit of idleness' as envisaged by Bertrand Russell, today many are healthier and experience a better quality of life right into old age. This 'quality of life' with age, however, is seen primarily in those who stay active and mobile[1].

Our approach to illness has changed drastically in the past 20 years. Even 10 years ago, patients with sciatica were often admitted for weeks of bedrest and traction. Now patients are out of bed within 24 h even after major surgery. Bedrest and its sequelae have become the enemy. The approach is to return to normal activity as soon as possible with 'relative' instead of 'strict' rest. Restoration of previous function is accomplished in subacute/acute rehabilitation centers with intensive physical therapy, psychological support and education.

Unfortunately, this 'exercise message' is impacting society too slowly. Obesity is on the increase in the USA despite public campaigns. Few adults exercise regularly; many start programs but few continue. We also know that less than 30% are ever counseled by their physician to exercise[2]. This is paramount to maintain compliance and motivation. In Australia, a television public relations campaign yielded better results, with respect to improved return to work rates after acute low back pain, than any prior physician management program. Public education was able to dispel myths and change patient expectations. Even mild or moderate physical activity can improve health at any age[3]. Improvements in energy level, mood and sleep, and a general sense of well-being are some of the most notable benefits of exercising for most adults (Table 1).

Table 1 Benefits of exercise for the elderly

Improvement in balance
Improvement in response time
Increase in muscle mass
Increase in bone mass
Increase in mental alertness
Improved immune function
Help to alleviate pain
Decrease in fracture risk
Helpful in obesity, diabetes, hypertension and
  hyperlipidemia

PHYSIOLOGY OF SARCOPENIA

The loss of muscle strength that is seen in the elderly is directly related to impaired mobility, falls and functional decline. The evidence that exercise improves functional status is promising, but inconclusive, due to the dearth of randomized, controlled studies. Nonetheless, most studies suggest that exercise by itself can improve gait and balance, decrease pain associated with arthritis, improve bone mineral density and thus decrease fracture risk. Muscle weakness occurs as a direct result of the loss of physical activity, commonly seen in the elderly. A variety of mechanisms (e.g. medical illnesses, nutritional depletion, sedentary lifestyle and the aging process itself) may underlie the specific decline in physical performance[4].

The health benefits of appropriately prescribed long-term exercise (more than 12 weeks) in adults aged 65 and older include improvements in strength and endurance, and increase in muscle mass and functional capacity. Sarcopenia is the term used to describe the loss of skeletal muscle mass and the alterations in quality, one of the most important contributors to the limitations in physical performance in old age[5]. Sarcopenia can be minimized through a strength-training program. The positive effects are reflected in muscle fiber type, capillary density and aerobic capacity. Current data suggest that a cumulative amount of 30–50 min of daily exercise (e.g. walking, gardening, housekeeping) performed 3–5 days a week and one set of resistive exercises twice a week can produce marked health benefits. Even frail institutionalized seniors, including those with mild dementia and incontinence, respond favorably to an advanced exercise program[6].

Women in particular benefit from maintenance of bone mineral density and prevention of osteoporosis, decreased susceptibility to falls, and even breast cancer or some other chronic diseases[7]. Exercise training may help to reverse the malnutrition seen in patients with chronic renal failure, delay the progression of renal disease and help to reduce the fatigue commonly seen in cancer survivors[8,9].

Exercise throughout one's life span should be encouraged in order to maximize peak bone mass, reduce age-related bone loss, and maintain strength and balance. Although the effects of exercise on bone density later in life are small, epidemiological evidence suggests that being active can nearly halve the incidence of hip fractures in the elderly[10]. Increased weight-bearing with resistance exercises (Figure 1) improves bone density and combats the effects of osteoporosis.

The basis of normal muscular activity is beyond the scope of this review. However, a brief discussion of neuromuscular physiology in the aged is helpful. There are two muscle fiber types: aerobic and anaerobic. The aerobic (type one/red) fibers are important for endurance exercises, whereas anaerobic (types two A and B/white) fibers are important for strengthening exercises. There are three types of muscle contractions: an isotonic contraction, in which the force of contraction is constant but the rate is variable; an isometric contraction, in which the force remains constant but there is no muscle shortening; and an isokinetic contraction, in which the force of contraction is variable but the rate is constant. A muscle contraction can occur with shortening of fibers, referred to as a 'concentric contraction' or another in which the muscle lengthens as it contracts, termed an 'eccentric contraction'. The maximal strength of a muscle is at its 'resting length' where there is considerable overlap between the actin and myosin myofilaments[6]. Currently, there is no known optimal type of physical strengthening activity to enhance health.

Muscle fibers have a broad range of contractile properties to generate the full range of power required for various activities[11]. A recent study by Krivickas and colleagues[12] revealed that both age and gender affect shortening velocity, which may explain the impairment in muscle function that occurs with aging and the greater impairment in muscle function in older women versus older men. Because these gender differences occur in old age, possibly postmenopausal hormonal changes play a role; estrogen may affect calcium kinetics or myosin ATPase activity[13].

BENEFITS OF EXERCISE

The functional aerobic capacity or maximal oxygen uptake (VO_2max) defines the

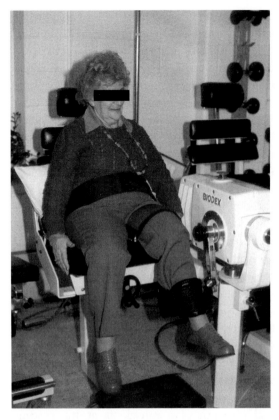

Figure 1 A 78-year-old female exercising on a Cybex machine in a physical therapy gym (reproduced with permission)

functional limit of the cardiovascular system. (Submaximal exercise performance is typically determined by the anaerobic threshold). A typical prescription for an aerobic training program consists of 30 min of continuous activity at a moderate intensity (50% of Vo_2 max) at least 3 days per week. In the case of frail elderly patients, even a modest walking program has been shown to improve aerobic fitness, reduce blood pressure, improve lipid profile, increase bone density and enhance mood[14].

Many older adults are often at increased risk for falls when performing activities of daily living that require dynamic postural control. Postural control deficits have been attributed to both age- and pathology-associated changes in spatial and temporal parameters associated with movements of the center of gravity (COG) within the stability region. Compared with younger adults, healthy older adults exhibit smaller voluntary COG excursions, reach maximal lean more slowly, and exhibit less postural control once they have achieved maximal lean[6,15]. Dynamic postural control is even further compromised as a result of an underlying pathology and/or deconditioning[11]. Both exercise and combined weight loss and exercise regimens lead to improvements in pain, disability and performance[16]. Biomechanical data suggest that exercise combined with diet may have an additional benefit in improved gait compared to exercise alone.

There now exists a wealth of data demonstrating that physical activity and exercise may ameliorate disease and delay decline in function in the geriatric population. Sedentary persons who improve their physical fitness are less likely to die of cardiovascular disease than are those who remain sedentary[17]. Older patients with cardiovascular disease are not aggressively referred to cardiac rehabilitation programs, due to concerns regarding orthopedic fragility, hemodynamic risk and life expectancy. However, most studies indicate that these older patients derive the same magnitude of improvement in functional capacity as their younger counterparts[18].

Endurance training can help to maintain and to improve cardiovascular function as measured by Vo_2 max, cardiac output, and arteriovenous oxygen difference. After cardiac rehabilitation, the elderly had significant improvements in exercise capacity (i.e. metabolic equivalents; METs), body mass indices, per cent body fat, high-density lipoprotein cholesterol, and low-density lipoprotein cholesterol but not total cholesterol[19].

Low intensity, habitual physical activity (≥ 5 h per week of activity) is a sufficient stimulus to enhance blood lipid and lipoprotein profiles in the elderly. Compared to less active individuals they had a better lipid profile. Older individuals with higher levels of cardiorespiratory fitness, regardless of their physical activity, showed lower levels of fasting insulin, triglycerides, total cholesterol, total to high-density lipoprotein cholesterol ratio, low-density lipoprotein and lower waist circumference[20].

After a cardiac rehabilitation program the elderly make significant improvements in estimated aerobic capacity: peak V_{O_2}, anaerobic threshold, total function scores and total quality of life scores[21]. A moderate-intensity home-based combined walking and resistance program for patients with class II to III heart failure is safe and effective in reducing symptoms and improving quality of life[14]. In a study of a group of 456 70-year-olds, unadjusted mortality at 6-year follow-up was significantly greater for subjects reporting no physical activity compared to those walking as little as 4 h weekly[22]. Thus, regular physical activity confers increased survival in the aged and is the basis for encouraging older people to engage in regular, moderate physical activity.

Even less physical activity than is currently recommended (two to 12 times per month, 0.5. to 2 h per week) is likely to improve the cardiovascular risk profile (lower systolic blood pressure, resting heart rate and body mass index)[23]. The very old are also likely to benefit from exercise. The effects of a twice-weekly, 6-month, progressive walking program for women in their ninth decade of life suggested that the training group showed lower resting and working heart rates, and increased activity[24]. In addition, morale improved as well. Any training program would have to be continued on a long-term basis to maintain the training-related benefits; these benefits were lost within 1 year if the training program was not maintained[25].

Motivational factors regarding the elderly patient's willingness to participate in exercise programs need to be addressed. In general, education and exercise history correlate positively with exercise, while perceived physical frailty and poor health may provide the greatest barrier to exercise adoption and adherence in the elderly[26]. The findings suggest that many older women feel physically vulnerable, are unsure about their actual risks and benefits in exercise settings and, in the face of uncertainty, report medical reasons as to why they should be excused from fitness-promoting exercise[27]. Reasons for not participating in a 'jogging program' include engaging in another aerobic program (i.e. walking), having a health condition that prevented jogging, and jogging as too uncomfortable[28]. Clearly, special precautions for the older patient are indicated and include attention to hydration and nutrition, underlying orthopedic and cardiopulmonary disorders and environmental factors. Exercise programs geared towards the elderly require appropriate modification.

FACTORS INFLUENCING ADHERENCE

Stimulating elderly patients to participate in exercise programs can be enhanced with group programs that incorporate friends and family. A recent article by Resnick and Spellbring[29] indicated that there were six major factors that influenced adherence to an exercise program for older adults: beliefs about exercise; benefits of exercise; past experiences with exercise; goals; personality; and unpleasant sensations associated with exercise. Interventions included teaching older adults about the benefits of exercises, establishing appropriate goals, and decreasing unpleasant and increasing pleasant sensations associated with exercise. In a study of adults aged 65 and older, predictors of both initiation and maintenance of physical activity were younger age, moderate to excellent health and the patient's belief that physical activity was important to his/her health. Forty per cent said that their physician was an important influence.

BARRIERS

Barriers to exercise cited included exercise accessibility and availability. There is evidence that even a home-based resistive exercise program (using elastic bands of varying thickness) can have both a high rate of adherence and achieve significantly improved lower extremity strength, improved tandem gait, and reduction in physical and overall disability at the 6-month follow-up[30]. Even a self-paced resistance training and walking exercise program can improve neuromotor performance and functional capacity, and this is a simple, safe, effective and cost-efficient model. Strength training has been shown to improve both physiologic and psychologic parameters including: positive and negative mood; trait anxiety; and perceived confidence in physical capability. No effects were noted in the patients' cognitive functioning[31]. There is potential for long-term health-care cost savings from a publicly funded moderate exercise program.

Recently, there has been a growth of 'aquatic' therapy programs, which take place in a pool and are geared towards older individuals. While the weight-independent attributes of this form of exercise are clear, the clinician needs to be aware of the decrements in respiratory and cardiovascular parameters that have been noted in young individuals immersed in water up to the neck. These decrements become more pronounced with exercise and include a decrease in maximal oxygen consumption and heart rate in deep water immersion compared with running on land. Currently, there is a lack of knowledge regarding the use of this form of exercise in frail elderly individuals[32].

Insulin resistance develops with aging, the mechanisms being multifactorial. Aging is associated with an increase in body weight; abdominal fat associated with hyperinsulinemia and visceral adiposity is correlated with insulin resistance as well. Modifications of the changes in body composition with aging by diet and exercise training could delay the onset of insulin resistance. The improvements in glucose metabolism after body weight loss and exercise training may be attributed to reduction of total and central body fat and changes in skeletal muscle blood flow[33].

Creatine plays an important role in cellular energy metabolism and potentially has a role in protein metabolism. Creatine monohydrate supplementation has been shown to result in an increase in skeletal muscle total and phosphocreatine concentration, to increase fat-free mass and to enhance high-intensity exercise in young healthy men and women. Recent evidence has also demonstrated a neuroprotective effect of creatine monohydrate supplementation in animal models of Parkinsons's disease, Alzheimer's disease, amyotrophic lateral sclerosis and after ischemia. In the elderly there is no evidence of a beneficial effect with respect to muscle mass and/or function after supplementation with creatine monohydrate[34]. Studies using different types of hormone supplementation have shown interesting and encouraging effects on skeletal muscle mass and function[35]. The potential risks with both growth hormone and androgen treatment are not known.

WHAT TYPE OF EXERCISE IS BENEFICIAL IN THE ELDERLY?

Walking

Gait patterns change with aging. Balance depends on the integrity of the visual, vestibular, proprioceptive input as well as sensory and motor integration. Muscles must rapidly adapt to change and co-ordinate with flexible joints. All of the above deteriorate with age. Seniors often rely on one system to compensate for inadequacy in others (e.g. relying on vision to compensate for loss of proprioception in feet). With age, gait slows (with longer stance and shorter steps), and there is greater sway standing or walking. Osteoporosis with kyphosis shifts the center of gravity forward, exacerbating the tendency to fall forward with any misstep. Cadence and stride length also decrease, leading to less propulsive power and momentum[11].

Exercise does not need to be of high intensity to be beneficial. Walking is the easiest, most convenient, most inexpensive and safest way to exercise. Walking works for anyone, at any time. Walking is aerobic but can be as strenuous or gentle as required. The risk of injuries is low, because walking is low impact and self-regulated. It is safe even in elderly cardiac patients, diabetics and arthritics. As little as three times a week for 20–40 min per walk is healthy. Patients can be counseled to start with a 10-min walk, two times a week and increase. A Harvard study involving nurses between 40 and 65 years of age showed that a walking program was inversely associated with the risk of coronary events and that even older, sedentary women lowered their risk. Walking more than 3 h per week or exercising vigorously for 1.5 h decreased the risk of cardiac problems by 40%[36]. Geriatric patients start off at a disadvantage, having lower endurance, joint muscle problems and fear. They are often fiscally restricted. Sensible shoes with laces, flexible soles with good shock absorbers and leather uppers with good arch supports are recommended. Patients should walk on smooth surfaces and avoid uneven terrain. Canes are excellent to decrease weight bearing on painful hips and knees, or to increase stance support (cane used on unaffected side).

In the fit elderly, the formula for targeted heart rate is as follows:

Targeted heart rate is 220 − age = maximum heart rate (the fastest acceptable heart rate) by X

where X varies with desired exercise: X is 80% for 'aerobic conditioning'; X is 60% for 'moderate conditioning'; and X is 40% for 'low-intensity workout'.

Prior to walking (whether it be fast or slow), a warm-up of 5 min, with calf and quad stretches, hamstring and side stretching, is necessary to prevent sprains. Targeted heart rate is checked after 5–10 min of getting into stride. After 20–40 min of walking, a cool-down with a 5-min slow-down follows.

An alternative to traditional walking for patients is aquatic exercise[37]. This is becoming available with pool classes for the elderly. In water, there is no stress or strain on arthritic joints. 'Water walkers' are used to ensure buoyancy, prevent drowning and alleviate anxiety. These foam flotation devices hold the patients around the waist. Stretching and aerobic programs can be easily facilitated.

Stationary cycling is another alternative. Bicycles are now relatively inexpensive and fit into most homes or apartments. It is recommended that cycling be performed for 25 min with a 5-min warm-up and cool-down. Seat height can be adjusted to decrease knee flexion ($< 10°$ at the lowest point of rotation of the pedal).

Exercise is an important modality of treatment for all chronic diseases of aging. Research has shown that 2–3 days per week of strengthening exercise can reduce disuse atrophy and age-related morbidity. Mental health benefits and improvements in immune function are well cited. Several trials have compared improved nutrition with exercise to delineate cost effectiveness. A trial comparing deconditioning versus improved nutrition of nursing home residents (mean age 87) over 10 weeks[38] showed that nutritional supplements had no affect on outcome, while muscles and strength increased by more than 100% in those who underwent exercise training. Stair climbing and thigh girth also improved.

Resistance exercise

The American College of Sports Medicine (ACSM) recommends that resistance parameters for the elderly should include one set of

8–10 repetitions that train all the large major muscle groups. This would include gluteals, quadriceps, hamstrings, pectoralis major, latissimus dorsi, deltoids and the abdominals. Each set of exercises should involve 8–10 repetitions and be performed 2–3 times a week[39]. Examples of such resistance exercises would include chest press, shoulder press, triceps extension, biceps curls, pulleys, lower back exercises, and abdominal crunches. For patients exercising at home, Theraband (Therex) exercising using different resistances can work well (color coded). Weights can be substituted by using canned foods such as soda and soup, which are equivalent to 1-lb (0.45-kg) weights. Patients interested in an overall reconditioning, resistance program can select a weight easily lifted through full range of motion, with good form for a minimum of eight repetitions. If this is not possible, the individual may switch to a lower weight to start with. As abilities improve and the repetitions becomes easier (able to perform more than 12 repeats), each weight can be increased by 5%. Customizing exercises through repetition maximums (RMs) (one RM is the maximum weight an individual can lift once) standardize exercises and document progress. A single set of exercises to fatigue with weight loads to 50% of one RM is as effective as multiple set programs performed in gymnasiums. It is recommended that for upper body work, 30–40% of one RM is undertaken and 50–60% for hips and legs[39,40].

Weight machines may be safer than free weights because of problems with posture and stability, low back pain, low vision and possibly dropping weights. Further, machines can be reset to restrict range of motion to a painfree arc. Caution: most machines are poorly designed ergonomically; physical therapy supervision is recommended.

Alternative exercise: yoga and Tai Chi

Yoga is a mind/body awareness type of exercise, which concentrates on deep breathing relaxation and meditation. Yoga suitable for older subjects includes Leyenger, Kripaki, Kundalini and Viniyoga schools[41]. Yoga encompasses stretching joints, increasing blood flow and isometric exercises to tone muscles and to improve standing balance. To date, there is limited outcome-based research on yoga.

The literal translation of yoga is 'union between mind and body' and was described in India 5000 years ago. Studies have shown that patients on a yoga program have shown significant overall regression of coronary arteriosclerosis (documented by arteriography), compared to controls who continued to show progress of disease. Deep breathing exercises, lowering blood pressure and decreasing levels of cortisol (stress hormone) and stretching the body provide better drainage of the lymphatic system and bronchi. Postures build muscle tone and improve balance and co-ordination. Yoga has been shown to decrease electromyogram (EMG) muscle activity by 58% during rest. Subjects who practice yoga can achieve higher work rates with a reduced oxygen consumption per unit work[40].

Tai Chi (or Tai Chi Chuan) is a form of gentle exercise and meditation that has been recommended for older adults with a variety of chronic illnesses. Tai Chi is an old martial art, which consists of slow, rhythmic, purposeful physical movements of the body, accompanied by breathing and mental control of balance. This is a no impact exercise, all the movements being graceful and controlled throughout range of motion of each joint. It can also be performed in a sitting or a semi-reclined position for patients who find it difficult to stand. Ankle and hip strategies such as used in conventional physical therapy for fall prevention are continually facilitated. Tai Chi is often performed in a group setting, which provides socialization and support. A cross-sectional study of 39 elderly patients practicing Tai Chi Chuan found that postural stability was improved in dynamic but not static balance. Those who regularly practice

Tai Chi perform better with challenged tasks than controls[42]. Based on this, it was felt that Tai Chi could be an excellent intervention for frequent fallers[43]. A 34% higher V_{O_2} peak compared to controls and higher skin blood flow was noted[44]. Tai Chi or Tai Chi Chuan is gaining momentum and popularity as an excellent geriatric group exercise.

PRECAUTIONS

Exercise prescribing for individual geriatric patients may be based on the following principles[14,17,19,21,23,39,40]:

(1) Cardiac patients should exercise at lower intensities, that is 40% maximum heart rate. Lower-intensity exercise may be compensated with increased repetitions (e.g. repetitions of 10–15 instead of 8–10).

(2) Neurological patients such as those with stroke or Parkinson's disease, who have fatigue limitations and thereby higher energy costs, should also exercise at lower intensities. Sitting exercise can be incorporated instead of standing to prevent falls in those with balance dysfunction.

(3) With progressive neurologic conditions such as ALS (Lou Gherig's disease), exercise is cautioned to avoid further exhaustion of the already compromised anterior horn cells.

(4) Exercise is contraindicated in myasthenia gravis because of early fatigue of neuromuscular junctions with repetitive exercise. Exercising inflamed muscles as in polymyositis or dermatomyosis can exacerbate the clinical condition.

(5) Musculoskeletal complications such as rheumatoid arthritis, bursitis or osteoarthritis require care and lower-intensity, low-impact exercises, only in pain-free range of motion.

(6) When uncontrolled, hypertension is a contraindication; blood pressure should be checked in all physical therapy centers prior to commencement of programs. Exercising while hypertensive can be dangerous.

(7) Medications (such as sedatives, tranquilizers, antidepressants, antihypertensives) should be reviewed. Furthermore, a cardiovascular and neurologic evaluation prior to starting an exercise program is appropriate. Patients with gait disturbances or cardiovascular problems may need to start their exercise programs in a supervised setting such as a physical therapy center. Exercise treadmill testing can be used to screen for high-risk individuals and to set an optimum target for heart rate intensity[40].

(8) Amputees face problems with standing and dynamic balance, and higher energy costs are required for simple ambulation, with risk of falls. Emphasis should encompass upper extremity exercises (e.g. upper extremity ergometers for aerobic reconditioning). Lower-extremity strengthening can be achieved with walking or swimming (swim prostheses are available). Amputees may have widespread vascular problems and should be screened accordingly.

Figure 2 shows a simple exercise program suitable for all seniors developed by the physical therapy department at St Vincent's Hospital, New York. This combination of exercise and stretches strengthens and improves balance. It is safe, easy, cheap, effective and an excellent way to start.

CONCLUSION

Both empiric and scientific data show that individuals who begin exercise even late in life can have numerous health benefits. Contrary to popular belief, the frail elderly can benefit from both resistance exercises and aerobic reconditioning, and the risk of injury is

Sitting:

1. Ankle pumps: Move ankles up and down.

2. Knee extension: Straighten knee in order to raise foot.

3. Walk in place.

4. While raising arms, take a deep breath. Exhale while bringing arms down.

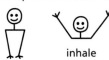

inhale

Standing: Hold on to a table or chair while performing the following exercises.

1. Move leg straight out to the side. Repeat 10 times with the left and
   10 times with the right.

2. Move leg back while keeping knee straight. Repeat 10 times with the left and
   10 times with the right.

Figure 2   A home exercise and conditioning program. Reproduced with permission from St Vincent's Hospital and Medical Center, Physical Therapy Department, New York City

relatively low (even in osteoarthritis). To date, most exercise protocols have focused on strength training. Research is needed to correlate other types of exercises with improvement in activities of daily living and function. It is now thought that any exercise is better than none (even walking slowly). We know that constant counseling and support are required by the medical community to maintain exercise programs. An exercise program does not have to be complicated. A simple sheet given to the patient, rubber bands, or even food cans substituting for weights can be effective. Benefits of simple exercises include better balance, faster response time, increased bone mass and better mental alertness.

References

1. Loefler ISP. 65 years of mobile life for all? *J R Soc Med* 2001;94:418–19
2. Wee C. Physical activity counseling in primary care. *J Am Med Assoc* 2001;236: 717–19
3. Marijkie JM, Chin A, de Jong N. Physical exercise and/or enriched foods for functional improvements in frail, independently living elderly: a randomized controlled trial. *Arch Phys Med Rehabil* 2001;82:811–17
4. Earles DR, Judge JO, Gumarson OT. Velocity training induces power specific adaptations in highly functional older adults. *Arch Phys Med Rehabil* 2001; 82:872–7
5. Westerterp KR. Daily physical activity and aging. *Curr Opin Clin Nutr Metab Care* 2000;3:485–8
6. Lieberman JS, Pugliese GN, Strauss NE. Skeletal muscle: structure, chemistry and function. In *Downey & Darling's Physiological Basis of Rehabilitation Medicine*. Woburn, MA: Butterworth–Heinemann, 2001:67–79
7. Curl WW. Aging and exercise: are they compatible in women? *Clin Orthop* 2000; 372:151–8
8. Castaneda C, Grossi L, Dwyer J. Potential benefits of resistance exercise training on nutritional status in renal failure. *J Renal Nutr* 1998;8:2–10
9. Schwartz AL. Patterns of exercise and fatigue in physically active cancer survivors. *Oncol Nurs Forum* 1998;25:485–91
10. Rutherford OM. Is there a role for exercise in the prevention of osteoporotic fractures? *Br J Sport Med* 1999;33:378–86
11. Blaszczyk JW, Lowe DL, Hanseb PD. Ranges of postural stability and their changes in the elderly. *Gait Posture* 1994; 2:11–17
12. Krivickas LS, Suh D, Wilkens J, *et al*. Age and gender-related differences in maximum shortening velocity of skeletal muscle fibers. *Am J Phys Med Rehabil* 2001:80: 447–55
13. Shepard RJ. What is the optimal type of physical activity to enhance health? *Br J Sports Med* 1997;31:277–84
14. Oka RK, De Marco T, Haskell WL, *et al*. Impact of a home-based walking and resistance training program on quality of life in patients with heart failure. *Am J Cardiol* 2000;85:365–9
15. Schieppati M, Hugon M, Grasso M, Nardone A, Galante M. The limits of equilibrium in young and elderly normal subjects and in parkinsonians. *Electroencephalogr Clin Neurophysiol* 1994;93: 286–98
16. Messier SP, Loeser RF, Mitchell MN, *et al*. Exercise and weight loss in obese older adults with knee osteoarthritis: a preliminary study. *J Am Geriatr Soc* 2000;48: 1062–72
17. Christmas C, Andersen RA. Exercise and older patients: guidelines for the clinician. *J Am Geriatr Soc* 2000;48:318–24
18. Sarwar R, Beltan-Niclos B, Rutherford OM. Changes in muscle strength, relaxation rate, and fatiguability during the human menstrual cycle. *J Physiol* 1996; 493:267–72
19. Braith RW, Vincent KR. Resistance exercise in the elderly person with cardiovascular disease. *Am J Geriatr Cardiol* 1999; 8:63–70
20. Dvorak RV, Tchernof A, Starling RD, *et al*. Respiratory fitness, free living physical activity, and cardiovascular disease risk in older individuals: a doubly labeled water study. *J Clin Endocrinol Metab* 2000;85: 957–63
21. Lavie CJ, Milani RVJ. Disparate effects of improving aerobic exercise capacity and quality of life after cardiac rehabilitation in young and elderly coronary patients. *Cardiopulm Rehabil* 2000;20:235–40
22. Stressman J, Maaravi Y, Hammerman-Rozenberg R, Cohen A. The effects of physical activity on mortality in the Jerusalem 70-year-olds longitudinal study. *J Am Geriatr Soc* 2000;48:499–504

23. Mensink GB, Ziese T, Kok FJ. Benefits of leisure-time physical activity on the cardiovascular risk profile at older age. *Int J Epidemiol* 1999;28:659–66

24. Hamdorf PA, Penhall RK. Walking with its training effects on the fitness and activity patterns of 79–91 year old females. *Aust N Z J Med* 1999;29:22–8

25. Morio B, Barra V, Titz P, *et al*. Benefit of endurance training in elderly people over a short period is reversible. *Eur J Appl Physiol* 2000;81:329–36

26. Rhodes RE, Martin AD, Taunton JE, *et al*. Factors associated with exercise adherence among older adults. An individual perspective. *Sports Med* 1999;28:397–411

27. O'Brien CS. 'My heart couldn't take it': older women's beliefs about exercise benefits and risks. *J Gerontol* 2000;55:283–94

28. Vitulli WF, Malek JM. Assumptions about fitness and exercise among elderly persons. *Percept Mot Skills* 1997;84:671–4

29. Resnick B, Spellbring AM. Understanding what motivates older adults to exercise. *J Gerontol Nurs* 2000;26:34–42

30. Jette AM, Lachman M, Giorgetti MM, *et al*. Exercise – it's never too late: the strong-for-life-program. *Am J Public Health* 1999;89:66–72

31. Tstsumi T, Don BM, Zaichkowsky LD, Delizonna LL. Physical fitness and psychological benefits of strength training in community dwelling older adults. *Appl Human Sci* 1997;16:257–66

32. Chu KS, Rhodes EC. Physiological and cardiovascular changes associated with deep water running in the young. Possible implications for the elderly. *Sports Med* 2001; 31:33–46

33. Ryan AS. Insulin resistance with aging: effects of diet and exercise. *Sports Med* 2000;30:327–46

34. Tarnopolsky MA. Potential benefits of creatine monohydrate supplementation in the elderly. *Curr Opin Clin Nutr Metab Care* 2000;3:497–502

35. Marijhe JM, Chin AP, Dynke de Jong, *et al*. Physical exercises and/or enriched foods for functional improvement in frail, independently living elderly. *Arch Phys Med Rehabil* 2001;82:811–17

36. Manson JE, Hu F, Rich-Edwards JW, *et al*. A prospective study of walking as compared with vigorous exercise in the prevention of coronary heart disease in women. *N Engl J Med* 1999;341:650–8

37. Heyneman CA, Premo DE. A water walkers exercise program for the elderly. *Public Health Rep* 1992;107:213–16

38. Fiatorone MA, O'Neil EF, Ryan ND, *et al*. Exercise training and nutritional supplementation for physical frailty in very elderly people. *N Engl J Med* 1994;330: 1769–75

39. Richard M. Pump it up with geriatric strength building; higher intensities produce better results. *Adv Dir Rehabil* 2000; 9:49–50

40. Rooney EM. Exercise for older patients: why it's worth your effort. *Geriatrics* 1993;48:68–77

41. Taylor MJ, Majundmar M. Incorporating yoga therapeutics into orthopaedic physiological therapy. In Galantino ML, Iglarsh ZA, Richardson JK, eds. *Orthopaedic Physical Therapy Clinics of North America: Complementary Medicine*. WB Saunders, 2000:341–59

42. Bottomley JM. The use of Tai Chi as a movement modality in orthopaedics. In Galantino ML, Iglarsh ZA, Richardson JK, eds. *Orthopaedic Physical Therapy Clinics of North America: Complementary Medicine*. WB Saunders, 2000:361–73

43. Wong AM, Yin-Chou L, Shih-Weic, *et al*. Coordination exercise and postural stability in elderly people: effect of Tai Chi Chuan. *Arch Phys Med Rehabil* 2001;82:608–12

44. Wang JS, Cheng L, Wong MK. Tai Chi Chuan training to enhance microcirculatory function in healthy elderly men. *Arch Phys Med Rehabil* 2001;82:1176–80

9 The pharmacology of aging

Lisa C. Hutchison, PharmD, MPH, BCPS

INTRODUCTION

The most common cause of iatrogenic illness in hospitalized elderly patients is adverse drug events, which cause 10–15% of hospital admissions in patients aged 60 and older[1,2]. In addition, 65% of nursing home residents experienced adverse drug events in a 4-year period[3]. In the ambulatory population, the costs of medication-related illnesses and death are estimated to be US $177.4 billion annually[4,5]. Although this study was not limited to the elderly, the average older person consumes 4.5 prescriptions and two over-the-counter medications concurrently and therefore a significant proportion of this figure[6].

A basic understanding of epidemiology, physiologic changes in the elderly and medication pharmacology leads us to develop some simple guidelines for medication use to limit the risk of adverse drug reactions in the elderly. Diligent application of these guidelines by each member of the health-care team can help reduce this significant morbidity and mortality.

PHARMACOEPIDEMIOLOGY

The umbrella category of adverse drug events (ADEs) is defined as any event, whether intentional or not, that produces an adverse outcome as a result of medication use[7]. This broad category includes both expected and unexpected outcomes, preventable and non-preventable events and intentional suicides. The definition of adverse drug reactions (ADRs) is less broad but still inclusive of side-effects of a medication, both common and rare. Generally, ADRs are considered non-preventable injuries caused by a pharmaceutical or herbal product and are a subset of ADEs. A medication error is the failure of a planned action involving a medication to be completed or the use of a wrong plan involving a medication to achieve an aim[2]. It is any preventable event that may cause or lead to inappropriate medication use or patient harm[8]. Medication errors include prescribing, dispensing, or administration errors. Even if an error does not actually cause harm or an ADE, it is tracked in an effort to identify potential system breakdown points so that they may be improved to prevent future errors that are injurious.

With these distinctions in definition it becomes easier to interpret data reported in the many studies on medication safety in the elderly. ADRs account for approximately 5% of all hospital admissions[9,10], and the elderly are two to three times more likely to experience an ADR than are other adults during a hospitalization. In a meta-analysis of 39 studies of ADRs excluding medication errors, 27% of the variance for rate of ADRs causing hospital admission was related to age[10]. ADEs may be attributed to disorders that are common among the elderly such as falls, anorexia, constipation, cognitive impairment or urinary retention. When the medication culprit is not identified, misdiagnosis and prescription of additional medications will occur, compounding the adverse event.

Medication errors are also more common among elderly patients, primarily because these patients are on more medications. Also, they frequently receive cardiovascular agents, the medications most often associated with medication errors. After controlling for these factors, no difference was seen in one study evaluating medication errors in hospitalized patients. Among hospital patients, 28% of ADEs are usually judged to be preventable. In one teaching hospital, the overall error rate was 3.13 per 1000 orders written. Of these, 1.81 per 1000 orders (or 58%) were judged to be significant errors[2].

Implementation of computerized physician order entry, increased prescribing knowledge, early recognition, reduced unnecessary drug use, increased use of pharmacists, geriatric dosing guidelines and geriatric labeling information have proved to reduce the rates of medication errors[11]. With ADRs, we must take a different approach. Since, by definition, these events are not preventable, we will not be able to stop their occurrence. However, by analyzing trends for particular medications and high-risk patients or situations, a heightened awareness will steer us to exert more caution. This caution will translate into more conservative use of high-risk medications and closer monitoring in high-risk patients or situations.

PHARMACOKINETIC CHANGES IN THE ELDERLY

The most important differences for medication use in the elderly relate to the pharmacokinetic alterations common in this population. Some ADEs are directly related to use of medications at a dose or frequency consistent with known pharmacokinetic parameters in young adults, but inconsistent with pharmacokinetic parameters in the elderly. A thorough understanding of physiologic changes that occur with aging explains many of the resulting pharmacokinetic alterations.

Absorption

Alterations in gastric acid acidity, gastric emptying and intestinal motility are observed with increasing age[12]. However, these changes produce minimal effects on absorption of oral medications. A delay in time to reach maximum concentration and a lower maximum concentration are seen, but the total amount of medication absorbed is unchanged. Therefore, the overall bioavailability of medications used for chronic conditions is generally unaffected.

For acute situations, such as may be seen with analgesics, the slower absorption is occasionally associated with a slower onset of action. This rarely causes a significant clinical problem. Conversely, an enteric coated medication may lose its protective coating in the stomach due to the higher pH, thus causing a more rapid onset, and perhaps adverse effects, as in the case with aspirin or bisacodyl. Enteric coated medications should be taken on an empty stomach in patients with a mild to moderate achlorhydria and avoided in patients with a stomach pH approaching neutral.

The extraction rate for medications by the liver after absorption is dependent upon the splanchnic blood flow. This flow is reduced in the elderly, which leads to an increased bioavailability for medications that generally have a high first-pass extraction. Medications such as verapamil and propranolol have lower effects due to low bioavailability; effects may be enhanced with age due to decreased extraction and improved bioavailability.

Percutaneous absorption of medications has not been studied in the elderly. However, one would expect some alterations for transdermal patches, due to the changes in collagen and fat layers. In addition, the adhesives used with transdermal patches may cause more damage with removal in the elderly, due to the lack of skin elasticity.

Distribution

As one ages, the body composition tends to change. A relative decrease in total body water and lean body mass is coupled with an increase in body fat[12]. As a result, the volume of distribution of water-soluble drugs, such as aminoglycosides, is reduced and smaller doses are required to achieve a therapeutic response. Alternatively, drugs that are lipophilic appear to have a larger volume of distribution relative to body weight. Once the body has a large store of a lipophilic medication, the drug's half-life will be prolonged if clearance is held constant. This relationship is:

Equation 1

$$\text{Elimination half-life } (T_{1/2})$$
$$= \frac{0.693 \times \text{volume of distribution}}{\text{clearance}}$$

A second confounding factor with distribution of medication in the elderly involves serum albumin. In healthy ambulatory elderly patients, serum albumin levels are not decreased and no change with medication distribution is anticipated[13]. However, in the face of malnutrition or chronic disease, significant decreases in serum albumin are observed. Drugs that are highly protein bound will have fewer binding sites and their free fraction in the serum will be increased. The free fraction is more directly related to the activity of the medication than to the total serum concentration (free and unbound combined). This becomes particularly important for medications that are more than 90% protein bound and have low rates of clearance.

One such medication that fits this pattern is phenytoin[13]. In cases where a low serum albumin is documented, measurement of the free phenytoin concentration is a better correlate to therapeutic or toxic effects. Other medications are similarly affected, but free drug concentration measurements are not routinely available. In these circumstances, lower initial doses and small dosage increases are justified in order to prevent an increased risk for toxicity. Table 1 lists medications commonly used in the elderly which are

Table 1 Medications with significant potential for problems related to protein binding in the elderly

Medications	Per cent protein bound
Cardiovascular	
Benazaprilat	95.3
Digoxin	25
Enalaprilat	40–60
Nicardipine	95
Warfarin	99
Central nervous system	
Diazepam	98
Etomidate	76
Flurazepam	97
Lorazepam	85
Meperidine	65–75
Nitrazepam	85
Phenytoin	90–95
Triazolam	89
Valproic acid	80–90
Musculoskeletal	
Diflunisal	> 90
Ibuprofen	90–99
Naproxen	> 90
Salicylic acid	50–80
Other	
Acetazolamide	95
Ceftriaxone	85–95
Furosemide	> 90
Theophylline	40

highly protein bound or documented to have altered binding in the elderly.

Metabolism

The liver primarily functions, in pharmacokinetic terms, to turn lipophilic molecules into hydrophilic ones. Hepatic metabolism occurs through one of two major groups of reaction referred to as Phase I and Phase II pathways (Table 2)[12,14]. Phase I reactions include oxidation and reduction. The elderly have reduced activity of Phase I pathways. The risk for toxicity is compounded in that medications that undergo Phase I reactions are frequently transformed into active metabolites. The effects of both parent drug and active metabolite become even more difficult to predict. When the active metabolites subsequently

Table 2 Hepatic drug metabolism in the elderly

Phase I reactions			Phase II reactions		
Oxidation		Reduction	Conjugation		
Hydroxylation	Dealkylation	Nitroreduction	Glucuronidation	Sulfation	Acetylation
Alprazolam*	Amitriptyline*	Citalopram	Acetaminophen	Acetaminophen	Procainamide*
Barbiturates	Chlordiazepoxide*	Nitrazepam	Lorazepam		
Carbamazepine*	Diazepam*		Oxazepam		
Ibuprofen	Flurazepam*		Valproic acid		
Imipramine*	Diphenhydramine		Zaleplon		
Desipramine	Fluoxetine*				
Nortriptyline	Lidocaine*				
Phenytoin	Meperidine*				
Propranolol*	Quazepam*				
Quinidine	Sertraline				
Risperidone*	Theophylline				
Warfarin	Tramadol*				
	Venlafaxine*				

*Active metabolites

require renal elimination, another variable is introduced into the equation. Diazepam and chlordiazepoxide are two medications that undergo Phase I reactions into the active metabolites lorazepam and oxazepam, respectively. As these chemical moieties are useful as medications in their own right, use of the parent compounds requires management of it and the active metabolite.

The activity of the Phase II pathways are generally maintained in the elderly. These include glucuronidation, acetylation and sulfation. These reactions tend to produce inactive metabolites, so medications eliminated through Phase II reactions are preferred in this age group[12].

Excretion

Although some elderly people maintain relatively good renal function, decreases in renal mass and blood flow cause most elderly patients to have a decrease in glomerular filtration rate (GFR). This is especially evident in patients with diabetes and/or hypertension. As the GFR drops, so does the excretion of water-soluble medications. With chronic dosing, an increased serum concentration occurs

due to the decreased clearance and increase in elimination half-life (refer to Equation 1). Therefore, proper dosing of renally eliminated drugs requires consideration of the patient's decrease in GFR.

According to some authorities, the best clinical measure of GFR is a 24-hour urine collection for a calculation of clearance with a serum creatinine measured simultaneously[15]. However, this approach is costly, time-consuming and inconvenient for the patient. In addition, its accuracy in the elderly has been questioned. A simple approximation of the creatinine clearance can be calculated from patient demographics utilizing the Cockcroft–Gault formula:

Equation 2

Creatinine clearance in males (ml/min)

$$= \frac{140 - (\text{age in years}) \times (\text{lean body weight in kg})}{(\text{serum creatinine in mg/dl}) \times 72}$$

Creatinine clearance in females (ml/min)
$$= (\text{creatinine clearance in males}) \times 0.85$$

Other formulas may also be appropriate, but the Cockcroft–Gault equation is the most widely accepted, and utilized in many package inserts for medication dosing. Commonly

Table 3 Medications commonly dosed using creatinine clearance estimates

Medication class	Medication
Antigout drugs	allopurinol, colchicine
Antimicrobial agents	acyclovir, aminoglycosides, carbapenems, famciclovir, fluconazole, fluoroquinolones, penicillins, sulfonamides, tetracycline, valcyclovir, vancomycin
Cardiovascular drugs	atenolol, digoxin, procainamide, some ACE inhibitors
Central nervous system drugs	amantadine, gabapentin, lithium, meperidine, rimantidine
Endocrine drugs	chlorpropamide, glipizide
Gastrointestinal drugs	H$_2$ blockers

ACE, angiotensin converting enzyme

used medications dosed via creatinine clearance estimates are shown in Table 3.

A few caveats must be kept in mind when utilizing this equation. First, actual body weight should be used if the patient's lean body mass is calculated to be above actual body weight. Second, the patient's muscle mass is the site of creatinine production. If the patient has lost significant amounts of muscle mass due to immobility or malnutrition, the serum creatinine will be low and the creatinine clearance will be overestimated. Some experts have suggested a conservative approach of always rounding a low serum creatinine up to 1 mg/dl in order to avoid this risk of overestimation[16]. This has not been studied adequately to make it widely accepted. Lastly, the patient's height and weight are often not available. In this situation, one may estimate lean body mass inaccurately and other alternative equations to estimate creatinine clearance should be used, such as the Jelliffe formula:

Equation 3

$$\text{Creatinine clearance in males (ml/min/1.73 m}^2)$$
$$= \frac{98 - 0.8 \, (\text{age} - 20)}{(\text{serum creatinine in mg/dl})}$$

$$\text{Creatinine clearance in females (ml/min/1.73 m}^2)$$
$$= (\text{creatinine clearance in males}) \times 0.90$$

Drug clearance at other sites

The majority of medications are cleared via the liver through metabolism or the kidney through excretion. However, other sites of clearance sometimes become important with specific medications or patients. Biliary excretion of parent drug and metabolites in the feces may be altered in patients with hepatitis, cirrhosis or cholestasis. Drug metabolism can occur at sites other than the liver including the kidney, gastrointestinal tract, lung, skin, blood and brain[17]. No change in the function of these alternative sites of clearance has been identified specifically for the elderly patient.

PHARMACODYNAMIC CHANGES IN THE ELDERLY

Pharmacodynamics has been defined as the effect of a drug at its receptor site. This new area of investigation focuses on pharmacologic responses associated with genetic differences usually found concentrated in different ethnic populations[12,14]. However, one change has been documented that is associated with aging. The concentration of β-adrenergic receptor sites decreases with age when measured in different age groups. Hence the effects of inhaled β-adrenergic agonists were blunted in older subjects as compared to younger. Likewise, β-adrenergic blocking agents exert less effect in lowering blood pressure or heart rate.

Medications that cause orthostatic hypotension are frequently problematic in the elderly due to a change in baroreceptor activity[18]. The patient's ability to adapt to a sudden change in pressure at the site of the baroreceptors by vasoconstriction of blood vessels is impaired. Anticholinergic medications also appear to have exaggerated adverse effects secondary to receptor site changes. As more studies are completed, many alterations in response to medications given to older patients will be better explained.

DRUG INTERACTIONS

Drug interactions can attenuate or accentuate a medication's therapeutic or adverse effect in a patient. Close scrutiny of a patient's medication profile is necessary to identify and avoid serious and problematic drug interactions of all types: drug–drug, drug–disease and drug–food interactions. While drug–drug interactions are the most studied, all three types interplay in each patient's medical care. Table 4, which identifies some of the most common and significant drug interactions, may be referenced for further information.

Drug–drug interactions

Pharmacokinetic parameters of a medication can be affected by other medications. Absorption interactions usually involve adherence of a substance such as a cation to the drug molecule, thus preventing the medication from being absorbed in the gastrointestinal tract. Highly protein bound drugs (see Table 1) can be displaced from their protein binding sites by other medications, resulting in distribution changes[13]. Renal excretion is altered when medications that undergo renal secretion compete for that secretory mechanism or if glomerular filtration is reduced. However, the most recognized drug–drug interactions involve hepatic metabolism through the cytochrome P450 (CYP) system.

Most substrates undergo metabolism by a specific enzyme, but each enzyme can metabolize many different compounds[19]. These enzymes are classified into three main enzyme families – CYP1, CYP2 and CYP3 – with many subfamilies and individual enzymes in each family. An induction of an enzyme will result in decreased serum concentrations and therapeutic effect of a medication, while inhibition will result in supratherapeutic levels and associated toxicities, unless the substrate can undergo metabolism or excretion by an alternative pathway. Inhibition and induction of drug metabolism may involve more than one CYP family and is usually dose dependent for the inducer/inhibitor.

Drug–disease interactions

Because diseases may affect the organs involved in drug absorption, distribution, metabolism and excretion, drug–disease interactions may occur. Hypertension reduces the GFR over time, reducing excretion of hydrophilic drugs. Cirrhosis can reduce hepatic metabolism of lipophilic drugs, decreased extracellular fluid reduces the volume of distribution of hydrophilic drugs and achlorhydria impairs absorption of acid-dependent medications. Also, drugs can worsen the signs and symptoms of some diseases. The use of non-steroidal anti-inflammatory agents, which seems ubiquitous, may exacerbate congestive heart failure, elevate blood pressure, worsen renal insufficiency or cause delirium in dementia[20].

Drug–nutrient interactions

Drug–nutrient interactions encompass both interactions with food and interactions with dietary supplements such as vitamins, herbs and homeopathy. Most drug–food interactions affect absorption, for example as a reduction or an increase in bioavailability.

Table 4 Some important drug interactions in the elderly

Drug/drug class	Drug/disease/food
ACE inhibitors	potassium-sparing diuretics
Fluoroquinolones	antacids, dairy products sucralfate
Digoxin	diuretics (both potassium-sparing and -losing) antacids quinidine
Anticholinergic drugs	benign prostatic hypertrophy glaucoma constipation dementia
Warfarin	many herbal remedies aspirin, non-steroidal anti-inflammatory agents green leafy vegetables, liver cholestyramine, colestipol fluoroquinolones co-trimoxazole amiodarone fluoxetine
Carbidopa/Levodopa	high-protein meals pyridoxine dopamine antagonists (antipsychotic agents) buspirone
Non-steroidal anti-inflammatory agents	diuretics ACE inhibitors hypertension congestive heart failure
Theophylline	cimetidine erythromycin rifampin
Selegiline	antidepressants
Tricyclic antidepressants	antiarrythmic agents orthostatic hypotension (see Anticholinergic drugs above)
Lipophilic benzodiazepines	calcium channel blockers macrolides grapefruit juice nefazodone

ACE, angiotensin converting enzyme

Some significant examples include fluoro-quinolones with dairy products, resulting in reduced absorption; carbidopa/levodopa absorption decreased when ingested with proteins; absorption of lipophilic medications increased following a high fat meal[21]. Fat in food may also influence the time-release mechanism of some sustained release medications. Alternatively, vitamin K-containing foods such as greens or liver can reduce effectiveness by interfering with warfarin's mechanism of action. Gingko, ginger and garlic may each exert an independent effect on platelets, exaggerated to the point of hemorrhage in a patient on warfarin, while goldenseal may cause increased clotting and would offset warfarin's therapeutic effect[22].

DRUGS REQUIRING SPECIAL CARE

Prescription medication

Non-pharmacologic approaches should be used when possible in older patients, because of their increased susceptibility to adverse events from medications. When medication must be used, side-effect potential must be weighed heavily into the risk–benefit evaluation. Beers has identified a set of medications that should be avoided in the elderly. These medications are labeled so for several reasons. First, the elderly are at an increased risk for ADEs from these agents. Second, these agents, particularly cardiovascular and central nervous system drugs, are commonly prescribed in the elderly population due to their increased incidence of disease in these systems. The Health Care Financing Administration used this list along with other resources in crafting its potential drug therapy problem indicators used in long-term care facilities[24]. Since long-term care surveyors will scrutinize their use, clear documentation must rationalize the risk–benefit of these medications. Table 5 presents the medications with the most severe ADEs, states why they can be problematic in the elderly, and gives some suggested alternatives.

Over-the-counter and herbal remedies

A group of agents often overlooked in the elderly are over-the-counter (OTC) medications and herbal remedies. When questioned about medication use, many older (and younger) patients neglect to mention use of these readily accessible items. They may not consider them to be medications, or they may have concern over the reaction of health-care providers. Although relatively safe, herbal and OTC medications can present problems. First, duplication can occur with prescription medications when patients are taking acetaminophen, antihistamines, decongestants, non-steroidal anti-inflammatory agents or histamine blocking drugs, increasing the risk for overdose and ADEs. Second, adverse drug interactions may occur, and have been documented between prescription drugs, OTC medications and herbal remedies[22]. Warfarin, for example, has been identified to interact with ginseng, garlic, ginger, *Gingko biloba* and feverfew, causing an increase in prothrombin time. A further word of caution concerning herbal products is required. Since manufacturing processes and scrutiny follow rules for food and not drugs, it is difficult to assure standardization of products across manufacturers and, sometimes, batches. This makes predicting possible patient response or risk for interactions even more difficult. Lastly, adverse pharmacoeconomics can occur if patients spend limited resources on these agents rather than on pharmaceuticals. One study on alternative therapy revealed that consumers in the USA spent $5.1 billion on herbal remedies and $3.3 billion on high-dose vitamins[25].

Polypharmacy

Polypharmacy is a term difficult to define. Most clinicians would say, 'I know it when I see it'. The key issues are that no medication should be used without an indication and that no duplication of therapy should occur. One could also add that, if side-effects develop, they should be addressed through changing medication or altering the dose rather than by adding additional medication, if possible. Polypharmacy frequently occurs in the elderly because of multiple disease states being treated by multiple physicians. If one primary care physician cannot be the only individual prescribing medications for a patient, then the next best alternative is for the patient to have one primary pharmacy. In this way, computerized checking for all potential drug–drug interactions and duplication of therapy is possible[11].

Table 5 Problematic medications in the elderly

Medication	Adverse drug event	Alternatives
Drugs to be avoided in the elderly		
Pentazocine	confusion, hallucinations	codeine, morphine, oxycodone
Long and medium acting benzodiazepines (flurazepam, diazepam, chlordiazepoxide)	extremely long half-life in the elderly, producing sedation and increased risk of fractures due to falls	lorazepam, zolpidem, oxazepam at low doses
Anticholinergic tricyclic antidepressants (amitriptyline, doxepin)	strong anticholinergic and sedating properties increasing risk for falls, constipation, and confusion	sertraline, citalopram, trazadone
Disopyramide	strong anticholinergic and negative inotropic properties	other antiarrhythmic agents
Barbiturates when used for sedation	increased and prolonged sedation	zolpidem, oxazepam
Meperidine	active metabolite accumulates in renal insufficiency, causing confusion, hallucinations, and seizures	morphine, oxycodone
Chlorpropamide	prolonged half-life increases risk for hypoglycemia	glipizide, glyburide
Dicyclomine, propantheline, and belladonna alkaloids	high anticholinergic properties increase risk for delirium	low-dose metoclopramide for upper gastrointestinal tract-related disease
Ticlopidine	risk for neutropenia	aspirin, clopidogrel
Drugs with special precautions		
Antihypertensives	risk for falls due to orthostatic hypotension	β-adrenergic blockers and thiazide diuretics preferred (monitor electrolytes) angiotensin converting enzyme inhibitors and calcium channel blockers also effective (avoid verapamil due to constipation)
Digoxin	potassium and fluid homeostasis, anorexia, delirium, heart block	avoid doses over 0.125 mg daily
Warfarin	bleeding risk is higher	frequent monitoring of prothrombin time and international normalized ratio check for drug–drug interactions for every additional drug added
Antibiotics (see Table 3)	accumulation of drug due to decreased renal function	adjust dose for creatinine clearance
Antipsychotic agents	sedation, cardiovascular effects, anticholinergic effects, tardive dyskinesia	select atypical antipsychotics (risperidone, quetiapine, olanzapine). Haloperidol can be used for acute agitation at low doses

Table 6   Optimal prescribing principles for older adults

Review medications regularly
Identify a current indication for each medication
Discontinue medications without an indication
Assess whether any current medications are contributing to symptoms or signs of illness

Before adding a new medication
Maximize the use of non-pharmacologic interventions
Evaluate for potential drug interactions or allergies
Dose at the lowest effective dose to minimize the risk for side-effects
Adjust the dose for pharmacokinetic changes (body composition, renal function, hepatic function)

Avoid risk for adverse drug events and prescribing errors
Write legibly or electronically
Add the purpose of the medication in the Sig (i.e. for pain, for blood pressure)
Communicate with interdisciplinary care team and patient/caregivers

Educate the patient/caregiver on the medication
Indication for use
Proper administration technique
Daily regimen
Expected therapeutic benefit
Side-effect potential
Monitoring requirements

Evaluate contributors to non-compliance
Avoid complex regimens and dosing schedules
Use proper dosage forms and packaging for physical disabilities (dysphagia, arthritis)
Select lower-cost medications or over-the-counter medications when possible
Assess understanding of therapy (cognitive impairment, poor hearing or vision)
Consider pill boxes, calendars, reminder systems when needed

POOR COMPLIANCE/ADHERENCE

Another practical issue for patients of any age is that of compliance or adherence to therapy. Numerous factors can contribute to non-compliance. In the elderly patient on a fixed income, cost is a primary concern. Until Medicare includes a prescription benefit, this will continue to be a leading factor in non-compliance[26]. Even then, we may see patients unable to afford their medications depending upon the restrictions put into place. Medication costs are unknown to most physicians. However, if patients ration out their medications in order to make them last longer, the medication risk–benefit evaluation has to include costs as a risk. One important option is that most major pharmaceutical companies have a patient assistance program. They can be identified through the pharmaceutical sales representative or the website: needymeds.com.

Second, the number of medication doses per day can contribute to non-compliance. It becomes difficult to manage the therapy when the number of drugs per day exceeds six, the number of doses exceeds 12 and the schedule is more frequent than twice daily. The prescriber must strive to simplify the regimen to improve compliance[27].

Some patients may not be compliant due to social and behavioral perceptions. If they are not convinced the medication would cure or prevent progression of a disease, or if they do not feel they are susceptible to the disease, many patients will not adhere to the prescribed therapy. The elderly perceive themselves as nearing the end of life and may not believe its length or quality can be altered. When asymptomatic conditions such as hypertension, hyperglycemia, hypercholesterolemia or osteoporosis are being treated, the patient disavows their existence or seriousness. Effective communication between the patient and the health-care team can identify these attitudes and methods to overcome them when they are inappropriate.

Although the list of factors contributing to non-compliance is long, one last item pertaining to the elderly should be noted. Fifty per cent of patients over the age of 85 have some form of cognitive impairment. This may cause them to forget whether they have taken doses of medication each day, thus putting them at risk to overdose, or underdose, essential medications. They may not understand the instructions given to administer the medication with or without food, the frequency or the indication. On the surface, the patient may be able to hide this from their physician. Even patients with intact cognition can have misconceptions about their drug therapy. One method to identify these problems is use of the Indian Health Service Model for patient counseling[28]. In this model, the educator asks the patient three questions to counsel them on medication use:

(1) What has your physician told you this medication is for?

(2) How did your physician tell you to take this medication?

(3) What did your physician tell you to expect?

These questions are used to identify what the patient understands about the indication for use, the dosing and administration regimen, and the therapeutic or adverse effects to be anticipated. The educator can then fill in the gaps or correct any misconceptions. If cognitive impairment is evident, alternative arrangements for medication administration through a caregiver can be made.

SUMMARY

Prescribing for the older patient is a complicated proposition due to their reduced residual capacity, number of diagnoses and lack of resources. Certainly, as people age, they grow more different rather than more alike. If the physician/clinician follows recommended guidelines, most adverse effects can be avoided or reversed quickly, and the patient will have a longer or better quality of life. Table 6 lists the principles of optimal prescribing practices for our elderly.

References

1. Leape LL, Brennan TA, Laird NM, *et al*. The nature of adverse events in hospitalized patients: results of the Harvard Medical Practice Study II. *N Engl J Med* 1991;324:377–84

2. Anon. Errors in health care: a leading cause of death and injury. In Kohn LT, Corrigan JM, Donaldson MS, eds. *To Err Is Human: Building a Safer Health System*. Washington, DC: National Academy Press, 2000:26–48

3. Cooper JW. Probable adverse drug reactions in a rural geriatric nursing home population: a four-year study. *J Am Geriatr Soc* 1996;44: 194–7

4. Johnson JA, Bootman JL. Drug-related morbidity and mortality: a cost-of-illness model. *Arch Intern Med* 1995;155:1949–56

5. Ernst FR, Grizzle AJ. Drug-related morbidity and mortality: updating the cost-of-illness model. *J Am Pharm Assoc* 2001;41:192–9

6. American Society of Consultant Pharmacists. The Silent Epidemic. *www.ascp.com/medhelp/silentepic.shtml*

7. Nadzam DM. A systems approach to medication use. In Cousins DD, ed. *Medication Use: A Systems Approach to Reducing Errors*. Oakbrook Terrace, IL: Joint Commission on Accreditation of Healthcare Organizations, 1998:5–17

8. Cousins DD. Defining medication errors. In Cousins DD, ed. *Medication Use: A Systems Approach to Reducing Errors*. Oakbrook Terrace, IL: Joint Commission on Accreditation of Healthcare Organizations, 1998: 39–56

9. Einarson TR. Drug-related hospital admissions. *Ann Pharmacother* 1993;27:832–40

10. Lazarou J, Pomeranz BH, Corey PN. Incidence of adverse drug reactions in hospitalized patients: A meta-analysis of prospective studies. *J Am Med Assoc* 1998;279: 1200–5

11. Rothschild JM, Bates DW, Leape LL. Preventable medical injuries in older patients. *Arch Intern Med* 2000;160:2717–28

12. Hammerlein A, Deredorf H, Lowenthal DT. Pharmacokinetic and pharmacodynamic changes in the elderly: clinical implications. *Clin Pharmacokinet* 1998;35:49–64

13. Grandison MK, Boudinot FD. Age-related changes in protein binding of drugs: implications for therapy. *Clin Pharmacokinet* 2000; 38:271–90

14. Lamy PP. Physiological changes due to age: pharmacodynamic changes of drug action and implications of therapy. *Drugs Aging* 1991;1: 385–404

15. Sawyer WT, Canaday BR, Poe TE, *et al.* Variables affecting creatinine clearance prediction. *Am J Hosp Pharm* 1983;40:2175–80

16. Lindeman RD. Changes in renal function with aging: implications for treatment. *Drugs Aging* 1992;2:423–31

17. Dharmarajan TS, Ugalino JT. Understanding the pharmacology of aging. In Krumm B, Dreger D, eds. *Hospital Physician: Geriatric Medicine Board Review Manual.* Wayne City, PA: Turner White Comms, 2001;1:1–12

18. Lipsitz LA. Orthostatic hypotension in the elderly. *N Engl J Med* 1989;321:952–7

19. Hansten PD. Drug interacations and interferences: cytochrome P450 enzyme interactions. In Anderson PO, Knoben JE, Troutman WG, eds. *Handbook of Clinical Drug Data*, 9th edn. Stamford, CT: Appleton & Lange, 1999: 823–7

20. Leipzig RM. Pharmacology and appropriate prescribing. In Cobbs EL, Duthie EH, Murphy JB, eds. *Geriatrics Review Syllabus*, 4th edn. Dubuque, Iowa: Kendall/Hunt Publishing Comp, 1999:30–5

21. Dharmarajan TS, Tota R. Appropriate use of medications in older adults. *Fam Pract Recertif* 2000;22:29–38

22. Miller LG. Herbal medicinals: selected clinical considerations focusing on known or potential drug–herb interactions. *Arch Intern Med* 1998;158:2200–11

23. Beers MH. Explicit criteria for determining potentially inappropriate medication use by the elderly. *Arch Intern Med* 1997;157: 1531–6

24. Clark TR, ed. Nursing home survey procedures and interpretive guidelines: a resource for the consultant pharmacist. In *Federal Indicators.* Alexandria, VA: American Society of Consultant Pharmacists, 1999; Appendix N

25. Eisenberg DM, Davis RB, Ettner SL, *et al.* Trends in alternative medicine use in the United States, 1990–1997: results of a follow-up national survey. *J Am Med Assoc* 1998;280: 1569–75

26. Owens NJ, Larrat EP, Fretwell MD. Improving compliance in the older patient: the role of comprehensive functional assessment. In Cramer JA, Spilker B, eds. *Patient Compliance in Medical Practice and Clinical Trials.* New York: Raven Press, 1991:107–19

27. Larrat EP, Taubman AH, Willey C. Compliance-related problems in the ambulatory population. *Am Pharm* 1990;NS30:18–23

28. Gardner M, Boyce RW, Herrier RN. Pharmacist–patient consultation program. US Public Health Service/Indian Health Service, 1996; Unit 1:1–38

10 Geriatric nutrition

T.S. Dharmarajan, MD, FACP, AGSF, and Ajit J. Kokkat, MD

AGING AND NUTRITION WORLDWIDE

We are faced with the problems of an aging society. Life expectancy has increased worldwide; at age 65, life expectancy in years is 16.5 in Japan, 15.6 in Greece, 15.0 in the USA, 13.9 in the UK and 13.9 in Argentina[1]. Older age is associated with co-morbidity, with nutritional problems no exception. Caloric consumption varies internationally and dietary habits differ. For instance, intake of daily calories per capita is 2921 for Japan, 3775 for Greece, 3642 for the USA, 3593 for France and 3242 for Canada[1]. Only the Greeks eat more calories per capita than Americans. Fish consumption is higher in countries with higher life expectancy, e.g. Japan[1]. Nutrition is a key element affecting health and quality of life; it also influences morbidity and mortality.

NUTRITION AND THE AGING PROCESS

Aging is associated with a decrease in lean body mass and total body water, with an increase in total body fat[2]. Often, decreased appetite and food intake are observed; attributes of the 'anorexia of aging' include medications, reduced postprandial hunger response, diseases such as dementia and depression, poor dentition, delayed gastric emptying and many others. Age alone is seldom the basis. Older adults are plagued with dental disease and ill-fitting dentures, further limiting food consumption[2,3]. Olfactory changes result in diminished smell sensation with the olfactory threshold increasing by 50% by the ninth decade, leading to poor smell recognition[4,5]. The ability to detect and discriminate between sweet, sour, salty and bitter tastes deteriorates, with salt and bitter tastes more affected than sweet[4,5]. Decreased basal salivary flow leads to a dry mouth; medications and disease are more often the basis. Older individuals tend to appreciate and respond to thirst much less than the younger age group, predisposing to dehydration, particularly in situations where there is fluid loss (e.g. fever, diarrhea) or lack of access to water (e.g. immobility). Dysphagia is not a part of normal aging and warrants evaluation, especially for neuropharyngeal causes such as cerebrovascular accident or Parkinson's disease. Gastric acid peptic activity is generally preserved with alterations the result from atrophic gastritis or medications. Gastric emptying time is seldom affected to a significant degree by the aging process alone. Absorption of nutrients from the small intestine is generally preserved. Of note is the fact that vitamin D receptors are down-regulated, leading to alterations in calcium and vitamin D absorption (Table 1).

NUTRITIONAL REQUIREMENTS

Food guide pyramids have been modified to address the special needs of the elderly. Fewer, nutrient-dense choices have been focused on in each food group. The adequate intake of fluids (approximately 2 liters daily)

Table 1   The aging gut and nutrition

Oral cavity, taste and smell
Less efficient chewing
Decreased basal secretion of saliva; stimulated flow unchanged
Olfactory thresholds elevated; ability to discriminate odors reduced
Reduced recognition of sweet, sour, salt, and bitter taste
Tooth discoloration and wear, noticeable gingival recession

Stomach
No significant change in basal and stimulated acid secretion*
Reduced gastric mucosal blood flow
Gastric emptying time generally normal*

Intestine
Splanchnic blood flow reduced
No change in absorption of fats and carbohydrates
Vitamin D receptor responsiveness diminished
Transport and absorption of calcium impaired
No change in orocecal transit time

Liver and pancreas
Hepatic blood flow decreased
Albumin synthesis preserved
Pancreatic exocrine function unchanged

*Alterations may be seen due to disease or medications

Table 2   Selected nutrient requirements in older adults. From references 6, 8 and 35

Nutrient	Daily requirement
Carbohydrate	55–60% of total calories
Protein	0.8 g/kg
Fat	< 30% of total calories
Cholesterol	300 mg
Water	30 ml/kg
Fiber	25–30 g
Vitamin A	600–700 μg retinol equivalents
Vitamin B_1	1 mg
Vitamin B_6	1.3 mg
Vitamin B_{12}	2.4 μg
Vitamin C	100 mg
Vitamin D	15 μg
Vitamin E	30 IU
Vitamin K	50 μg/kg
Folic acid	400 folate equivalents (240 μg)
Calcium	1200 mg, 1500 mg (postmenopausal)
Magnesium	420 mg (men), 320 mg (women)
Iron	10 mg
Zinc	12 mg

and fiber has been emphasized. A flag at the top of the pyramid highlights the need for vitamins D and B_{12}, and calcium[6] (Table 2). Vegetarians can avoid protein deficiency by using soya protein, which is nutritionally equivalent to protein from animal sources; deficiencies in vitamins B_{12} and D, iron and zinc are common[7]. Phytates found in whole grain and soya products, and oxalic acid found in spinach inhibit iron absorption. On the other hand, studies have shown that vegetarian diets are associated with lower risk for obesity, constipation, coronary artery disease and hypertension[7].

Carbohydrates, proteins, and fats

Previous US recommended dietary allowances based on a ratio of total energy expenditure to resting energy expenditure of 1.5 underestimated the amount of energy expended by older adults during physical activity; a ratio of 1.75 may be more appropriate[6]. Current energy recommendations are in the range of 2000–2400 kcal/day, adjustable for the average daily energy expenditures and physical activities[6]. Average daily caloric needs are 30 kcal/kg body weight; carbohydrates are the primary energy source, accounting for 55–60% of total energy requirements[8].

Protein requirements for elderly subjects range from 0.78 to 0.91 g/kg per day, suggesting that probably 0.8 g/kg per day is adequate[6]. Dietary fat intake can be limited to 30% of the total caloric intake without creating a negative impact on nutrient balance[9]. Attempts should be made to decrease dietary cholesterol and saturated fatty acid intake, while increasing polyunsaturated fats.

Vitamins

Folic acid deficiency is common in the elderly and has assumed significance due to the causative relationship of high blood levels of homocysteine and low folate levels. Vitamin B_6 which is also involved in homocysteine metabolism is frequently deficient in this age group[6]. Vitamin B_{12} requirements do not change with age; however, malabsorption of protein bound B_{12} (the form occurring naturally in food) from diminished acid peptic activity (related to disease or medication) can lead to deficiency. High vitamin C levels have been associated with decreased prevalence of senile cataracts, higher levels of high-density lipoprotein cholesterol and reduced incidence of coronary artery disease[6]. Supplemental β-carotene may actually increase the incidence of lung cancer in heavy smokers instead of having a beneficial effect on oncologic or vascular disease. Vitamin A toxicity is more common in older adults, due to increased vitamin A absorption from the gut and decreased plasma clearance of retinyl esters and chylomicron remnants by the liver[6]. Osteomalacia is common, as a result of diminished exposure to sunlight, poor skin synthesis of vitamin D, decreased intestinal absorption (altered receptor activity) and decreased hydroxylation of vitamin D in both kidney and liver[6]. Further, vitamin D intake may be poor unless foods are fortified with the vitamin, as in some countries. Vitamin D requirements are 400 IU daily[8]. High circulating vitamin E levels have been linked to improved immune status, protection and stabilization of membranes, lower prevalence of cancer and cataracts, and slowed progression of Alzheimer's disease; but at doses more than 100 IU/day, vitamin E must be viewed as a drug[6]. In the elderly, ongoing antibiotic therapy, malabsorption and high vitamin K clearance rates can result in deficiency of vitamin K, manifesting as abnormal prothrombin time[9].

Minerals and trace elements

Calcium intake along with adequate vitamin D intake is necessary to prevent bone mineral loss in the geriatric population. Serum ferritin is a marker for iron stores but difficult to interpret in the presence of inflammation, when levels rise (acute phase reactant). Absorption of iron appears unaffected by aging. Iron deficiency should prompt aggressive investigation

as to the cause, especially blood loss from the gastrointestinal tract. Phosphorus deficiency can occur in the elderly, facilitated by the frequent use of aluminum-containing antacids. Hypophosphatemia is associated with osteomalacia, cardiomyopathy, and hematological and muscle disorders[9]. Magnesium deficiency in the elderly usually arises from alcoholism, uncontrolled diabetes, loop diuretic use or inadequate intake[9].

Water

Fluid intake is necessary to replace physiological losses, ensure better digestion and intestinal function, and preserve renal clearance. Russell and co-workers proposed that fluid or water intake should be equal to or greater than 2 liters/day to prevent dehydration[6]. Older subjects are less able to conserve salt and water and their thirst response is blunted. This phenomenon is even more pronounced in individuals with cerebral disease[10]. In institutionalized patients, daily fluid intake of 30 ml/kg body weight is a standard prescription, with a minimum intake of 1500 ml/day, unless contraindicated, e.g. in heart failure[8]. The amount must be increased based on demands – as in dermal, renal and gastrointestinal losses. Although evidence-based documentation is not readily available, one recommendation to manage chronic constipation is adequate intake of water[10]. However, increased fluid intake can lead to increased urine volume, resulting in nocturia with resultant insomnia and urinary incontinence, a major inconvenience in this age group. Therefore, fluid intake should be individualized.

Fiber

Dietary fiber is a term for plant products resistant to digestion by gut enzymes in the human ileum. Insoluble fiber includes cellulose, hemicellulose and lignin, which bind water five to seven times their dry weight,

Table 3   An approach to nutritional assessment

History and physical examination
Is there any unintentional weight loss or gain (> 10% in 6 months or > 5% in 1 month)?
Enquire about recent or chronic illness
Review all medications – prescription and over-the-counter
Ask about alcohol use
Assess dietary intake
Examine for signs of nutritional deficiency

Anthropometric measurements
Height and weight
Body mass index (BMI) = $\dfrac{\text{weight in kg}}{(\text{height in m})^2}$ normal 24–27

Mid-arm circumference measures skeletal muscle mass
Triceps and subscapular skinfolds measure subcutaneous fat

Biochemical and hematologic parameters
Albumin: normal level > 3.5 g/dl, half-life 18–21 days
Prealbumin: normal level > 15 mg/dl, half-life 2–3 days
Transferrin: normal level > 200 mg/dl, half-life 8–10 days
Absolute lymphocyte count: < 1500/mm^3 suggests PEU
                           < 800/mm^3 indicates severe malnutrition
Cholesterol: < 160 mg/dl indicates undernutrition
              < 130 mg/dl associated with poor prognosis

Diagnostic studies (individualize)
Metabolic panel, thyroid function tests, urinalysis
Iron, folic acid and vitamin B$_{12}$ levels
Chest radiograph, tuberculin skin test, anergy panel
Specific assessments when needed (e.g. screening for cancer, depression, infection)

PEU, protein energy undernutrition

resulting in larger, softer stools[9]. Soluble fiber includes pectin, mucilages and gums that adsorb less water, and are degraded in the large bowel by bacteria, releasing short-chain fatty acids, resulting in flatulence. Soluble fiber can reduce the rate of glucose absorption and may decrease the plasma cholesterol levels in hypercholesterolemic patients by 10–15%[9]. Daily fiber intake should range from 25 to 30 g along with adequate water. Natural sources are preferred over synthetic fiber. Examples of natural sources are raw fruits and vegetables, whole-grain products and legumes; psyllium is available in synthetic powder and wafer forms.

THE NUTRITIONAL ASSESSMENT

Nutritional assessment involves detailed history taking, physical examination, measurement of body weight, anthropometrics, serum proteins, and hematologic and immune parameters. Dietary intake may be determined by diet history, 24-h recall, food records or food frequency questionnaires[11]. Memory impairment in geriatric patients interferes with dietary recall; physical disability can make recording food intake difficult. Anthropometrics include measurement of height, weight, body and limb circumferences, skinfold thicknesses and body mass index (Table 3). Interpretation of anthropometric data is difficult in the elderly, due to the lack of standardized measurement techniques, alteration in height and posture with aging, and few age-based normograms available[11]. Loss of height over the life span in men may be 2.9 cm, in women 4.9 cm. Changes with aging can also mimic malnutrition. The healthy elderly can exhibit lymphopenia and anergy to intradermal antigens, reducing the utility of these nutritional indicators[2]. The commonly used biochemical marker for malnutrition is serum albumin, with levels below 3.5 g/dl generally regarded as suggestive of protein energy undernutrition (PEU). While albumin is an excellent parameter, the longer half-life (2–3 weeks) compared to prealbumin (2–3 days) makes the latter a better but more expensive indicator of early malnutrition[8,11]. Cytokine release from acute stress or injury results in reduced synthesis and increased catabolism of albumin; hepatic disease and renal loss lead to lower levels[12]. Serum transferrin, another marker, has a half-life of about 9 days. An absolute lymphocyte count of $<1500/mm^3$ suggests PEU; counts below $800/mm^3$ indicate severe malnutrition, provided other causes of lymphopenia have been excluded[11]. Increased mortality is noted at both extremes of cholesterol level, low and high; levels under 160 mg/dl indicate undernutrition and levels below 130 mg/dl are associated with poor prognosis[8,9].

The mini nutritional assessment

The mini nutritional assessment (MNA) is a validated screening tool that provides a rapid assessment of nutritional status in older adults. It is composed of simple measurements and questions needing 10 min for completion[13]. There are two parts to the MNA. The first involves screening and inquires about food intake, weight loss, mobility, recent illness, neuropsychological problems and calculation of body mass index. If the screening score indicates possible PEU, the next part is administered. This portion assesses environment, medications, pressure ulcers, dietary habits, selected protein-rich foods, fruit and vegetable intake, fluids, need for assistance with meals, self-assessment of nutritional status and measures mid-arm and calf circumferences[13]. The maximum possible score is 30 points. Depending on the total scores, subjects are assigned into three categories: normal (24–30 points), risk of malnutrition (17–23.5 points) and frank malnutrition (less than 17 points)[8]. Vellas and colleagues found the MNA to have a sensitivity of 96%, specificity of 98% and predictive value of 97%[13].

MALNUTRITION

Protein energy undernutrition

The prevalence of PEU in the hospitalized elderly has been reported to range from 30 to 61% with associated prolonged hospitalization, increased mortality and complications such as infections and pressure ulcers[12]. Older adults hospitalized from a long-term care facility are more likely to have PEU than their counterparts from the community, perhaps attributable to the increased co-morbidity, polypharmacy, and increased dependency in activities of daily living[12]. Early nutritional screening and prompt intervention is recommended when PEU is suspected. Malnutrition in the elderly commonly results from diminished food intake, attributed to multiple factors such as cognitive and physical impairments, anorexia, poverty, limited access to food, inappropriate food choices and restrictive diets[2]. Risk factors that suppress appetite and pose barriers to eating should be looked for[14] (Table 4).

If the gastrointestinal tract is functional, it should be the route to deliver nutrition, as the health of the gut is improved by the presence of food within. Starvation for more than 5 days results in atrophy of the intestinal villi. Rapid feeding in this situation overwhelms the absorptive capacity of the gut, resulting in diarrhea[14]. Peripheral alimentation is useful while enteral nutrient delivery is gradually resumed. While hypoalbuminemia is the hallmark of PEU, other causes such as liver disease, protein-losing enteropathy, and renal and dermal protein losses should be considered. Depression may be a cause and often evades diagnosis.

Megesterol acetate therapy for 12 weeks can improve appetite and well-being in

Table 4   Factors contributing to protein energy under-nutrition

Barriers to feeding
Oral or dental disease, lack of assistance with feeding, inappropriate food consistency, strict meal schedules, poor eyesight, taste alteration, poor motor co-ordination

Social factors
Poverty, ethnic preferences, restrictive diets, social isolation, elder abuse

Medications
Antibiotics, anticholinergics, digoxin, antihypertensives, oral iron supplements and many others.

Neuropsychiatric
Dementia, delirium, depression, late-life paranoia

Interference with eating
Congestive heart failure, malabsorption syndromes, diabetic gastroparesis, dementia, dysphagia

Increased energy needs
Cancer (gastrointestinal, breast, lung), infections (pneumonia, urosepsis, tuberculosis, HIV), chronic obstructive pulmonary disease, wounds, burns, fractures

geriatric patients with low body weight or weight loss[15]. Human growth hormone, a potent endogenous anabolic hormone, enhances wound healing and helps maintain lean body mass when given parenterally, but complications such as hyperglycemia, hypercalcemia and fluid retention may ensue[16]. Injection of slow-release testosterone leads to a modest increase in anabolic activity with attendant risks including hirsutism, mood changes, gynecomastia and potentiation of prostate cancer[16]. Oxandrolone, a testosterone analog, combined with adequate calorie and protein intake, results in weight gain primarily in the lean mass compartment[16]. Cyproheptadine has been shown to stimulate appetite.

Obesity

Obesity results from a complex interaction between psychological, genetic, and environmental factors or disease. Body mass index (weight in kilograms divided by height in meters squared) is used to define overweight and obesity. Overweight is defined as a body mass index of 27.3 kg/m^2 in women and 27.8 kg/m^2 in men, while obesity is 30 kg/m^2 or more[17]. Prevalence of obesity in the elderly is on the increase, especially in men. The proportion of overweight American men aged 60–74 years increased from about 20% in 1960 to 40% in 1991[17]. Leptin, a protein produced by adipocytes, normally regulates feeding behavior and energy balance. Decreased sensitivity of the brain to leptin may play a role in obesity[2]. Overweight is associated with increased risk of osteoarthritis of hips and knees, breast and colon cancer, coronary heart disease and diabetes. Weight reduction programs in the elderly should help attain a modest weight loss. Whether caloric restriction is instituted or drug intervention undertaken, efforts should be made to preserve bone and muscle in the face of weight loss, by aerobic and resistance exercises.

Enteral versus parenteral nutrition

When oral intake is not possible for any reason, alternative means of feeding becomes a consideration; decision-making entails clinical judgement and ethical concerns on the part of the patient, surrogate and health-care provider. Tube feeding is often resorted to; nasogastric tubes are the choice for short-term feeding and percutaneous endoscopic gastrostomies for long-term enteral support. A detailed chapter on tube feeding appears elsewhere in this text.

Parenteral nutrition is indicated in patients who are not candidates for enteral support. Total parenteral nutrition (TPN) involves the use of hypertonic solutions tolerated only when delivered to large venous vessels; peripheral parenteral nutrition (PPN) contains lower concentrations of dextrose and amino acids, failing to meet nutritional requirements unless lipid infusions are supplemented. Peripherally inserted central lines can be used for TPN, avoiding complications of central catheter placement such as pneumothorax, arterial

Table 5 Effects of drugs on nutrition. From references 19 and 20

Effect	Drug
Absorption of nutrients	
Vitamin B_{12} deficiency from inhibition of gastric acid secretion	acid lowering agents
Hepatotoxicity leading to malabsorption of fats and fat-soluble vitamins	alcohol
Hypophosphatemia due to formation of non-absorbable phosphates	aluminum antacids
Hypokalemia from gastrointestinal loss of potassium	laxatives
Iron deficiency secondary to mucosal hemorrhage	indomethacin
Metabolism of nutrients	
Osteomalacia from altered vitamin D metabolism	anticonvulsants
Vitamin B_6 deficiency due to inhibition of pyridoxal kinase	isoniazid
Excretion of nutrients	
Chelation of minerals such as copper and zinc	penicillamine
Renal excretion of calcium, magnesium, and potassium	diuretics
Folic acid displacement from plasma protein-binding sites	aspirin
Drug effects on appetite	
Anorexia	alcohol, digoxin, hydralazine
Hyperphagia	glucocorticoids, anabolic steroids, cyproheptadine
Dysgeusia	lithium, captopril, methimazole
Xerostomia	clonidine, antihistamines, tricyclic antidepressants

puncture and hemorrhage[18]. Energy and protein content should be estimated based on patient requirements and electrolytes should be tailored for the underlying disease. Trace elements and vitamins excluding vitamin K (interferes with warfarin) are added to prevent micronutrient deficiencies. Older adults on TPN are prone to develop complications and require close monitoring. Fluid overload, hyperglycemia and hypoglycemia may occur and should be looked for. Line infections may be prevented by the use of single-lumen catheters and aseptic line care. Abnormal liver function tests from steatosis may result from carbohydrate overfeeding. Alongside parenteral nutrition, enteral feeding even in small amounts can prevent changes in the gut and reduce cholestasis.

SPECIAL CONSIDERATIONS

Drug–nutrient interactions

Older adults typically consume several prescribed and over-the-counter medications.

Cardiovascular drugs are the most commonly prescribed medications for the elderly in Europe (percentage of cardiac drug prescriptions for patients over the age of 65 was 68 in the UK, 59 in Germany, 60 in the Netherlands and 57 in Belgium[19]). More than 60% of older adults use non-prescription drugs regularly, especially analgesics, antihistamines, antacids, and nutrient supplements. Drug–nutrient interactions can take many forms, some of which are described below (Tables 5 and 6)[20]. Antacids containing aluminum bind phosphate in the gut, reducing its absorption, and predisposing to hypophosphatemia[2]. Phenytoin alters vitamin D metabolism via induction of hepatic enzymes, adversely affecting calcium homeostasis[2]. Diuretics through renal tubular effects lead to loss of sodium, potassium, calcium and magnesium[11]. Corticosteroids can inhibit calcium absorption and alter glucose metabolism, causing osteoporosis and hyperglycemia[11]. Mineral oil laxatives inhibit fat-soluble vitamin absorption, leading to deficiency[11]. Anorexia and dysgeusia can

Table 6   Effect of food on drug therapy. From references 19 and 20

Effect of food	Drug affected
Absorption of drugs	
Competition with amino acids for same transport mechanism	levodopa
Drug absorption reduced by food	hydrochlorothiazide, captopril, phenytoin
Drug absorption delayed by food	digoxin, glipizide, theophylline
Drug absorption increased by food	carbamazepine, diazepam, lithium
Distribution of drugs	
Free fatty acids can displace drugs from binding sites on albumin	diazepam
Hypoalbuminemia results in increased free drug concentrations	warfarin
Metabolism of drugs	
Grapefruit juice inhibits metabolism by cytochrome P450	cyclosporine, nifedipine
High protein diets increase drug clearance	theophylline
Nutritional supplements and drug therapy	
Megadoses of vitamin E potentiate anticoagulant effect of warfarin	warfarin
Large doses of vitamin C inhibit warfarin anticoagulant effect	warfarin
High-dose folic acid supplements can decrease phenytoin levels	phenytoin

result from various medications, e.g. angiotensin converting enzyme (ACE) inhibitors and anticholinergic agents. High protein intake can decrease levodopa absorption from the gut. The consumption of green leafy vegetables, a good source of vitamin K, counteracts the anticoagulant effect of warfarin.

Food security

Food security entails access to enough food that is safe, nutritionally adequate and obtained through normal channels. Poverty is common in the geriatric population, limiting ability to purchase nutritious food; physical disability, common in this age group, interferes with the procurement and preparation of meals. Lack of transportation and stores in the proximity contribute to food insecurity[21]. Older adults are more frequently admitted to the hospital when their refrigerators are empty[22]. Health professionals should encourage nutrition assistance programs to include older adults in their outreach efforts. The Nutrition Screening Initiative introduced in the USA in 1990 provides a multidisciplinary approach to nutrition screening, intervention (social services, oral health, mental health, medication use, nutrition education and nutrition support), increased public awareness and increased government funding for research in nutrition[2]. Significant differences in the knowledge of nutrition exist in England between sociodemographic groups. Men appeared to have lower awareness than women, and knowledge declined with lower educational and socioeconomic status[23]. Comprehensive interdisciplinary care management including older adults, their families and caregivers can improve outcomes effectively[21].

Dietary supplements and herbal remedies

Dietary supplements are products intended to supplement the diet that contain one or more of the following: vitamins, minerals, herbs or other botanicals, amino acids and appetite stimulants[24]. Examples are calcium, used to prevent osteoporosis and folic acid to prevent neural tube defects. Vitamin E may play a role in prevention of cataract formation, age-related macular degeneration, Alzheimer's disease and Parkinson's disease, atherosclerosis and coronary heart disease[21]. Ascorbic acid, vitamin A and zinc are important for wound healing[21]. Physicians must enquire about herbal supplements; top-selling 'herbs' include ginseng, echinacea, *Gingko biloba*, garlic and St John's wort[24]. Many herbs including gingko, garlic and St John's wort can lead to bleeding tendencies, and are dangerous when taken with warfarin.

Nutrition and the vascular system

High blood levels of homocysteine have been correlated with vascular damage, including coronary artery disease, cerebrovascular disease and peripheral vascular disease[25]. Folate, vitamin B_6 and vitamin B_{12} are involved in homocysteine metabolism; deficiency leads to elevated levels[25]. Hyperhomocysteinemia also occurs in hypothyroidism and chronic renal failure, and levels increase with age[26]. The beneficial effect of vitamin E on atherosclerosis may be explained by modulation of immune and inflammatory cell interaction with endothelial cells, and the inhibition of platelet aggregation, smooth muscle cell proliferation and low-density lipoprotein oxidation[27].

Abnormal cholesterol levels in the elderly are assuming significance. High cholesterol levels correlate with an increased incidence of atherosclerotic heart disease. Reduced absorption and increased excretion of cholesterol can be achieved by decreasing saturated fats in the diet and increasing fiber intake[28]. Diets rich in fresh fruit and salad vegetables protect against cardiovascular disease[29].

The current cholesterol guidelines do not recommend an upper age cut-off to limit treatment for high cholesterol levels. Dietary recommendations are combined with exercise as the initial step prior to considering drug therapy. In this regard food sources of fiber, such as green leafy vegetables, beans, broccoli, and asparagus, not only provide fiber, but also dietary folate which appears associated with a reduced risk of cardiovascular disease[30]. A recent study from New Zealand interestingly demonstrated that calcium supplementation in postmenopausal women (for fractures) resulted in a beneficial effect on HDL cholesterol as compared with placebo[31].

Nutrition and pressure ulcers

Predictors of pressure ulcer development include compromised nutrition status, low body weight, low cholesterol and total lymphocyte counts, anemia and reduced dietary protein intake[32]. Low serum albumin also results from loss of protein through exudates from pressure ulcers. Nutritional status correlates with pressure ulcer healing[32]. Although zinc supplementation in the absence of true deficiency is controversial, replacement is indicated where deficiency is suspected[32]. Vitamin C, iron, manganese and copper are necessary for collagen synthesis and integrity; deficiency of any of these factors interferes with wound healing[32]. Ascorbic acid administration in the presence of deficiency has been shown to reduce pressure ulcer surface area. Adequate protein intake ensures anabolism, while supplying adequate non-protein calories to meet energy demands and prevent catabolism. Dietary iron should exceed the age-specific recommended dietary allowance (RDA) to allow for losses from ulcer exudates[32].

Nutrition and cognition

Cellular and molecular oxidative injuries play a role in the pathogenesis of neurodegenerative diseases of the brain and antioxidant vitamins may limit the extent of neuronal injury. Antioxidants may protect against injury to cell organelles, membranes and molecules via free radicals released during cell metabolism. These antioxidants include glutathione, selenium, carotenoids and vitamins E, C, and A. Vitamins E and C supplements have been shown to protect against vascular dementia and improve cognition[33]. Thiamine deficiency, frequently seen with alcohol abuse, can result in neurologic injury; deficiency of folate and vitamin B_{12} can cause cognitive impairment.

Table 7 Ten commandments of geriatric nutrition

(1) Enhance food enjoyment with flavors and colors
(2) Ask about alcohol use
(3) Avoid restrictive diets
(4) Drink adequate fluids
(5) Include protein-rich foods in the diet
(6) Consume fruits, vegetables, and fortified grain products
(7) Ensure adequate intake of calcium, folic acid, and vitamins D and B_{12}
(8) Use dietary supplements judiciously
(9) Use fiber to prevent constipation
(10) Conduct periodic medication review

Nutrition and the bone

Calcium homeostasis depends on a finely tuned endocrine system. Vitamin D acts by increased intestinal absorption of calcium, decreased renal calcium and phosphate loss, and increased bone resorption of calcium. Age-related loss of bone calcium affects both sexes, leading to osteoporosis, with increased risk of fractures. Postmenopausal osteoporosis (type 1) and age-related osteoporosis (type 2) are two distinct clinical entities[34]. Calcium intake is generally low in older adults. Vitamin D deficiency is common from a variety of mechanisms, as stated earlier. Further, several older subjects tend to avoid dairy products because of a high prevalence of lactose intolerance. A negative calcium balance results from the low calcium intake and vitamin D deficiency, stimulating parathyroid hormone secretion. The resultant secondary hyperparathyroidism leaches calcium from the bones, increasing the risk of fractures. Nursing home residents supplemented with vitamin D and calcium showed a much lower cumulative probability of hip fracture than those not supplemented[26]. Dairy products and fortified food are good sources of calcium. A total calcium intake of 1200–1500 mg inclusive of food and supplementation is recommended[8].

SUMMARY

Nutritional assessment should be a routine part of the evaluation of older adults. Malnutrition is common and often goes unrecognized. Much can be done to prevent and treat various nutritional disorders, but this should not be at the expense of quality of life with the use of restrictive diets (Table 7)[35,36]. A team approach involving the physician, nurse, nutritionist and social worker will go a long way to achieve the goal of optimizing nutrition in the geriatric population.

References

1. Miller DK, Morley JE, Rubenstein LZ. An overview of international aging and nutrition. In Morley JE, Glick Z, Rubenstein LZ, eds. *Geriatric Nutrition*, 2nd edn. New York: Raven Press, 1995:1–4
2. Refai W, Seidner DL. Nutrition in the elderly. *Clin Geriatr Med* 1999;15:607–25
3. Christensen GJ. The inevitable maladies of the mature dentition. *J Am Dent Assoc* 2000;131:803–4
4. Kaneda H, Maeshima K, Goto N. Decline in taste and odor discrimination abilities with age, and relationship between gustation and olfaction. *Chem Senses* 2000;25:331–7
5. Dharmarajan TS, Pitchumoni CS, Kokkat AJ. The aging gut. *Practical Gastroenterol* 2001;25:15–27
6. Russell RM, Rasmussen H. The impact of nutritional needs of older adults on recommended food intakes. *Nutr Clin Care* 1999; 2:164–76
7. Walter P. Effects of vegetarian diets on aging and longevity. *Nutr Rev* 1997;55:S61–8
8. Dharmarajan TS, Kathpalia RK. A review of geriatric nutrition. In Dreger D, Krumm B, eds. *Hospital Physician Geriatric Board Review Manual*. Wayne, PA: Turner White Communications, 2000;1:1–12

9. Bidlack WR, Wang W. Nutrition requirements of the elderly. In Morley JE, Glick Z, Rubenstein LZ, eds. *Geriatric Nutrition*, 2nd edn. New York: Raven Press, 1995: 25–49

10. Lindeman RD, Romero LJ, Liang HC, *et al.* Do elderly persons need to be encouraged to drink more fluids? *J Gerontol* 2000;55: M361–5

11. Chandra RK, Imbach A, Moore C, *et al.* Nutrition of the elderly. *Can Med Assoc J* 1991;145:1475–87

12. Kamel HK, Karcic E, Karcic A, *et al.* Nutritional status of hospitalized elderly: differences between nursing home patients and community-dwelling patients. *Ann Long-term Care* 2000;8:33–8

13. Vellas B, Guigoz Y, Garry PJ, *et al.* The Mini Nutritional Assessment and its use in grading the nutritional state of elderly patients. *Nutrition* 1999;15:116–22

14. Sullivan DH. Undernutrition in older adults. *Ann Long-term Care* 2000;8:41–6

15. Yeh SS, Wu SY, Lee TP, *et al.* Improvement in quality of life measures and stimulation of weight gain after treatment with megesterol acetate oral suspension in geriatric cachexia: results of a double-blind, placebo-controlled study. *J Am Geriatr Soc* 2000; 48:485–92

16. Chang DW, DeSanti L, Demling RH. Anticatabolic and anabolic strategies in critical illness: a review of current treatment modalities. *Shock* 1998;10:155–60

17. Harris T. Weight and age: paradoxes and conundrums. In Hazzard WR, Blass JP, Ettinger WH Jr, *et al.*, eds. *Principles of Geriatric Medicine and Gerontology*, 4th edn. New York: McGraw-Hill, 1999: 967–72

18. Wallace JI. Malnutrition and enteral/parenteral alimentation. In Hazzard WR, Blass JP, Ettinger WH Jr, *et al.*, eds. *Principles of Geriatric Medicine and Gerontology*, 4th edn. New York: McGraw-Hill, 1999:1455–69

19. Blumberg J, Couris R. Pharmacology, nutrition, and the elderly: interactions and implications. In Chernoff R, ed. *Geriatric Nutrition*, 2nd edn. Gaithersburg, MD: Aspen Publishers, 1999:63–83

20. Dharmarajan TS, Kumar A, Pitchumoni CS. Drug–nutrient interactions in older adults. *Pract Gastroenterol* 2002;26:37–55

21. Weddle DO, Fanelli-Kuczmarski M. Position of the American Dietetic Association: nutrition, aging, and the continuum of care. *J Am Diet Assoc* 2000;100:580–95

22. Boumendjel N, Herrmann F, Girod V, *et al.* Refrigerator content and hospital admission in old people. *Lancet* 2000;356:563

23. Parmenter K, Waller J, Wardle J. Demographic variation in nutrition knowledge in England. *Health Educ Res* 2000;15:163–74

24. Radimer KL, Subar AF, Thompson FE. Nonvitamin, nonmineral dietary supplements: issues and findings from NHANES III. *J Am Diet Assoc* 2000;100:447–54

25. Appel LJ, Miller ER, Jee SH, *et al.* Effect of dietary patterns on serum homocysteine: results of a randomized, controlled feeding study. *Circulation* 2000;102:852–7

26. Rosenberg IH. Nutrition and senescence. *Nutr Rev* 1997;55:S69–77

27. Meydani M. Effect of functional food ingredients: vitamin E modulation of cardiovascular diseases and immune status in the elderly. *Am J Clin Nutr* 2000;71:1665S–8S

28. Ellegard L, Bosaeus I, Andersson H. Will recommended changes in fat and fiber intake affect cholesterol absorption and sterol excretion? An ileostomy study. *Eur J Clin Nutr* 2000;54:306–13

29. Cox BD, Whichelow MJ, Prevost AT. Seasonal consumption of salad vegetables and fresh fruit in relation to the development of cardiovascular disease and cancer. *Public Health Nutr* 2000;3:19–29

30. Bazzano LA, He J, Ogden LG, *et al.* Dietary intake of folate and risk of stroke in US men and women. NHANES I Epidemiologic Follow-up Study. *Stroke* 2002;33: 1183–89

31. Reid IR, Mason B, Horne A, *et al.* Effects of calcium supplementation on lipid concentrations in normal older women: a randomized controlled trial. *Am J Med* 2002;112:343–7

32. Osterweil D, Wendt PF, Ferrell BA. Pressure ulcers and nutrition. In Morley JE, Glick Z, Rubenstein LZ, eds. *Geriatric Nutrition*, 2nd edn. New York: Raven Press, 1995:335–42

33. Masaki KH, Losonczy KG, Izmirlian G, *et al*. Association of vitamin E and C supplement use with cognitive function and dementia in elderly men. *Neurology* 2000; 54:1265–72

34. Lindeman RD. Mineral requirements. In Chernoff R, ed. *Geriatric Nutrition*, 2nd edn. Gaithersburg, MD: Aspen Publishers, 1999:63–83

35. Carter WJ. Macronutrient requirements for elderly persons. In Chernoff R, ed. *Geriatric Nutrition*, 2nd edn. Gaithersburg, MD: Aspen Publishers, 1999:13–26

36. Thomas DR, Morley JE. Nutritional assessment and indicators of undernutrition in the elderly. *Res Staff Physic* 2002;48: 47–55

11 Tube feeding in the older adult

T.S. Dharmarajan, MD, FACP, AGSF, and Dilip Unnikrishnan, MD

INTRODUCTION

Changing demographics have resulted in an aging population the world over, characterized by frailty and co-morbidity. Notable is the high prevalence of dementia with its associated nutrition-related issues. In advanced dementia, individuals often fail to make appropriate food choices or feed on their own, at times even with assistance. If an older individual is not able to maintain acceptable oral intake, alternative means of feeding become a consideration, the choices usually being parenteral or enteral nutrition. Parenteral nutrition is a temporary approach, expensive and attended by its specific complications. Enteral feeding via a tube is the modality increasingly used under such circumstances to maintain adequate nutrition, although its utility and advantages have been the subjects of controversy.

INDICATIONS FOR TUBE FEEDING

Enteral feeding is preferred for providing nutrient support in patients with a functioning gastrointestinal tract, when they are unable to eat or drink in the normal manner. Deglutition is impaired in neurodegenerative diseases such as Alzheimer's disease or Parkinson's disease, and cerebrovascular disorders such as stroke[1]. Further, demented patients with poor oral intake and malnutrition have associated illnesses such as pressure ulcers, dehydration and infections, with increased caloric requirements[2,3]. Prevention of aspiration pneumonia in the presence of dysphagia is another commonly cited, but poorly substantiated, indication[4,5]. In other instances, tube feeding has been initiated to improve patient comfort, prolong survival or tide over an acute illness[6,7]. Financial considerations, including the need to transfer patients to a chronic care facility, and caregiver convenience have appeared to influence decisions[6–9]. Often, religious beliefs and values guide the caregiver to accept tube feeding as a means of providing food and nutrition to an older individual. Some common indications and contraindications to tube feeding are listed in Table 1.

MAKING THE DECISION

When non-oral means of feeding is a consideration, a comprehensive nutritional evaluation is indicated. This includes anthropometric measurements including serial weights, body mass index and mid-arm circumference, biochemical nutritional parameters including total protein, albumin, prealbumin, total cholesterol, total lymphocyte count, transferrin and measures of immunologic function (anergy testing)[1]. Patients with significant weight loss (more than 5% weight loss in 1 month or 10% in 6 months), weights significantly lower

Table 1 Indications and contraindications for tube feeding. From references 2, 4, 12, 16, 19

Indications
Severe dysphagia
Protein energy malnutrition
Mechanical causes (strictures, malignancies)
Delirium or coma
Anorexia, not amenable to other measures
Malabsorption (inflammatory bowel disease)
Recurrent aspiration (unproven benefit)
Gastrointestinal decompression
Inability to eat (ventilator-dependent)

Contraindications
Absolute
   Intestinal obstruction
Relative
   ischemic bowel (severe)
   continuing gastrointestinal bleeding
   acute pancreatitis
   high-output gastric fistulas
   severe hypomotility

Table 2 Discussion with the surrogate on tube feeding: a useful checklist for decision-making. From references 3, 4, 10, 20, 24, 28

(1)   Is the decision made based on knowledge of the patient's expressed wishes?
(2)   Were alternatives considered (including option of withholding tube feeding)?
      Meticulous hand feeding, evaluation of dentition, modification of food consistency, assessment of food preferences, review of medications, environmental manipulations
(3)   Were dietary restrictions removed?
(4)   Did the discussion emphasize that tube feeding:
      (a)   does not prolong survival
      (b)   does not prevent aspiration
      (c)   does not prevent pressure sores
      (d)   does not improve functional status or quality of life
      (e)   does not necessarily improve nutritional parameters
(5)   Was it made clear that discomfort and complications may result from tube placement and feeding?
(6)   Have surrogate's concerns about tube feeding, including issues of thirst and hunger at the end of life, been satisfactorily addressed?

than ideal body weight and requiring assistance with feeding are considered at high risk[10]. A search to identify reversible factors such as depression, thyroid disease, gastrointestinal malignancy and disordered dentition is reasonable. Socioeconomic factors and food availability need to be assessed. Unnecessary dietary restrictions, medications and food preferences are evaluated and modified to improve oral intake[3,10]. When dysphagia is suspected, a formal speech and swallow evaluation should be performed; modified barium swallow or videoflouroscopy helps assess the nature and degree of dysphagia[3].

It is important to document the need for feeding tube placement including evaluation for dysphagia, physical examination and laboratory indicators, discussions with a multidisciplinary team and assessment of the risks and benefits from the planned procedure[3,10]. Surveys have shown that the decision to begin tube feeding is most often made during hospitalization for an acute illness[7]. The health-care provider often initiates the discussion; the patient and/or surrogate makes the decision influenced by medical, ethical, moral and religious values, hoping for an

improvement in nutrition, longevity and overall well-being of the patient[7]. The discussion should be honest and meaningful with no assurances from the health-care provider of undue expectations (Table 2).

FEEDING TUBES

Commonly available modalities for tube feeding include nasogastric, percutaneous endoscopic gastrostomy (PEG) and jejunostomy. A comparison of the three is provided in Table 3. Gastrostomy tubes placed endoscopically or surgically have become the preferred method, because of lower procedure-related and long-term complications.

Nasogastric tubes

Nasogastric tubes are ideal for short-term gastric access and are placed easily at the bedside. The tube is lubricated, and advanced carefully to a predetermined distance (40–45 cm); the position is confirmed by air insufflations and

Table 3 Comparison of percutaneous endoscopic gastrostomy (PEG) with other modalities of tube feeding. From references 11, 14, 15, 20, 30

	PEG	Nasogastric	Jejunostomy
Duration of feeding	long term (months–years)	short term (days–weeks)	long term (months–years)
Placement of tube	involves a specialist	easy	involves a specialist
Patient comfort	better tolerated	low	better tolerated
Complications			
specific	clogging infection leakage	nasal ulceration frequent replacement esophageal stricture	clogging, diarrhea infection leakage
general*	(see below)	(see below)	(see below)
Risk of aspiration	present	present	present
Bolus feeding	possible	possible	difficult
Treatment failure†	low	high	moderate

*For PEG and jejunostomy – skin infections, hematomas, wound dehiscence, bleeding, diarrhea (infectious and non-infectious), tube migration. Rarely: necrotizing fasciitis and myositis, erosion into pleural cavity, peritonitis, septicemia, bowel perforation, gastrocolocutaneous fistula
†Treatment failures include malposition, displacement or blockage of tube, with loss of feeding time

radiologically prior to use[2,11]. Nasogastric tubes incur discomfort and risk dislodgement. Hence care to anchor the tube to the nose with tape is essential. Accidental tracheal placement of the tube is more common with altered mentation and impaired gag reflexes[11]. Nasogastric tubes are not used for more than 3–4 weeks, due to risk of mucosal erosions, infections and esophageal strictures. They are most helpful in acute illnesses such as stroke or delirium, when recovery is expected within a short period, and the tube remains in place for only a few days.

Percutaneous endoscopic gastrostomy

Gastrostomy tubes can be placed surgically, endoscopically or radiologically[12]. Introduced in 1980 by Gauderer and colleagues, PEG has since become the mainstay for enteral feeding[6,13]. More than 100 000 gastrostomy tubes are placed in the USA every year, mostly in patients with dementia[6,8]. Compared to surgical gastrostomy, PEG has the advantages of not requiring prolonged anesthesia in the older individual, a short procedure time, fewer complications, lower cost and improved

cosmetic benefits[14]. Complications are few, with a procedure-related mortality of less than 2% in most studies[4,13].

The procedure is usually performed under intravenous sedation; the site is chosen by transillumination and indentation of the gastric wall by finger pressure at the site. Contraindications for PEG include intestinal obstruction, ascites, coagulopathy, peritonitis, conditions that preclude endoscopic access to the stomach, and when the gastric wall cannot be approximated to the abdominal wall for any reason[15].

Jejunostomy

Jejunostomy tubes are usually placed surgically, although recently they have been placed endoscopically as well. Placed distal to the ligament of Trietz, jejunostomy tubes were thought to decrease the incidence of aspiration events, although this was never proved conclusively[16]. These tubes are smaller in caliber and hence prone to clogging or kinking, with resultant loss of feeding time[16]. An increased incidence of diarrhea may occur, as the feeds are administered directly into the small intestine.

Table 4 Summary of some commonly used tube feeding formulas

Indication	Product and description
Routine use	Isocal, Osmolyte isotonic, low residue, 1 cal/ml, calories from CHO 50%, fat 37%, protein 13%
Diabetes	Choice DM, Glucerna isotonic (360–375 mOsm/kg), low CHO content (30–35% cal)
Motility disorders	Jevity, Ultracal, FiberSource isotonic, fiber (5–14 g fiber/l), calories from CHO 50%, fat 33%, protein 17%
Predialysis	Suplena low protein (30 g/l), low electrolytes, hyperosmolar (600 mOsm/kg), 2 cal/ml
Dialysis	Nepro, Magnacal Renal higher protein (70 g/l), low electrolytes, hyperosmolar (635 mOsm/kg), 2 cal/ml
Hypervolemia	Deliver 2.0 2 cal/ml, low sodium content, 40% calories as CHO 40%, fat 45%, proteins 15%
Respiratory disease	Pulmocare, Respalor moderate CHO, 1.5 cal/ml, calories from CHO 28–39%, fat 41–55%
Hepatic disease	NutriHep 50% branched chain amino acids, hyperosmolar, useful in hepatic encephalopathy

CHO, carbohydrates; cal, calories

THE PRESCRIPTION

The tube feeding prescription is tailored to individual needs, and titrated to meet the daily requirements of calories and essential nutrients[17]. Tube feeding formulas contain water, carbohydrates, fats, proteins, electrolytes and micronutrients. The patient status, taking into consideration activity, co-morbidity (renal, hepatic or pulmonary function, gut motility disorders, diabetes, hydration, febrile or catabolic states) along with nutritional assessment will determine requirements.

Tube feeding formulas

Several formulations for tube feeding are available in the market. Standard formulas provide 1 kcal/ml caloric value, have an osmolarity between 280 and 350 mOsm/l, 50–55% carbohydrates, 15–20% proteins, 30% fat and 70–85% water[16]. Products designed for specific co-morbid conditions vary in proportions of constituents[16]. A list of the commonly used formulas and their characteristics is detailed in Table 4. Preparations rich in fiber are available for gastrointestinal motility disorders. Products for diabetics contain relatively more fat and simple sugars, while low-protein, high-carbohydrate formulas with appropriate electrolytes are used in predialysis settings. Patients with respiratory illnesses may benefit from the use of low-carbohydrate, high-fat products to minimize carbon dioxide generation[16]. Products (high in branched-chain amino acids and low in aromatic amino acids) are available for hepatic encephalopathy, while formulas with high (2 kcal/ml) caloric value are options in fluid-restricted states such as congestive heart failure[2].

Water requirements

Most isotonic preparations contain 70–85% water, lower in hypertonic formulations. Typical requirements for water are 30–35 ml/kg per day; the requirements are higher during febrile illness and with ongoing losses such as diarrhea or vomiting. In general, adequate fluids should be administered to maintain a daily urine output of 1.2–1.5 liters[18]. Water can also be administered as boluses; currently available feeding pumps can be programmed to deliver a desired volume at predetermined intervals.

The role for supplements

Supplements to tube feeding may be added in the form of proteins (Promod, Casec), carbohydrates (Polycose) or fats (medium-chain triglyceride oils, Lipisorb), and help meet nutrient or caloric requirements[19]. Most tube feeding formulations are fortified with vitamins and trace elements, sufficient to meet daily requirements when administered in amounts of 1.5–2 l/day[20].

Feeding rate: bolus or continuous?

Tube feeds can be administered as continuous or bolus feeds. Isotonic feeds can be started at full strength; hypertonic feeds are usually diluted with water (50% by volume) and altered to full strength in 24 h[2]. For continuous feeds, the feeding is initiated at a rate of 20 ml/h and increased by 20–40 ml every 8–12 h to meet daily requirements[11,16]. Patients able to maintain some oral intake during the day can be supplemented by tube feeding at night. Bolus feeding (larger feed volume over a short time) is useful in ambulatory patients and at times for caregiver convenience; in this case the feeding pattern mimics normal intake.

The head end should be elevated to 30–45° during continuous feeding and for at least half an hour following bolus feeding to decrease the risk of aspiration[16]. Gastric residuals should be checked frequently on initiation of feeds and prior to increasing the rate of infusion, to check tolerance to feeds. Residuals are checked while the infusion is in progress for continuous feeds, and an hour after cessation of feeding for bolus administration. In general, a residual less than 150 ml or less than twice the rate of continuous feeds is considered acceptable[11,21].

ADMINISTRATION OF MEDICATIONS

The patient on tube feeding is typically on multiple medications requiring administration via the tube. Medicines are usually crushed and dissolved in a solvent prior to administration. Medications are the most common basis for tube clogging; periodic flushes with water (30–50 ml) will minimize the problem[2]. Drug–drug interactions, altered bioavailability, and drug–nutrient interactions are possible in this setting. Long-acting preparations lose their properties when crushed and need to be replaced by alternative preparations. Interactions of medications with nutrients (e.g. levodopa/carbidopa with dietary proteins) may require that feeds be withheld for some time after administration of certain medications[22].

COMPLICATIONS

Immediate complications from insertion of PEG tubes are rare and relate to the procedure, such as perforation or bleeding. Short-term complications are usually local, affecting the area around the tube insertion, while long-term use is associated with dislodgement of the tube and complications related to the feed itself (Table 5).

Local

These include infection around tube insertion site, hematomas, wound dehiscence and leakage of feeds. Frequent inspection of the tube insertion site and cleansing is recommended. Rarely, colonic perforation, gastric leakage and peritonitis result; the distal tip of the feeding tube may migrate and result in small intestinal obstruction.

Mechanical

Nasogastric tubes are uncomfortable and are often pulled out by the cognitively impaired patient, requiring replacement and an increased use of restraints[14]. Dislodged PEG tubes can be reinserted if the tube has been in position for over 2 weeks and the patient is evaluated soon after dislodgement. The position of the tube should always be checked

Table 5 Complications encountered with tube feeding and management. From references 15, 17, 20, 21, 30

Complication	Monitoring and management
Diarrhea	slow infusion rate. If bolus, change to continuous feeding
	use isosmolar or diluted formulas
	consider fiber-containing preparations
	review medications for possible etiology
	rule out infection
Nausea, bloating, vomiting	rule out tube migration
	check gastric residuals
	consider low-fat, lower osmolar preparations
High gastric residuals	rule out obstruction, ileus
	slow infusion rate
	consider promotility agents
Metabolic and electrolyte	
hypo- and hypernatremia	adjust water intake, evaluate for diarrhea, review medications
hypo- and hyperglycemia	tailor content of feed and antidiabetic medications
potassium and phosphorus	review medications, evaluate for diarrhea, alter tonicity of feeds
Aspiration pneumonia	elevate head end to 30–45° during and immediately after feeds
	monitor gastric residuals
	anticipate higher risk with impaired gag reflex, prior aspiration

radiologically prior to use for feeding. Medications or hypertonic formulas may clog tubes[22]. Clogging is minimized by periodic flushes during continuous feeds, before and after bolus feeds and following administration of medications. Smaller diameter jejunostomy tubes have a higher incidence of clogging and kinking.

Metabolic, electrolyte

Following initiation of tube feeding, monitoring is essential for abnormalities in serum glucose and electrolytes (sodium, potassium, magnesium and phosphorus)[2]. Alteration in biochemical values may be related to the formula, disease, water intake or medication. Hyperglycemia may warrant a change in carbohydrate content of the formula or addition of hypoglycemic agents. Hyponatremia may result from excessive water administration, diuretics, heart failure or diarrhea. Hypernatremia typically indicates febrile dermal losses or inadequate water intake. Hypo- and hypernatremia necessitate alteration in the amount of water administered.

Gastrointestinal

Complaints relating to the gastrointestinal tract are common in patients with tube feeding and include abdominal distension, nausea and vomiting, cramping and bloating, diarrhea and constipation[20]. Although some of these are related to the tonicity and content of feeds, concomitant use of medications or bacterial contamination of feeds or equipment might well be responsible. Most currently available formulas are lactose free, thus eliminating the problem of lactose intolerance[16]. Bags and tubes used for feeding must be changed daily, unused feeds beyond recommended 'hang periods' should be discarded and personal hygiene exercised in handling the equipment and feeds.

Abdominal cramps and bloating occur more with the use of hypertonic feeds, high fat content or bacterial contamination. The symptoms can be alleviated with diluted formulas or reduction in the rate of feeding[20]. Diarrhea in a patient on tube feeding should prompt search for an infection (*Clostridium difficile*), contamination of the feed or possible adverse drug reaction (e.g. sorbitol in elixirs)[16,19]. Slowing the rate of feeding, use of diluted feeds or addition of bulking agents can help. On the other hand, patients with constipation benefit from the use of high-fiber formulas, increase in water administration and intermittent use of stool softeners or laxatives to relieve symptoms.

When gastric residuals are high, the initial evaluation should exclude mechanical causes such as obstruction or ileus. Gastric emptying may be delayed with gastroparesis (diabetes) and use of anticholinergic medications. If no reversible or correctable factors are found, in the absence of obstruction, promotility agents such as metoclopramide or erythromycin may help improve gastric emptying.

Aspiration pneumonia

Although prevention of aspiration pneumonia has been cited as an indication for tube placement, the complication remains frequent and is associated with high mortality[2,14]. Data suggest the occurrence of aspiration events in over half the patients on PEG feeding. Bolus feeding, high gastric residuals, prior aspiration, history of pneumonia and presence of dysphagia are predisposing factors. Patients should be maintained at 30–45° head elevation during feeding and for 1 h after feeds to minimize this complication[19]. Use of slow continuous feeds in preference to large bolus feeds in high-risk individuals may help.

TUBE FEEDING AND OUTCOME IN DEMENTIA

There are indications that tube feeding in older adults with dementia has failed to meet the expectations prior to insertion of the tube[4,23,24]. Most studies note a 30-day mortality ranging from 4.1 to 28%[17]. The high mortality more likely reflects the severity of co-morbid illnesses present; in fact, many died even before completion of the initial evaluation for tube insertion[6,13,25]. Patients with pneumonia, cardiac failure or malignancy

had a higher mortality compared to those with malnutrition[26]. Overall, long-term survival following tube insertion ranged from 3 to 12 months, with an average of 7 months[25]; 63% of patients died in 1 year, up to 81.3% by 3 years[4,26].

An improvement in nutritional parameters has not been consistently observed following tube feeding[4,8]. Mechanical complications (tube dislodgement, clogging), diarrhea or acute illness result in loss of feeding time or increased demands, suggesting inadequate calorie and fluid intake. However, even in patients receiving adequate calories, loss of lean body mass and weight is evident. Aspiration pneumonia remains a leading cause of death in patients on enteral nutrition, although it is frequently cited as an indication to initiate tube feeding[4,6,23]. It is now believed that tube feeding does not prevent aspiration of oral secretions or regurgitation of gastric contents; it is suggested that the presence of the tube decreases lower esophageal sphincter pressure, increasing the risk of aspiration[27]. The use of jejunostomy tubes has not helped either. Attempts to improve healing of pressure sores by tube-feed mediated nutritional supplementation have not materialized[4,23].

Measures of functional independence, muscle strength or quality of life have not demonstrated significant improvement in functional status of nursing home residents on tube feeding (Table 6)[4,6,8,15,28]. Whether the comfort of the resident is improved with this feeding modality is also questionable. Thirst or hunger in terminally ill patients can be relieved with ice chips and lip lubrication; the placement of feeding tubes in such instances may potentially cause discomfort from nausea, bloating, diarrhea, increased use of restraints and cough[4,10,29]. A few studies from nursing homes suggest that careful oral feeding with adjustment of dietary consistency, medications, staff education, optimal environmental manipulation, swallowing reminders, facilitation techniques (chin stroking, gentle brushing) and use of supplements can improve

Table 6   Tube feeding in dementia: outcome data

Reference	Outcome
Callahan et al. (2000)[6]	16% died before baseline assessment, 1-year mortality 50%
	Improvement in nutritional and functional status rare
Grant et al. (1998)[26]	In 81 105 patients, hospital mortality 15.3%, 1-year mortality 63%; 3-year mortality 81.3% post-gastrostomy
Mitchell et al. (1997)[23]	Feeding tubes did not improve survival in 1386 nursing home residents with cognitive impairment over 24 months
Rabeneck et al. (1996)[27]	In 7369 patients, median survival after tube placement 7.5 months, 23.5% died during index hospitalization
Finucane et al (1996)[5]	Medline search suggested that feeding tubes do not prevent aspiration; some studies showed high rates of aspiration in tube-fed patients
Kaw et al (1994)[8]	No significant improvement in serum albumin and cholesterol levels
	No improvement in functional status during 18 months' follow-up
	Death attributed to aspiration in half the patients with pneumonia

Table 7   A summarized approach to enteral nutrition. From references 3, 10, 12, 23, 28, 32

Step I
Assess for weight loss
Evaluate nutritional indicators: anthropometric, biochemical, immunologic

Step II
Verify that caloric intake is adequate
Verify that the gastrointestinal tract is functional

Step III
Evaluate for cause of malnutrition
Assess swallowing, cognition, tests for malabsorption or other disease

Step IV
If nutrition can be provided by oral intake, consider supplements. Discontinue restricted diets
If not, consider enteral nutrition, provided gut is functional

Step V
Once decision has been made to initiate enteral nutrition:
Choose modality of tube feeding
  short term: nasogastric tube
  long term: percutaneous endoscopic gastrostomy (or jejunostomy)
Determine tube feeding prescription
  Calculate requirements, determine formula and rate
  Select continuous vs. bolus feeding

Step VI
Monitor weights, clinical status, and appropriate laboratory tests on a periodic basis
Assess for complications
Consider whether return to oral intake is possible

weight gain and nutritional parameters in malnourished elderly patients[4].

In the US, there are differences noted from State to State with regards to the use of tube feeding, often relating to the practices prevalent in the use of 'do not resuscitate' orders[31].

SUMMARY

Tube feeding used in appropriate selected situations can be an effective means of providing hydration, nutrition and medications. A summarized approach is provided in Table 7. However, data have not demonstrated consistent benefit in improving quality of life, function, long-term nutritional parameters or prolongation of survival. Ethical dilemmas and legal aspects cloud decision-making.

Nevertheless, the health-care provider must be aware of the fundamentals of enteral nutrition and its proper use in the geriatric population.

References

1. Refai W, Seidner DL. Nutrition in the elderly. *Clin Geriatr Med* 1999;15:607–25
2. Thomas DR. A complete primer on enteral feeding. *Ann Long-term Care* 2001;9:41–8
3. Cefalu CA. Appropriate dysphagia evaluation and management of the nursing home patient with dementia. *Ann Long term Care* 1999;7:447–51
4. Finucane TE, Christmas C, Travis K. Tube feeding in patients with advanced dementia: a review of the evidence. *J Am Med Assoc* 1999;13:1365–70
5. Finucane TE, Bynum JP. Use of tube feeding to prevent aspiration pneumonia. *Lancet* 1996;348:1421–4
6. Callahan CM, Haag KM, Weinberger M, *et al.* Outcomes of percutaneous endoscopic gastrostomy among older adults in a community setting. *J Am Geriatr Soc* 2000; 48:1048–54
7. Callahan CM, Haag KM, Buchanan NN, *et al.* Decision-making for percutaneous endoscopic gastrostomy among older adults in a community setting. *J Am Geriatr Soc* 1999;47:1105–9
8. Kaw M, Sekas G. Long-term follow-up of consequences of percutaneous endoscopic gastrostomy (PEG) tubes in nursing home patients. *Dig Dis Sci* 1994;39:738–43
9. Stuart SP, Tiley EH 3d, Boland JP. Feeding gastrostomy: a critical review of its indications and mortality rate. *South Med J* 1993; 86: 169–72
10. Braun UK, Kunik ME, Rabeneck L, Beyth RJ. Malnutrition in patients with severe dementia: is there a place for PEG tube feeding? *Ann Long-term Care*, 2001;9: 47–55
11. Dove DE, Sahn SA. The technique of administering enteral nutrition. Practical

pointers for ensuring correct placement, avoiding complications. *J Crit Illn* 1995;10: 881–8
12. Pfau PR, Rombeau JL. Nutrition. *Med Clin North Am* 2000;84:1209–30
13. Hull MA, Rawlings J, Murray FE, *et al.* Audit of outcome of long-term enteral nutrition by percutaneous endoscopic gastrostomy. *Lancet* 1993;341:869–72
14. Park RH, Allison MC, Lang J, *et al.* Randomised comparison of percutaneous endoscopic gastrostomy and nasogastric tube feeding in patients with persisting neurological dysphagia. *Br Med J* 1992;304: 1406–9
15. Kiyici N, Dharmarajan TS, Pitchumoni CS. Percutaneous endoscopic gastrostomy in the elderly: clinical and ethical aspects. *Practical Gastroenterol* 2001;25:12–23
16. DeWitt RC, Kudsk KA. Enteral nutrition. *Gastroenterol Clin North Am* 1998;27: 371–86
17. Dharmarajan TS, Unnikrishnan D, Pitchumoni CS. Percutaneous endoscopic gastrostomy and outcome in dementia. *Am J Gastroenterol* 2001;96:2556–63
18. Inadomi DW, Kopple JD. Fluid and electrolyte disorders in total parenteral nutrition. In Maxwell MH, Kleeman CR, Narins RG, eds. *Clinical Disorders of Fluid and Electrolyte Metabolism*, 4th edn. New York: McGraw Hill, 1987:945–66
19. Klein S, Fleming CR. Enteral and parenteral nutrition. In Feldman M, Scharschmidt BF, Sleisenger MH, *et al.*, eds. *Feldman: Sleisenger & Fordtran's Gastrointestinal and Liver Disease*, 6th edn. Philadelphia: WB Saunders, 1998:254–300
20. Chernoff R. Nutritional support for the elderly. In Chernoff R, ed. *Geriatric*

Nutrition: The Health Professional's Handbook, 2nd edn. Gaithersburg, MD: Aspen Publishers, 1999:420–7

21. Drickamer MA, Cooney LM Jr. A geriatrician's guide to enteral feeding. *J Am Geriatr Soc* 1993;41:672–9

22. Dharmarajan TS, Kumar A, Pitchumoni CS. Drug–nutrient interactions in older adults. *Practic Gastroenterol* 2002;26:37–55

23. Mitchell SL, Kiely DK, Lipsitz LA. The risk factors and impact on survival of feeding tube placement in nursing home residents with severe cognitive impairment. *Arch Intern Med* 1997;157:327–32

24. Dharmarajan TS, Unnikrishnan D. The art and science of tube feeding. *Postgrad Med* 2003;accepted for publication

25. Kobayashi K, Cooper GS, Chak A, *et al*. A prospective evaluation of outcome in patients referred for PEG placement. *Gastrointest Endosc* 2002;55:500–6

26. Grant MD, Rudberg MA, Brody JA. Gastrostomy placement and mortality among hospitalized Medicare beneficiaries. *J Am Med Assoc* 1998;279:1973–6

27. Rabeneck L, Wray NP, Petersen NJ. Long-term outcomes of patients receiving percutaneous endoscopic gastrostomy tubes. *J Gen Intern Med* 1996;11:287–93

28. Gillick M. When the nursing home resident with advanced dementia stops eating: what is the medical director to do? *J Am Med Dir Assoc* 2001;9:259–63

29. Slomka J. What do apple pie and motherhood have to do with feeding tubes and caring for the patient? *Arch Intern Med* 1995;155:1258–63

30. Grant JP. Percutaneous endoscopic gastrostomy. Initial placement by single endoscopic technique and long-term follow-up. *Ann Surg* 1993;217:168–74

31. Teno JM, Mor V, DeSilva D, *et al*. Use of feeding tubes in nursing home residents with severe cognitive impairment. *JAMA* 2002;287:3211–2

32. Li I. Feeding tubes in patients with severe dementia. *Am Fam Physician* 2002;65:1605–10

12 Perioperative medical management

T.S. Dharmarajan, MD, FACP, AGSF, *Dilip Unnikrishnan*, MD, *and* *Lekshmi Dharmarajan*, MD, FACP, FACC

INTRODUCTION

Surgical procedures are increasingly necessitated in older adults, due to the presence of co-morbidity in this age group. In 1996, based on estimates from the National Hospital Discharge Summary, more than 4.5 million elderly in the USA underwent in-patient surgery[1]. One in four surgical patients is over age 65; approximately half the geriatric population is predicted to require surgery during their lifetime[2,3]. Surgery is beneficial to varying degrees for cataracts, prostate hyperplasia, malignancies, degenerative joint disease and fractures, and is crucial in emergencies such as acute cholecystitis. In the past, the older adult was often considered unsuitable for surgery, with many surgeons reluctant to operate because of co-morbidities or advanced age alone[4]. Today, even high-risk procedures such as aneurysmal surgery are performed more frequently. In 1995, 75% of all postoperative deaths occurred in geriatric subjects[4]. The 30-day postoperative mortality in the elderly has dropped presently to 5–10%, much improved from earlier decades[5].

Today, age by itself is no longer considered a contraindication for surgery. However, physiologic changes from aging may diminish functional reserves and decrease the ability to respond to stress. Co-morbidity, polypharmacy and psychological factors all influence the perioperative state and recovery.

Successful surgery in the older adult may help attain near previous levels of functional independence and improve the quality of life. Perioperative management involves the identification and modification of risk factors to optimize goals.

ROLE OF THE PRIMARY PHYSICIAN: THE CONCEPT OF 'CLEARANCE'

The concept of 'clearance for surgery' is a misnomer, misrepresenting the process of preoperative medical management. The role of the physician is to evaluate the patient, identify co-morbid processes, assess risks and benefits of surgery, offer corrective measures for remediable factors, indicate and optimize irreversible conditions and utilize available indices to offer an objective 'risk stratification'. Intraoperative care is provided if and when requested, and the patient is followed postoperatively to ensure an optimal medical status and outcome. Throughout perioperative care, a co-ordinated approach between the physician, surgeon and anesthesiologist is vital.

PREPARING FOR SURGERY

History and physical examination

A focused history and detailed physical examination is the initial step in evaluation. For many, the preoperative period may be the first opportunity for a comprehensive medical assessment. The history is obtained from the patient or caregiver and should include current and past illnesses and hospitalizations, a comprehensive review of medications (oral, topical, ophthalmic and over-the-counter medicines including supplements and herbs), history of prior surgery or anesthesia and alcohol or tobacco use[6]. Excessive alcohol or benzodiazepine use may require monitoring for evidence of withdrawal symptoms and be treated accordingly. A history of rheumatoid arthritis may require imaging studies of the neck; information is provided to the anesthesiologist for precautions to prevent atlantoaxial subluxation during intubation[7].

Laboratory investigations and other tests

The choice and extent of laboratory testing is guided by the history, physical examination and co-morbid conditions[6]. Laboratory testing is generally not indicated unless an abnormal result is likely to change patient management[6,8]. Routine preoperative tests (often guided by the institutional policy) include hemoglobin/hematocrit, white blood cell count, tests for renal function (blood urea nitrogen and serum creatinine), glucose, electrolytes and, if indicated, bleeding and coagulation parameters (platelet count, prothrombin time, activated partial thromboplastin time) and urine analysis. Sometimes tests for liver function, thyroid function and drug levels are obtained to guide perioperative management. Recently performed test results should be obtained and needless repetition avoided[9]. Blanket ordering of unnecessary profiles increases the statistical possibility of obtaining abnormal results. The legal liability of not ordering a test is less than ordering a test and failing to act on an abnormal result[10].

A chest X-ray and electrocardiogram are generally recommended in older adults because unsuspected abnormalities may be present in this age group; abnormalities are found in up to a quarter of routine electrocardiograms[11]. Specific tests are tailored for assessment of co-morbid conditions, e.g. an echocardiogram in cardiac failure or pulmonary function tests prior to lung resection.

The optimum hemoglobin or hematocrit for surgery is not well defined. In the older adult with cardiac or pulmonary disease, especially with anticipated blood loss during surgery, a hemoglobin of 10 g/dl and/or hematocrit of 30% is desirable[12]. An older patient with heart or lung disease, with a shorter life expectancy, requiring prolonged surgery with blood loss, is more likely to benefit from transfusion as opposed to a younger patient with little co-morbidity and longer life expectancy.

ASSESSMENT OF RISK

General factors

Age

Although advanced age is included in perioperative risk indices, it is not *per se* a contraindication for surgery[13]. Goldman's criteria and Detsky's modified multifactorial index state age (over 70 years) as an independent risk factor for predicting perioperative death, while the American College of Cardiology (ACC)/American Heart Association (AHA) list advanced age as a minor risk factor[4,8,14,15] (Table 1). The American Society of Anesthesiology (ASA) scale found age to play very little role amongst the different classes, suggesting that other factors are more important than age itself[4]. Aging is, however, associated with a decrease in functional reserves, and along with co-morbid illnesses increases the likelihood of complications perioperatively. The mortality risk in an 80-year old patient undergoing major surgery is around 5% compared to less than 2% in younger adults[4,16]. When both age and co-morbidity are considered, the latter is a better predictor of outcome.

Table 1 Clinical predictors of increased perioperative cardiovascular risk (myocardial infarction, congestive heart failure, death)

Major
Unstable coronary syndromes
  recent myocardial infarction[*] with evidence of important ischemic risk by clinical symptoms or non-invasive study
  unstable or severe[†] angina (Canadian class III or IV)[‡]
Decompensated congestive heart failure
Significant arrhythmias
  high-grade atrioventricular block
  symptomatic ventricular arrhythmias in the presence of underlying heart disease
  supraventricular arrhythmias with uncontrolled ventricular rate
Severe valvular heart disease

Intermediate
Mild angina pectoris (Canadian class I or II)
Prior myocardial infarction by history or pathological Q waves
Compensated or prior congestive heart failure
Diabetes mellitus

Minor
Advanced age
Abnormal ECG (left ventricular hypertrophy, left bundle branch block, ST-T abnormalities)
Rhythm other than sinus (e.g. atrial fibrillation)
Low functional capacity (e.g. inability to climb one flight of stairs with a bag of groceries)
History of stroke
Uncontrolled systemic hypertension

ECG, electrocardiogram. [*]The American College of Cardiology National Database Library defines *recent* myocardial infarction as > 7 days but ≤ 1 month (30 days). [†]May include 'stable' angina in patients who are unusually sedentary. [‡]Campeau L. Grading of angina pectoris. *Circulation* 1976;54:522–3
Reproduced with permission. ACC/AHA Guidelines for the Perioperative Cardiovascular Evaluation for Noncardiac Surgery. *J Am Coll Cardiol* 1996;27:910–48. Copyright 1996 by the American College of Cardiology and American Heart Association, Inc.
Note: The 2002 ACC/AHA guidelines have added the following clinical predictors[23]:
    Major predictors include 'Acute or recent myocardial infarction'
    Intermediate predictors include 'Renal insufficiency'

Functional status

Good preoperative functional status, assessed by evaluating activities of daily living (ADL) and instrumental activities of daily living (IADL), reflects better postoperative recovery and capability of participating in rehabilitation measures. The ability to leave home and return on one's own twice weekly appears a favorable functional status indicator[4]. Functional status limitation in men increased surgical risk nearly 10 times in one study[4]. Baseline functional status helps determine postoperative goals and level of rehabilitation services[1,7]. Preoperative ADL scores predict 1-year survival in patients with hip fractures[4].

The Dripps' ASA physical status classification, initially reported in 1941, has been helpful in evaluating the general status of the patient and perioperative risk[4]. The scale divides patients into five groups; class I, healthy; class II, mild systemic disease; class III, severe systemic disease, although not incapacitating; class IV, incapacitated from life threatening illness; and class V, moribund, unlikely survival even with surgery. The ACC/AHA guidelines for cardiac evaluation use the Duke Activity Status Index to assess functional risk. Functional status is expressed in metabolic equivalents (MET), with 1 MET being equivalent to the oxygen consumption of a 70-kg, 40-year-old man in the resting state (3.5 ml/kg per min)[8].

Cognition

The preoperative cognitive status predicts postoperative complications and functional recovery. The Mini Mental Status Examination of Folstein and Folstein is a commonly used tool to evaluate cognition. Dementia is associated with a higher incidence of perioperative complications, postoperative delirium and prolonged hospitalization compared to those with intact cognition[1,6,13]. The mortality was increased in patients with dementia by 52%, when compared to patients without dementia, in one study[4]. Depression, overt or masked, is common in the elderly and contributes to significant morbidity[11].

Nutrition

Mortality, morbidity and duration of hospitalization are increased in the malnourished patient[17]. Anthropometric measurements and laboratory parameters (serum albumin, serum cholesterol, total lymphocyte count) are used to assess nutritional status, with prealbumin a measure of recent change[18]. Serum albumin less than 3.5 g/dl is associated with a four-fold increase in complications and a six-fold increase in mortality[4]. Attempts to improve nutrition by aggressive enteral or parenteral measures are unrewarding and sometimes associated with increased complications from therapy[4,17]. Hence, postponement of surgery for the sole purpose of improving nutrition is not generally recommended[4].

Evaluation of organ/system involvement

Cardiovascular

Ischemic heart disease is the single best predictor of postoperative cardiac complications[4]. The association of cardiovascular factors and perioperative complications was studied by Goldman and colleagues[14] and subsequently by Detsky et al.[15]. Goldman's criteria give more significance to myocardial infarction within 6 months, S_3 or elevated jugular venous pressure and rhythm other than sinus (includes more than five premature ventricular beats), while Detsky's criteria give greater importance to critical aortic stenosis, myocardial infarction within 6 months, class III/IV angina, recent pulmonary edema (within 1 week) and emergency surgery. Both indices do not attribute age (over 70 years) to be a significant risk factor[9,14,15,19,20]. Initially published in 1996, and subsequently updated in 2002, the ACC/AHA guidelines for cardiovascular evaluation prior to non-cardiac surgery offer a comprehensive preoperative cardiac assessment (Table 1)[8,21-24]. The American College of Physicians guidelines (1997) in general parallels the recommendations of the ACC/AHA[1,20].

The stepwise approach used in the ACC/AHA guidelines is based on clinical risk predictors, prior cardiac evaluation, functional status and surgical risks[8,23,24]. Acute myocardial infarction (within 7 days of documented event), recent myocardial infarction (7 days to 1 month), unstable angina, severe valvular disease, decompensated heart failure and significant arrhythmias are major clinical predictors (Table 1)[8,23,24]. Functional status is assessed using the Duke Activity Status Index; perioperative risk is increased when unable to meet a 4-MET energy demand[8,24]. Ability to climb a flight of stairs, run a short distance, walk on level ground at 4 miles/h or play golf equals an energy expenditure of 4–10 METs[8,23,24]. In the elderly, co-morbid states such as vascular insufficiency, amputation or neuromuscular disease can limit functional status[6]. In these instances, the level of activity may be inadequate to manifest symptoms of angina or dyspnea requiring non-invasive testing to elicit evidence of cardiac disease. Patients who had recent coronary revascularization (within 5 years) or coronary evaluation (angiogram or stress test within 2 years) and are asymptomatic do not need further workup. Surgical risk depends on the type of surgery and associated hemodynamic

Table 2 Cardiac risk* stratification for non-cardiac surgical procedures

High (reported cardiac risk often > 5)
Emergency major operations, particularly in the elderly
Aortic and other major vascular
Peripheral vascular
Anticipated prolonged surgical procedures associated with large fluid shifts and/or blood loss

Intermediate (reported cardiac risk generally < 5)
Carotid endarterectomy
Head and neck
Intraperitoneal and intrathoracic
Orthopedic
Prostate

Low[†](reported cardiac risk generally < 1)
Endoscopic procedures
Superficial procedures
Cataract
Breast

*Combined incidence of cardiac death and non-fatal myocardial infarction
†Does not generally require further preoperative cardiac testing
Reproduced with permission. ACC/AHA Guidelines for the Perioperative Cardiovascular Evaluation for Noncardiac Surgery. *J Am Coll Cardiol* 1996;27:910-48. Copyright 1996 by the American College of Cardiology and American Heart Association, Inc.

stress[8,23]. Surgical procedures are stratified into high, intermediate and low risk (Table 2). Emergency surgery is not delayed to complete preoperative evaluation; the risk of invasive testing may exceed that of the proposed non-cardiac surgery[24].

Those with minor or no clinical predictors generally do not need testing unless associated with poor functional status (less than 4 METs) and scheduled for a high-risk surgical procedure[8,23]. When clinical predictors are intermediate, patients with (a) poor functional status (< 4 METs) and (b) good functional status (> 4 METs) and requiring a high-risk surgical procedure, benefit from non-invasive testing and postponement of surgery until cardiac status is stabilized[8]. Dipyridamole thallium and dobutamine stress echocardiography are particularly useful for patients with intermediate risk[19,22]. Negative predictive values of myocardial perfusion tests for myocardial infarction or cardiac death are approximately 99% as opposed to low positive predictive values[8,21,22]. The results may be used to make decisions for or against further invasive testing. Individuals with high-risk clinical predictors should be considered for invasive cardiovascular evaluation prior to elective surgery.

Recent coronary events, decompensated congestive heart failure and arrhythmias are considered risk factors in all studies. Surgery within 3 months of myocardial infarction carries a risk of 8–30% for perioperative infarction or death, decreasing to 3.5–5% when surgery is performed 6 months or more after a myocardial infarction[4]. However, the ACC/AHA guidelines in 2002 seem to avoid separating the post-myocardial infarction period into 3- and 6-month intervals; despite inadequate data, they recommend a 4–6-week wait post-myocardial infarction prior to elective surgery if a stress test does not demonstrate residual myocardium at risk[23].

Symptomatic valvular stenosis carries high perioperative risk of cardiac failure or hypotension and should be evaluated and treated as in the non-operative setting. Options for treatment include percutaneous valvotomy or valve replacement[8]. Regurgitant lesions are generally tolerated better perioperatively and can be stabilized with intensive therapy and monitoring[8]. Valvular disease is an indication for endocarditis prophylaxis.

Congestive heart failure carries increased perioperative morbidity; the etiology of cardiac failure should be determined and medical treatment optimized prior to surgery. Cardiomyopathy is associated with risk of perioperative cardiac failure and requires postoperative observation. The presence of arrhythmias should prompt evaluation for drug toxicity, cardiopulmonary disease or metabolic abnormalities[8]. Pulmonary artery catheterization is not routinely recommended, but is helpful in patients with severe coronary artery disease, recent myocardial infarction with congestive heart failure, cardiomyopathy or significant valvular heart disease undergoing high-risk procedures[8,9,21,23]. In general, the indications for pacemaker insertion and percutaneous transluminal coronary angioplasty (PTCA) are similar to the ACC/AHA task force guidelines in the nonoperative setting[8,23,24]. Post-PTCA elective surgery may be delayed for 1 week to allow healing of vessel injury, and at least 2 weeks, preferably 4–6 weeks, post-stent insertion; this is to allow re-endothelization to occur[23].

Hypertension

Uncontrolled hypertension is a significant risk factor; elective surgery should be postponed if systolic and diastolic blood pressures are higher than 180 and 110 mmHg, respectively[22,23,25,26]. Antihypertensive medications should not be withheld and must be given in the morning of surgery with a small amount of water. β-Blockers are particularly useful in the surgical setting, as they oppose catecholamine-induced side-effects[7]. β-Blockers and clonidine should not be abruptly discontinued and may be administered by parenteral or transdermal routes, respectively, to prevent rebound hypertension[8].

Calcium channel blockers have sometimes been associated with increased postoperative bleeding.

Pulmonary

Age-associated changes in the respiratory system may predispose to increased perioperative complications. The PaO_2 decreases with age, although $PaCO_2$ remains normal; the response to hypoxia and hypercapnia, however, is diminished[2]. The closing volume increases linearly with age, increasing the risk for atelectasis[2]. Resting values for oxygen uptake, and right atrial, pulmonary artery and pulmonary capillary wedge pressures are not changed in the older asymptomatic individual[2]. Cough reflexes are impaired, and a ventilation perfusion mismatch occurs at the lung bases, the basis for early mobilization after surgery.

Obesity, chronic lung disease, smoking, prolonged anesthesia and repeat surgery in 1 year are predictors of pulmonary complications after surgery[4,13,27]. Upper abdominal procedures are more likely to compromise diaphragmatic function and increase complications compared to those on the lower abdomen or pelvis[1,27,28]. Patients should be counseled to stop smoking, with maximum beneficial effects when this is discontinued at least 8 weeks prior to elective surgery[25,29,30]. Routine pulmonary function testing (PFT) is not required in all patients. Uncontrolled asthma or chronic obstructive lung disease, history of heavy smoking and pneumonectomy are indications for PFT[7,11]. Vital capacity less than 50% predicted, forced expiratory volume in 1 s (FEV_1) less than 2 litres and hypoxia or hypercapnia suggest increased perioperative risk[4]. Opiates and benzodiazepines can compromise respiratory function in the older adult and increase risk of hypoxia[2]. Preoperative instructions on respiratory maneuvers, chest physiotherapy and appropriate use of antibiotics and bronchodilators may help minimize postoperative pulmonary complications[29,30].

Table 3 Medications and surgery

Administer in the morning of surgery
  antihypertensives
  antiepileptics
  antiarrhythmics
  bronchodilators

Withhold on a temporary basis, prior to surgery
  antiplatelet agents (aspirin, non-steroidal
    anti-inflammatory drugs)
  anticoagulants (heparin, warfarin)

If necessary, consider switching in the perioperative
  period
  oral to parenteral or transdermal preparation
  oral hypoglycemics to insulin

Consider initiating
  antibiotics for endocarditis prophylaxis
  antibiotics for wound prophylaxis or infection
  prophylaxis for deep vein thrombosis
  steroids, if adrenal suppressed
  β-blockers, if indicated
  intravenous dextrose solution for diabetics

After surgery
  resume prior medications with appropriate revision

From references 3, 4, 6, 7, 13, 24, 25, 27, 31, 32

Renal

An age-related but variable decline in renal function, at the rate of about 1% per year from the third decade, determines the pharmacokinetics of anesthetic or other medications that are renally excreted in the older adult[2]. Further, the sarcopenia of aging may be the reason for a normal or only slightly raised serum creatinine even with significant renal impairment. Creatinine clearance calculated by the Cockroft–Gault equation is a better assessment of renal function than serum creatinine measurement alone in this age group. Baseline renal insufficiency, left ventricular dysfunction and a rising serum creatinine are risk factors for postoperative renal failure[4]. Prerenal factors (hypotension, blood loss, inadequate hydration) are often the basis for worsening renal function following surgery. However, obstructive causes and tubular damage from ischemia or drugs should nevertheless be excluded.

Diabetes mellitus

In diabetics, blood glucose needs to be monitored pre-, intra- and postoperatively for adequate control[1]. Oral hypoglycemics are preferably switched to insulin prior to surgery. Half the usual dose of long-acting insulin is administered in the morning of surgery and dextrose containing intravenous fluids initiated[25]. Intermittent subcutaneous administration or continuous intravenous infusions of insulin are options for control of hyperglycemia[1].

MEDICATIONS AND SURGERY

Revision of regimen

The older adult is likely to be on multiple prescription and over-the-counter medications; these should be reviewed (Table 3). Antiepileptic, bronchodilator, cardiovascular, antihypertensive and diabetic medications are usually continued to the day of surgery, and administered on the morning of surgery along with a sip of water[6,24,27]. Medications that cannot be taken orally may be substituted to appropriate parenteral choices[27]. Diuretics are preferably withheld on the day of surgery[13]. If on a steroid equivalent of 20 mg of prednisone or more for over a week in the prior 6 months, stress-dose steroids, equal to 50 mg of hydrocortisone, are administered every 6–8 h for 2–3 days and tapered off[3]. The traditional dose of 100 mg hydrocortisone every 8 h with prolonged taper is considered high, as the physiological stress amount of cortisol peaks around 150 mg/day and quickly returns to baseline. A consensus paper has recommended using a dose of 25 mg for 1 day, 50–75 mg/day for 1–2 days, and 100–150 mg/day for 2–3 days, based on whether the surgical procedure is minor, moderate or major respectively[31]. While many patients on long-term steroids may be adrenal suppressed, it is difficult to perform an adrenocorticotrophic hormone stimulation test in most patients, especially in emergency situations[32]. Hence the practice is to give stress steroid doses, although evidence is anecdotal[32].

Perioperative β-blockers are effective in preventing intraoperative and postoperative myocardial ischemia and reducing the incidence of death from cardiac causes, benefits extending for several weeks after surgery[7,9,19,20,26]. If at least 7 days are available prior to surgery, the goal would be to titrate the dose of β-blockers to a resting heart rate of 60 per minute[33]. Drugs for congestive heart failure, such as angiotensin converting enzyme inhibitors and diuretics, should be continued. Patients on nitroglycerine are continued on the medication, although the role for intravenous nitroglycerine has not been conclusively shown[8]. Appropriate revisions of the medication regimen must be made in the post-operative period, based on the clinical status and the ability of the patient to resume oral intake.

Endocarditis prophylaxis

Valvular disease requires antibiotic prophylaxis prior to surgery. In mitral valve prolapse, the presence of thickened valves and regurgitant flow are indications[7]. Endocarditis prophylaxis is based on standard AHA guidelines.

Antibiotic prophylaxis for surgery

Surgical wounds are classified into clean, clean contaminated or contaminated (dirty) depending on whether mucosal barriers are broken, presence of inflammation or infection (pus) and if there has been a break in aseptic technique. Cardiac, vascular, neurologic and ocular procedures are considered clean. Procedures on the gastrointestinal tract, biliary tract and head and neck surgery are clean contaminated (cross mucosal barrier, gastrointestinal spillage), while ruptured viscus or trauma surgery (presence of infection, infected urine or bile, gross gastrointestinal spillage) are

termed contaminated[4]. Clean contaminated procedures require only antibiotic prophylaxis, while contaminated surgery needs prophylaxis and extended treatment for several days[4]. Antibiotics are usually administered 0.5 h before the procedure and re-dosed if surgery is prolonged, to attain adequate tissue concentration[4]. The choice of antibiotic is best left to the operating team, usually selected based on procedure, expected organisms and antibiotic sensitivity reports in the institution.

Perioperative anticoagulation

The elderly individual is likely to be on aspirin or warfarin for treatment of coronary or cerebral vascular disease, atrial fibrillation or deep vein thrombosis (DVT); the risks of discontinuing anticoagulation should be weighed against the benefits of diminished bleeding. Withholding four doses of warfarin is usually sufficient to normalize the International Normalized Ratio (INR), but prothrombin time and INR are best checked to confirm adequate levels prior to surgery[34,35]. For emergency surgery, fresh frozen plasma or vitamin K can be used to reverse warfarin effects. Administration of vitamin K is not the choice prior to elective surgery, since a therapeutic response will be delayed on resuming oral anticoagulation. If at high risk for thromboembolism (prosthetic valves, recent DVT), intravenous heparin may be used when oral anticoagulation is discontinued, stopped 6 h prior to the procedure and restarted 12 h after surgery or later, based on the presence or absence of bleeding complications[34]. If intravenous anticoagulation is contraindicated in patients at risk for DVT and/or pulmonary embolism, placement of a vena cava filter may be considered. Aspirin and non-steroidal anti-inflammatory drugs (NSAIDs) are stopped 5–7 days prior to surgery, to decrease the risk of bleeding from platelet dysfunction[35]. Elective surgery is generally avoided in the first month following an acute venous or arterial thromboembolism[34,35].

Perioperative anticoagulation entails the use of subcutaneous heparin, low-molecular-weight heparin or warfarin[9,35]. Risk factors for DVT include age over 40 years, previous history of DVT or pulmonary embolism, extensive pelvic, abdominal or neurosurgery, malignancy, orthopedic surgery and immobility from spinal injury or stroke[25,35]. Subcutaneous heparin can be started 2 h prior to surgery and continued at 8- to 12-h intervals at a dose of 5000 units subcutaneously[35]. Withholding anticoagulation prior to surgery is based on the nature of the procedure, the type of anesthesia (e.g. bleeding from spinal anesthesia) and the preferences of the surgeon. Intermittent pneumatic calf compression or elastic stockings may be additionally used in high-risk situations or as an alternative when anticoagulation is contraindicated. DVT prophylaxis is usually begun before surgery and continued post-operatively until adequate ambulation is achieved.

RISKS RELATED TO TYPE OF SURGERY

Emergency surgery carries a high risk[20]. Mortality in emergency surgical procedures in the elderly may be as high as 20% compared to 1.9% for elective surgery[4]. A diagnosis of surgical emergency is often delayed in the older adult due to atypical presentations; conversely, surgery may at times be postponed with an expectation that conservative medical treatment will be effective. Morbidity and mortality are increased while stabilizing medical illnesses. Body cavity surgery also carries higher risk, compared to surgery elsewhere[19,20].

ANESTHESIA

Both regional and general anesthesia are associated with comparable outcomes, the choice being individualized depending on co-morbidity[5,16]. Some studies support the use of regional anesthesia when at risk for thromboembolic disease and general anesthesia if at risk for hypotension[5]. Nonetheless, it is generally accepted that there is no one best myocardial protective anesthetic technique, with the choice of anesthesia best left to the anesthesiologist[8,22,24].

THE POSTOPERATIVE PERIOD

Follow-up by the physician in the postoperative period is as important as preoperative evaluation. Complications such as delirium are missed in up to 50% of affected patients, suggesting a need for closer observation to recognize and treat complications. Medications withheld during the immediate preoperative phase may have to be restarted; on the other hand, medications are also a cause of delirium and non-essential drugs should be discontinued. Early mobilization helps reduce the incidence of complications such as pressure sores, urinary retention and pulmonary atelectasis, and prevents deconditioning. Weakness of neck extensors and antigravity leg muscles occurs within days of impaired mobility and limits independent transfer and ambulation[18]. In addition, discharge from the acute care facility should be anticipated and planned in collaboration with a multidisciplinary team.

Delirium

Postoperative delirium is common in the older adult (up to 73% in hospitalized patients), contributing to significant morbidity and mortality[2,16,18,36]. The incidence is almost three times higher in those over age 75, compared to the 65–75 age group[18]. Delirium increases in-hospital mortality by 15–30%, coupled with inability to return to independent living[16]. Risk factors in the perioperative period include infection, urinary retention, medications, constipation, electrolyte disturbances and sleep disorders. Delirium is particularly common in the pre- and post-surgical settings with hip fracture[37]. Antihistamines, narcotics, antiemetics,

NSAIDs and anticholinergic medications are well recognized causes[18]. Meperidine and its metabolite normeperidine accumulate in older adults with renal impairment and may cause delirium or seizures. Pre-existing dementia is a risk factor for postoperative delirium, contributed in part by non-availability of eyeglasses or hearing aids, disruption of sleep and use of restraints[1,16]. The delirious patient is unable to co-operate for rehabilitation and is at risk of complications from restraints. Treatment includes identification and correction of inciting factors. Environmental factors such as noisy monitors or bright lighting in intensive care units may predispose to development of delirium.

Fever

Infections of the urinary tract, lower respiratory tract and surgical wounds are causes of fever in the postoperative patient. Urinary tract infections are the most common, particularly following catheterization, and require treatment if symptomatic. Pneumonia carries the highest mortality, up to 27% in some studies[4]. Fever could also result from the surgical procedure, thrombophlebitis, medications and other non-infectious complications. Judicious use of antibiotics for prophylaxis, sterile surgical techniques, early removal of urinary catheters or other lines and improved pulmonary toilet help decrease postoperative infections.

Pain

Narcotic analgesics may contribute to delirium, constipation, ileus, hypoventilation or hypotension in the older adult[18]. NSAIDs carry the risk of gastrointestinal bleeding and renal toxicity. Patient-controlled analgesia is the therapeutic standard for postoperative pain, although its value is hindered in the older adult because of impaired cognition[24,33]. Adequate pain management may decrease postoperative catecholamine secretion, thus decreasing predisposition cardiac ischemia. Optimal analgesia also encourages mobilization and rehabilitation, reduction of hospital stay and recovery of overall functional status[23].

Cardiovascular complications

In those patients with suspected cardiac disease, an electrocardiogram is recommended in the immediate postoperative period and at 48 h. The highest risk for cardiovascular events is the first 24 h after surgery, with most infarctions occuring in the first 2 days[9,13]. Cardiac events may be asymptomatic; an evaluation is prompted in those with hypotension, arrhythmias or unexplained delirium[9]. Cardiac enzymes are measured in those at high risk and not routinely[8,9,22]. Recognition of postoperative myocardial infarction or cardiac ischemia is important, as these carry a risk of reinfarction or cardiac death[8,23,24,26].

Pulmonary complications

Pneumonia is common in the postoperative period, with high mortality. Poor oropharyngeal reflexes, the presence of a nasogastric tube, altered mentation and malnutrition are associated with respiratory complications. Sterile respiratory equipment, pulmonary exercises and improved nutritional support can decrease the incidence of pneumonia. Other pulmonary complications include atelectasis, adult respiratory distress syndrome, respiratory failure and pulmonary embolism[28]. Early mobilization improves gas exchange and minimizes complications. Helpful measures include pain control, bronchodilator therapy, chest physiotherapy and lung expansion maneuvers such as incentive spirometry or intermittent positive pressure breathing[29,30].

Urinary retention

Short-term use of urinary catheters in the perioperative period is acceptable, but prolonged use beyond 72 h is associated with urinary infections. Urinary retention is particularly common after hip surgery and is managed with temporary catheterization. Medications that predispose to urinary retention (e.g. analgesics, anticholinergic agents) should be considered as possible etiology.

SUMMARY

Surgical procedures are increasingly performed in older adults. A co-ordinated approach between physician, surgeon, anesthesiologist and consultant can help achieve meaningful risk assessment, amelioration of at least some problems and improved surgical outcome. Surgery should never be denied on the basis of age alone. The goals are to improve function and enhance quality of life.

References

1. Wertheim WA. Perioperative risk. Review of two guidelines for assessing older adults. American College of Cardiology and American Heart Association. *Geriatrics* 2000;55:61–6

2. Oskvig RM. Special problems in the elderly. *Chest* 1999;115(5 Suppl):158–64S

3. Francis J. Perioperative management of the older adult. In Hazzard WR, Blass JP, Ettinger WH Jr, *et al.*, eds., *Principles of Geriatric Medicine and Gerontology*, 4th edn., New York: McGraw-Hill, 1999: 203–25

4. Thomas DR, Ritchie CS. Preoperative assessment of older adults. *J Am Geriatr Soc* 1995;43:811–21

5. Lien CA. Regional versus general anesthesia for hip surgery in older patients: does the choice affect patient outcome? *J Am Geriatr Soc* 2002;50:191–4

6. Litaker D. Preoperative screening. *Med Clin North Am* 1999;83:1565–81

7. Clark E. Preoperative assessment. Primary care work-up to identify surgical risks. *Geriatrics* 2001;56:36–40

8. Eagle KA, Brundage BH, Chaitman BR, *et al.* Guidelines for perioperative cardiovascular evaluation for noncardiac surgery. Report of the American College of Cardiology/American Heart Association Task Force on Practice Guidelines (Committee on Perioperative Cardiovascular Evaluation for Noncardiac Surgery). *J Am Coll Cardiol* 1996; 27:910–48

9. Lefevre F, Arron MJ, Chadha V, Cohn SL. A cost-effective approach to periperative care for the primary care physician. *J Clin Outcomes Man* 2000;7:43–52

10. Macpherson DS. Preoperative laboratory testing: should any tests be 'routine' before surgery? *Med Clin North Am* 1993;77: 289–308

11. Muravchick S. Preoperative assessment of the elderly patient. *Anesthesiol Clin North Am* 2000;18:71–89

12. Carson JL, Willett LR. Is a hemoglobin of 10 g/dL required for surgery? *Med Clin North Am* 1993;77:335–47

13. Miller DL. Perioperative care of the elderly patient: special considerations. *Cleve Clin J Med* 1995;62:383–90

14. Goldman L, Caldera DL, Nussbaum SR, *et al.* Multifactorial index of cardiac risk in noncardiac surgical procedures. *N Engl J Med* 1977;297:845–50

15. Detsky AS, Abrams HB, McLaughlin JR, *et al.* Predicting cardiac complications in patients undergoing non-cardiac surgery. *J Gen Intern Med* 1986;1:211–19

16. Liu LL, Leung JM. Predicting adverse postoperative outcomes in patients aged 80 years or older. *J Am Geriatr Soc* 2000;48: 405–12

17. Perioperative total parenteral nutrition in surgical patients. The Veterans Affairs Total Parenteral Nutrition Cooperative Study Group. *N Engl J Med* 1991;325:525–32

18. Hirsch CH. When your patient needs surgery: how planning can avoid complications. *Geriatrics* 1995;50:39–44

19. Holly TA, Ockene IS. Preoperative consultation. In Alpert JS, ed. *Cardiology for the Primary Care Physician.* New York: Mosby, 1996:11–18

20. Palda VA, Detsky AS. Perioperative assessment and management of risk from coronary artery disease. *Ann Intern Med* 1997; 127:309–28

21. Eagle KA, Brundage BH, Chaitman BR, *et al.* Guidelines for perioperative cardiovascular evaluation for noncardiac surgery: an abridged version of the report of the American College of Cardiology/American Heart Association Task Force on Practice Guidelines. *Mayo Clin Proc* 1997;72: 524–31

22. Karcic AA, Rizvon MK. Perioperative cardiovascular evaluation. Step-by-step approach to risk assessment and follow-up care. *Postgrad Med* 2000;108:127–8, 131–4, 140–2

23. Eagle KA, Berger PB, Calkins H, *et al.* ACC/AHA guideline update for perioperative cardiovascular evaluation for non cardiac surgery – executive summary: a report of the American College of Cardiology/American Heart Association Task Force on Practice Guidelines (Committee to Update the 1996 Guidelines on Perioperative Cardiovascular Evaluation for Noncardiac Surgery). *J Am Coll Cardiol* 2002;39:542–53

24. Eagle KA, Brundage BH, Chaitman BR, *et al.* Guidelines for perioperative cardiovascular evaluation for noncardiac surgery. Report of the American College of Cardiology/American Heart Association Task Force on Practice Guidelines. Committee on Perioperative Cardiovascular Evaluation for Noncardiac Surgery. *Circulation* 1996;93:1278–317

25. Pompei P. Preoperative assessment and perioperative care. In Cassel CK, Cohen HJ, Larson EB, eds. *Geriatric Medicine,* 3rd edn., New York: Spring-Verlag, 1997: 189–200

26. Martin DE, Shanks GE. Strategies for the preoperative evaluation of the hypertensive patient. *Anesthesiol Clin North Am* 1999;17:529–48

27. Noble DW, Kehlet H. Risks of interrupting drug treatment before surgery. *Br Med J* 2000;321:719–20

28. Ferguson MK. Preoperative assessment of pulmonary risk. *Chest* 1999;115(5 Suppl): 58–63S

29. Mohr DN, Lavender RC. Preoperative pulmonary evaluation. Identifying patients at increased risk for complications. *Postgrad Med* 1996;100:241–4, 247–8, 251–2

30. Smetana GW. Preoperative pulmonary evaluation. *N Engl J Med* 1999;340:937–44

31. Shaw M. When is perioperative 'steroid coverage' necessary? *Cleveland Clin J Med* 2002;69:9–11

32. Mandell BF, Lance VL. Taking it to the bar: medicolegal ramifications of perioperative steroid coverage. *Cleveland Clin J Med* 2002;69:7–8

33. Fleisher LA. Perioperative evaluation of the patient with hypertension. *J Am Med Assoc* 2002;287:2043–6

34. Kearon C, Hirsh J. Management of anticoagulation before and after elective surgery. *N Engl J Med* 1997;336:1506–11

35. Martin R. Perioperative approach to the anticoagulated patient. *Anesthesiol Clin North Am* 1999;17:813–30

36. Karanikolas M, Swarm RA. Current trends in perioperative pain management. *Anesthesiol Clin North Am* 2000;18:575–99

37. Samuels SC, Evers MM. Delirium: pragmatic guidance for managing a common, confounding and sometimes lethal condition. *Geriatrics* 2002;57:33–8

13 Surgery in the elderly

Nanakram Agarwal, MD, MPH, FRCS, FACS, *and*
Ravinder K. Annamaneni, MD, FRCS

INTRODUCTION

Surgery in the elderly population is rapidly becoming a specialized field. The problems in geriatric patients are unique, involving alterations in physiology and also ethical and emotional issues. When managing older patients, the goal is not only to enhance survival but also to improve the quality of life and minimize suffering.

PHYSIOLOGY

In addition to age-related physiological changes in the respiratory system, vital capacity decreases approximately 75% after laparotomy. There is also an increase in dead space and a decrease in expiratory volumes and flow rate. The clinical effects of the physiologic changes are a gradual decrease in arterial Po_2, and an increased risk of atelectasis and pneumonia in the postoperative period. Postoperative pneumonia is associated with 15–20% of mortality in the geriatric patient. Preoperative exercise and incentive spirometry can decrease the postoperative complications in older patients, especially in smokers.

In general, the cardiac complication rate (i.e. arrhythmias, acute myocardial infarction, congestive heart failure and cardiac death) associated with general anesthesia and surgery should be approximately 0.2%. The presence of pre-existing cardiac disease, such as a recent myocardial infarction, increases the operative risk substantially. Better preoperative assessment and optimization has reduced this risk significantly.

There is a controversy about whether routine investigations for non-cardiac surgery are necessary in otherwise healthy patients. In the absence of any history or suspicion of cardiac disease based on a careful history and physical examination, a reasonable approach is not to subject the older patient routinely to unnecessary screening, other than a preoperative electrocardiogram. In the presence of potential or obvious cardiac disease, comprehensive evaluation is indicated[1].

Normal aging places the kidney at risk for injury during the perioperative period from ischemia and nephrotoxic drugs. Careful attention to the presence and control of predisposing conditions before surgery, appropriate dosing of nephrotoxic drugs and monitoring of the fluid status before, during and after the procedure are indicated.

Normal 'physiologic' aging is characterized by a gradual loss of reserve capacity. During periods of stress (such as a surgical procedure), the elderly may not meet the increased demand. This loss of reserve capacity is the single most important factor that decreases the patient's ability to tolerate surgery. It is imperative that the surgeon identifies those at increased risk for complications and considers alternative modalities of surgical treatment, such as minimally invasive surgery.

GASTROINTESTINAL SURGERY

Pharyngeal and esophageal surgery

During the evaluation for suspected esophageal disease, it should be borne in mind that older patients are susceptible to all disorders common in younger adults; some esophageal disorders are uniquely associated with age and must be specifically considered to avoid missed or delayed diagnosis (e.g. Zenker's diverticulum, cervical osteophyte and dysphagia due to aortic compression) accurate diagnosis may be difficult because symptoms of esophageal disease may be obscured or attributed to other co-existing disorders, e.g. chest pain due to esophageal spasm or gastroesophageal reflux, which may mimic coronary artery disease.

In patients aged 85 years and older, 15% describe some symptoms of swallowing dysfunction. Motility problems in the cricopharyngeous muscle can result in Zenker's diverticulum. Specifically, failure of the cricopharyngeal muscle to relax results in a herniation of mucosa above this muscle and below the thyropharyngeal muscle. Therapy for this condition must be individualized. In the presence of isolated upper sphincter dysmotility, cervical esophagomyotomy below the diverticulum with or without diverticulectomy can be performed. Successful treatment of pharyngoesophageal diverticulae in elderly debilitated patients can be achieved by endoscopic methods.

Achalasia is a disorder of esophageal motility, characterized by an aperistaltic esophagus, an elevated pressure of the lower esophageal sphincter (LES) and often incomplete LES relaxation with swallowing. Treatment options include pneumatic dilatation, which has a failure rate of 15–40%. Successful surgical outcome can be achieved by either thoracoscopic or laparoscopic surgery with minimal morbidity.

In addition to heartburn, older patients with gastroesophageal reflux can present with laryngitis, chronic cough, bronchitis, asthma and aspiration. Ordinarily patients refractory to medical treatment are referred for surgery. Before operative repair is considered, the presence of gastroesophageal reflux should be evaluated by endoscopy, 24-h pH monitoring and esophageal manometry. Successful repair by Nissen fundoplication has been reported in patients up to 71 years of age. Recently, similar success has been accomplished with the laparoscopic approach[2].

Esophageal cancer resection in the aged is a complicated problem because of the low surgical cure rate and high morbidity and mortality rates. Older patients are at increased risk for pulmonary, nutritional and anastamotic complications. After aggressive control of respiratory and nutritional status in the perioperative period, esophagectomy can be performed safely in older patients. The data from the recent literature suggest that age should not be a factor in the selection of treatment for carcinoma of the esophagus or cardia. No statistical difference was noted in the operative mortality rate, although the 30-day mortality was higher in the elderly (7.2%) than in the young (3%). Esophagectomy for carcinoma of the esophagus can be carried out with acceptable risk in the elderly[3,4].

Gastric surgery

Typically, in the geriatric population, peptic ulcer disease is associated with vague symptomatology. Pain is less commonly a presenting feature. More than 50% of elderly patients present with a complication as their first symptom, with melena the most frequent presentation[5]. The majority of gastric ulcers occur late in life, with a poorer outcome. Nearly two-thirds of peptic ulcer-related deaths arise from complications of gastric ulcers, and much of this increase in mortality can be attributed to delay in surgical treatment. The majority present with acute upper gastrointestinal hemorrhage from erosive gastritis, duodenal and gastric

Table I Mortality and morbidity rates by age for different surgical procedures

Surgery	Mortality ( )		Morbidity ( )		Reference no.
	< 70 years	> 70 years	< 70 years	> 70 years	
Esophagectomy	2.4	5.3	32.6	37.6	3
Gastrectomy	0.46	3	21.2	33.7	10
Laparoscopic cholecystectomy	0	0	6	18	13
Liver resection	1	5	50	51	16
Pancreaticoduodenectomy	2	4	32	33	18
Colectomy	5.0	1.7	30	39	22

ulcers. Early endoscopy is essential for diagnosis, assessing prognosis and instituting appropriate therapy. Endoscopic hemostatic ulcer therapy in patients with high-risk peptic ulcers (acute bleeding and non-bleeding visible vessel) decreases rebleeding and operation rate by 75% and mortality rate by 40%[6]. In a prospective randomized study, the mortality was 4% for early surgical therapy and 15% in the initial non-operative group. Early elective operation after initial endoscopic hemostasis is indicated: first, in the presence of co-morbid disease and/or hemodynamic instability with a visible vessel in the ulcer crater, or a large posterior duodenal ulcer or a large lesser curvature ulcer; second, in recurrent ulcer bleeding while hospitalized; and third, with a total blood transfusion exceeding 5 units[7].

Over the past decades the incidence of perforated peptic ulcer has declined in the young and men, but has risen among the elderly and women. About one of four ulcer perforations can be attributed to the use of non-steroidal anti-inflammatory drugs. A lethal outcome is 3.6 times as likely with perforated gastric ulcer when compared with perforated duodenal ulcer. The delay prior to surgical treatment is the most important determinant for mortality, complication rates and hospital costs. Patients with clinical peritonitis and suspected perforation should be operated upon without time-consuming evaluations[8].

Gastric carcinoma is predominantly a disease of older people today, with two-thirds of

cases occurring over age 65. More than one-quarter of patients have a history of gastric ulcer. Endoscopy and four-quadrant ulcer biopsy is a must in all elderly patients with gastric ulcer; early surgical intervention is indicated with unhealed, partially healed or recurrent gastric ulcer. Gastric resection provides the most effective therapy in terms of both cure and palliation[9].

Bittner and colleagues[10] recently compared the results of total gastrectomy for carcinoma of the stomach in 163 patients older than 70 years with those of 217 younger patients (Table 1). The presence of concomitant medical disease increased the risk for morbidity and mortality. Young patients without concomitant disease had a morbidity rate of 17%, and if they had concomitant disease the rate was 28%. The rates were similar in the older patients, at 21% and 31%, respectively. The authors attributed the improved operative results for gastric cancer to better preoperative management of concomitant disease, improved preoperative and postoperative nutrition, better operative technique, standardized preoperative antibiotics and prophylaxis for thromboembolic complications[10]. In well-selected cases, total gastrectomy with *en bloc* resection of invaded organs can be performed safely even in the elderly[11].

A frequently performed operation on the stomach in the elderly is gastrostomy. The indication is usually prolonged enteral nutrition in patients with dysphagia following a stroke, or patients with dementia, head and neck cancers, severe gastroesophageal reflux with aspiration, or prolonged decompression for intra-abdominal malignancies. Although the Stamm technique has been a standard procedure for over a century, percutaneous endoscopic gastrostomy (PEG) is the procedure of choice today.

Open gastrostomy is usually performed in those unable to undergo PEG because of the presence of obstructing pharyngeal or esophageal lesions and severe contractures. Complications from the procedure include peritonitis, wound infection and gastrointestinal bleeding, aspiration pneumonitis, tube migration and persistence of a gastrocutaneous fistula after tube removal. Complications unique to improper PEG placement include gastrocolic and gastroenteric fistulae.

Gallbladder and hepatic surgery

With aging, the incidence of gallstones increases. Gallstone disease in the older individual is different, in that the male/female ratio equalizes, the presentation is more acute and complication rates are higher. The reasons for increased incidence of gallstones are decreased metabolism of cholesterol with increased secretion into bile and diminished synthesis of bile acid by the liver. Decreased motility and reduced ejection fraction of the gallbladder promotes stasis and stone formation.

The presentation is typically late and as an emergency with complications, with higher morbidity and mortality rates. Whereas elective cholecystectomy has associated morbidity and mortality rates of 28% and 0.8%, respectively, emergency surgery is associated with rates of 66% and 19%, respectively[12]. Laparoscopic cholecystectomy has become the gold standard for symptomatic gallstone disease. The advantages of laparoscopic cholecystectomy over open cholecystectomy include less pain, shorter hospitalization and rapid return to usual activity. Most significant is the low rate of respiratory complications[13].

This approach is also applicable to acute cholecystitis[14].

Endoscopic sphincterotomy is safe for the management of complicated gallstone disease in the elderly. For common bile duct stones, endoscopic retrograde cholangiopancreatography with papillotomy has been advocated by some as the only therapy needed. The use of endoscopic retrograde cholangiopancreatography and percutaneous gallbladder drainage, to convert an emergency situation to an elective one, followed by subsequent cholecystectomy is an effective way of decreasing the morbidity and mortality in the frail geriatric patient.

Hemangiomas and cysts are the usual benign lesions in the elderly, the clinical significance being to distinguish these from metastatic lesions. Hepatocellular carcinoma is the most common primary liver malignancy. Surgical resection is the primary modality of treatment for cure. Morbidity and mortality rates after hepatic resection are comparable in young and old, indicating that surgery should not be avoided on the basis of age alone[15,16].

Metastases from gastrointestinal tract primary tumors are the most common type referred for resection. Tumors of the liver are 20 times more likely to be metastatic disease rather than primary cancers. Patients undergoing resection have a 30% 5-year survival rate compared to 0% for those who do not undergo resection. In one study, 5-year survival rates for patients with primary tumor resection were between 18% and 76%, with no differences noted between younger and older patients[17].

Pancreatic surgery

Acute pancreatitis causes significant morbidity in the geriatric population. Gallstones are the most common basis, followed by alcohol. Other causes of acute pancreatitis include operative trauma, endoscopic retrograde cholangiopancreatography (ERCP) and ischemia, especially with cardiac and aneurysmal surgery.

In the elderly, acute pancreatitis may manifest as a mild illness with pain as the predominant symptom and few abdominal signs. The morbidity and mortality rates from acute pancreatitis are higher in this age group. Most authors consider age above 55 years as a significant risk factor for death. Laparoscopic cholecystectomy with either preoperative ERCP or intraoperative cholangiography can be performed for gallstone pancreatitis during the same hospital admission without significantly increased risk, regardless of age.

Pancreatic adenocarcinoma increases steadily with age, from 14 cases per 100 000 for those 50–59 years to 115 cases per 100 000 for individuals older than 80 years[18]. Although Whipple's original procedure carried a high mortality rate (20–25%), studies in the mid- to late 1980s showed that the operation could be performed with lower (2–5%) mortality. For well-selected patients and in experienced hands, this complicated procedure is safe even in those over 70 years[19].

Appendicitis

Older patients present atypically with minimal abdominal discomfort. Absence of initial fever, and leukocytosis, are probably the result of a depressed immune response. Anatomically, the appendix in aged individuals is usually atrophic with decreased lymphatic tissue, which may contribute to a more rapid progression of the inflammatory process and earlier perforation. Perforations are more common among older patients than younger patients (35% vs. 13%) and are associated with treatment delay[20]. Delays in presentation, diagnosis and eventual treatment result in higher morbidity and mortality rates.

Even though it is estimated currently that only 5–10% of all patients with appendicitis are in the geriatric age group, they account for more than 50% of the deaths associated with appendicitis. A delay from the onset of symptoms to operation of more than 37 h was associated with a 72% perforation rate compared with 41% in those operated on before 37 h[21]. Early diagnosis and aggressive intervention are therefore vital for successful management.

Colorectal surgery

Colonic diseases increase in incidence as age progresses. More than 50% of the overall population has colonic pseudodiverticulae by age 80. In the elderly, diverticular disease presents with marked phlegmonous inflammation, colonic obstruction and fistulization resulting in increased morbidity and mortality. Complications of diverticular disease include bleeding and perforation, which needs surgical intervention if a conservative approach fails. Patients with free perforated diverticulitis require emergency resection of the sigmoid colon, proximal end colostomy of the descending colon and stapled closure of the rectum (Hartmann's procedure). Diverticular abscess is best managed initially by percutaneous drainage followed by elective sigmoid colectomy with primary anastomosis. In selected complicated patients (stricture and fistula) resection and primary anastomosis is performed, with low morbidity and mortality[22].

Sigmoid volvulus is believed to increase in frequency after age 60 because of increased mobility of the redundant sigmoid colon about its elongated mesentery. Risk factors for sigmoid volvulus include chronic constipation and institutionalization. Non-operative detorsion with flexible sigmoidoscopy is the initial treatment of choice, with a mortality of 0%. Emergency surgery is indicated for gangrene and for failure of non-operative decompression[23].

There is a decrease in rectal sphincter tone, pressures and rectal sensation with aging. These result in disorders of defecation, specifically incontinence and impaction. Other dysmotilities in the rectum include

Table 2 Mortality (%) by type of surgery in common surgical procedures

Surgery	Elective	Emergency	Reference no.
Cholecystectomy	0.8	19	12
Colectomy	3	21	24
Abdominal aortic aneurysm repair	8.6	59	29
Hernia repair	0	10	36

internal intussusception and rectal prolapse. Low anterior resection, rectopexy, or local transanal excision have acceptable morbidity and mortality.

Ischemic colitis can be acute or chronic, with reversible or irreversible ischemic changes. Initial treatment is usually conservative, but if the changes are progressive surgical exploration must be performed for resection of ischemic bowel.

The incidence of colonic cancer increases with age. Although the overall incidence of colonic neoplasia in the USA is 17 per 100 000 population, in men and women older than 85 years the incidence is 239 cases per 100 000 population. Concomitant medical disease is more important than chronological age in predicting the postoperative outcome for colonic surgery[24]. The clinical presentation influences outcome. A high percentage needs emergency surgery, which translates to more complicated disease and higher mortality. In those over the age of 80, Spivack and co-workers found that the mortality rate of elective resection was 3% and for emergency resection was 21%[25]. Once again, an emergency situation was a more influential factor than the patient's chronological age.

Surprisingly, cancer in the elderly is frequently treated poorly, with the percentage of patients receiving definitive treatment declining with increasing age. Following surgery for colorectal cancer, 5-year survival was related to stage and type of operation and not to age. The risk of 5-year mortality for stage I patients was 0.214 times the risk faced by stage IV patients, and the risk of

mortality after resection was roughly a third of the risk after palliative colostomy or non-surgical treatment. Age should no longer be perceived as a 'risk factor' in decision making; rather, associated medical conditions need to be optimized (Table 2)[26]. With recent advancement in minimally invasive surgery, laparoscopic colectomy is performed with increasing frequency and encouraging results. Earlier oral intake and earlier discharge from the hospital with no difference in morbidity were observed in laparoscopic assisted colectomy compared to open colectomy[27].

CARDIOTHORACIC AND VASCULAR SURGERY

Cardiac surgery is generally well tolerated in the elderly, with good functional outcome and long-term performance status following surgery[28].

Under elective conditions and with well-managed concomitant disease, vascular surgery can be both safe and effective. In 1994, Perler reviewed the results, pooled from seven studies of repair of ruptured abdominal aortic aneurysms in 176 patients older than 65[29]. The survival rate from ruptured aneurysms was 59%. On the other hand, in a review of 834 patients aged 65–80, pooled from ten studies, the mortality rate from elective aneurysm repair was 8.6%. Unfortunately, despite the safety of elective surgery, patients are still treated conservatively, due to an incorrect assumption that the operative mortality in this group is unacceptably high. The decision to proceed with elective abdominal aortic aneurysm should be based on the size of the aneurysm and the physiologic age of the patient rather than chronological age. In a medically stable patient it is recommended to perform elective repair for abdominal aortic aneurysm larger than 5 cm in diameter. For smaller aneurysms serial ultrasound examinations should be conducted every 6 months, with planned elective repair if the size increases more than 0.5 cm between examinations or reaches 5 cm in diameter.

A similar situation prevails in the case of carotid artery disease. Octogenarians are not referred for operation despite several studies suggesting that endarterectomy is safe, carries minimal mortality and prevents strokes. Perler noted a stroke rate from surgery of 2.8% in the age group of 65–80 and mortality rate of 2.4%. Survival after endarterectomy in patients older than 80 years is similar to that for the general population[29]. Indications in the octogenarian include high-grade carotid occlusive lesions, hemispheric symptoms and well-controlled concomitant disease.

Limb salvage operation is indicated for ischemic rest pain, non-healing ulcers and frank gangrene. In a study of 262 patients 80 years of age or older undergoing lower extremity arterial reconstruction, the 30-day perioperative mortality rate was 2.3% and the limb salvage rate at 5 years was 92%. The postoperative residential status and ambulatory function scores remained the same or improved in 88% and 78% of patients, respectively. Lower extremity arterial reconstruction even in the very elderly preserves not only the limb but also residential status and ambulatory function[30].

Placement of transluminal endovascular stents has been used successfully to treat thoracic aneurysms, abdominal aortic aneurysms, peripheral aneurysms, aortoiliac occlusive disease and femoropopliteal occlusive disease, especially in high-risk elderly patients with minimal morbidity. The procedures can be performed under local anesthesia with intravenous sedation.

HEAD AND NECK SURGERY

Thyroid

As age progresses, the incidence of thyroid nodules increase. Exposure to ionizing radiation increases the incidence of thyroid cancers. Because radiation treatment for benign diseases such as tonsillitis, hemangiomas, thymic enlargement and lymphadenopathy has not been practiced for many years, most patients with these entities are now in the older age group. Tissue diagnosis preoperatively by fine needle aspiration testing is mandatory. Anaplastic thyroid carcinoma and thyroid lymphoma are both treated non-operatively. Thyroid surgery in the elderly is usually well tolerated. Thyroid carcinoma carries a higher mortality rate, suggesting that older adults present later in the course of the disease, are more susceptible to metastatic spread of cancer, or have more malignant variants.

Parathyroids

There is a higher prevalence of hyperparathyroidism, especially the sporadic type, in the elderly. It is believed that up to 1.5–3% of hospitalized geriatric persons may have this disease. Operative intervention for primary hyperparathyroidism is safe and usually successful. The reported morbidity rates are 8–18% and mortality rates 0–2%, with cure rates of 99.5%.

BREAST SURGERY

Breast cancer incidence and mortality increase with advancing age. Half of all breast cancers occur in woman older than 65 years of age. The incidence of breast cancer in patients older than 65 years is 322 cases per 100 000 population compared to 60 cases in patients younger than 65 years[31].

The patient care evaluation survey for breast carcinoma conducted by the Commission on Cancer of the American College of Surgeons reflected that several differences exist in the detection, diagnostic methods, stage at diagnosis, treatment approaches and outcome of breast cancer in the elderly woman compared with younger women[32]. Stage at diagnosis appears to be more advanced in the elderly. Overall disease-specific survival was worse in the elderly, but when analyzed by stage, was significantly different for only certain stages. Similarly, the Canadian study suggested that less aggressive patterns of care are provided to older patients with breast cancer independent of co-morbidity. This could explain, at least in part, the sustained poor results in this population[33].

Morbidity and mortality rates from mastectomy are low. In a study by Morrow, who reviewed eight studies with patients ranging from older than 65 years to older than 80 years, the mortality rate ranged from 1 to 4.5%, and the morbidity rate was between 7% and 20%[34]. A false perception that breast cancer in the elderly is a slow, relatively benign process may predispose the physician to treat the disease less aggressively. The results of good surgical and adjunctive therapy for elderly women are as good as those for younger women. It is not appropriate to deny older patients therapies that will decrease the frequency of recurrence and improve their overall quality of life.

Elderly patients typically present with clinically palpable lesions. Co-morbid illnesses usually preclude operative intervention, and simple local control of the disease should then be the goal of therapy. A tissue diagnosis can be established with bedside fine needle aspirate or core needle biopsy, and the treatment can then be individualized. Significant improvement in the local control and lower recurrence rates can be achieved by wide excision. Tamoxifen therapy alone can be used for these frail patients. Multiple trials have demonstrated response rates from 10% to 50%, and failure rates between 23% and 58%[35]. The response to treatment usually takes more than 12 months.

For patients older than 70 years, tamoxifen is frequently administered regardless of the node or receptor status, and axillary lymph node dissection may therefore not be necessary. Local control of the axillary area in these patients can be achieved by including this area in the port of radiation.

HERNIA REPAIR

The incidence of abdominal wall hernia in the elderly age group is approximately 13 per 1000 people. Of all hernias, 70% are inguinal, 10% ventral, 6% femoral, 3% umbilical and 1% esophageal hiatal. Although 85% of all groin hernias occur in men, 84% of femoral hernias occur in women[36]. Repair of a groin hernia can be performed as an out-patient procedure with either epidural anesthesia or local anesthesia with intravenous sedation, with low mortality even in the presence of co-morbidities. The technique of tensionless mesh plug hernioplasty, in which a preformed mesh plug is placed into the defect and an on-lay patch is placed over the repair, reduces the dissection of tissue and operation time. This procedure is well tolerated as an out-patient procedure even in the frail elderly patient, and the recurrence rate is low.

Even in patients over age 80 with significant co-morbidity, elective repair can be performed with near zero mortality and morbidity (as low as 5%). In contrast, emergency hernia repair carries significant morbidity (> 50%) and mortality (8–14%), largely because of bowel incarceration on presentation, and up to 30% of patients requiring intestinal resection. Unfortunately, 15–20% of herniorrhaphies in older patients in the USA and UK are performed for incarceration and small bowel obstruction[37].

TRAUMA AND EMERGENCY SURGERY

Age-related changes lead to diminished peripheral vision, impaired hearing, decreased stability of gait, an increased likelihood of syncopal episodes and increased tendency to fracture. Accidents are the fifth leading cause of death in people older than 65, and falls constitute two-thirds of these accidental deaths[38].

After the age of 80 years, falls are the most common form of fatal injury[39]. The mortality following trauma in patients older than 65 years is 27% when compared to younger patients, in whom it is 14%. The Major Trauma Outcome Study from the American College of Surgeons has also shown that, when controlled for severity of injury by the injury severity score, survival is lower in patients of 65 years or more in every group of trauma.

Head trauma in the elderly individual carries a high mortality rate. Older patients take longer to recover from head trauma than younger patients and require more intensive rehabilitation. Special consideration needs to be given to the elderly, in the form of monitoring systemic perfusion through the use of invasive monitoring and intracranial perfusion with a cranial pressure-monitoring device.

Burn injuries are another common cause for morbidity in elderly patients, and comprise approximately 8–10% of total trauma. The elderly are at risk for burns because of impaired vision, decreased reaction time, depressed alertness and decreased pain sensation. In general, burns over 40% of total body surface area in older individuals suggest a poor prognosis, due to concomitant medical disease: burn wound sepsis and multisystem failure.

Several reports have suggested that emergency surgery carries significant mortality and morbidity in the elderly population. Higher complication rates result for identical diseases compared to the young, due to delay in presentation, diagnosis and treatment. Some illnesses are more severe in the elderly, such as peptic ulcer, and appendiceal, colonic and gallstone disease. Early referral for elective management of treatable disease, a high index of suspicion in patients with abdominal pain and early surgery are some of the ways to ensure a favorable outcome and maintain a good quality of life for the patient.

SURGERY IN THE NURSING HOME PATIENT

At the age of 65 years, 10–20% of individuals are expected to become dependent on others for one or more basic activities of daily living including bathing, dressing, transfers and eating. This proportion increases to 25% at 75 years and 50% at 85 years. Many of these patients will need chronic nursing care. Several studies have shown that approximately 43% of people older than 65 years are expected to enter nursing homes before they die.

A recent study on nursing home patients has suggested that, while decubitus care, stoma and enteral tube care made up a large proportion (33%) of surgical referrals, common surgical diseases of the abdomen, breast and vascular system still accounted for 55% of consultations. In patients undergoing major abdominal and vascular procedures, there was a higher complication rate than in those undergoing lesser procedures (18% vs. 6%), but there was no difference in the 30-day mortality rate (10% vs. 6%) or the 18-month actuarial survival rate (33% vs. 32%), respectively[40]. Multivariate analysis for the risk of death revealed that the overall survival was adversely affected primarily by the presence of coronary artery disease (relative risk (RR) 3.27), dementia (RR 2.39) and age older than 70 (RR 2.03), and unaffected by the need for surgery, the magnitude of the procedure performed, sex, the number of co-morbid conditions or medications or whether a preoperative 'do not resuscitate' (DNR) order was written. While the overall survival of these frail elderly patients is poor, surgical procedures do not influence overall survival, and can be performed with reasonable outcome.

SUMMARY

As the population ages, more older patients will present for treatment of surgical disease. The frailty of this population and anticipated increased use of nursing homes will bring forth a new population with different medical goals and expectations. The goal of surgical treatment in the frail elderly patient may be basically similar to that of a normal healthy patient; the ultimate goals of such therapy are quite different. Although we still focus on maximizing life span, social and ethical issues and the quality of life become more important. When treating patients in the later years of life, our focus must shift from maximizing survival to maximizing the quality of life, maintaining dignity and minimizing suffering.

These different goals should not mean that aggressive surgical therapy is not indicated in the healthy or frail older adult patient. Emergency surgery carries a high mortality. In contrast, in this era of excellent perioperative care and less invasive surgical techniques, elective surgery is safe in the healthy or even the frail elderly. Use of newer techniques in the field of interventional radiology and aggressive endoscopic procedures can convert emergency situations to elective ones. However, early referral for elective management of a treatable disease is imperative for ensuring a favorable outcome.

Research over the past several decades regarding the perioperative risk in elderly patients suggests that advanced age *per se* only minimally increases the operative risk as compared to the risk of the disease process. Educating patients, family members and internists about the role and risks of surgical procedures, dealing with issues such as withdrawal or withholding support, and issues of enforcing DNR orders in the operating room should most certainly be co-ordinated between the surgeon, physician and anesthesiologist.

References

1. Zenilman M. Surgery in the elderly. *Curr Probl Surg* 1998;35:99–179
2. Khajanchee YS, Urbach DR, Butler N, *et al.* Laparoscopic antireflux surgery in the elderly. *Surg Endosc* 2002;16:25–30
3. Ellis HF Jr, Williamson WA, Heatley GJ. Cancer of the esophagus and cardia: does age influence treatment selection and surgical outcomes? *J Am Coll Surg* 1998;187:345–51
4. Poon RTP, Law SYK, Chu KM, *et al.* Esophagectomy for carcinoma of the esophagus in the elderly. Results of current surgical management. *Ann Sur* 1998;227:357–64
5. McCarthy DM. Acid peptic disease in the elderly. *Clin Geriatr Med* 1991;7:231–54
6. Kolkman JJ, Meuwissen SG. A review on treatment of bleeding peptic ulcer: a collaborative task of gastroenterologist and surgeon. *Scand J Gastroenterol Suppl* 1996;218:16–25
7. Cochran TA. Bleeding peptic ulcer: surgical therapy. *Gastroenterol Clin North Am* 1993;22:751–78
8. Svanes C. Trends in perforated peptic ulcer: incidence, etiology, treatment, and prognosis. *World J Surg* 2000;24:277–83
9. Sawyers JC. Gastric carcinoma. *Curr Probl Surg* 1995;32:103–78
10. Bittner R, Butters M, Ulrich M, *et al.* Total gastrectomy: updated operative mortality and long-term survival with particular reference to patients older than 70 years of age. *Ann Surg* 1996;224:37–42
11. Kim JP, Kim SJ, Lee JH, Kim SW, Choi MG, Yu HJ. Surgery in the aged in Korea. *Arch Surg* 1998;133:18–23
12. Houghton PWJ, Jenkinson LR, Donaldson LA. Cholecystectomy in the elderly: a prospective study. *Br J Surg* 1985;72:220–2

13. Magnuson TH, Ratner LE, Zenilman ME, Bender JS. Laparoscopic cholecystectomy: applicability to the geriatric population. *Am Surg* 1997;63:91–96

14. Lo CM, Lai EC, Fan ST, *et al.* Laparoscopic cholecystectomy for acute cholecystitis in the elderly. *World J Surg* 1996;20:983–6

15. Hanazaki K, Kajikawa S, Shimozawa N, *et al.* Hepatic resection for hepatocellular carcinoma in the elderly. *J Am Coll Surg* 2001;192:38–46

16. Fong Y, Blumgart LH, Fortner JG, Brennan MF. Pancreatic or liver resection for malignancy is safe and effective for the elderly. *Ann Surg* 1995;222:426–37

17. Takenaka K, Shimada M, Higashi H, *et al.* Liver resection for hepatocellular carcinoma in the elderly. *Arch Surg* 1994;129:846–50

18. Reila A, Zinsmeister AR, Melton LJ III, *et al.* Increasing incidence of pancreatic cancer among women in Olmsted County, Minnesota, 1940–1988. *Mayo Clin Proc* 1992;67:839–45

19. Hannoun L, Christophe M, Ribeiro J, *et al.* A report of forty-four instances of pancreaticoduodenal resection in patients more than seventy years of age. *Surg Gynecol Obstet* 1993;177:556–60

20. Kraemer M, Franke C, Ohmann C, Yang Q. Acute appendicitis in late adulthood: incidence, presentation, and outcome. Results of a prospective multicenter acute abdominal pain and a review of the literature. *Langenbecks Arch Surg* 2000;385:470–81

21. Lau WY, Fan ST, Yiu TF, Chu DW, Lee JM. Acute appendicitis in the elderly. *Surg Gynecol Obstet* 1985;161:157–60

22. Wong WD, Wexner SD, Lowry A, *et al.* Practice parameter for the treatment of sigmoid diverticulitis – supporting documentation. *Dis Colon Rectum* 2000;43:290–7

23. Peoples JB, McCafferty JC, Scher KS. Operative therapy for sigmoid volvulus. Identification of risk factors affecting outcome. *Dis Colon Rectum* 1990;33:643–6

24. Boyd JB, Bradford B Jr, Watne AL. Operative risk factors of colon resection in the elderly. *Ann Surg* 1980;192:743–6

25. Spivak H, Maele DV, Friedman I, Nussbaum M. Colorectal surgery in octogenarians. *J Am Coll Surg* 1996;183:46–50

26. Agarwal N, Leighton L, Mandile MA, Cayten CG. Outcomes of surgery for colorectal cancer in patients age 80 years and older. *Am J Gastroenterol* 1990;85:1096–101

27. Delgado S, Lacy AM, Valdecasas JC, *et al.* Could age be an indication for laparoscopic colectomy in colorectal cancer? *Surg Endosc* 2000;14:22–6

28. Khan JH, McElhinney DB, Hall TS, Merrick SH. Cardiac valve surgery in octogenarians improving quality of life and functional status. *Arch Surg* 1998;133:887–93

29. Perler BA. Vascular disease in the elderly patient. *Surg Clin North Am* 1994;74:199–216

30. Pomposelli FB Jr, Arora S, Gibbons GW, *et al.* Lower extremity arterial reconstruction in the elderly: successful outcome preserves not only the limb but also residential status and ambulatory function. *J Vasc Surg* 1998;28:215–25

31. Yancik R, Ries LG, Yates JW. Breast cancer in aging women: a population-based study of contrasts in stage, surgery, and survival. *Cancer* 1989;63:976–81

32. Busch E, Kemeny M, Fremgen A, *et al.* Patterns of breast cancer care in the elderly. *Cancer* 1996;78:101–11

33. Herbert-Croteau N, Brisson J, Latreille J, *et al.* Compliance with consensus recommendations for the treatment of early breast carcinoma in elderly women. *Cancer* 1999;85:1104–13

34. Morrow M. Breast disease in elderly women. *Surg Clin North Am* 1994;74:145–61

35. Robertson J, Ellis I, Elston C, *et al.* Mastectomy or tamoxifen as initial therapy in operable breast cancer in elderly patients: 5 year follow up. *Eur J Cancer Clin Oncol* 1992;28A:908–10

36. Nyhus LM, Bombeck CT, Klein MS. Hernias. In Sabiston DC, ed. *Textbook of surgery*, 14th edn. Philadelphia: WB Saunders, 1991:1134–49

37. Rosenthal RA. Small bowel disorders and abdominal wall hernia in the elderly patient. *Surg Clin North Am* 1994;74: 261–91

38. Rubenstein LZ. Falls in the elderly: a clinical approach (Topics in Primary Care Medicine). *West J Med* 1983;138:273–5

39. Scwab CW, Kauder DR. Trauma in the geriatric patient. *Arch Surg* 1992;127:701–6

40. Zenilman ME, Bender J, Magnuson TH, Smith GW. General surgical care in the nursing home patient: results of a dedicated geriatric surgery consult service. *J Am Coll Surg* 1996;183:361–70

14 Physical medicine and rehabilitation in older adults

Maria de Araujo, MD, *and Mario Nelson*, MD

DEFINITION OF TERMS

Rehabilitation is defined as the development of a person to the fullest potential consistent with his or her impairment and environmental limitations.

Impairment, disability and handicap definitions according to the World Health Organization are provided in Table 1[1]. Physicians have recognized the benefits of early ambulation and that unnecessary bedrest and immobility lead to physiologic changes in persons who are chronically sick, aged or disabled and are particularly susceptible to the adverse effect of immobilization. Immobility reduces the functional reserve of the musculoskeletal system and functional capacity of the cardiovascular system, resulting in weakness[2]. Early rehabilitation intervention may prevent deconditioning, maximize function and improve quality of life in older adults, the main goal being to help achieve independence. The patient and the caregiver must be involved in decision making in regard to his or her management.

THE REHABILITATION TEAM MEMBERS AND THEIR ROLES

To minimize the risk of a debilitating hospital stay, the integration of an interdisciplinary and/or multidisciplinary team into hospital care may help ensure that patients will

Table 1 Definitions according to the World Health Organization, reference 1

Term	Definition
Impairment	any loss or abnormality of function
Disability	any restriction resulting from an impairment of the ability to perform an activity, which is considered normal for a person
Handicap	any disadvantage resulting from impairment or disability that limits or prevents the fulfillment of a role that is normal for an individual

embark on an early mobilization program and that the rehabilitation plans and goals are properly formulated. Geriatricians and physiatrists (specialists in physical medicine and rehabilitation) are often members of interdisciplinary teams, while most primary care physicians function in the multidisciplinary setting. The interdisciplinary team members (Table 2) meet periodically to discuss management, progress and discharge planning. The physician evaluates the medical and functional deficits of the patient, and designs a plan for treatment based on the potential for rehabilitation and goal setting, with the help of team members. If an older patient lives alone and has memory deficits, an occupational therapist may help with home evaluation, to determine whether it is safe

Table 2 The rehabilitation team members and their roles

Team member	Roles
Physician	evaluates the medical and functional deficits
	designs a plan for treatment based on the potential for rehabilitation
Patient and caregiver	participate in goal setting, plan for treatment and carry out instructions given by team members
Physical therapist	further assesses the strength, range of motion, balance and co-ordination
	evaluates the need for mobility aids
	performs exercise training
	applies modalities (e.g. heat, cold, electrical stimulation)
Occupational therapist	evaluates activities of daily living, cognition, safety and assistive devices (e.g. splints, wheelchairs)
Speech therapist	evaluates speech, language and swallowing abilities; helps improve communication skills and swallowing adaptation mechanisms
Rehabilitation nurse	attends to the patient's needs
	ensures that patients practice skills acquired during therapy
	ensures proper bed position and skin care
Social worker	provides counseling (coping with disability, finance, equipment and/or need for placement)
	facilitates patient's discharge
Audiologist	performs audiometric studies
	evaluates need for hearing aids
Dietitian	evaluates nutrition needs; advises type of diet

to discharge the patient home, and, in co-ordination with a physical therapist, assess the need for health aids.

Many patients have difficulty in coping with a new disability and may need the intervention of a psychologist. Depression is common in older adults with rehabilitation needs, and may necessitate the intervention of a geriatric psychiatrist. Orthotists and prosthetists play a role in providing devices to improve function. The social worker should provide counseling and assess financial, equipment and environmental issues to help patients and caregivers cope with disability. The recreation therapist encourages participation in the rehabilitation program and improves motivation for leisure activity.

Family members, environment modifications and home care services make an impact on choice of the location to provide rehabilitation to the older adult. All members of the rehabilitation team are responsible for the education of patients and family about the risks for pressure ulcers, and implementation of preventive measures. Co-morbid conditions, such as urinary tract infection, confusion and depression may interfere with rehabilitation. Avoiding prolonged immobilization, chronic use of indwelling catheters and unnecessary medications may reduce the risk of some of these problems.

Visual impairment is a major factor contributing to loss of balance and risk for falls. In patients with diabetes, especially with peripheral neuropathy, visual impairment further decreases independence in ambulation. Caregivers are instructed to inspect the diabetic feet for skin damage, which leads to advanced lesions (ulcers). Properly fitting shoes, modified to distribute pressure, will prevent ulceration in insensate feet. Hearing loss in patients older than 65 years may be significant. Audiometric evaluation is offered and a hearing aid provided. Older adults are sometimes reluctant to use hearing aids, however, due to uncomfortable fit and sound distortion. Adaptation techniques for vision, hearing and communication impairments, and also for assistive devices, will encourage independence.

AGING AND THE MUSCULOSKELETAL SYSTEM

Normal aging has an effect on skeletal muscle, in both structure and function: muscle mass decreases, strength diminishes, the rate of contraction slows and the resistance to fatigue is reduced[3]. Muscle endurance relative to maximum strength does not appear to diminish with age. The loss of muscle mass has been related to a reduction in the total number of muscle fibers or a reduction in size of type II fibers[4]. The decline of muscle strength may be due to reduction in the number of functioning motor units and change in the pattern of activity, leading to disuse of certain muscles. It may be reversible if the older adult is physically active. Stiffness is usually present due to changes in the connective tissues of tendons, ligaments, joint capsules and muscles. In the bone there are changes in the pattern of bone deposition and resorption, leading to osteoporosis.

REHABILITATION OF COMMON GERIATRIC DISORDERS

Deconditioning

Effects of prolonged bed rest and immobilization are commonly encountered by the physiatrist, in the hospital and skilled nursing facility, resulting in deconditioning. Changes in musculoskeletal, cardiovascular, neuropsychological and skin systems, among others, lead to complications, especially in older adults. Some of these changes may be minimized by judicious prescription of bedrest[5], or may be reversible through a comprehensive rehabilitation program.

Musculoskeletal system

Prolonged immobilization decreases muscle strength and endurance. Lack of joint mobility leads to restriction in the periarticular connective tissue, and shortening of tendons and muscles, causing contracture of joints. This mainly involves the hips and knees, as these joints are kept flexed when lying in bed or sitting for a prolonged time. Several changes occur in bone as a result of decreased muscular activity, lack of stress on the bones and complex endocrine and metabolic reactions, leading to osteoporosis.

Cardiovascular system

Bedrest increases the resting pulse rate; following bedrest there is a more pronounced increase in the heart rate with exercise[6]. Orthostatic hypotension, also common after bedrest, may be in part due to intravascular volume depletion, compounded by an increase in venous pooling in the lower extremities.

Immobilization is a risk for thrombotic complications from stasis due to reduced muscular pumping of blood from the lower extremities and increased blood viscosity.

Central nervous system

Prolonged inactivity and confinement causes intellectual deficit and emotional disturbances, probably due to sensory deprivation, decreased motor activity, poor balance and loss of co-ordination. Peripheral neuropathy may occur in elderly patients, especially those with diabetes and end-stage renal disease as well as those on chemotherapy. When confined to bed or a chair, these individuals should be monitored for signs of compression neuropathy[7].

Integumentary system

Changes in skin lead to increased risk of breakdown when exposed to continuous pressure, moisture and shearing forces. Altered mental status, from disease or medication, increases this risk. Frequent changing of the position of patients while in bed, relief of pressure, good skin care and toileting, and proper transfer technique will help prevent skin breakdown.

Management

Although the adverse effects of immobilization do not spare any age or gender, the geriatric population is particularly vulnerable. Prevention of complications of bedrest and immobilization is one of the goals in rehabilitation. Proper positioning in bed and avoiding placement of pillows under the knees will minimize flexion contracture of knees and hips. Instruction is given for early mobilization, active range of motion exercises and to lie prone to stretch the joints, a few times a day. If the patient has weakness, passive range of motion should be performed. Splinting may be used to position a joint in a functional position, if there is a risk for contracture of a particular joint, such as in 'foot drop'. Standing (during transfers) and sitting (in a chair) may prevent some of the cardiovascular deconditioning. Wrapping of the lower extremities helps prevent pooling of blood in the legs and minimizes orthostasis. Exercise training serves as a physiologic stimulus that increases energy metabolism of the active muscle and, proportionally, cardiovascular function[8]. The successful application of acute exercises to enhance orthostatic stability, daily endurance exercise to maintain aerobic capacity, or specific resistance exercises to maintain musculoskeletal integrity constitute effective rehabilitation management of patients deconditioned after prolonged bedrest[9].

Arthritis

A common complaint in the elderly population is joint pain secondary to 'arthritis'. Many patients think that it is normal to have pain in the joints with age. Osteoarthritis is the most common form of arthritis in older adults, but it should not be considered a normal feature of aging, as changes found in cartilage from asymptomatic older subjects are quite different from those seen in osteoarthritic cartilage[10]. Osteoarthritis of the knee impacts on daily activities, such as dressing, transferring and walking, and pain may cause sleep disturbances[11]. Prolonged immobilization and inactivity to avoid pain leads to decreased range of motion of the painful joint. The elderly often resist using a needed assistive device, such as a cane or walker, due to concern about looking disabled. The consequences of inactivity exacerbate the problems associated with aging and arthritis, increasing the risk for functional dependence[12]. Quadriceps and gluteus medius muscle weakness is prevalent in patients with osteoarthritis of the knee and hip, respectively. Current treatments focus on pain management and improvement of function[13], through a comprehensive rehabilitation program, consisting of modalities such as heat, cold and electrical stimulation, range of motion and strengthening exercises, instruction in energy and joint conservation techniques and education in behavior modification. Studies of community-dwelling older adults with symptomatic knee osteoarthritis show improvements in physical performance, pain and disability after participating in either an aerobic or a resistance exercise program[14]. Assistive devices should be used for ambulation.

Total joint replacement is indicated when advanced arthritis causes severe pain and functional limitation that does not respond to conservative treatment, including analgesics, non-steroidal anti-inflammatory drugs and physical therapy[15]. Hip and knee are the common joints replaced. Rehabilitation should start on the first day after surgery, including range of motion and strengthening exercises of key muscles, progressing to transfers and ambulation training with a walker. Most surgeons utilize continuous passive motion machines for patients with knee replacement to maintain good range and decrease edema. Early mobilization of the limbs will help reduce the risk of deep vein thrombosis.

Stroke

Stroke is the most common vascular neurological disorder of the elderly. Processes affecting the blood vessels include thrombosis, embolism, rupture of a vessel, vasculitis and hypertensive arteriosclerotic change[16]. Stroke is associated with significant morbidity and mortality. Psychosocial and environmental factors play a role in disability seen in stroke[17].

In-patient rehabilitation programs appear to facilitate recovery following a stroke, although the effect upon neurologic improvement is controversial. Treatment of stroke patients in a dedicated unit has demonstrated advantages over general neurologic or medical wards, in terms of decreased mortality and reduced length of stay[18]. Improvement after stroke, from neurological recovery, usually occurs in the first few months, with improvement of function, and better quality of life. The patient's capabilities and prior level of functioning should be assessed, and measurable goals established with the patient and caregiver. Post-discharge out-patient treatment helps further improvement in mobility[19].

Rehabilitation should begin as soon as the patient has stabilized, usually on the first or second day after onset of the stroke. The environment is very important; patients should be taken to the gym for therapy, a measure that improves motivation. Kitchen evaluation may help determine the ability of the patient to function at home. Therapy started in the acute stage in the hospital will continue at home, in the out-patient department, in the acute rehabilitation facility or in long-term care settings. The functional status of the patient and the type of social support available helps determine the appropriate setting for therapy. During the acute stage, the patient should be monitored for swallowing deficits. The speech therapist will work with the nutritionist, nurses and family to ensure appropriate diet and precautions during feeding to prevent aspiration, and to minimize the risk of skin breakdown, contractures and decrease in endurance. Visual field and sensory deficits interfere with the rehabilitation process, and if identified early allow the therapist to incorporate adaptation techniques. Lack of motivation for engaging in rehabilitation may be due to depression. Counseling and discussion of the disease process with patient and family may be of help.

As motor function returns, synergistic movements may appear (patient unable to isolate joint movements). If the lower extremity presents with flexor synergism, as the patient tries to stand up, the hip and knee will flex and the patient will be unable to stand. Usually an extension synergism is present; here, an ankle–foot orthosis may be prescribed if there is difficulty in control of the ankle during walking, to improve gait and safety. Most older patients will need a walking aid following a stroke.

Communication and swallowing disorders in addition to bladder and bowel incontinence, are factors contributing to institutionalization.

Parkinson's disease

Parkinson's disease is a degenerative brain disorder with peak incidence between the ages of 60 and 70 years. The etiology of Parkinson's disease is usually idiopathic, but encephalitis, arteriosclerosis, anoxia, trauma or drug factors may be contributory[20]. The common manifestations include tremor, rigidity, bradykinesia, loss of flexibility, postural changes, gait disturbances, dysarthria and dementia. The gait may be slow and shuffling, with loss of associated arm movements.

Physical therapy plays a role in management, to prevent contractures, and to maintain strength, good posture and safe ambulation. Cognitive stimulation and speech training are part of the rehabilitation program. Studies suggest that patients with Parkinson's disease on exercise programs improved gait, grip strength and motor co-ordination for tasks requiring fine control and spine flexibility[21,22]. Strength can be gained through resistance training, as in other older adults[23].

Amputation

Rehabilitation of the geriatric amputee requires special consideration. Associated medical problems, such as cardiac failure, end-stage renal disease and arthritis, among others, complicate rehabilitation.

Peripheral vascular disease, from arteriosclerosis and diabetes, accounts for 90% of the amputations in the elderly. Morbidity and mortality are increased with amputation, the higher mortality being seen during the first few postoperative years, especially among above-the-knee amputees[24]. The outcome has improved with better amputation level selection and surgical technique.

Amputation in most cases helps regain function that had been limited by ulcers, tissue necrosis and pain.

Consultation with the rehabilitation team prior to surgery facilitates a better outcome, with instructions in proper bed positioning, avoiding placement of pillows under the knee and range of motion exercises to prevent contracture (of hip and knee) which may interfere with fitting of the prosthesis.

Strengthening and co-ordination exercises may be started prior to surgery, if tolerated. The elderly amputee will need assistive devices for ambulation; stronger upper extremities will facilitate their use.

After surgery the patient should be mobilized as soon as possible, to prevent deconditioning from bedrest. Stump management, training of the amputee, with or without a prosthetic replacement and wheelchair mobility, are part of the rehabilitation process. Postoperative training is initiated at the bedside on the first day after surgery, starting with bed mobility activities and progressing to transfers and ambulation between parallel bars. It is important for the patient to become ambulatory indoors prior to discharge from the hospital. Stump wrapping will shape the stump and reduce edema. The patient and family should be instructed in safety precautions and care of the other limb.

An evaluation for equipment needed at home should be made before discharge. Management of pain is an important issue, and should not be neglected. After the loss of a limb, the remaining part may be associated with a phantom sensation (feeling that the amputated limb is present) and/or phantom pain (actual sensation of pain in the missing limb)[25]. Firm bandaging, massage and percussion of the stump and the use of a prosthesis usually helps improve phantom sensation. The phantom pain requires aggressive management.

When evaluating an amputee for a prosthesis many factors are considered. Adequate cognition helps maximize the benefit from prosthetic rehabilitation, given that rehabilitation involves learning many skills, including gait training and care and maintenance of the prosthesis[26]. Cardiac function should be monitored during training, as many elderly patients suffer from coronary artery disease, hypertension, diabetes and peripheral vascular disease. Diabetics may have visual and sensory impairments, which can make ambulation training difficult. Fluctuating edema of the lower extremities will affect the fitting of the prosthesis. The ability to don and doff the prosthesis, the presence of contractures and the ability to transfer and ambulate all influence the fitting of the prosthesis. The concurrence of dual disabilities in the same patient, such as hemiplegia and lower extremity amputation, is increasingly being recognized as a significant rehabilitation challenge[27], since even a mild residual hemiparesis impacts on rehabilitation[28].

Fitting a prosthesis

The components of the prosthesis should be chosen carefully to ensure proper fitting and function. The socket should be carefully fabricated to have total contact. The suspension should be simple and safe to use. There are many types of prosthetic foot; the one commonly used is the SACH foot (solid

Table 3 Environmental factors contributing to falls

Poorly illuminated rooms and stairs
Scatter rugs
Slippery floors; wet surfaces
Thick pile carpets
Lack of handrails
Low toilet seats
Low, soft chairs
Loose appliance cords
Improperly placed furniture
Improper storage in shelves and closets
Water heater temperature

Table 4 Mobility aids

Standard cane
Increases base of support
Made of aluminum (adjustable) and wood
For proper fitting, measure from the tip of the cane to the
    patient's great trochanter

Quad cane
Increases base of support further
Measured as for standard cane

Walker
Maximum support
The patient's elbow should be flexed 20° when standing
    with the walker

Platform walker
A platform is added to a walker to facilitate hand grasp
    and elbow position

ankle, cushion heel) because of its low cost and durability. Patients wearing a prosthesis minimize energy expenditure by altering their rate of ambulation. Above-knee amputation will require more energy expenditure than below-knee amputation. Preservation of the knee joint improves gait and decreases energy consumption[29]. With a comprehensive rehabilitation program, many elderly amputees should be able to walk functionally.

Fractures

Fractures remain a common cause of morbidity in the geriatric population. Risk factors include frequent falls due to impaired balance, lower extremity weakness, postural instability, visual loss, osteoporosis and sensory deficits in addition to environmental factors (Table 3). Falls may cause head trauma, soft tissue injury, severe lacerations and hip fractures[30]. Deterioration of quality of life and prolonged hospital stay are major issues after hip fractures[31]. Rehabilitation management starts early with goals to minimize immobility and regain function. Mobility and range of motion exercises, started on the first day, progress to transfers, ambulation and activities of daily living training, as tolerated.

ASSISTIVE DEVICES

Assistive devices are used to improve function, safety and mobility of the individual with impairments. Since many patients may be relatively inactive in the acute care setting, functional assessment and recommendations on mobility aids should be part of discharge planning[32]. Ambulatory aids increase the area of support, improve balance, reduce lower limb pain and provide sensory feedback[33]. The types of mobility aid (Table 4) needed depend on the extent of balance and weight-bearing assistance needed by the patient. Stability when walking depends on the location of the center of gravity. Canes used in the hand opposite the lower extremity with muscular weakness or joint pathology provide a normal pathway for the center of gravity[34]. Crutches are usually not used by older adults, as they may cause loss of balance and falls. The energy cost (oxygen consumption) of ambulating with crutches, compared to normal walking, is twice as great[35]. An elderly patient in need of more support than a cane should use a walker. Walkers provide maximum support for the patient and wheels can be placed to the walker's front legs to facilitate movement of the walker, for patients with decreased balance and function of the upper extremities.

Wheelchairs (Table 5) should provide mobility to patients, be safe to negotiate and

Table 5 Factors to consider in wheelchair prescription

Durability
Ease of folding to transport and store
Proper placement of brakes and seat belt for safety
Size
  to fit patients
  to adapt to environment
Types of wheelchair
  rigid frame
  folding wheelchair
  motorized (battery powered)
  standard weight
  ultra-lightweight
  reclining
Cushions
  foam
  gel filled
  air filled

Table 6 Bathroom equipment

Grab bars
Tub seat
Hand-held shower
Raised toilet seat
Mobile commode
Skid strips for tub

require minimal assistance from others. Most wheelchairs are constructed of aluminum, which makes it durable and somewhat light. Adjustment of the wheels can improve positioning and, in the case of patients with hemiplegia, low-placed wheels allow the user to reach the floor and propel the wheelchair with the functional foot. Patients prone to orthostatic hypotension often benefit from reclining or semireclining chairs. Reclining chairs add weight, width and bulk and make transport more difficult. Elevating legrests can be used to help minimize dependent edema. Armrests are available in fixed and detachable full and desk lengths. The full-length armrests provide more area for resting of the arm or for pushing the body forward in a transfer. Desk-length armrests extend forward only partially, and allow the user to

slide the knees under a desk. Wheel locks are an important safety mechanism. For patients with cognitive deficits the brakes can be placed in the rear of the chair, to be activated only by an attendant. Motorized wheelchairs provide more independence to patients with weakness and poor endurance, but are heavier and difficult to transport. Motorized scooters are a good choice for persons who can ambulate and perform most activities of daily living, but lack endurance to ambulate long distances and to use a manual wheelchair. They are helpful in advanced rheumatoid arthritis, degenerative joint disease, cardiac disease, multiple sclerosis and polio, among others.

The most important prescribing considerations in all cases include the diagnosis, clinical status, environment and social support. When discharging patients home, equipment recommendations will help improve safety and function at home. Bathroom equipment (Table 6) would make the patient more independent and safe. Patients with difficulty in ambulation benefit from a bedside commode. Hospital beds should be rarely prescribed, as patients find it difficult to get up from this bed, encouraging inactivity.

References

1. World Health Organization. *International Classification of Impairments, Disabilities and Handicaps*. Geneva, Switzerland: WHO, 1980

2. Halar EM, Bell KR. Immobility, physiological functional changes and effects of inactivity on body functions. In DeLisa JA, Gans BM, eds. *Rehabilitation Medicine Principles and*

Practice, 3rd edn. Philadelphia: Lippincott-Raven, 1998:1015–34

3. Carter WJ. Effect of normal aging on skeletal muscle. *Phys Med Rehab State Art Rev* 1990;4:1–7

4. Alonso JA, Cote LJ. Biology of aging in humans. In Downey JR, Myers SJ, Gonzalez EG, *et al.*, eds. *The Physiological Basis of Rehabilitation Medicine*, 2nd edn. Boston: Butterworth-Heinemann, 1994:689–704

5. Harper CM, Lyles YM. Physiology and complications of bed rest. *J Am Geriatr Soc* 1998;36:1047–54

6. Downey RJ. Physiology of bed rest. In Downey JA, Myers SJ, Gonzales EG, *et al.*, eds. *The Physiological Basis of Rehabilitation Medicine*, 2nd edn. Boston: Butterworth-Heinemann, 1994:448–54

7. Buschbacher RM. Deconditioning, conditioning and the benefits of exercise. In Braddom RL, ed. *Physical Medicine & Rehabilitation*, 1st edn. Philadelphia: WB Saunders, 1996:687–708

8. Halar EM. Physical inactivity a major risk factor for coronary heart disease. Physical medicine and rehabilitation. *Clin North Am* 1995;6:55–67

9. Convertino VA, Bloomfield SA, Greenleaf JE. An overview of the issues: physiological effects of bed rest and restricted physical activity. *Med Sci Sports Exerc* 1997;29:187–90

10. Fife RS. Osteoarthritis. In Klippel JH, Weyand CM, Wortmann RL, eds. *Primer on the Rheumatic Disease*, 11th edn. Atlanta, GA: Arthritis Foundation, 1997:216–17

11. Wilcox S, Brenes GA, Levine D, *et al.* Factors related to sleep disturbance in older adults experiencing knee pain or knee pain with radiographic evidence of knee osteoarthritis. *J Am Geriatr Soc* 2000;48:1241–51

12. O'Grady M, Fletcher J, Ortiz S. Therapeutic and physical fitness exercises prescription for older adults with joint disease: an evidence-based approach. *Rhem Dis Clin North Am* 2000;26:617–46

13. McKinney RH, Ling SM. Osteoarthritis: no cure, but many options for symptom relief. *Cleve Clin J Med* 2000;67:665–71

14. Ettinger WH Jr, Burns R, Messier SP, *et al.* A randomized trial comparing aerobic exercise and resistance exercise with a health education program in older adults with knee osteoarthritis: the Fitness Arthritis and Seniors Trial (FAST). *J Am Med Assoc* 1997;277:25–31

15. Goldstein J, Zuckerman JD. Selected orthopedic problems in the elderly. Geriatric rheumathology. *Rheum Dis Clin North Am* 2000;26:593–616

16. Kawalick M, Lerer A. Stroke syndromes: medical management of the elderly stroke patient. *Phys Med Rehabil State Art Rev* 1989;3:469–77

17. Gresham GE, Phillips TF, Wolf PA, *et al.* Epidemiologic profile of long-term stroke disability: the Framingham Study. *Arch Phys Med Rehabil* 1979;60:487–91

18. Ruff RM, Yarnell S, Marinos JM. Are strokes patients discharged sooner if inpatient rehab services are provided seven v six days per week? *Am J Phys Med Rehabil* 1999;78:143–6

19. Paolucci S, Grasso MG, Antonucci G, *et al.* Mobility status after inpatient stroke rehabilitation: 1 year follow-up and prognostic factors. *Arch Phys Med Rehabil* 2001;82:2–8

20. Gersten JW. Rehab for degenerative diseases of the central nervous system. In Kottke FJ, Stillwell GK, Lehmann JF, eds. *Krusen's Handbook of Physical Medicine & Rehabilitation*. Philadelphia: WB Saunders, 1982:699–706

21. Palmer SS, Mortimer JA, Webster DD, *et al.* Exercise therapy for Parkinson's disease. *Arch Phys Med Rehabil* 1986;67:741–5

22. Schenkman M, Cutson TM, Kuchibhatla M, *et al.* Exercise to improve spinal flexibility and function for people with Parkinson's disease: a randomized, controlled trial. *J Am Geriatr Soc* 1998;46:1207–16

23. Scandalis TA, Bosak A, Berliner JC, *et al.* Resistance training and gait function in patients with Parkinson's disease. *Am J Phys Med Rehabil* 2001;80:38–43

24. Brown PS. The geriatric amputee. Rehabilitation and the aging population. *Phys Med Rehabil State Art Rev* 1990;4:67–76

25. Wikoff EK. Preprosthetic management. Prosthetics. *Phys Med Rehabil State Art Rev* 1994;8:61–72

26. Phillips NA, Mate-Kole CC, Kirby L. Neuropsychological function in peripheral vascular disease. Amputee patients. *Ach Phys Med Rehabil* 1993;74:1309–14

27. Varghese G, Hinterbuchner C, Mondal P, *et al.* Rehabilitation outcome of patients with dual disability of hermiplegia and amputation. *Arch Phys Med Rehabil* 1978; 59:121–3

28. O'Connell PG, Gnatz S. Hemiplegia and amputation: rehabilitation of the dual disability. *Ach Phys Med Rehabil* 1989;70: 451–5

29. Waters R, Perry J, Antonelli D, *et al.* Energy cost of walking amputees: the influence of level of amputation. *J Bone Joint Surg* 1976;58-A:42–6

30. Twersky JI. Falls in the nursing home. *Clin Fam Pract* 2001;3:653–66

31. Randell AG, Nguyen TV, Bhalerao N, *et al.* Deterioration in quality of life following hip fracture: a prospective study. *Osteoporos Int* 2000;11:460–6

32. Graham D, Newton RA. Relationship between balance abilities and mobility aids in elderly patients at discharge from an acute care setting. *Physiother Res Int* 1999;4: 293–301

33. Hennessey WJ, Johnson EW. Lower limb orthosis. In Braddom RL, ed. *Physical Medicine & Rehabilitation.* Philadelphia: WB Saunders, 1996:333–58

34. Lehmann JF. Gait analysis: In Kottke FJ, Stillwell GK, Lehmann JF, eds. *Krusen's Handbook of Physical Medicine & Rehabilitation*, 3rd edn. Philadelphia: WB Saunders, 1982:86–101

35. Fisher SV, Patterson RP. Energy cost of ambulation with crutches. *Arch Phys Med Rehab* 1981;62:250–6

15 Pain assessment and management

J. Elizabeth Whiteman, MD

Pain is a common symptom in the geriatric population. Pain remains a difficult problem in the elderly, and is often unrecognized and undertreated[1]. The prevalence of pain is high. Unrelieved pain may also contribute to other symptoms such as depression, sleep disturbance and functional limitations, aside from significant distress to the patient and caregivers[2].

Pain assessment in older adults is often difficult and other factors should be addressed. Multiple medical problems and symptoms can complicate the evaluation. Cognitive function is important in the management of pain. Older persons have a higher risk of side-effects to medications and treatments. Pain can be effectively managed in older patients and should be a focus in symptom management in this population.

PATHOPHYSIOLOGY

Types of pain

Understanding the classification of pain may help the clinician select treatment and determine prognosis. There are two general classes of pain: nociceptive and neuropathic. Nociceptive pain results from the stimulation of pain receptors. It can be visceral or somatic and can arise from tissue injury, inflammation or mechanical deformation and usually responds well to common analgesics. Neuropathic pain results from a pathophysiologic process involving the peripheral or central nervous system (CNS). This type of pain often responds to non-conventional analgesics such as antidepressants and anticonvulsants. Mixed pain syndromes have unknown or multiple mechanisms; treatment is more difficult.

Age-related changes

Age-related changes in pain perception have been observed. Elderly patients may present with painless myocardial infarctions and abdominal catastrophes. Anatomic and neurochemical changes associated with aging alter pain perception. Sensory changes result from a reduction in Pacini's corpuscles, and Meissner's and Merkel's discs. However, the number of free nerve endings does not change with aging. In the peripheral nervous system the myelinated fibers have slower conduction, and there are reduced numbers of unmyelinated fibers. The CNS has loss of neurons in the cortex, midbrain and brainstem. These changes may account for alterations in pain sensitivity[3]. Drug distribution is another factor to consider in the older patient. Most analgesics are dependent on hepatic metabolism and the cytochrome P450 system[4].

ASSESSMENT

There are no biological markers or measurements that reflect the intensity or character of

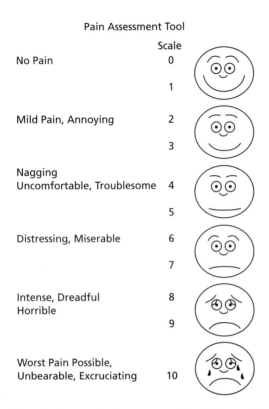

Pain Assessment Tool

	Scale	
No Pain	0	
	1	
Mild Pain, Annoying	2	
	3	
Nagging Uncomfortable, Troublesome	4	
	5	
Distressing, Miserable	6	
	7	
Intense, Dreadful Horrible	8	
	9	
Worst Pain Possible, Unbearable, Excrucicating	10	

Figure 1 Pain scales. Figure reproduced with permission from *Intellicard Symptom Management Algorithms, A Handbook for Palliative Care*, Second Edition. Linda Wrede-Seaman, MD, Medical Director, Providence Hospice of Yakima, Yakima WA

pain. The most accurate and reliable measure is the patient's report[5]. Accurate assessment is important for identifying the source of the pain and planning the best mode of treatment. Older patients often tend to under-report pain. They may have multiple medical problems which make the assessment more difficult. Cognitive impairment in the patient makes it difficult to assess pain fully. Often family, caregivers and other health providers are helpful in the evaluation.

History and physical examination

Assessment needs to start with a thorough history. Questions should relate to when, what, where and how the patient describes the pain. Any treatments tried in the past and

any medical history should be reviewed. Any other descriptions of the pain should be documented. Documentation of the limitations or psychological impact of pain on the patient should be assessed. The physical examination should concentrate on the musculoskeletal and nervous systems. Assessment of the psychological and cognitive status of the patient is important in pain assessment and for management.

Pain instruments

Pain scales help categorize and quantify symptoms. There are several to choose from. However, little information is available on the use of these scales in the geriatric population. Pain should be addressed initially and on follow-up visits to monitor and control symptoms. Unidimensional (pain rating only) and multidimensional (pain rating and how pain affects daily activities, mood, etc.) scales (approaches) can both be helpful in the geriatric population. The Geriatric Pain Measure was developed to evaluate the validity and reliability of a multidimensional pain assessment instrument for older people[6]. It incorporates daily function and reliably assesses pain. In elderly patients who have significant physical or cognitive limitations, unidimensional pain scales are more helpful (Figure 1).

Pain scales are simple to use and rely on patient report. In a visual analog scale, faces, numbers or colors are used to represent different levels of pain. In cognitively impaired or delirious patients assessment can be more difficult. Often much of the information needs to come from the clinician's visual assessment of the patient. Grimacing, moaning or agitation may be signs of pain. Most geriatric patients with mild to moderate cognitive impairment are able to report pain reliably[7,8].

In the aged, other limiting factors can complicate management. Vision or hearing impairment can limit assessment. Functional limitations, weakness and severe cognitive dysfunction make use of pain scales difficult. A tool used for measurement must be appropriate for the patient and should always be used consistently in subsequent evaluations.

TREATMENT

World Health Organization pain scale

The World Health Organization recommendations for pain base medication choices on the intensity of pain[9]. The recommendations are designed in a stepwise manner.

The scale does not imply that one treatment has to fail before another is tried. When the pain is severe it should be treated accordingly with strong opioids. Also, adjuvant drugs may be used early in pain management. When combined, using appropriate dosing guidelines, these are highly effective. Any patient with pain that impairs functional status or quality of life should receive analgesic medications[10]. All analgesics carry some risk, but if used properly can be safe and effective.

Routes of administration

One should start with the least invasive route of administration. Some drugs are available via a variety of routes (subcutaneous, intramuscular, intravenous, transcutaneous, sublingual and rectal). Patients who tolerate oral medications should initially receive medication by mouth. It is the most convenient route and produces relatively stable blood levels. Drug effects are usually seen in 30 min to 2 h. For those unable to swallow or who have gastrointestinal obstruction, the rectal route may be the next least invasive. Many of the opiods have a rectal formulation. The drugs given rectally may have delayed or limited absorption, because they partially bypass hepatic metabolism[11].

Parenteral routes are used for patients who need rapid analgesia, or who need high doses that are difficult to administer orally or rectally. Routes are intravenous, intramuscular and subcutaneous. Bolus injections achieve the most rapid onset; however, patients receive poor pain control, with toxicity at peak onset and risk of breakthrough pain. Repeated intramuscular bolus injections are painful and offer no pharmacologic advantage[12]. Subcutaneous infusion is less painful and an indwelling subcutaneous needle may be helpful to reduce the discomfort of repeated injections.

Continuous infusion is much preferred and can achieve steady states of pain control. Both intravenous and subcutaneous routes can be used. Continuous infusions reduce the problem of the bolus effect. Many devices also allow the patient to administer bolus infusion for breakthrough pain. Subcutaneous infusion can be administered by a 25–27-gauge butterfly needle, left under the skin for up to a week[13]. In ambulatory patients, devices are available to provide continuous infusion. Dosing with subcutaneous infusion can produce blood levels similar or equivalent to intravenous infusion[14]. Limitations of subcutaneous infusions are slower onset and lower peak effect[15]. Subcutaneous infusion volumes may be up to 10 ml/h. Volumes greater than this are poorly absorbed and can be painful.

Other routes of administration include transdermal, sublingual and submucosal. Fentanyl is the only opioid available for transdermal application at this time. Sublingual absorption is possible with any opioid; however, bioavailability is poor if the drug is not highly lipophilic[16]. Sublingual preparations are limited and even the absorption of morphine is limited in the sublingual route. For sublingual or buccal administration in less conscious patients, much of the drug is slowly swallowed and the drug does get absorbed. Fentanyl has been formulated in a transmucosal preparation for premedication and breakthrough pain. A transdermal patch is also available for chronic pain management. The transdermal patch is sometimes more convenient and can be changed every 72 h.

Table 1 Non-opioid agents

Drug	Dose	Preparations
Salicylates		
Aspirin	325–650 mg every 6 h	tablets, suppositories, suspensions
Non-steroidal		
Ibuprofen	200–800 mg every 6–8 h	tablets, suspensions
Naproxen	500 mg every 12 h	tablets, suspensions
Sulindac	150–200 mg every 12 h	tablets
Indomethacin	25–50 mg every 8–12 h	capsules, suspensions, suppositories
Trilisate	500–1500 mg every 12 h	tablets, suspensions
Ketorolac	10 mg every 4–6 h	tablets, intravenous/intramuscular
Cyclo-oxygenase-2 inhibitors		
Celecoxib	100–200 mg every 12 h	capsules
Rofecoxib	12.5–50 mg in 24 h	tablets, suspensions
Miscellaneous		
Acetaminophen	325–1000 mg every 6 h	tablets, suppositories, suspensions
Tramadol	50–100 mg every 6 h	tablets

Dosing

Timing the medication is important. Short-acting rapid-onset medication should be available for episodic pain. For continuous pain, medications need to be provided around the clock. A steady state of analgesia needs to be attained. Controlled-release preparations can be used to achieve a steady state, with a short-acting pain reliever for breakthrough pain as needed.

ANALGESICS

Non-opioid analgesics

These are listed in Table 1.

Acetaminophen

Acetaminophen is one of the safest analgesics for the elderly with mild to moderate pain. It has a lower incidence of side-effects and better tolerance in most patients. While it has no anti-inflammatory activity, it is helpful in musculoskeletal and osteoarthritis pain[17]. It is safer than non-steroidal anti-inflammatory drugs (NSAIDs) and can also be used with other medications for chronic pain. Acetaminophen is dosed up to 1000 mg four times a day. Overdose can result in irreversible hepatic necrosis. The maximum daily dose should not exceed 4000 mg[18]. Caution should be used in patients who consume high doses, other combination products, or excessive alcohol.

Non-steroidal anti-inflammatory agents

NSAIDs are potent inhibitors of prostaglandin synthesis. NSAIDs work by reducing inflammation, decreasing direct pain perception, and via central effects on pain as well[19]. Classic NSAIDs work on the cyclo-oxygenase pathway that converts arachidonic acid to prostaglandins[20]. Cyclo-oxygenase (COX) 1 and COX 2 are the two forms of the enzyme. COX 1 is present in most organ systems and plays a role in normal blood flow to the kidneys, liver and gastric mucosa, and also affects platelet aggregation. Common side-effects with prolonged use are gastro-intestinal ulceration and renal dysfunction[21,22]. COX 2 is the enzyme mainly responsible for inflammation. Newer NSAIDs are more selective in inhibiting COX 2, and therefore have less organ toxicity, but similar effect in pain relief and inflammation[23]. These drugs

Table 2 Approximate equianalgesic doses of commonly used opioids. Adapted from reference 51

Drug	Parenteral	Enteral	Onset (min)	Duration (h)	Half life (h)
Morphine	10 mg	30 mg	15–30	3–7	2–4
Codeine	130 mg	200 mg	15–30	4–6	3
Fentanyl	0.1 mg		7–8	1–2	2–6
Fentanyl TM*		0.5TM	5–15	5–15	2–4
Hydrocodone	N/A	30 mg	10–20	4–8	3–4
Hydromorphone	1.5 mg	7.5 mg	15–30	4–5	2–3
Oxycodone	N/A	20 mg	15–30	2–5	3–4
Propoxyphene	N/A	130 mg	30–60	4–6	6–12
Meperidine	75 mg	300 mg	10–45	2–4	3–4
Methadone	10 mg	20 mg	30–60	4–8	15–120

*Fentanyl TM is transmucosal fentanyl; see specific dosing guidelines

do, however, have a ceiling effect and limited potency for pain relief.

The non-specific COX inhibitors are appropriate for short-term use especially in inflammatory conditions such as gout, calcium pyrophosphate arthropathy and acute flare-ups of rheumatologic disease. They may also help with headache, cramping and mild to moderate pain. A large number of NSAIDs are now available; individual drugs vary with respect to anti-inflammatory activity. They are non-habit forming and can be given orally, intravenously or intramuscularly. A few topical preparations with limitations in pain and inflammatory effect are available[24].

High doses of NSAIDs should be avoided for long-term use in the elderly, as there is a risk for gastrointestinal bleeding, renal impairment and bleeding from platelet dysfunction[22,25]. The use of misoprostol, H_2 blockers and proton pump inhibitors are only partially helpful in reducing adverse effects on the gastrointestinal tract. Renal function may already be impaired in the elderly, and caution is needed with use of any NSAID. Drug interactions may also be a problem. The potential advantages are the reduction of inflammation, cancer pain and bone pain, and use as an adjuvant with other drugs. Constipation, sedation and other CNS side-effects are uncommon, making them useful for moderate to severe pain or as adjuvant therapy.

Opioids

Opioids are very useful for the treatment of pain in advanced disease, particularly for moderate to severe pain. There are a variety of formulas available (Table 2). Opioid is a term for medications that interact with the opioid receptors in the body. Many receptors are present throughout the brain and spinal cord. Opioids work as an agonist at the opioid receptors, resulting in decreased perception of pain. Opioids have no ceiling to their analgesia. They relieve all types of pain regardless of the pathophysiology. The elderly may be more sensitive to the pain-relieving properties of opioids compared to younger people[26,27]. The prolonged half-life and altered pharmacokinetics of opioid drugs produce relief with smaller doses than in younger people. This has been shown to be true in postoperative as well as chronic cancer pain[28].

The only contraindication to opioid use is a history of hypersensitivity. True hypersensitivity would be a rash, wheezing and edema due to histamine release. Allergies are most common to morphine derivatives. A synthetic opioid, one without dyes or preservatives, may then be tried, as the prevalence of allergic reactions is much lower. Opioids have the potential to cause cognitive disturbances, respiratory depression and constipation in the elderly. These side-effects occur in a dose-dependent fashion; if pain persists with few effects the dose can be escalated. Respiratory depression is a consequence that is poorly understood. Careful titration of an opioid to analgesic doses for pain relief is rarely associated with induced respiratory depression and iatrogenic death[29]. Tolerance to these side-effects usually develops in a few days and patients return to a fully alert status and cognitive function. Until tolerance develops, patients need to be instructed not to drive and to take caution against falls or other accidents. Once tolerance has developed, patients can return to their normal activities and may even experience improved physical function once pain is relieved.

Gastrointestinal side-effects need to be monitored. Constipation is a side-effect that should be assessed and managed when starting opioids. Patients should be instructed to increase fluid intake, maintain activity and use stool softeners and laxatives routinely. Prior to use of stimulant laxatives, fecal impaction should be excluded; suppositories or enemas help with bowel evacuation. Nausea from opioids can also be an issue. Antiemetics such as prochlorperazine, chlorpromazine haloperidol, and antihistamines are commonly used to help alleviate nausea. Many of these agents, however, have their own side-effects, including movement disorders, anticholinergic side-effects and delirium, requiring caution in the elderly. Build-up of toxic metabolites needs to be continually considered with opioid analgesia. The active metabolite of morphine is morphine 6 glucuronide. It is dependent on hepatic function and can accumulate in renal insufficiency. In an opioid-naive elderly patient, smaller doses of morphine should be started initially. Normeperidine, the metabolite of meperidine, accumulates in renal failure, causing CNS side-effects such as delirium and seizures. Meperidine is not recommended for chronic pain. Mixed agonist–antagonist agents such as butorphanol, nalbuphine and pentazocine have limited efficacy and may cause acute withdrawal symptoms in patients who are using pure agonist opioids[30].

Tolerance, dependence and addiction

Clinicians who prescribe opioids need to understand the terms tolerance, dependence and addiction. Tolerance is a pharmacologic phenomenon. The definition of tolerance is diminished effect of a drug associated with constant exposure over time. Tolerance is difficult to predict in opioids. Patients usually develop tolerance to drowsiness and respiratory depression before they develop tolerance to analgesia. More recent studies on opioids in the management of arthritis pain noted that tolerance was not often significant[31]. Many patients remain stable for years without developing significant tolerance to the analgesic effects.

Dependence is also a pharmacologic phenomenon. Dependence is also seen in many drug classes such as corticosteroids and β-blockers. Drug dependence occurs after the patient has been exposed to a drug for a period of time. Dependence is present when patients experience uncomfortable side-effects when the drug is abruptly withheld. It is difficult to predict, and varies with dose and time of drug exposure and is different with individual opioid compounds. Symptoms associated with dependence and withdrawal include anorexia, nausea, diaphoresis, tachycardia, elevated blood pressure and low-grade fever. Worse are skin mottling, gooseflesh and autonomic crisis. Tapering off opioids slowly over a few days can control these symptoms. In severe cases clonidine can control serious autonomic side-effects.

Addiction is a behavioral problem. People develop a compulsive or overpowering drive to take a drug in order to experience psychological effects. The craving compulsion drug use continues despite the negative physical and social consequences. Addicted patients often have erratic behavior, which can be in the form of buying, selling or procuring drugs on the street; the craving is for benefits other than pain relief. Other medical, social and economic factors play large roles in addictive behavior[32,33].

Pseudoaddiction should not be confused with addiction. Hoarding of medication, persistent or worsening pain complaints, frequent office visits or requests for dose escalations associated with unrelieved pain is pseudo-addiction. True addiction is rare among patients taking opioid analgesics for medical reasons. Fear of addiction and side-effects should not justify failure to treat pain adequately, especially in those patients near the end of life. Clinicians need to be cautious of the misconception that the need for increasing doses of a drug is due to tolerance, rather than progression of the disease. Patients' symptoms and disease progression should be followed closely and pain treated accordingly.

Fear of addiction is a major barrier to pain management in the elderly[31]. Fears by both clinicians and patients have been overinfluenced by social pressures to reduce illegal drugs used by patients for psychological rather than medical reasons. Many clinicians are intimidated by the regulations of controlled substances by state and federal authorities as well as medical state license boards. These issues may be contributory in patients who seek suicide rather than enduring pain. Many organizations such as the American Medical Association, the American College of Physicians and the American Geriatrics Society have released position statements supporting comfort and control of pain in patients near the end of life[34-36]. Clinicians have an obligation to provide comfort, pain relief and dignity for patients.

Dosing

Morphine is most often used as the measure for dose equivalence. Preparations include oral tablets in both short- and long-acting preparations. Liquid morphine in short-acting and immediate-release formulas is used for breakthrough pain. Also available are commercially prepared long-acting sprinkles. Fentanyl is available intravenously, as a transmucosal lozenge and a patch. The transdermal fentanyl patch is ideal for patients who cannot swallow or are not able to tolerate other opioids. The patch has a reservoir that deposits fentanyl subcutaneously, reaching a steady state in 48–72 h. It is effective, safe and relatively well tolerated in patients with cancer[37]. Transdermal application can also lead to constipation and sedation, but possibly a better quality of life due to the convenience. Patients should be cautioned on proper application and use (Table 3)[38].

Oral transmucosal fentanyl citrate (Actiq®) is fentanyl on an applicator that patients can rub on the oral mucosa for rapid absorption of the drug. It is useful for breakthrough pain or prior to maneuvers such as dressing changes. Pain relief usually starts within 5 min[39,40].

Levorphanol and methadone are potentially useful drugs. They have a longer duration of action with need for less frequent dosing. The potential for drug accumulation and risk for sedation may be less ideal in older adults. Hydromorphone (Dilaudid®) and oxycodone are alternatives available as tablets, liquids and suppositories. Hydromorphone will soon be available in a long-acting formula as well. They are synthetic opioids and can be used when patients have a true allergic reaction to morphine, side-effects from morphine metabolites, or poor renal function with risk of accumulation of metabolites.

Combinations of opioid preparations are also available. Opioid–acetaminophen or opioid–anti-inflammatory combinations can mean fewer pills to swallow and the benefit of an adjuvant type of pain medication. The doses of acetaminophen and anti-inflammatory agents need to be monitored for potential side-effects and toxicity.

Table 3 Fentanyl dosing and patient instructions (Durogesic® patch)

Transdermal fentanyl patch/oral morphine[†]

25 µg/h, 7.5 mg every 4 h
50 µg/h, 15 mg every 4 h
75 µg/h, 22.5 mg every 4 h
100 µg/h, 30 mg every 4 h

Onset of action 24–48 h
Change patch every 72 h

Place on upper body in clean, dry, hairless place
Choose a different site when placing a new patch
Remove old patch and fold sticky sides together, flush down the toilet
Wash hands after handling
Do not use heat over location of patch; this can lead to increased amounts of medication released
Do not cut patches; this alters drug delivery mechanism
Caution in opioid-naive and elderly patients

---

*Adapted from package insert, Fentanyl Transdermal Sytem, Janssen 2001
[†]From reference 38

ADJUVANT MEDICATIONS

A variety of other medications not formally classified as analgesics are helpful in certain situations (Table 4). 'Adjuvant' analgesic drugs are used in addition to opioids or other drugs but can be used as the primary pain relievers in certain cases. These agents usually work together with other traditional drugs and non-pharmacologic pain strategies to relieve pain. The potential risk for side-effects remains in older adults and hence the need to use low doses and monitor closely.

Antidepressants

Antidepressants have been the most widely studied class of non-analgesic medication for pain. Tricycle antidepressant analgesic effects appear to be related to the inhibition of norepinephrine and serotonin in the brain[41]. In diabetic neuropathy a randomized placebo-controlled trial indicated that desipramine and amitriptyline were effective in the treatment of symptoms. Fluoxetine was no better than placebo[42]. Desipramine may be a better choice to use in geriatrics, because of the lower side-effect profile compared to amitriptyline.

Side-effects from the anticholinergic properties cause dry mouth, blurred vision, constipation, urinary retention and confusion. These can be bothersome in the elderly and therefore these drugs are not commonly recommended. Selective serotonin reuptake inhibitors (SSRI) have had mixed results. While SSRI antidepressants have a much lower side-effect profile, most show no improvement in relief of pain.

Antiseizure medications

Antiseizure medications are known to relieve the neuropathic pain in trigeminal neuralgia. Antiepileptic drugs such as dilantin, tegretol and valproic acid may be helpful in diabetic neuropathy and other neuropathic pain, but because of side-effects, the risk may outweigh the benefit. Sedation, confusion and tremor can be detrimental to the quality of life. Gabapentin is effective for the treatment of diabetic and post-herpetic neuropathy[43,44]. It has a significant benefit on pain and a low side-effect profile. Patients usually experience some sedative effects; starting at low doses and escalating up helps develop a tolerance to the drowsiness. The usual effective dose is 900–3600 mg/day in three divided doses. Slow titration and monitoring are necessary.

Table 4 Adjuvant drugs

Drug class	Dose	Routes	Indications	Side-effects
Antidepressants				
Amitriptyline	10–25 mg	po	neuropathic pain	anticholinergic,
Nortriptyline	10–25 mg	po		orthostasis
Desipramine	10–25 mg	po		
Anticonvulsants				
Clonazepam	0.5–1 mg qd-tid	po	neuropathic pain	sedation
Carbamazepine	100 mg qd-tid	po		leucopenia, thrombocytopenia
Gabapentin	100 mg qd-tid	po		sedation, ankle swelling
Corticosteroids				
Dexamethasone	2–4 mg qd-qid	po/iv/sq	cerebral edema, bone metastases, neuropathic pain, cord compression	steroid psychosis, gastrointestinal bleeding, osteoporosis
Prednisone	15–30 mg tid-qid	po		
Local anesthetics				
Lidocaine	5% ointment, 5% liquid, patch 5% for 12 h	topical qid	localized pain postherpetic neuralgia	localized erythema
Capsaicin	0.025–0.075% cream	topical qid		burning
Emla® cream or disc	2.5 g	1 h before procedure		
Bisphosphonates				
Pamidronate	60–90 mg	iv over 24 h	bone pain, metastases	pain flare
Etidronate	5–10 mg/kg	iv/po	Paget's disease	
Risedronate	30 mg qd × 2 months	po	Paget's disease	esophageal irritation
Calcitonin	25–200 IU/day	sq/nasal	bone pain	hypersensitivity

qd, everyday; tid, three times a day; qid, four times a day; po, orally; iv, intravenously; sq, subcutaneously

Local anesthetics

Local anesthetics have also been shown to relieve neuropathic pain. Topical preparations for localized pain can be helpful. Topical preparations of lidocaine or Emla® (a mixture of lidocaine and prilocaine) cream can be used to premedicate an area prior to an invasive procedure. Lidocaine is also available as a topical patch that relieves pain and is worn for up to 12 h a day. Topical administration includes aspirin and non-steroidal preparations.

Corticosteroids

Corticosteroids inhibit prostaglandin synthesis and reduce edema[45]. They are helpful in the treatment of neuropathic pain, and bone pain due to metastasis. Side-effects can be fluid retention, gastrointestinal related and hyperglycemia. Neuropsychological effects including delirium, and withdrawal symptoms may be severe if the medication is stopped suddenly. Chronic use causes Cushing's syndrome, osteoporosis, myopathy and skin changes.

Calcitonin and bisphosphonates

For the chronic pain of osteoporosis, calcitonin has had mixed results. More recently it was shown that calcitonin and bisphosphonates could help the pain associated with metastatic bone disease[46,47], and may be beneficial in multiple myeloma and Paget's disease.

Table 5 Non-pharmacologic measures to alleviate pain

Method	Benefits	Risks
Education	patient information	none
Psychological		
relaxation	diversion from pain	not full relief
distraction		use accordingly
hypnosis		adjuvant to pharmacologic measures
Exercise	muscle stretch and reconditioning	injury or inflammation if not skilled
Meditation	relaxation	none
Music therapy	relaxation, diversion	none
Alternative therapy		
acupuncture	endorphin release	bleeding, nerve pain less
acupressure	endorphin release	than with use of needles
aromatherapy		
Other		
transcutaneous electrical nerve stimulation	nociceptive pain	skin irritation
biofeedback		may need prolonged training

ANESTHETICS AND SURGICAL APPROACHES

Many anesthetic and surgical approaches to pain are available. Spinal opioid administration is used in cases of acute perioperative pain and with chronic pain when oral methods fail. External or internal implanted pumps offer opioids directly to the spinal opioid receptors. In patients with localized pain not controlled by other measures neurolytic blockade can reduce pain temporarily. Sympathetic blockade can be helpful in cases of visceral pain, but requires skill.

Trigger-point injections have been widely used for myofacial pain syndromes. Local injection of trigger points followed by stretching and massage usually shows some improvement. Results of ice massage or vapocoolant spray followed by exercise and physical therapy can show similar results[48].

Continuous drug infusions are effective in providing steady state drug levels. Implantable pumps are available to deliver intravenous, subcutaneous, intrathecal and epidural injections. Continuous infusion is useful in severe pain and needs to be individualized for appropriate use. Patients who have chronic pain that is poorly controlled should be referred to pain specialty clinics for evaluation.

NON-DRUG STRATEGIES

Non-drug strategies can be used alone or in combination with appropriate analgesic medication. The elderly can be candidates for a broad range of modalities, many with few side-effects. These methods can enhance pain control (Table 5).

Education is important, providing information on types of pain, instruments to measure pain and appropriate use of analgesic medication. Non-drug strategies can also be taught for use at home. Studies have shown that education alone significantly improves pain management[49,50].

The transcutaneous electrical nerve stimulation (TENS) unit can help in chronic pain management. Electrodes are placed in the painful area and nerve stimulation is set as continuous or pulsatile bursts. The results vary but are useful in musculoskeletal nociceptive pain as well as neurogenic pain from nerve compressions or neuropathies. Biofeedback may also play a role in non-invasive pain management.

Psychological interventions include relaxation techniques, distraction, biofeedback and hypnosis. These techniques focus on enhancing healthy behavior and are used along with analgesics. Fear, anxiety, agitation and depression are common with pain symptoms and add to discomfort. Biofeedback is used to help with relaxation, but limited data are available. Antidepressants and anxiolytics may be used as adjuvants in pain management and also help reduce the psychological symptoms.

Many use alternative types of therapy, including acupuncture, acupressure, supplements and vitamins. Used as a form of pain relief, acupuncture may release endorphins that relieve pain. Several supplements and vitamin formulas are available, but these should be used with caution, as there are no explicit data available. Although there is little information on the effectiveness of these treatments, patients should be able to discuss options with their physician. The potential for drug interactions must be minimized.

Exercise, meditation, music and touch therapies are helpful in getting a patient to focus on other stimuli. Exercise helps by adding strength and endurance. Relaxation is the main goal and helps in pain management.

PAIN AND SUFFERING

Pain and quality of life are important issues that affect many patients. Pain is a symptom and its origin can be multifactorial. The patient's physical, psychological, social and spiritual being affects quality of life. It is also important to inquire about other factors that may play a role. The physician or health-care provider needs to be involved in the total care of the patient.

CONCLUSION

Views of pain management in the elderly have changed over the past few years. There are higher expectations from patients, families and health-care advocates concerning adequate treatment of pain. Optimal pain control depends on comprehensive assessment and close monitoring of the older patient. Pain may be controlled by the use of medications, but a multifactorial approach is needed, especially in patients with chronic pain and multiple medical problems, who have a higher risk of side-effects. The goal is resolution of pain and improvement in quality of life.

References

1. Bernabei R, Gambassi G, Lapane K, *et al.* Management of pain in elderly patients with cancer: SAGE Study Group. Systemic Assessment of Geriatric Drug Use via Epidemiology. *J Am Med Assoc* 1998;279: 1877–82
2. Ferrell BA. Pain management in elderly people. *J Am Geriatr Soc* 1991;39:64–73
3. Gibson SJ, Helme RD. Age differences in pain perception and report: a review of physiological, psychological, laboratory and clinical studies. *Pain Rev* 1995;2:111–37
4. Gloth M. Pain management in older adults: management and treatment. *J Am Geriatr Soc* 2001;49:188–99

5. Turk DC, Melzac R. The measurement of pain and assessment of people experiencing pain. In Turk DC, Melzack R, eds. *Handbook of Pain Assessment*. New York: Guilford Press, 1992:135–51
6. Ferrell BR, Stein W, Beck J. The Geriatric Pain Measure: validity, reliability and factor analysis. *J Am Geriatr Soc* 2000;48: 1669–73
7. Weiner DK, Peterson BL, Logue P, *et al.* Predictors of self-report in nursing home residents. *Aging Clin Exp Res* 1998;10: 441–20
8. Parmelee AP, Smith BD, Katz IR. Pain complaints and cognitive status among

elderly institutional residents. *J Am Geriatr Soc* 1993;41:517–22.

9. World Health Organization. *Cancer Pain Relief, with a Guide to Opioid Availability, Cancer Pain Relief and Palliative Care,* 2nd edn. Report of the WHO Expert Committee, WHO Technical Report Series, No. 804. Geneva, Switzerland: WHO, 1996

10. AGS Panel on Chronic Pain in Older Persons. The management of chronic pain in older persons. *J Am Geriatr Soc* 1998; 46:635–51

11. Hanning CD. The rectal absorption of opioids. In Benedetti C, Chapman CR, Givon G, eds. *Advances in Pain Research and Therapy,* vol. 14. New York: Raven Press, 1990:259–69

12. Hanks GW, de Conno F, Ripamonti C, *et al.* Morphine in cancer pain: modes of administration. *Br Med J* 1996;312:823–6

13. Coyle N, Cherney N, Portenoy RK. Subcutaneous opioid infusions in the home. *Oncology* 1994;8:21–7

14. Waldman CS, Eason JR, Rambonul E, Hanson GC. Serum morphine levels, a comparison between continuous subcutaneous infusions and intravenous infusions in post operative patients. *Anesthesia* 1984; 39:768–71

15. American Pain Society. *Principles of Analgesic Use in the Treatment of Acute Pain and Cancer Pain.* Glenview, IL: American Pain Society, 1999

16. Weinberg DS, Inturrisi CE, Reidenberg B, *et al.* Sublingual absorption of selected opiod analgesics. *Clin Pharmacol Ther* 1988;44:335–42

17. Bradley JD, Brandt KD, Katz BP, *et al.* Comparison of an antiinflammatory dose of ibuprofen, an analgesic dose of ibuprofen and acetaminofen in the treatment of patients with osteoarthritis of the knee. *N Engl J Med* 1991;325:87–91

18. Sandler PP, Smith JC, Weinberg CR, *et al.* Analgesic use and chronic renal disease. *N Engl J Med* 1989;320:1238–43

19. Roth SH, Merits and liabilities of NSAID therapy. *Rheum Dis Clin North Am* 1989; 15:479–98

20. Cryer B, Feldman M. Cyclooxygenase-1 and cyclooxygenase-2 selectivity of widely used non steroidal anti-inflammatory drugs. *Am J Med* 1998;104:413–21

21. Allison MC, Hewatson AG, Torance CJ, *et al.* Gastrointestinal damage associated with the use of non steroidal anti-inflammatory drugs. *N Eng J Med* 1992;327:749–54

22. Griffin MR, Piper JM, Daugherty JR, *et al.* Nonsteroidal antiinflammatory drug use and increased peptic ulcer disease in elderly persons. *Ann Intern Med* 1991;144:257–63

23. Bell GM, Schnitzer TJ. Cox 2 inhibitors and other NSAIDs in the treatment of pain in the elderly. *Clin Geriatr Med* 2001; 17:489–502

24. Radermacher J, Hentsch D, Scholl MA, *et al.* Diclofenac concentrations in synovial fluid and plasma after cutaneous application in inflammatory and degenerative joint disease. *Br J Clin Pharmacol* 1991;31:537–41

25. Gurwitz JH, Avoron J, Ross-Degnan D, Sipsitsz LA. Non steroidal anti-inflammatory drug associated azotemia in the very old. *J Am Med Assoc* 1990;264:471–5

26. Kaiko RF. Age and morphine analgesia in cancer patients with post operative pain. *Clin Pharmacol Ther* 1980;28:823–6

27. Bellville WJ, Forrest WH Jr, Miller E, Brown BW Jr. Influence of age on pain relief from analgesics: a study of post-operative patients. *J Am Med Assoc* 1971; 217:1835–41

28. Kaiko RF, Wallenstein SL, Rogers AG, *et al.* Narcotics in the elderly. *Med Clin North Am* 1982;66:1079–89

29. Dahl JL. Effective pain management in terminal care. *Clin Geriatr Med* 1996;12:279–300

30. Hoskin PJ, Hanks GW. Opiod agonist antagonist drugs in acute and chronic pain states. *Drugs* 1991;41:326–44

31. Portenoy RK. Opiate therapy for chronic non cancer pain. Can we get past the bias? *Am Pain Soc Bull* 1991;1:4–7

32. Jaffe JH. Drug addiction and drug abuse. In Gillman AG, Goodman LS, Rall TW, Murad F, eds. *Goodman and Gillman's The Pharmacological Basis of Therapuetics,* 7th edn, New York: Macmillan, 1985: 532–81

33. Melzack R. The tragedy of needless pain. *Sci Am* 1990;262:27–33

34. AGS Ethics Committee. The care of dying patients: a position statement. *J Am Geriatr Soc* 1995;43:577–8

35. Council on Scientific Affairs, American Medical Association. Good care of the dying patient. *J Am Med Assoc* 1996;275: 474–8

36. American College of Physicians and the ACP Ethics and Human Rights Committee. *Ethics Manual*, 4th edn. *Ann Intern Med* 1998;128:576–94

37. Sion P, Moulin D, Hays H. A clinical evaluation of transdermal therapuetic system fentanyl for the treatment of cancer pain. *J Pain Symptom Manage* 1998;16:102–11

38. Storey P. More on the conversion of transdermal fentanyl to morphine. *J Pain Symptom Manage* 1995;10:581–2

39. Fine PG, Steisand JB. A review of oral transmucosal fentanyl citrate: potent, rapid and non invasive, opioid analgesia. *J Palliat Med* 1998;1:55–63

40. Fine PG. Clinical experience with Actiq (oral transmucosal fentanyl citrate) for the treatment of cancer pain. *Todays Therapeutic Trends: J New Dev Clin Med* 1999; 17:1–11

41. Max MB. Antidepressants and analgesics. In Fields HL, Leibeskind JC, eds. *Progress in Pain Research and Management*, vol 1. Seattle: IASP Press, 1994:229–46

42. Max MB, Lynch SA, Muir J, *et al*. Effects of desipramine, amitriptyline and fluoxetine on pain in diabetic neuropathy. *N Engl J Med* 1992;326:1250–6

43. Backonja M, Beydoun A, Edward KR, *et al*. Gabapentin for the symptomatic treatment of painfull neuropathy in patients with diabetes mellitus: a randomized controlled trial. *J Am Med Assoc* 1998;280:1831–6

44. Rowbotham M, Harden N, Stacey B, *et al*. Gabapentin for the treatment of post herpetic neuralgia: a randomized controlled trial. *J Am Med Assoc* 1998;280:1837–42

45. Watanabe S, Bruera E. Corticosteroids as adjuvant analgesics. *J Pain Symptom Manage* 1994;9:442–5

46. Mystakidou K, Befon S, Hondros K, Kouskouni E, Vlahos L. Continuous subcutaneous administration of high dose salmon calcitonin in bone metastasis: pain control and beta-endorphin plasma levels. *J Pain Symptom Manage* 1999;18:323–30

47. Purohit OP, Anthony C, Radstene CR, *et al*. High dose intravenous pamidronate for metastatic bone pain. *Br J Cancer* 1994;70:554–8

48. Ferrell BA. Pain management. In Hazzard W, Blass J, Ettinger W, *et al*., eds. *Principles of Geriatric Medicine and Gerontology*, 4th edn. New York: McGraw-Hill, 1999:428–30

49. Ferrell BR, Rhiner M, Ferrell BA. Development and implementation of a pain education program. *Cancer* 1993;72(11 Suppl): 3426–32

50. Rhiner M, Ferrell BR, Ferrell BA, Grant MM. A structured non drug intervention program for cancer pain. *Cancer Pract* 1993; 1:137–43

51. Hanks G, Cherney N. Opioid analgesic therapy. In Doyle D, Hanks G, MacDonald N, eds. *Oxford Textbook of Palliative Medicine*, 2nd edn. Oxford: Oxford University Press, 1998:334

16 Hospice and palliative care

Michelle L. Moehl, MD, and Ronald S. Schonwetter, MD

Success in medicine is generally measured by cure, and death is often seen as failure – with the blame at times being placed on the physician, medications, or even the patient. Effective care of patients at the end of their lives requires a shift in the focus and goals of care. Just as a patient can achieve success in life, a successful death can also be obtained.

As the availability of medications and treatments that prolong life has increased, the expectation of cure has grown. Patients are frequently kept alive through circumstances not previously imagined. Even with these advances in medical therapies, the fact remains that every person will die and most will die of a disease process. The curative model of medicine has made it harder for physicians, patients and their families to accept this inevitable endpoint. As the culture of medicine has become more specialized, the emphasis on care of the whole person (and not just a particular organ system) has declined. In response, hospice was developed to provide end-of-life care for the whole person and their family.

A study involving focus groups consisting of nurses, social workers, chaplains, hospice volunteers, physicians, patients and bereaved family members clarified the components of a 'good death'[1]. This study confirmed the importance of pain and symptom management, decision-making and patient autonomy, preparation for death and completion – four themes found in the palliative literature. It also identified two new themes: contributions to others and affirmation of the whole person. Physicians' ideals for a good death centered mostly on medical needs, while the patients placed as much importance on psychosocial and spiritual needs as on physical needs[1]. In order to care for the whole person, it is necessary to acknowledge their psychosocial and spiritual needs, as well as their physical symptoms and disease process.

HOSPICE CARE

Cicely Saunders opened the first modern hospice center (St Christopher's Hospice) in London in 1967. The emphasis was on symptom control and care of terminally ill patients' and families' psychosocial needs through an interdisciplinary team approach. In 1974, the first hospice in the USA opened in New Haven, Connecticut. Funded by the National Cancer Institute, it served as a model of home care for the terminally ill and their families[2]. Subsequently, the Tax Equity and Fiscal Responsibility Act of 1982 authorized Medicare to reimburse hospices for care of terminally ill patients.

The goal of hospice is to provide a comfortable end of life while attending to the patients' and families' physical, emotional and spiritual needs. Hospice promotes the idea that death is a natural part of life that should be neither hastened nor postponed. Emphasis is placed on maximizing quality of life and providing comfort care. Bereavement services are provided to family members after the patient's death.

Although the majority of hospice care is provided in the home setting, patients may also receive care in nursing homes, assisted living facilities, hospice homes and acute hospital settings if needed. Respite services are also available for up to 5 days. According to Medicare guidelines, hospice provides medications and equipment related to the primary terminal diagnosis.

When a patient's primary physician considers the patient to have a terminal disease process with a life expectancy of less than 6 months, a referral can be made to hospice. Patients generally are assigned to interdisciplinary teams, which may consist of a physician, nurses, counselors, home health aids and clergy. Home visits are provided based on the needs of the patient. The patient, family and interdisciplinary team work together to develop reasonable goals for the patient's remaining time. The condition of each patient is reviewed regularly to determine whether changes are needed in therapy and to ensure eligibility of the patient. Because the art of predicting survival length is inexact, a patient's condition may occasionally improve and that patient may no longer qualify for hospice care. At that point, the patient could be discharged from hospice; they may be re-enrolled in the future.

In the USA in 2001, about 775 000 patients received hospice care from over 3200 hospice organizations operating in all 50 states, Puerto Rico and Guam. In 2000, 87% of patients were over the age of 65, and the average length of stay was 48 days (median 25 days)[3]. In 2000, of the nearly 2.4 million patients who died in the USA, 50% died in a hospital. However, about 7% of patients enrolled in a hospice died in a traditional hospital[3]. Despite the large number of patients dying in hospitals, almost half of hospitals surveyed in one study did not offer end-of-life, pain management, or hospice services[4].

PROGNOSTIC INDICATORS

Determination of the point at which a disease process becomes a terminal illness, during which the focus of care may emphasize palliation rather than cure, is difficult. Perhaps because it is generally easier to prognosticate in patients with cancer or perhaps because patients with non-cancer illnesses were not considered terminal even with advanced disease, the majority of early hospice patients had cancer as their primary diagnosis. In part, to assist with determination of eligibility for hospice care and to increase access to hospice care, guidelines were developed to identify patients with non-cancer diagnoses who might have a life expectancy of less than 6 months should the disease follow its usual course. These guidelines, however, have not been empirically tested and serve only as a general suggestion. Some of the common prognostic guidelines are provided in Table 1.

In a prospective study involving patients with end-stage breast, gastrointestinal, or lung cancer, the factors that correlated most strongly with decreased length of survival included liver metastases, moderate-to-severe co-morbidity, weight loss of > 8.1 kg in the previous 6 months, serum albumin < 3.5 g/dl, lymphocyte count $< 1 \times 10^9$, lactate dehydrogenase > 618 U/l and clinical estimate of survival by treating physicians of less than 2 months. The only symptoms that significantly correlated with decreased survival length were nausea and vomiting[5].

PALLIATIVE CARE

The goal of palliative care is described by its Latin origin *pallium* meaning a cloak or cover[6]. Managing bothersome symptoms in patients with chronic progressive illnesses, maximizing quality of life and relieving suffering are its objectives. In contrast to hospice care, the provision of palliative care is not limited to the last 6 months of life. It can

Table 1   Prognostic indicators

Heart disease
New York Heart Association Class IV congestive heart failure, despite optimal treatment with vasodilators and
   diuretics
Supporting documentation: ejection fraction < 20%, resistant symptomatic arrhythmias, history of cardiac arrest,
   unexplained syncope, embolism to brain of cardiac origin, or concomitant HIV

Chronic obstructive pulmonary disease
Disabling dyspnea at rest
Poor responsiveness to bronchodilators resulting in decreased functional capacity
Evidence of progression of disease (increasing visits to emergency department/hospital)
Po_2 < 55 mmHg, or oxygen saturation < 88% on supplemental oxygen, or Pco_2 > 50 mmHg
Supporting documentation: FEV_1 < 30% predicted, decrease of FEV_1 > 40 ml/year, right heart failure secondary
   to pulmonary disease, unintentional weight loss > 10% of body weight over 6-month period, or resting
   tachycardia > 100/min

Dementia
Inability to ambulate, dress and bathe without assistance
Urinary and fecal incontinence
No meaningful verbal communication or speech < 6 words
Stage seven or below on Functional Assessment Staging Scale
One of the following in past year: aspiration pneumonia, pyelonephritis, septicemia, multiple stage
   3 or 4 decubitus ulcers, recurrent fever after antibiotics, weight loss of > 10% over past 6 months or albumin
   < 2.5 g/dl.

Failure to thrive
Documentation of a terminal condition
Nutritional impairment with body mass index < 22 kg/m²
Functional disability represented by a Palliative Performance Scale of ≤ 40

---

be provided from the onset of the diagnosis of a chronic progressive illness. Curative care does not necessarily end at the point that palliative care begins. Symptom management can be achieved while the search for a reversible cause is performed. However, at times an underlying cause may not be identified, or curative treatment may not be desired or feasible.

Pain management

One of the most distressing symptoms for both patients and their families is pain. Insufficient pain management may be due to inadequate pain assessment, reluctance to prescribe opioids and poor training in pain management[7].

In order to achieve the best treatment of pain, it is helpful to determine the etiology. Treatment strategies should be chosen based

upon the type and location of pain, the severity, co-morbid conditions and interactions with the patient's current medications, treatment side-effects and the patient's goals. Acute pain or exacerbation of chronic pain should be assessed with a comprehensive history and physical examination to seek the underlying cause.

The first well-known guidelines for pain control in patients with cancer were developed by the World Health Organization (WHO). The WHO developed an analgesic ladder for pain control with medication types recommended based upon pain severity[8]. Non-opioid pain medications (non-steroidal anti-inflammatory drugs (NSAIDs), acetaminophen, or aspirin) ± adjuvant are recommended for mild pain, while weak opioids (e.g. codeine, hydrocodone) ± adjuvant are suggested for moderate pain, and strong opioids (e.g. morphine, oxycodone,

Table 2   National Comprehensive Cancer Network (NCCN) guidelines for treatment of specific pain problems

---

Pain associated with inflammation
   trial of non-steroidal anti-inflammatory drugs (NSAIDs) or glucocorticoids
Bone pain without oncologic emergency (e.g. epidural cord compression or impending fracture)
   trial of NSAIDs or opioids
Local bone pain (e.g. rib pain)
   consider local radiation therapy or nerve block
Diffuse bone pain
   consider trial of bisphosphonates, hormonal therapy or chemotherapy for responsive tumors, glucocorticoids
   and/or systemic administration of radioisotopes in selected patients
   consider physical medicine evaluation
   for resistant pain consider invasive anesthetic (nerve blocks, spinal opioids and anesthetics), orthopedic or
   neurosurgical approaches
Nerve compression or inflammation
   trial of glucocorticoids
Neuropathic pain
   primarily burning pain:
      trial of antidepressant: start with low dose and increase every 3–5 days (e.g. nortriptyline, 10–100 mg/day;
      amitriptyline, 10–100 mg/day; doxepin, 10–100 mg/day; desipramine, 10–100 mg/day; venlafaxine,
      37.5–225 mg/day)
   primarily shooting pain:
      trial of anticonvulsant: start with low dose and increase every 3–5 days (e.g. gabapentin, 100–200 mg three
      times a day; carbamazepine, 100–400 mg twice a day)
      consider topical agents, e.g. local anesthetics or capsaicin. If results are unsatisfactory after a 2–3-week trial
      at a reasonable dose, consider referral to a pain service or to an anesthesiologist/neurosurgeon for an inva-
      sive procedure
Painful lesions that are likely to respond to antineoplastic therapies
   consider trial of radiation, hormones or chemotherapy

'These guidelines are a work in progress that will be refined as often as new significant data become available. The NCCN guidelines are a statement of consensus of its authors regarding their views of currently accepted approaches to treatment. Any clinician seeking to apply or consult any NCCN guideline is expected to use independent medical judgement in the context of individual clinical circumstances to determine any patient's care or treatment. The National Comprehensive Cancer Network makes no warranties of any kind whatsoever regarding their content, use or application and disclaims any responsibility for their application or use in any way.' 'These guidelines are copyrighted by the National Comprehensive Cancer Network. All rights reserved. These guidelines and illustrations herein may not be reproduced in any form for any purpose without the express written permission of the NCCN.'
Permission obtained

hydromorphone, fentanyl, or methadone) ± adjuvant for severe pain.

More recently the National Comprehensive Cancer Network (NCCN) published guidelines that contain multiple components for the assessment and treatment of cancer pain (Table 2). Recommendations include quantification of pain intensity, formal pain assessment, reassessment of pain intensity after therapy is initiated, psychosocial support and distribution of pertinent educational material[9].

The guidelines for the treatment of chronic pain in older patients set forth by the American Geriatric Society Panel recommend considering non-pharmacologic methods of pain control in addition to pharmacologic treatment. Non-pharmacologic therapies suggested include the following: patient education, self-help techniques, cognitive–behavioral therapies, exercise and physical or occupational therapy[10].

Acetaminophen is often the first-line medication for patients with mild pain, since it is relatively safe for the elderly. However, since acetaminophen is included with opioids in many pain medications, the dose must be monitored to prevent hepatotoxicity. The usual maximum dose is 4 g, but hepatotoxicity can occur at lower doses in patients with pre-existing liver disease.

NSAIDs are also common first-line agents, but must be used cautiously in the elderly. Side-effects include gastrointestinal hemorrhage, renal toxicity and hypertension[11,12]. Cyclo-oxygenase-2 (COX2) inhibitors seem to have similar analgesic effects[13] with less gastrointestinal toxicity[14] and a minimal anticoagulation effect. As with the majority of medications used in the elderly, 'start low and go slow' is a good principle.

Neuropathic pain may be less responsive to opioids than nociceptive pain (visceral or somatic). Some anticonvulsants and antidepressant agents are typically effective. Effective medication doses are usually less than the therapeutic level needed for the antidepressant or anti-epileptic effects.

The WHO[8], Agency for Health Care Policy and Research[15], American Geriatric Society[10] and NCCN[9] agree that, when cancer pain does not respond to non-opioid medication, opioids should then be considered.

In terminal patients, opioids should also be considered for non-malignant refractory pain. In elderly patients with terminal conditions, the pain should be decreased to an acceptable level with the lowest dose of medication possible to minimize adverse effects. Initial doses of opioids in the elderly should be 25–50% lower than usual starting doses, with each rescue dose at about 5% of the daily total opioid dose, given up to every 2 h as needed[16]. Although the side-effects of sedation and nausea generally resolve with continued use of opioids typically after 2–3 days, constipation is a very common side-effect, which does not improve. To prevent constipation, initiation of a bowel regimen should be considered when opioids are begun.

Constipation

Constipation is a symptom that commonly occurs in patients at the end of their lives. About 80% of hospice patients require prescriptions for laxatives[17]. Constipation can cause patients distress and may be associated with abdominal pain and distension, nausea and vomiting, decreased oral intake, urinary incontinence or delirium. Evaluation of constipation includes a brief history and physical examination including rectal examination for stool impaction and consideration of abdominal radiographs if the patient is at high risk for intestinal obstruction.

Since constipation is a very common side-effect of opioids, prophylactic measures should be considered at their initiation. Non-pharmacologic measures such as increased activity as tolerated, adequate fluid intake and increased fiber in the diet may be helpful, but often a stool softener and/or laxative is needed for a patient to avoid constipation.

When prophylactic measures fail, treatment should be aimed at the underlying problem or the predominant symptom. Hard stools usually respond better to stool softeners (lubricant, surfactant, saline or osmotic laxatives, or bulk-forming agents) while soft stools usually respond better to peristaltic stimulants (anthracenes, polyphenolics). A study of volunteers taking opioids suggested that a combination of stool softener and peristaltic stimulant was more efficacious with fewer side-effects than either alone[18]. When oral agents are not effective or not tolerated, enemas or suppositories should be considered.

Bowel obstruction

Ovarian and colorectal carcinomas are the most common malignancies associated with bowel obstruction; however, approximately 3% of all advanced cancers are complicated by bowel obstruction[19]. Intestinal obstruction can be caused by luminal obstruction, bowel wall infiltration, external compression, intra-abdominal adhesions, dysmotility secondary to carcinomatosis, or constipation/fecal impaction[19].

The traditional approach to a patient with bowel obstruction has involved surgical evaluation for removal of the obstructed portion of the gastrointestinal tract, or tumor debulking. However, patients at the terminal phases of their disease are often at high risk for surgical procedures. Nasogastric tube insertion has also been a common approach, but may not be as successful as was previously thought. Surgical literature has reported that obstructive symptoms were not relieved in 40–100% of patients undergoing emptying of the gastric contents[19].

There is growing support for use of gastrointestinal stents placed either endoscopically or radiographically[20,21]. When successfully placed, self-expanding stents placed radiographically relieved bowel obstruction in the majority of patients with a low risk of complications including colonic perforation, peritonitis and death[22].

Pharmacologic measures have shown promising results in the treatment of bowel obstruction. The antisecretory agent octreotide appears to decrease vomiting in the majority of patients[23,24], decrease nasogastric tube output[24] and possibly provide total relief of obstructive symptoms. A prospective randomized trial comparing scopolamine and octreotide in 17 inoperable patients with bowel obstruction concluded that both medications were associated with pain relief and removal of nasogastric tubes[25]. Octreotide had a more rapid reduction of gastrointestinal secretions. Parenteral hydration (over 500 ml/day) was also associated with decreased nausea and drowsiness[25].

Opioids and antiemetics are useful in relieving symptoms of pain and nausea[19]. Prokinetic agents can be useful in partial obstruction but may exacerbate symptoms in complete obstruction. Corticosteroids may decrease the inflammatory response, edema and nausea[19].

Nausea and vomiting

Nausea and vomiting are common symptoms in patients with terminal cancer[26]. These symptoms can be highly distressing to patients and can contribute to decreased quality of life. Optimal management includes medication targeted at the etiology, and alteration in factors that trigger nausea and vomiting. Non-pharmacologic approaches include relaxation techniques, distraction, fresh air, reducing prior triggers, avoiding foods with strong odor or sweet, salty, fatty, or spicy foods, and eating food at room temperature[27].

There are multiple etiologies of nausea and vomiting, with different emetic stimuli, sites of action and neurotransmitter receptors. Determination of the cause of the nausea and/or vomiting is the first step in initiating optimal treatment. Subsequently, therapy can be targeted at that specific cause. Medications directed at the receptor-specific causes of nausea and vomiting were successful in 93% of patients in one study[28]. Selected antihistamines acting at the vomiting center are usually effective when the stimulus involves the central nervous system. Phenothiazines and haloperidol are dopamine receptor antagonists that act at the chemoreceptor trigger zone and are often useful in nausea and vomiting due to medications and biochemical disorders. Prokinetic agents such as metoclopramide can be effective in gastric stasis-induced nausea and vomiting[28].

Dyspnea

Dyspnea, the subjective sensation of shortness of breath, occurs commonly in terminally ill patients. The etiology of dyspnea is usually multifactoral, involving mechanical, biochemical, vascular and psychogenic elements. Symptoms often do not correlate with objective measures[29]. Evaluation of dyspnea should be done in the context of the underlying disease process while treating initially to provide symptomatic relief. Treatment should also be aimed at the underlying cause in concordance with the patient's wishes. Reversible causes of dyspnea (e.g. pneumonia, pneumothorax, anemia, fluid overload, pleural effusion, or pericardial effusion) should be sought. If no reversible cause is found or primary treatment is not tolerated or desired, measures to relieve dyspnea symptoms alone should continue. Sometimes non-pharmacologic measures, such as relaxation therapy, breathing exercises, cool air and a calming presence may also be helpful[30]. Opioids can be considered for first-line treatment of the sensation of dyspnea. Opioids decrease respiratory distress by altering the perception of breathlessness, decreasing ventilatory response to hypoxia and hypercapnia, and reducing oxygen consumption[31]. Although systemic morphine is helpful in relief of dyspnea, nebulized morphine has not been shown to be better than nebulized saline for shortness of breath in randomized controlled trials[32]. However, several case reports have shown the beneficial effects of nebulized morphine on dyspnea[33–35]. Other medications that should be considered for treatment of dyspnea symptoms include corticosteroids, albuterol and benzodiazapines.

COMMUNICATING GOALS

In general, characteristics associated with higher likelihood of not wanting cardiopulmonary resuscitation include older age, female sex, diagnosis of cancer, dependence on activities of daily living and belief that prognosis is poor[36]. To the surprise of many physicians, the SUPPORT trial demonstrated that health professionals are not very proficient at predicting patient's end-of-life preferences[37]. Therefore, in order to provide treatment consistent with the patient's desires, it is helpful to determine the patient's philosophy for end-of-life care. Although Living Wills and advance directives have done much to increase awareness of end-of-life decision-making, their wording is often vague and difficult to apply to specific situations. On the other extreme, some advance directives give too many choices and

are overly specific – making their completion very difficult due to terminology and situations that are difficult to understand. One study revealed that patients often have misunderstandings about medical treatments such as mechanical ventilation even after discussion of advance directives[38]. It is also important to ask patients whether they have advance directives, because these are often completed without physician consultation or knowledge[39]. Even if a patient has completed advance directives, they are often not transported from the nursing home when a patient is hospitalized[40]. Although somewhat controversial, some studies have suggested that advance directives may not have accomplished their original goals exemplified by the following: no effect on resuscitation decisions[41]; no decrease in use of general medical treatments[42]; no reduction in costs[42,43]; and little increase in discussion between patients and doctors on end-of-life issues[42].

Although advance directives have not yet shown their full potential, they are still valuable as a way to encourage patients to discuss their values with the physician and their loved ones and to help the patient feel in control at a time when they are vulnerable[44,45]. Studies support the fact that patients want to discuss advance directives with their primary physician[46,47] and they prefer the physician to initiate that discussion[48]. One study reported that, when elderly patients were provided with evidence-based outcome data about prognosis after cardiopulmonary resuscitation, they often changed their preference for it[49]. A review of clinical trials of interventions designed to affect end-of-life care concluded that 'educational interventions aimed at physicians, using specific educational and motivational techniques, backed up by suitable organizational change, achieved increased use of patient preferences in decision-making'[40]. Studies also suggest that physician education reduces use of life-sustaining treatments[40].

The Patient Self-Determination Act of 1991 requires that health-care facilities receiving Medicare payments inform all patients about advance directives and ask whether patients have completed them. Often, this question is one of many on a preadmission form for the hospital. Ideally, the approach to initiation of advance directives should be individualized. If possible, the first discussion should occur when the patient is an out-patient at a time when he or she is relatively stable. The physician should approach the topic in a gentle manner with words that are easily understandable. It is valuable to determine under what circumstances a patient would view life as no longer worth living and then guide the patient to make decisions based upon that perspective. It is also helpful for the patient to designate a health-care surrogate to make health-care decisions if the patient is unable to speak for him/herself.

NUTRITION AND HYDRATION IN TERMINALLY ILL PATIENTS

The issue of when to withhold or withdraw artificial nutrition and hydration in terminally ill patients is controversial. Because eating and drinking are viewed as necessary and beneficial in healthy patients, it is often assumed that food and fluid provide the same advantage to terminally ill patients. Several studies, however, suggest that artificial nutrition and hydration may not prolong life and may actually hasten death. The data from the SUPPORT trial suggests that, although nutritional support in critically ill patients improves survival in coma, enteral feeding and hyperalimentation are associated with decreased survival in acute renal failure and multiorgan system failure with sepsis[50]. Additionally, patients with cirrhosis or chronic obstructive pulmonary disease are likely to have decreased survival with tube feeding[50]. The effect of dehydration on terminally ill patients remains largely unknown. Although thirst and dry mouth are common in dying patients, these symptoms have shown little correlation with fluid status and can be improved with sips of water and oral care[51,52]. Animal and human case studies suggest that caloric- and fluid-deprived subjects at the end of life do not experience distress, because of the analgesic effects of released opioids and ketones[53,54]. However, some researchers suggest that dehydration can be associated with terminal agitation and advocate the use of hypodermic fluid infusion[55].

A common misconception is that percutaneous endoscopic gastrostomy (PEG) tubes reduce the risk of aspiration. However, a reduction in aspiration pneumonia and mortality has not been clinically demonstrated[56]. In fact, one series of nursing home residents with feeding tubes placed for swallowing and chewing problems found a higher 1-year mortality rate compared to matched controls[57].

It is commonly thought that intravenous hydration increases the quantity of respiratory secretions. However, a study assessing the relationship between respiratory tract secretions, thirst and dry mouth in patients near death not receiving artificial hydration showed that, although the majority of patients reported dry mouth and sensation of thirst, those symptoms did not correlate with level of hydration[51]. Contrary to prior anecdotal evidence, there was not a statistically significant relationship between hydration level and respiratory secretions[51].

Although the option to withhold or withdraw artificial nutrition and hydration in terminally ill patients is still viewed as unethical by some health-care professionals and families[58], it has gained support over the past two decades. In 1983, the presidential commission on biomedical ethics determined that artificial nutrition and hydration were not needed in all cases and thus were not an automatic requirement for patients[59]. Additionally, the American Medical Association classified artificial nutrition and hydration as 'life-prolonging medical treatment' in 1986[60]. The legal right to withhold or withdraw artificial nutrition and hydration was determined in the Cruzan case, which noted that artificial nutrition and hydration should be viewed the same as other medical treatments.

CONCLUSION

With the growth of hospice and palliative care programs as well as the increase in research and education in end-of-life issues, care of terminally ill patients and their families will continue to improve. Attention must be given to the multiple causes of suffering among patients near the end of life, with emphasis on psychosocial, spiritual and physical factors. Effective end-of-life care is best provided with an interdisciplinary team working to achieve a patient's goals determined after discussion with the health-care team. We should continue to maximize quality of life among the terminally ill and allow them a dignified, comfortable and peaceful end of life.

References

1. Steinhauser KE, Clipp EC, McMeilly M, et al. In search of a good death: observations of patients, families, and providers. Ann Intern Med 2000;132:825–32

2. Berry ZS, Lynn J. Hospice medicine. J Am Med Assoc 1993;270:222–3

3. Facts and figures on hospice care in America. National Hospice and Palliative Care Organization website: www.nhpco.org September 2002

4. White KR. Hospital provision of end-of-life services: who, what, and where? Med Care 2002;40:17–25

5. Vigano A, Bruera E, Jhangri G, et al. Clinical survival predictors in patients with advanced cancer. Arch Intern Med 2000;160:861–8

6. Twycross R. General topics. In Twycross R, ed. Introducing Palliative Care, 2nd edn. New York: Radcliffe Medical Press, 1997:2

7. Von Nostrand JF, Cleeland CS, Gonin R, et al. Physicians' attitudes and practice in cancer pain management: a survey from the Eastern Cooperative Oncology Group. Ann Intern Med 1993;119:121–6

8. WHO. Cancer Pain Relief: With a Guide to Opioid Availability, 2nd edn. Geneva: World Health Organization, 1996

9. National Comprehensive Cancer Network. Guidelines for cancer pain. Oncology 2000; 14:135–50

10. AGS Panel on Chronic Pain in Older Persons. The management of chronic pain in older persons. J Am Geriatr Soc 1998; 46:635–51

11. Wolfe MM, Lichtenstein DR, Singh G. Gastrointestinal toxicity of nonsteroidal anti-inflammatory drugs. N Engl J Med 1999;340:1888–99

12. Whelton A, Hamiliton CW. Nonsteroidal anti-inflammatory drugs: effects on kidney function. J Clin Pharmacol 1991;31:588–98

13. Ehrich EW, Dallob A, De Lepeleire I, et al. Characterization of rofecoxib as a cyclooxygenase-2-specific isoform inhibitor and demonstration of analgesia in dental pain model. Clin Pharmacol Ther 1999;21: 943–53

14. Lanza FL, Rack MF, Simon TJ, et al. Specific inhibition of cyclooxygenase-2 with MK 0966 is associated with less gastroduodenal damage than either aspirin or ibuprofen. Aliment Pharmacol Ther 1999;13:761–7

15. Jacox A, Carr DB, Payne R, et al. Management of Cancer Pain: Clinical Practice Guideline Number 9. AHCPR Publication No. 94-0592. Rockville, MD: Agency for Health Care Policy and Research, US Department of Health and Human Services, Public Health Service, 1994

16. Abrahm JL. Advances in pain management for older adult patients. Clin Geriatr Med 2000;16:269–311

17. Rousseau PC, Disease-a-month. J Hosp Palliat Care 1995;41:769–844

18. Sykes NP. A volunteer model for the comparison of laxatives in opioid-related constipation. J Pain Symptom Manage 1996;11: 263–69

19. Baines MJ. The pathophysiology and management of malignant intestinal obstruction. In Doyle D, Hanks GWC, MacDonald N, eds. *Oxford Textbook of Palliative Medicine*. Oxford: Oxford University Press, 1998: 526–34

20. Dhir V, Gopal S, Saikia TK, *et al*. Palliation of malignant colonic obstruction by self-expandable metal stent. *Indian J Gastroenterol* 2000;19:86–7

21. Coco C. Use of a self-expanding stent in the palliation of rectal cancer recurrences. A report of three cases. *Surg Endosc* 2000;14:708–11

22. Camunez F, Echenagusia A, Simo G, *et al*. Malignant colorectal obstruction treated by means of self-expanding metallic stents: effectiveness before surgery and in palliation. *Radiology* 2000;216:492–7

23. Riley J, Fallon M. Octreotide in terminal malignant obstruction of the gastrointestinal tract. *Eur J Palliat Care* 1994;1:23–5

24. Mangili G, Franchi M, Mariani A, *et al*. Octreotide in the management of bowel obstruction in terminal ovarian cancer. *Gynecol Oncol* 1996;61:345–8

25. Ripamonti C, Mercadante S, Groff L, *et al*. Role of octreotide, scopolamine butylbromide, and hydration in symptom control of patients with inoperable bowel obstruction and nasogastric tubes: a prospective randomized trial. *J Pain Symptom Manage* 2000;19:23–34

26. Grond S, Zech D, Diefenbach C, *et al*. A prevalence and pattern of symptoms in patients with cancer pain: a prospective evaluation of 1635 cancer patients referred to a pain clinic. *J Pain Symptom Manage* 1994;9:372–82

27. Enck RE. *The Medical Care of Terminally Ill Patients*. Baltimore: Johns Hopkins University Press, 1994:11–156

28. Lichter I. Results of antiemetic management in terminal illness. *J Palliat Care*, 1993;9:19–21

29. Mahler DA, Rosiello RA, Harver A, *et al*. Comparison of clinical dyspnea ratings and psychophysical measurements of respiratory sensation in obstructive airway disease. *Am Rev Respir Dis* 1987;135:1229–33

30. Twycross R. Symptom management – respiratory symptoms. In Twycross R, ed. *Introducing Palliative Care*, 2nd edn. New York: Radcliffe Medical Press, 1997:95–8

31. Bruera E, Macmillan K, Pither J, *et al*. Effects of morphine on the dyspnea of terminal cancer patients. *J Pain Symptom Manage* 1990;5:341–4

32. Noseda A, Curpiaut JP, Markstein C, *et al*. Disabling dyspnea in patients with advanced disease: lack of effect of nebulized morphine. *Eur Respir J* 1997;10:1079–83

33. Farncombe M, Chater S. Case studies outlining use of nebulized morphine for patients with end-stage chronic lung and cardiac disease. *J Pain Symptom Manage* 1993;8:221–5

34. Tanaka K, Shima Y, Kakinuma R, *et al*. Effects of nebulized morphine in cancer patients with dyspnea: a pilot study. *Jpn J Clin Oncol* 1999;29:600–3

35. Zeppetella G. Nebulized morphine in the palliation of dyspnea. *Palliat Med* 1997;11: 267–75

36. Convinsky KE. Communication and decision-making in seriously ill patients: findings of the SUPPORT project. The Study to Understand Prognoses and Preferences for Outcome and Risk of Treatments. *J Am Geriatr Soc* 2000;48:s187–93

37. The SUPPORT principle investigators. A controlled trial to improve care for the seriously ill hospitalized patients: The Study to Understand Prognoses and Preferences for Outcomes and Risks of Treatments (SUPPORT). *J Am Med Assoc* 1995;274:1591–8

38. Fischer GS, Tulksy JA, Rose MR, *et al*. Patient knowledge and physician predictions of treatment preferences after discussion of advanced directives. *J Gen Intern Med* 1998;13:447–54

39. Teno J, Lynn J, Wegner N, *et al*. Advanced directives for seriously ill hospitalized patients: effectiveness with the patient self-determination act and the SUPPORT intervention. *J Am Geriatr Soc* 1997;45: 500–7

40. Hanson LC, Tulsky JA, Danis M. Can clinical interventions change care at the end of life? *Ann Intern Med* 1997;126:381–8

41. Kapp M, Mossman D. Measuring decisional capacity: cautions on the construction of a 'capacimeter'. *Psychol Pub Pol Law* 1996; 2:73

42. Gibson JMcI. National values history project. *Generations* 1990;14:s51–3

43. Kane RS, Burns EA. Cardiopulmonary resuscitation policies in long-term care facilities. *J Am Geriatr Soc* 1997;45:154

44. Singer PA, Martin DK, Lavery JV, *et al*. Reconceptualizing advance care planning for a patient's perspective. *Arch Intern Med* 1998;158:879–84

45. Martin DK, Thiel EC, Singer PA. A new model of advance care planning: observations from people with HIV. *Arch Intern Med* 1999;159:86–92

46. Edinger W, Smucker DR. Outpatients' attitudes regarding advanced directives. *J Fam Pract* 1992;35:650–3

47. Lo B, McLeod GA, Saika G. Patient attitudes in discussing life-sustaining treatment. *Arch Intern Med* 1986;146:1613–15

48. Johnston SC, Pfeifer MP, McNutt R. The discussion about advanced directives: patient and physician opinions regarding when and how it should be conducted. *Arch Intern Med* 1995;155:1025–30

49. Schonwetter RS, Walker RM, Kramer DR, *et al*. Resuscitation decision-making in the elderly: the value of outcome data. *J Gen Intern Med* 1993;8:295–300

50. Borum ML, Lynn J, Zhong Z, *et al*. The effect of nutritional supplementation on survival in seriously ill hospitalized adults: an evaluation of the SUPPORT data. Study to Understand Prognoses and Preferences for Outcomes and Risks of Treatments. *J Am Geriatr Soc* 2000;48(5 Suppl):s33–8

51. Ellershaw JE, Sutcliffe JM, Saunders CM. Dehydration and the dying patient. *J Pain Symptom Manage* 1995;10:192–7

52. McCann RM, Hall WJ, Groth-Juncker A. Comfort care for terminally ill patients: the appropriate use of nutrition and hydration. *J Am Med Assoc* 1994;l272:1263–66

53. Elliot J, Haydon D, Henry B. Anaesthetic action of esters and ketones evidence for an interaction with the sodium channel protein in squid axons. *J Physiol* 1984;354:407–18

54. Printz L. Terminal dehydration, a compassionate treatment. *Arch Intern Med* 1992; 152:697–700

55. Fainsinger RL, Bruera E. When to treat dehydration in a terminally ill patient? *Support Care Cancer* 1997;5:205–11

56. Ahronheim JC. Nutrition and hydration in the terminal patient. In Schonwetter RS, ed. *Clinical Geriatic Medicine*. Philadelphia: WB Saunders, 1996;12:379–91

57. Mitchell SL, Keily DK, Lipsitz LA. Does artificial enteral nutrition prolong the survival of institutionalized elders with chewing and swallowing problems? *J Gerontol Biol Sci Med Sci* 1998;53:207–13

58. Solomon MZ, O'Donnell L, Jennings B, *et al*. Decisions near the end of life: professional views on life-sustaining treatments. *Am J Pub Health* 1993;83:14–23

59. *President's Commission of the Study of Ethical Problems in Medicine and Biomedical and Behavioral Research: Deciding to Forego Life-sustaining Treatment*. Washington DC: US Government Printing Office, 1983

60. American Medical Association. *Current Opinions of the Council on Ethical and Judicial Affairs*. Chicago, IL: American Medical Association, 1986

17 Ethical and legal issues in nursing home care

Robert A. Norman, DO, MPH

OVERVIEW

I believe the task at hand is three-fold, a trilemma. First, we all must adhere to the federal and state laws. To avoid the risks of lawsuits, development of and adherence to clear, specific and appropriate policies and procedures, quality assurance and adequate documentation are a must. Second, the health-care professional must be allowed to provide humane, optimal and compassionate care, and not avoid responsibility because of fear of litigation. Third, and perhaps most important of all, the individual has the right, whenever possible, to make well-informed decisions about his or her own health.

As Loewy states, 'Physicians can give their patients facts ... can counsel them about risks and benefits, but ultimately it is the (rational and competent) patient who must decide (his or) her own fate.' Loewy further states that, 'by the same token, physicians cannot hold other moral agents hostage to their own belief system'[1].

Henderson points out there is a preferred use of 'resident' among nursing home staff. However, he states, 'such labeling masks the reality of institutional care as it is typically practiced. A person who has a chart kept on him or her, whose time is regulated by institutional convenience, and whose privacy is compromised by 'necessary' physical monitoring, such as vital signs, bowel habits, etc. – is a patient.' He uses the term 'patient' to

Table 1 Major principles of medical ethics

Autonomy
Respect for a person's right to self-determination regarding his/her life, body, mind and medical care

Beneficence
The obligation to do good and act in the best interests of others

Justice
The duty to treat individuals fairly and without discrimination, and to distribute resources in a non-arbitrary and fair manner

Non-maleficence
The obligation to avoid harm

Fidelity
The duty to keep promises

convey what he feels is the greater reality of institutional long term care[2].

The basic principles of nursing home medical ethics are noted in Table 1[3].

Table 2 lists common ethical issues in nursing home care[3]. The vast majority of nursing home residents have diminished functional capacities and/or cognitive impairments upon admission, and are therefore especially vulnerable and susceptible to having others make their decisions (paternalism). As Kapp points out, 'Life is a series of decisions waiting to be made. Many of these decisions become complex over time. And for each decision, there must be a decision maker.' He

Table 2 Common ethical issues in the nursing home

Ethical issues	Examples
Preservation of autonomy	Choices in many areas are limited in most nursing homes (see Table 3). Families, physicians, and nursing home staff tend to become paternalistic.
Quality of life	This concept is often mentioned in relation to decision making, but it is difficult to measure, especially among those with dementia. Agist biases can influence perceptions of nursing home residents' quality of life.
Decision-making capacity	Many nursing home residents are incapable or questionably capable of participating in decisions about their care. There are no standard methods of assessing decision-making capacity in this population.
Surrogate decision making	Many nursing home residents have not clearly stated their preferences or appointed a surrogate before becoming unable to decide for themselves. Family members may be in conflict, have hidden agendas, or be incapable of making or unwilling to make decisions.
Intensity of treatment	A range of options must be considered, including cardiopulmonary resuscitation and mechanical ventilation, hospitalization, treatment of specific conditions (e.g. infection) in the nursing home without hospitalization, enteral feeding, comfort and support care only.

continues by stating, 'Ordinarily, the person who will be most directly affected by a particular decision is the one who makes it. There are times, though, when that individual is not factually and legally capable of making and expressing difficult choices affecting his or her own life.'[4] The next step is one of great debate. Should the legal system be called in to empower one or more persons to make decisions on behalf of the incapacitated individual? What type of legal device should be used? How much intrusiveness into personal autonomy need occur? Decisions must be made on tough issues, such as involuntary commitment, guardianship, protective services, representative payees and powers of attorney. Each decision is filled with its own inherent problems and ethical dilemmas.

Table 3 provides an overview of the basic rights of nursing home residents. The Minimum Data Set (MDS), a part of every patient's admission record, has a specific section (Section AC, Customary Routine) dedicated to documenting residents' daily preferences related to the issue of individual rights. Although institutional policies and care routines determine most of these issues,

it is important to maximize these rights when determining the care of the patient.

DECISIONS TO LIMIT CARE

Among all of the issues, perhaps the most hotly debated involves decisions about treatment for dependent, frail, often cognitively impaired nursing home residents at the end of life. Loewy states, 'To limit access to healthcare for the elderly – rather than for those of whatever age who can no longer benefit from it – seems an arbitrary decision and one that, among other things, would clearly deny equal protection to an arbitrarily chosen group of people.' He goes on to state, 'A decision to limit care for all the elderly above a certain arbitrarily determined age should not (ethically speaking) even be considered before what constitutes waste is not communally defined and, as far as possible, eliminated. Society would be hard put to defend a decision to support young permanently vegetative or comatose patients (or to buy and use more than the medically essential technology) but to deny therapy to functioning persons merely because they had attained a particular chronological age.'[1]

Table 3   Basic ethical issues in daily care: the rights of nursing home residents

Access to and choice of medical and other health-related care
Opportunity to participate in resident and family groups (e.g. a Resident Council)
The right to non-disruptive care routines that account for individual preferences, e.g.
   bed and awakening times
   avoidance of routines that disrupt sleep
   choice of when to get dressed and what to wear
   freedom from unnecessary medications and physical restraints

Choices about eating
   freedom from unnecessary restrictive diets
   opportunity to eat non-institutionalized foods of preference when available
   right to eat at other than mealtimes, e.g. bedtime snacks

Opportunity and freedom to participate in activities, including activities outside the facility
The right to have visitors
The right to mange finances when capable
The right to security of personal property
The right to voice complaints and grievances
The right to privacy
   mail
   use of telephone
   bathroom and bathing
   non-intrusive roommate(s)
   confidentiality of medical and other records
   access to private area for appropriate sexual expression

Much of what happens to us is based on the 'natural lottery' of life – the destiny of our DNA[1]. The misfortune of some people in this world lands them in long-term care situations. Perhaps they have few family ties, are locked into wheelchair-only mobility, and are characterized by limited meaningful contact with others. We can simply ignore the problem by depositing our elderly and disabled in nursing homes, or we can choose to recognize the growing need to care for those souls spending perhaps their last days in physical and emotional confinement.

What is the patient's home?

The title nursing 'home' has legal and ethical implications. Statutes have been enacted in 32 states of the USA to ensure that terminally ill persons at home are not resuscitated against their will by emergency medical service teams[4]. Does the same apply to the nursing home? Is this not the patient's home? Does the fact that it is a form of communal group living erase the basic rights of a private individual?

Care of the dying patient

Key principles of caring for dying patients have been established by the American Geriatrics Society, outlined in Table 4[5]. In making decisions on limiting care, it is implied that the nursing home staff are willing and able to provide the care necessary for patients' comfort if they become subacutely ill. Substantial nursing time spent on prevention of skin breakdown, nutrition, hydration and suctioning is often needed. Transfer to an acute-care facility may be necessary if the patient's condition deteriorates.

Federal and state rules bear on many of these decisions, particularly those involving the intensity of nutrition and hydration.

Nursing home costs

In Florida, where I practice, the annual cost of insurance per nursing home bed has

Table 4   Key points in the American Geriatric Society's position statement on the care of dying patients

The care of the dying patient, like all medical care, should be guided by the values and preferences of the individual patient.

Palliative care of dying patients is an interdisciplinary undertaking that attends to the needs of both patient and family.

Care for dying patients should focus on the relief of symptoms, not limited to pain, and should be addressed by both pharmacologic and non-pharmacologic means.

Dying patients should be guaranteed access to comprehensive, interdisciplinary palliative care across the spectrum of care settings as part of any federal or state health-care reform plan, without care being conditional on the financial status of the patient.

Reimbursement policies should be modified to enhance the availability of palliative care.

Administrative and regulatory burdens that may serve as barriers to palliative care should be reduced.

Physicians, as well as other health-care professionals, at all levels of training should receive concrete, insightful and culturally sensitive instruction in the optimal care of dying patients.

The public, including out patients and out colleagues, needs to be educated regarding the availability of palliative care as an important and desirable option for dying patients.

Adequate funding for research on the optimal care of dying patients should be provided.

increased from under $300 per bed a few years ago to well over $3000 per bed in many nursing homes. Who or what is to blame? Unreasonable expectations of the patient or the patient's family? Greed? A poor grasp of the 'natural lottery'? The costs of lawsuits?

The insurance cost per bed is only one part of the costs directly related to legal pressures. Each nursing home owner and administrator has to be prepared to deal with the myriad problems that can occur.

Through economies of scale, the nursing home 'chains' can decrease their per bed insurance costs. In similar fashion to the stand-alone drugstore or bookstore, it is difficult for the 'Ma and Pa' single nursing home to stay afloat in the chain business mentality of the early 21st century.

ADVANCE DIRECTIVES

The actual term is 'Advanced Proxy Plan'. Few patients with diseases such as advanced dementia complete advance directives. Those documents that do exist are usually quite general and do not provide adequate guidance for specific medical interventions. A health-care proxy appointed by the patient or family member is almost always included in treatment decisions.

Disease-specific advance directives

Although most existing advance directives are generic, available for use in any health circumstance, particular conditions may warrant specificity. The Living Will of an AIDS patient might include information on pneumocystis pneumonia, toxoplasmosis of the central nervous system (CNS), dementia and cryptococcal meningitis. The Alzheimer's patient may choose to create a Living Will with competence to complete the advance directive, hospitalization, tube feeding and antibiotic therapy[6]. A person afflicted with chronic obstructive pulmonary disease may have a Living Will containing information with decision-making relevant to intubation and ventilation in case of acute respiratory failure. Metastatic cancer diagnosis may include Living Will information on cardiopulmonary

Table 5 Examples of levels of intensity of medical care that might be included in advance directives of nursing home residents

Cardiopulmonary resuscitation (CPR)
Mechanical ventilation (respirator care)
Care of intensive care unit (ICU)
Care in an acute hospital, but without CPR, respirator, or ICU care
Care in the nursing home only, including specific treatments when indicated (e.g. antibiotics, blood transfusions)
Comfort and supportive care only, with enteral ('tube') feeding if necessary for nutrition and/or hydration
Comfort and supportive care only, without enteral feeding

resuscitation, pain control, hospitalization and intensive care. A patient with hepatic cirrhosis may include information on blood transfusions, intensive care and emergency surgery to stop hemorrhage[7].

The disease-specific advance directives have several advantages over a generic directive, including an easier selection process due to a narrow selection of choices, more relevance to their particular condition and more exact prognostic information[8]. Table 5 includes examples of levels of intensity[3].

RESTRAINTS

What are restraints? Restraints are any devices or objects that the individual cannot easily remove and that restrict freedom of movement or normal access to his or her body. Examples include belts, vests, shoulder harnesses, geriatric chairs with tray tables, pelvic/arm/leg restraints, tightly tucked bedsheets and wheelchair safety bars[9].

Full bedrails are considered restraints if they prevent a resident's egress from the bed. Significant numbers of nursing home residents have been injured or died from inappropriately used bedrails.

Restraints should never be used as a means of controlling wandering or elopement[10]. The proper use is for therapeutic intervention to treat a patient's medical condition after obtaining informed consent, and only after less restrictive devices have been tried[9]. Restraints include the use of psychoactive medications, which can bring on potential side-effects in an older, frail population. The Omnibus Reconciliation Act guideline states: 'The resident has the right to be free from any physical or chemical restraint imposed for purposes of discipline or convenience, and not required to treat the resident's medical symptoms. Each resident's drug regimen must be free from unnecessary drugs which is defined by excessive dose, excessive duration, duplicate therapy, inadequate indications for its use or the presence of adverse consequences which indicate the dose should be reduced or discontinued.'

LEGAL AND ETHICAL ISSUES FOR THE NURSING HOME STAFF

Although the facility malpractice insurance generally covers the medical director, the doctor serving as director still works in the shadow of the potential litigation hammer. Given the nature of the nursing home business, it is a difficult job at best. The medical director is expected to provide coverage 24 h a day, 365 days a year. The task of overseeing the medical care of the patients is enough of a challenge; the medical director is often ill-equipped to handle the ethical and legal issues that arise. The Director of Nursing, nursing staff and other nursing home workers must attempt to do the best job possible given the institutional demands and workload. Sometimes the nursing home provider serves as a musician on the Titanic, knowing that the patient will go down (as we all must someday) but providing comfort. At other times, the worker needs to be aggressive in his or her efforts to keep the patient alive. All of this must be done in good faith and with good intentions, while working under the legal radar screen.

Biomedical ethics committee

In an ideal world, all nursing homes would have a biomedical ethics committee, filled with physicians, administrators, social service directors, community members, clergy and lawyers. Most nursing homes, however, do not have these resources. Options include joining with other nursing homes to form a committee or adopting the local medical and legal society's guidelines.

Biomedical ethics committees should be involved in education of staff, residents and families; development of guidelines, policies and procedures to handle ethical dilemmas; quality assurance activies that ensure adherence to policies, guidelines and procedures; and self-education about medical ethical principles and dilemmas.

I do not believe the biomedical ethics committee should make decisions on individual cases. In most situations, there is a lack of expertise, time restraints may come into play and the group should not take the decision-making process away form the resident or his or her loved ones. In rare circumstances when conflicts cannot be resolved in any other way, the committee can be involved rather than the court system. A neutral person, preferably a trained ethicist, can help mediate if the resident, family or physician cannot come to a mutual agreement[3].

ELDER ABUSE

A recent report (31 July 2001) from Cox News Service stated, 'More than 30 percent of U.S. nursing homes were cited for physical, sexual or verbal abuse of residents over a two-year span' according to congressional investigators. The study noted that 5283 nursing facilities had been written up by state inspectors in 1999 and 2000 for violations that often resulted in injuries to residents. The report, based on annual inspection results of the nation's 17 000 nursing homes, found a dramatic increase in citations for mistreatment nationwide since 1996[11]. The findings may be a result of better detection and enforcement, but also may reflect an actual increase in cases of abuse.

The article describes numerous horror stories on elder abuse. In Florida, a nursing home staff member took a call light button from a resident and placed it out of reach. The patient wet the bed due to the inability to acquire a bedpan. More severe cases of abuse included physical attacks on residents by staff in Illinois, Oklahoma and Ohio homes, and sexual assaults on frail female residents in Texas and California homes by male residents. Hundreds of cases of verbal abuse have been reported.

The federal government has been studying nursing home mistreatment for more than 15 years. Congress passed major reforms in 1987. However, a steady stream of investigation continues to turn up serious problems in the estimated 1.5 million nursing home residents.

The abusive treatment is blamed on many factors, including a severe nursing shortage, low staff salaries, a high turnover of nursing home workers (sometimes exceeding 100% a year) and poor screening of workers. The aides, who perform the majority of hands-on care, are often provided with only a few weeks of training and paid similarly to fast-food workers.

The American Health Care Association is calling on Congress for federal money to recruit, train and pay nursing home staff. The Bush administration has announced a new effort to provide accurate ratings of nursing homes, replacing systems that have been shown to be unreliable due to shifting conditions inside homes and uneven inspections by states.

TEACHING AND RESEARCH IN LONG-TERM CARE

I believe the nursing home has not been utilized enough for teaching purposes. Undergraduate and graduate students can find a wealth of knowledge in these settings, both from studying the rehabilitative, psychological and socioeconomic aspects of caring for patients as well as simply talking to the patients, who account for thousands of years of collective wisdom. Trainees in geriatric medicine should be given specific knowledge and skill objectives for their clinical rotations.

Along the way, we must be diligent about our boundaries when doing the important task of research. As Joel Savishinsky pointed out, 'While the growth in long-term care has also led to an increase in practical, policy-oriented, and theoretical research on institutions, there has not been a lot of attention given to the ethical issues that researchers themselves face in the conduct of their studies.'[12]

If nursing home care is to be improved, research involving well-designed studies demonstrating effective methods of managing common conditions is of great importance.

SUMMARY

Kapp, in his essay on 'Proposals for Improvement', suggests that, 'First and most fundamentally, physicians must possess and exhibit a high degree of compassion and empathy for the viccisitudes – medical, legal, and combined – sometimes encountered by their older patients. Instead of invariably and indomitably striving for and expecting to achieve a miraculous scientific cure, breakthrough, or remission in every clinical experience, the physician in many cases must come to realize and emphasize instead the palliative, caring, supportive purposes of medical intervention, the quality-of-life-enhancing opportunities that challenge the physician who is caring for a patient of advanced years.' Kapp continues his powerful writing by stating (page 254), 'The zero-sum ideology of medicine, in which there is clear victory or defeat, must be put aside in favor of a much broader spirit of compassionate sustenance as a valid role of medicine.'[4]

I have focused on crucial ethical and legal issues in nursing home care and suggested strategies for dealing with them. I hope ethical and legal decisions will live at the bedside and not be battled in court; the right of residents to make their own decisions should take center stage. Living under the constant fear of legal liability and the microscope of cost containment, we face an uphill battle. Informed health-care professionals, families and patients must come together in fertile dialog to make good decisions. The more we understand the complex world of ethical and legal issues in nursing home care, the greater the opportunity to serve the best interests of our patients.

WEB RESOURCES

Aging with Dignity http://www.agingwithdignity.org
This organization, which acts as an advocate for elderly patients and their caregivers, has made available to the public an advance directive called Five Wishes, which is valid in 34 states and the District of Columbia.
American Academy of Family Physicians http://www.familydoctor.org/handouts/003.html
Choice in Dying http://www.choices.org
Healthwatch http://www.cbs.healthwatch.com
These sites offer reliable, high-quality patient information about advance directives.
Educating Physicians on End-of-Life Care (EPEC) http://www.ama-assn.org/ethic/epec/index/htm
Module 1 of the EPEC curriculum provides a helpful model for talking with patients about end-of-life issues.

Growth House, Inc.   http://www.
growthhouse.org/
This site is a gateway to Web-based resources
on end-of-life care topics.
Living Wills and Values History Project
http://www.euthanasia.org/vh.html
The values history is an advance planning
document that addresses patients' values and
attitudes.

The Medical Directive http://www.
medicaldirective.org
This advance planning instrument was originally published in a JAMA article: Emanuel
LL, Emanuel EJ. The Medical Directive. A
new comprehensive advance care document.
J Am Med Assoc 1989;261:3288–93

References

1. Loewy EH. *Textbook of Healthcare Ethics*. New York: Plenum Press, 1996:280,259
2. Henderson JN. The culture of care in a nursing home: effects of a medicalized model of long term care. In Henderson JN, Vesperi M, eds. *The Culture of Long Term Care. Nursing Home Ethnography*, 221
3. Ouslander JG, Osterweil D, Morley J. *Medical Care in the Nursing Home*. New York: McGraw-Hill, 1991:444–445
4. Kapp MB. *Geriatrics and the Law*. New York: Springer Publishing Co, 1999: 101,184
5. American Geriatrics Committee. The care of dying patients: a position statement from the American Geriatrics Society. *J Am Geriatr Soc* 1995;43:577–8
6. Volicer L. Management of severe Alzheimer's disease and end-of-life issues. In *Clinics in Geriatric Medicine, Alzheimer's Disease and Dementia*. Philadelphia: WB Saunders, 2001:387
7. Emmanuel E, *et al*. A detailed examination of advanced directives. *Patient Care* 2000; Nov 15:92–108
8. Singer PA. Disease-specific advance directives. *Lancet* 1994;344:594–6
9. Weinberg AD. *Risk Management in Long-term Care*. New York: Springer Publishing Co, 1998;20–21
10. Johnson SH. The fear of liability and the use of restraints in nursing homes. *Law, Med Health Care* 1990;18:263–73
11. Cox News Service. Study: 30% of nursing homes cited. Reported in the *St Petersburg Times*, 31 July 2001
12. Savishinsky J. In and out of bounds: the ethics of respect in studying nursing homes. In Henderson JN, Vesperi M, eds. *The Culture of Long Term Care, Nursing Home Ethnography*, 105

18 Elder abuse

Bhavesh S. Patel, MD, and William Lewis, MSW, CSW

INTRODUCTION

The problem of abuse in our society is more widespread than thought by many health-care professionals[1]. Unlike child abuse, awareness of elder abuse among health providers is less clear[1,2]. Even though it is a serious problem in domestic as well as institutional settings, elder abuse has been slow in gaining the attention of health-care professionals and the community[1]. For clinicians, abuse should be considered as an illness and, if not considered in the differential diagnosis, will probably not be identified[3]. The following will summarize the growing problem of elder abuse including its definitions, risk factors, epidemiological data, detection and management.

HISTORY OF ELDER ABUSE

Rosenblatt and Lachs stated that early documentation of family violence dates back to the biblical account of Cain and Abel[4]. Elder abuse has been recorded since the 19th century, but not brought to the forefront until 1980, when it was addressed by the US House Select Committee on Aging. In 1973, the Older Americans Act established the Adult Protective Services (APS). In the UK, elder abuse began to receive attention in the late 1970s after reports of 'granny bashing' in the British media[4].

DEFINITIONS

Definitions and terminology of elder abuse vary tremendously among researchers and

Table 1 Nationwide reporting of elder abuse in the USA. From reference 9

Year	Number of reports
1986	117 000
1987	128 000
1988	140 000
1990	211 000
1991	213 000
1993	227 000
1994	241 000
1996	293 000

the laws of different states[5-7]. In 1987, the American Medical Association's Council on Scientific Affairs defined elder abuse as an act or omission that results in harm or threatened harm to the health or welfare of an elderly person[8]. The literature also shows a lack of consensus on the definition of neglect[5]. Neglect is characterized by withholding physical, psychological or financial resources that the older person needs to be happy and healthy[9]. Many authorities prefer to avoid the terms 'abuse' and 'neglect' and favor instead the terms 'inadequate care of the elderly' or 'mistreatment of the elderly', which includes acts of both omission and commission[7]. Federal definitions of elder abuse, neglect and exploitation were presented for the first time in the 1987 amendments to the Older Americans Act as guidelines for identifying the problem and not for enforcement purposes[9].

Table 2   Types of elder abuse. From references 1, 2, 6 and 11

Physical abuse
Use of physical forces that may result in bodily injury, physical pain or impairment

Sexual abuse
Non-consensual sexual contact of any kind with an elderly person

Emotional abuse
Infliction of anguish, pain or distress through verbal or non-verbal acts

Financial/material exploitation
Illegal or improper use of an elder's funds, property, or assets

Neglect
Refusal or failure to fulfil any part of a person's obligations or duties to an elderly person

Self-neglect
Behavior of an elderly person that threatens the elder's health or safety

Abandonment (violations of rights)
Desertion of an elderly person by an individual who has physical custody of the elder or
   by a person who has assumed responsibility for providing care to the elder

Table 3   Risk factors of elder abuse. From references 2, 15 and 16

Victim-related	*Caregiver-related*
Female sex	Use of alcohol or illegal drugs
Advanced age	History of abuse as a child
Dependence on caregiver	Shared living with the victim
Social isolation (risk for financial abuse)	Inexperience at providing care
Living with someone	Unrealistic expectations
(risk for physical and verbal abuse)	Overwhelming situation
Behavioral disorders	Psychiatric diseases
Physical and cognitive impairments	Economic or other stress
Dementia (risk for sexual abuse)	History of violent behavior

EPIDEMIOLOGIC FEATURES

The true national incidence and prevalence of elder abuse is unknown. Each year approximately 10% of the geriatric population are abused, with 4% experiencing moderate to severe forms of abuse[10]. Some experts believe that only one out of 14 domestic elder abuse incidents (excluding self-neglect) comes to the attention of authorities[7]. The National Center on Elder Abuse (NCEA) conducted a study on elder abuse and collected data from the APS and state units on aging. It was found that between 1986 and 1996 there was a steady increase in reporting of domestic elder abuse nationwide, with an increase of 150% during that period (Table 1).

The study also revealed that the median age of a victim was 77.9 years and the most common form of abuse in the domestic setting was neglect, followed by physical abuse, financial abuse, and other types. The majority of elder abuse victims were female. However, over the past few years, the gender gap has narrowed[11]. In the study, 66.4% of the victims were White, 18.7% were Black, 10.4% were Hispanics, and Native Americans/Pacific Islanders were less than 1%. In 1990, the majority of perpetrators were male (54.7%) but by 1996 there was no significant gender predominance. Adult children were found to be most frequent abusers of the elderly, followed by other family members and spouses[11]. Abuse that occurs in institutional

Table 4 Observations suggestive of elder abuse. From references 1, 6 and 7

Poor supervision by the caregiver
Delays in seeking medical care
Unexplained injuries
Missed medical appointments
Inconsistent histories between the caregiver and a patient
Discrepancy between the laboratory findings and the history
Implausible or vague explanations
Reluctance to answer questions
Recurrent admissions
Presentation of a frail patient without a designated caregiver
Attempts to prevent interaction between the patient and health-care providers
Fear of the caregiver
Living arrangement not compatible with assets
Unexplained withdrawals from a bank account

settings should be a concern of physicians as well. At present little information is available on elder abuse in institutions[1,7].

TYPES OF ELDER ABUSE

Many authors define four types of elder abuse: physical, emotional, financial and neglect[12–14]. The NCEA defines seven different types of elder abuse: physical, sexual, emotional, financial, neglect, abandonment and self-neglect[11]. Examples of physical abuse include hitting, grabbing, pushing, slapping or causing bodily injury. Sexual abuse includes indecent exposure, touching the genitals, breast, anus, mouth or attempts at penetration of the vagina. Emotional abuse involves threatening violence, humiliation, bullying, blaming, intimidating, name-calling or isolation of the elderly. Financial exploitation includes misappropriating money, forcing to change the will, or denying an elder the right to access personal funds. Examples of neglect include failure to provide food, shelter, clothing, medical care, hygiene and person care, or inappropriate use of medications. Abandonment (violations of rights) includes denial of privacy or participation in decision-making about health, marriage and/or other personal

issues. Self-neglect involves refusal to seek help despite having difficulties in performing activities of daily living (ADL) and instrumental activities of daily living (IADL)[1,2,6,11]. For definitions of elder maltreatment, see Table 2.

RISK FACTORS

Risk factors are different for each type of abuse and are related to the setting in which abuse might occur[2]. In general for the victim, risk factors are chronic diseases, functional impairments, cognitive impairment and social isolation. For the abuser, they are substance abuse, psychiatric disorder, history of violence and dependence on the victim[15]. Other risk factors are listed in Table 3[2,15,16]. Factors leading to elder abuse in institutions include staff with a high level of personal or job stress and low job satisfaction of the primary caregiver[1].

ASSESSMENT OF ELDER ABUSE

Identification of maltreatment is often difficult and relies on precise observation, history-taking skills and physical examination[6]. The American Medical Association (AMA) recommends that physicians ask geriatric patients about abuse routinely, even in the absence of signs and symptoms[17]. Organizations such as the Joint Commission on Accreditation of Healthcare Organization (JCAHO), the American College of Emergency Physicians (ACEP), the NCEA and the AMA have recommended protocols or objective criteria to identify victims of elder abuse[6,17]. Many assessment tools have been developed to evaluate elder maltreatment, but none has yet been validated. Observations suggestive of domestic elder abuse are shown in Table 4. Suggestive features of abuse in institutional settings include theft of money, oversedation, poor hygiene, substandard care, unexplained weight gain or loss, wrongful death, untrained or insufficient staff, unsanitary conditions and sexual assault.

Table 5 Questions to obtain information about elder abuse. From references 1, 6 and 7

General questions for victims
Do you feel safe where you live?
Who prepares your meals?
Who handles your checkbook?

Specific questions for victims
Does anyone try to hurt you or are you afraid of anyone at home?
Do you have frequent disagreements with your caregiver?
When you disagree, what happens?
Have you been slapped, punched or kicked?
Do you have to wait long for food or medicine?
Have you been made to stay in your room for a long time?
Have you been threatened or yelled at?
Has anyone touched you inappropriately?
Is your money stolen from you, or used inappropriately?

Questions for caregivers
What is it like caring for the patient?
What obligations do you have outside the home?
Do you ever lose control while caring?
Do you feel overwhelmed sometimes?
Any specific factors causing stress?
Do you understand the patient's illness, needs and prognosis?

A careful history is crucial in screening for possible maltreatment, and one should become familiar with the interviewing process[7]. It is very important that both patient and caregiver are interviewed together and separately during an evaluation. Demonstrating empathy, having a non-judgemental approach and understanding the caregiver's burden can increase willingness to discuss the problem, thereby yielding more information[7,18] (Table 5).

Health-care providers may want to start with general questions, followed by specific questions. It is recommended that confrontation be avoided during the data acquisition phase of an evaluation[7,18]. Victims of elder abuse do not always present with dramatic physical manifestations. Therefore, the physician must stay vigilant during the physical examination[1]. Signs may correlate poorly with reports of physical abuse[18]. In a review of 36 cases of emergency-department records, neglect was a more common manifestation of abuse than injury[19]. The most common physical injuries were unexplained bruises, lacerations, abrasions, head injuries and unexplained fractures. The most common clinical presentations of neglect were dehydration and malnutrition[19]. However, on an out-patient basis, the physician is more likely to encounter subtle forms of maltreatment in which neglect, psychological abuse or both may predominate[7] (Table 6)[1,6,7,20].

Finally, in the assessment of possible abuse and/or neglect, the physician should have some familiarity with the patient's financial and social resources, including availability of other members to assist the patient and offer financial help, if needed. This is of crucial importance when interventions are considered[7].

MANAGEMENT OF ELDER ABUSE

Management of elder abuse includes immediate care, long-term assessment, recognition of reporting barriers, and prevention. Every effort should be made to preserve the family and not just to rescue the victim from alleged abusers. Once maltreatment is suspected, the immediate concern would be the victim's safety. Hospitalization would be justified if the victim is in danger or requires assistance with ADL and medical needs[21]. Emergency shelter for older adults during an acute crisis may help until the situation can be evaluated and managed. If a person refuses any intervention and has the capacity to make that decision, his or her wishes should be honored[1,6]. In such cases, victims should be educated about the resources available for help. Victims should be made aware of the fact that abuse may escalate in the future and is unlikely to end without any intervention. A close follow-up plan should be established based on the individual's needs. For victims who do not have decision-making capacity, the court may need to appoint a guardian or conservator to make decisions about living

Table 6 Physical examination findings of elder abuse. From references 1, 6, 7 and 20

General appearance
Problems with hygiene, dressing, cleanliness, etc.

Skin and mucous membranes
Skin lesions (pressure ulcers, bruises, etc.) in various stages; poor skin turgor or other signs of dehydration; deficient care of established lesions

Head and neck
Hematoma on scalp; traumatic alopecia; lacerations and abrasions

Eye, nose and throat
Recent subconjuctival or vitreous hemorrhage; whiplash injuries from excessive shaking; deviated septum from repeated trauma

Oral cavity
Tooth fractures; oral venereal lesion or cigarette burns on lips

Chest
Welts; bruises or rib fractures

Abdomen
Unexplained rectal bleeding, bruises, spleen rupture or intra-abdominal hemorrhage

Pelvic
Unexplained vaginal bleeding; foreign bodies in vulva or rectum

Extremities
Signs of restraint use on the wrist and ankle, or immersion burns

Musculoskeletal system
Occult fractures, unexplained pain; gait disturbances

Neuro-psychiatric examination
Increasing or non-responding cognitive impairments; depressive symptoms; anxiety; delusions; hallucinations and behavioral problems

Imaging and laboratory tests
Multiple fractures in different stages of healing; low drug levels; lower levels of nutritional parameters or positive toxicological screening

arrangements and care[7]. Usually, the state APS participates prominently in this process.

The second priority is to contact the appropriate state agency directly or through local services[17]. The reporting of suspected abuse is mandatory in all states of the USA if the abuse occurred in an institution and in most states (42 states) if it occurred in the home. Individual state requirements on mandatory reporting of elder abuse can be

obtained from the NCEA. In more than three-quarters of the USA, the agency designated to receive reports is the APS; in the remaining states it is the state unit on aging[15].

Long-term assessment varies from case to case and requires the help of an interdisciplinary team. It includes education and counseling to patients, their families and caregivers. When a high burden of chronic diseases is causing abuse, respite or home care may improve the problem[1,7]. When psychiatric factors (in the abuser) are involved, such interventions become less useful and an alternative living arrangement may be required[7]. Employment assistance to the caregiver may decrease the incidents of financial abuse of the elderly. Barriers that would prevent reporting of future elder abuse must be identified and addressed. Victims keep silent very often about their abusive caregivers. This may be because of embarrassment in reporting their relatives or fear of nursing home placement. Patient's reluctance to report abuse suggests the need to empower older adults and to enhance their self-esteem[1,6,7].

Prevention of elder abuse is not well studied in research. Both the APS and area agencies on aging believe that professional and public awareness is vital to prevent abuse from occurring[6]. A physician or other healthcare professional may be the only person an abused victim has contacted. Recognizing and addressing the high-risk profile of victims and abusers can prevent elder maltreatment. It has been found that abused persons are at high risk of death. A large 13-year longitudinal study revealed that survival was 9% for abused victims when compared with 40% for non-abused controls[15].

MANDATORY REPORTING LAWS AND ELDER ABUSE

The Older Americans Act of 1976 established the Nursing Home Ombudsman Program to respond to the abuse and neglect of residents of long-term care facilities[7]. The

Table 7   Resource list of elder abuse. From references 6, 9, 20, 22 and 23

Eldercare Locator: 1-800-677-1116
National Center on Elder Abuse (NCEA):1225 I Street, NW, Suite 725, Washington DC 20005
   Phone: (202)-682-2470
   Fax: (202)-898-2583
   NCEA Website: http://www.elderabusecenter.org
US Administration on Aging: http://www.aoa.gov/
National Aging Information Center: http://www.aoa.dhhs.gov/naic
The National Council on the Aging: http://www.ncoa.org
National Association of State Units on Aging: http://www.nasua.org

reporting of suspected or confirmed abuse is mandatory in all states if the abuse took place in an institutional setting, as mentioned earlier. Mandatory reporting laws and reporting units vary from state to state for domestic abuse. Table 7 gives some telephone numbers and web addresses for reporting elder abuse. Health-care professionals should be familiar with laws in their geographical area regarding mandatory reporting, what must be reported, and consequences of not reporting or unfounded abuse after reporting.

The need for documentation

Accurate documentation of an event involving abuse is vital in management and for reporting. Health-care professionals should note the event using the patient's own words. Detailed documentation should include complete description of the injury, severity, duration, frequency and form of abuse. Pertinent physical examination, laboratory and radiological findings need to be addressed as well. Reporting of elder abuse is confidential and protected from litigation unless it was made maliciously[22,23].

CONCLUSIONS

The public health issue of elder abuse is still in its infancy and should evolve over time. Elder abuse occurs in many forms, and entails a high degree of suspicion for diagnosis. Clinicians should take a non-confrontational, non-judgemental and methodical approach with help from an interdisciplinary team to assess elder abuse. The health-care professionals should also consider the patients' perception and belief about what constitutes abuse in their culture. There is a need for systematic and prospective research in most areas of elder abuse including detection, management and preventive strategies. Health-care professionals and the public need to be increasingly aware of this major health issue and its prevention.

References

1. Clarke ME, Pierson W. Management of elder abuse in emergency department. *Emerg Med Clin North Am* 1999;17:631–44
2. Tinker A, McCreadie C. Elder abuse. In Tallis R, Fillit H, Brocklehurst JC, eds. *Geriatric Medicine and Gerontology*. New York: Churchill Livingston, 1998:1431–7
3. Lett JE. Abuse of the elderly. *J Fla Med Assoc* 1995;82:675–8
4. Rosenblatt DE, Lachs MS. Elder mistreatment. In Evans JG, Williams TF, Beattie BL, et al., eds. *Oxford Textbook of Geriatric Medicine*. New York: Oxford University Press, 2000:1164–9

5. Johnson TF. Elder mistreatment identification instruments: finding common ground. *J Elder Abuse Neglect* 1989;1:15–36

6. Kleinschmidt KC. Elder abuse. a review. *Ann Emerg Med* 1997;30:463–72

7. Lachs MS, Pillemer K. Abuse and neglect of elderly persons. *N Engl J Med* 1995;332: 437–43

8. Council on Scientific Affairs. Elder abuse and neglect. *J Am Med Assoc* 1987;257:966–71

9. Tatara T, Kuzmeskus L. *Elder Abuse in Domestic Setting. Elder Abuse Information Series, No.1 and 2.* Washington, DC: National Center on Elder Abuse, 1996–1997

10. Collins KA, Bernnett AT, Hanzlick R, *et al.* Elder abuse and neglect. *Arch Intern Med* 2000;160:1567–8

11. Tatara T, Kuzmeskus L. *Summaries of Statistical Data on Elder Abuse in Domestic Setting for FY 95 and FY 96.* Washington, DC: NCEA, 1997

12. McGuire P, Fulmer T. Elder abuse. In Cassel CK, Cohen HJ, Larson EB, *et al.*, eds. *Geriatric Medicine.* New York: Springer, 1999:855–9

13. Pillemer K, Finkelhor D. The prevalence of elder abuse: a random sample survey. *Gerontologist* 1998;28:51–7

14. Brewer RA, Jones JS. Reporting elder abuse: limitation of statutes. *Ann Emerg Med* 1989;18:1217–21

15. Breckman R. Elder abuse. In Beers MH, Berkow R, Bogin RM, *et al.*, eds. *The Merck Manual of Geriatrics.* Whitehouse Station, NJ: Merck Research Laboratories, 2000: 149–55

16. Fordyce M. Elder abuse. In Fordyce M, ed. *Geriatric Pearls.* Philadelphia: FA Davis, 1999;122–5

17. American Medical Association. *Diagnostic and Treatment Guidelines on Elder Abuse.* Chicago, IL: American Medical Association, 1992:4–37

18. Homer AC, Gilleard C. Abuse of elderly people by their carers. *Br Med J* 1990;301: 1359–62

19. Jones J, Dougherty J, Schelble D, *et al.* Emergency department protocol for the diagnosis and evaluation of geriatric abuse. *Ann Emerg Med* 1988;17:1006–15

20. Marshall CE, Benton D, Braizer JN. Elder abuse, using clinical tools to identify clues of mistreatment. *Geriatrics* 2000;55: 43–53

21. Gall JS, Szwabo PA. Psychological aspects of aging. In Cobbs EL, Duthie EH Jr, Murphy JB, eds. *Geriatrics Review Syllabus.* Dubuque, IA: Kendall-Hunt, 1999:23–9

22. Stiles MM, Koren C, Walsh K. Identifying elder abuse in the primary care setting. *Clin Geriatrics* 2002;10:33–41

23. Fulmer T. Elder mistreatment. In Cobbs EL, Duthie EH, Murphy JB, eds. *Geriatrics Review Syllabus*, 5th edn. Malden, MA: Blackwell Publishing, 2002:54–60

19 The older driver

Christina M. Davitt, MSN, GNP, and
Mary-Letitia Timiras, MD, FACP

INTRODUCTION

The role of the primary care provider is to maximize the older patient's potential for independent functioning while preserving safety. This can be especially challenging when decisions regarding elderly drivers need to be made. The policies governing older drivers are diverse in different states in the USA and in different countries[1]. The guidelines for physicians expected to guide patients and their caregivers in the matter of driving are inconsistent and diverse[2–4]. The debate of whether the patient's autonomy overrides their safety and the public's safety becomes critical when helping elderly patients and their families.

As geriatric persons comprise the fastest growing segment of the population, it would not seem surprising that the number of elderly drivers is continuously increasing[5]. This fact as well as the trend to move out of urban areas into suburbs or rural areas further accounts for the increased reliance on motor vehicles for transportation in the elderly. The availability of public or alternative transportation modes has failed to keep up with the demand in most communities, thus encouraging the use of private automobiles. Although it would seem logical that driving among urban dwelling elderly would be less of an issue because of the availability of public transportation, in fact the elderly are often too impaired by medical illnesses such as arthritis and heart disease to use the bus or the train.

THE OLDER DRIVER AND ACCIDENTS

Although the overall rate of motor vehicle crashes decreases after age 20, this rate increases for persons over age 65 if corrected for miles driven. Older drivers usually drive significantly fewer miles than younger ones, so it is important to correct for miles driven[6]. Having done so, the crash risk for drivers over 85 years of age is 2.5 times the average risk. Furthermore, the elderly have an increased risk of death from the same impact. Most crashes occur at intersections, particularly when making left turns against oncoming traffic. Older drivers have a greater likelihood of traffic violations usually involving right of way or sign errors. They are also less likely to reform bad habits after an accident, and continue to be a risk to others on the road[7].

PREDISPOSITION: PHYSIOLOGICAL AND/OR DISEASE RELATED

Chronologic age alone is not in and of itself a risk factor for hazardous driving[8]. There are many elderly drivers who can outdrive younger peers; but rather, a decline in functional status of the individual correlates with diminished driving abilities[9]. The decline is caused by a combination of physiologic changes that occur with aging and disease states that commonly affect aged individuals. One study suggested that the number of co-morbid conditions rather than

Table 1 Factors that may increase risk of adverse driving events

Physiologic changes
Visual
    presbyopia
    diminished visual acuity
    decreased visual fields
    decreased resistance to glare
Auditory
    presbycusis

Medical illnesses/drugs
Arthritis
Cardiovascular disease
Cerebrovascular disease
Dementia
Diabetes
Parkinson's disease
Sleep apnea
Alcohol
Medications (e.g. sedatives)

any specific one correlated with risk of adverse driving events[10].

Physiologic changes that occur with aging having the most impact on driving are mainly visual changes, although hearing loss (presbycusis) has also been implicated. Visual changes include decreased acuity, decreased field of vision, poor adaptation to change in light, heightened sensitivity to glare and deterioration in depth perception. Presbyopia diminishes the ability to see nearby objects such as dashboard gauges. The poor adaptation to light changes and sensitivity to glare make night-time driving more challenging. A study correlated impairment of field of view with increased crash risk in older drivers[11]. Although a decrease in reaction time is another physiologic change that occurs with age, it does not seem to play a significant role in crash risk. Possibly this is due to the older driver's ability to compensate for certain physical limitations; for example, by driving at slower speeds and avoiding dense traffic (Table 1).

Common disease states in the elderly that affect driving include: arthritis, dementia, Parkinson's disease, cardiovascular and cerebrovascular disorders, seizures and sleep disorders. Diabetics on insulin were at highest risk according to one study[12]. However, diabetics who are well controlled without hypoglycemic episodes do not appear to have driving difficulties. Coronary artery disease in and of itself also does not carry any increased incidence in crashes. Obviously any disease state that impairs mobility, control or limb strength will affect the driver's ability to maneuver the automobile safely.

MEDICATIONS AND RISK

The elderly, in general, take more medications than younger drivers, resulting in profound impact on driving ability[13,14]. The list of medications implicated in automobile crashes is extensive; however, certain classes of drugs are particularly troublesome. Any psychotropic or anticholinergic medications are high on the list of potential offenders. Benzodiazepines with long-acting metabolites and diphenhydramine are especially implicated[13,14]. Finally, the elderly are more susceptible to the effects of alcohol, which is well known to affect driving ability in all age groups.

MUSCULOSKELETAL FACTORS

Several studies have attempted to discover factors associated with an increase in motor vehicle crashes in an attempt to better evaluate the patient. One study identified the following factors associated with increased crashes in older adults: 40% or greater reduction in field of view, history of falls in previous 2 years, not on a daily β-blocker[15]. Another study demonstrated increased crash risk in individuals who had difficulty in copying a design on the Mini-Mental Status examination, walked fewer blocks and had foot abnormalities[16]. More recently, visual acuity worse than 20/40, limited neck rotation and poor performance on number calculations and visual attention tasks showed an increased risk of crashing[17]. There was a demonstrated increased risk in patients who complained of back pain, took non-steroidal anti-inflammatory drugs and exhibited poor performance on a free recall memory test[18]. These studies confirm the importance of visual and visual–spatial deficits as well as musculoskeletal abnormalities that inhibit range of motion.

Individuals with obvious musculoskeletal and/or mobility problems are more likely to adapt their driving or even curtail it if they feel it is appropriate. Likewise, individuals with visual limitations are also likely to modify their driving behavior, for example, by avoiding night-time or inclement weather driving. Individuals with dementia, however, are not likely to make appropriate adjustments in their driving habits, because of lack of insight regarding their cognitive deficits. Therefore, the health-care provider and caregivers are more likely to become involved in guiding such patients in deciding whether or not they should drive and in what circumstances.

SHOULD THE DEMENTED ADULT DRIVE?

The matter of whether or not demented individuals should drive provides the ultimate challenge for the health-care practitioner. Since dementia by definition involves deficits in several cognitive areas, including judgement and not just memory loss, it would seem worrisome for these individuals to be operating a vehicle where decisions are made on a continual basis. Some authorities do not recommend cessation of driving for individuals with 'mild dementia'[19–22]. Others recommend driving only under supervision (with a 'co-pilot')[23]. Some feel that all patients diagnosed with dementia should be evaluated by the Department of Motor Vehicles (DMV) in a formal manner[24,25]. In fact, the state of California requires physicians to report

demented patients to the DMV for further evaluation. Professional organizations such as the American Academy of Neurology and the American Academy of Psychiatry recommend that all patients with Alzheimer's disease be advised to stop driving completely[26].

REGULATIONS AND DRIVING

As alluded to earlier, the legal and governmental regulations concerning elder drivers vary from state to state. Most states do not have specific policies concerning demented patients. In most states, the physician is protected from liability issues if they report a patient to the DMV, in a few states they are not. Thus, the physician is frequently caught in a dilemma regarding patient confidentiality versus public safety. Furthermore, a demented patient may not care whether or not they have a valid license and will only stop driving if they have no physical access to an operational automobile. Occasionally, the family needs to get involved in managing the situation by disabling or removing the vehicle. It is often difficult, however, for families to stop their loved one from driving because of the consequent loss of independence for the senior and the increased burden on the family of providing transportation.

SCREENING AND EVALUATION

Is there a role for routine screening of older drivers? Some states require periodic visual and/or driving tests. One study showed the effectiveness of such screening[27]. Another compared motor vehicle crashes in two countries: one had screening and the other did not. They did not find any difference in the incidence of crashes[28]. There appears to be reluctance on the part of government to actively involve itself in this matter. Many seniors feel threatened by any limitations made on their primary mode of transport. In fact, there is an increased incidence of

Table 2 Evaluation of the older driver

Complete history and physical examination
Driving history
Visual acuity and field assessment
Joint range of motion, including neck
Gait and balance evaluation
Mental status examination
Driving simulation by an occupational therapist

depression among seniors who have stopped driving for whatever reason[29].

Therefore, there is an increasing reliance on the health-care provider to guide patients and their families in making decisions regarding the driving status of elders. Based upon current knowledge, it would be reasonable, in addition to a history and physical examination, to make some determination of visual limitations, range of motion limitations of neck and major joints, gait and balance abnormalities and, finally, mental status deficits. It is clear that a driving history should be taken in all individuals who undergo a geriatric assessment[30] (Table 2).

A comprehensive driving history would include any incidents, time, location and details of when the patient drives as well as comments from passengers or other observers. Additional help could be obtained from a formal driving test carried out by facilities that specialize in these evaluations; these services are usually associated with a physical or occupational therapy program[31]. In view of the importance of driving to the patient's independence and well-being, as well as the risk to society from impaired drivers, the health-care provider should attempt to maximize every patient's ability to drive safely[32].

References

1. Retchin SM. The older driver. In Pathy MS, ed. *Principles and Practice of Geriatric Medicine*, 3rd edn. New York: John Wiley & Sons, 1998:153–64
2. Reuben DB, Traines M, Silliman RA. The aging driver, medicine, policy, and ethics. *J Am Geriatr Soc* 1988;36:1135–42
3. Miller DJ, Morley JE. Attitudes of physicians toward elderly drivers and driving policy. *J Am Geriatr Soc* 1993;41:722–4
4. Berger JT, Rosner F, Kark P, et al. Reporting by physicians of impaired drivers and potentially impaired drivers. *J Gen Intern Med* 2000;15:667–72
5. Retchin SM, Anapolle J. An overview of the older driver. *Clin Geriatr Med* 1993;9:279–91
6. Bedard M, Stones MJ, Guyatt GH, et al. Traffic-related fatalities among older drivers and passengers: past and future trends. *Gerontologist* 2001;41:751–6
7. Messinger-Rapport BJ. How to assess and counsel the older driver. *Cleveland Clin J Med* 2002;69:184–92
8. Carr D, Jackson RW, Madden DJ, et al. The effect of age on driving skills. *J Am Geriatr Soc* 1992;40:567–73
9. Reuben DB. Assessment of older drivers. *Clin Geriatr Med* 1993;9:449–57
10. Forrest KY-Z, Bunker CH, Songer TJ, et al. Driving patterns and medical conditions in older women. *J Am Geriatr Soc* 1997;45:1214–18
11. Owsley C, McGwin G, Ball K. Visual processing impairment and risk of motor vehicle crash among older adults. *J Am Med Assoc* 1998;279:1083–8
12. Koepsell TD, Wolf ME, McCloskey L, et al. Medical conditions and motor vehicle collision injuries in older adults. *J Am Geriatr Soc* 1994;42:695–700
13. Weiler JM, Bloomfield JR, Woodworth GG, et al. Effects of fexofenadine, diphenhydramine, and alcohol on driving performance. *Ann Intern Med* 2000;132:354–63
14. Hemmelgarn B, Suissa S, Huang A, et al. Benzodiazepine use and the risk of motor

vehicle crash in the elderly. *J Am Med Assoc* 1997;278:27–31

15. Sims RV, Owsley C, Allman RM, *et al*. A preliminary assessment of the medical and functional factors associated with vehicle crashes by older adults. *J Am Geriatr Soc* 1998;46:556–61

16. Marrottoli RA, Cooney LC, Wagner DR, *et al*. Predictors of automobile crashes and moving violations among elderly drivers. *Ann Intern Med* 1994;121:842–6

17. Marottoli RA, Richardson ED, Stowe MH, *et al*. Development of a test battery to identify older drivers at risk for self-reported adverse driving events. *J Am Geriatr Soc* 1998;46:562–8

18. Foley DJ, Wallace RB, Eberhard J. Risk factors for motor vehicle crashes among older drivers in a rural community. *J Am Geriatr Soc* 1995;43:776–81

19. Torbe JD, Waller PF, Cook-Flannagan CA, *et al*. Crashes and violation among drivers with Alzheimer's disease. *Arch Neurol* 1996;53:411–16

20. Fox GK, Bowden SC, Bashford GM, *et al*. Alzheimer's disease and driving: prediction and assessment of driving performance. *J Am Geriatr Soc* 1997;45:949–53

21. O'Neill D. Physicians, elderly drivers and dementia. *Lancet* 1992;339:41–3

22. Fisk JD. Ethical guidelines of the Alzheimer Society of Canada. *Can J Neurol Sci* 1998;25:242–8

23. Shua-Haim JR, Gross JS. The 'Co-pilot' driver syndrome. *J Am Geriatr Soc* 1996; 44:815–17

24. Reuben DB. Dementia and driving. *J Am Geriatr Soc* 1991;39:1137–8

25. Johansson K, Bronge L, Lundberg C, *et al*. Can a physician recognize an older driver with increased crash risk potential? *J Am Geriatr Soc* 1996;44:1198–204

26. Zuin D, Ortiz H, Boromei D, *et al*. Motor vehicle crashes and abnormal driving behaviours in patients with dementia in Mendoza, Argentina. *Eur J Neurol* 2002; 9:29–34

27. Levy DT, Vernick JS, Howard KA. Relationship between driver's license renewal policies and fatal crashes involving drivers 70 years or older. *J Am Med Assoc* 1995;274:1026–30

28. Hakamies-Blomquist L, Johansson K, Lundberg C. Medical screening of older drivers as a traffic safety measure – a comparative Finnish–Swedish evaluation study. *J Am Geriatr Soc* 1996;44:650–3

29. Marottoli RA, Mendes de Leon CF, Glass TA, *et al*. Driving cessation and increased depressive symptoms: prospective evidence from the New Haven EPESE. *J Am Geriatr Soc* 1997;45:202–6

30. Gallo JJ, Robok G, Wlesikar SE. The driving habits of adults aged 60 years and older. *J Am Geriatr Soc* 1999;47:335–41

31. Lloyd S, Cormack CN, Blais K, *et al*. Driving and dementia: a review of the literature. *Can J Occup Ther* 2001;68: 149–56

32. Carr DB. The older adult driver. *Am Fam Physician* 2000;61:141–6, 148

20 Geriatric nursing

Rosemarie Lifrieri, RN, C, MSN, MBA, CNA, and
Susan D. LaMonica, RN, C, MSN, MBA, CNA

INTRODUCTION

As the world ages and the population increases, so do the challenges facing nursing. The medical complexities, the lack of sufficient care facilities, the aging caregiver, the shortened acute care stays, and the declining recruitment to the nursing profession lead to a constant uphill battle to provide appropriate care for the geriatric population.

The 'baby boomers' are now starting to age. By 2050 in the USA, the population of seniors 65 and older will double and those 85 and over will quadruple. By 2020, the ratio of those over 65 to working adults will be one to four[1].

Nursing has come a long way since Florence Nightingale. Although her basic philosophy and caring techniques are still our core, nursing has broadened into a more elaborate and complex process. Florence Nightingale's contributions to the evolution of nursing as a profession were invaluable. Before she undertook her reforms, nurses were largely untrained personnel who considered their job a menial chore. Her efforts raised the stature of nursing to a profession with high standards and important responsibilities. 'The Nursing Process is a systematic, decision-making process that involves assessment (data collection), planning, implementation and uses evaluation and subsequent modification as feedback mechanisms that promote the ultimate resolution of the patient's nursing problem. The process as a whole is cyclic, the steps being interrelated, interdependent, and recurrent.'[2] The professional nurse's skills of assessment, planning, implementation and evaluation are the fundamental elements which allow the nurse to be the essential health-care provider for the geriatric patient. Our assessments and plans are now considered valuable data for the overall care plan for the geriatric patient. Nurses of the 21st century struggle with maintaining the traditional elements of nursing care. This becomes more difficult in a fast-paced, high-technology environment. Often, health-care providers forget the humanistic aspect of the person in relation to the disease. One needs always to be cognizant of the fact that nursing care may be one of the key elements for the successful recuperation of an elderly person who has been ill. A nurse is defined as a person, usually a woman, trained to care for the sick or the infirm under the direction of a doctor[3]. Nursing has brought many rewards and satisfactions to caregivers who choose to accept the challenge of nursing the elderly. The geriatric nurse is a unique and distinct professional. In much the same way as physicians determined the need for practitioners toward the specific care of the patient over the age of 65, nursing also started to educate professionals and students in the specialty of caring for the elderly. The school of thought professing that all adults, regardless of age, should be cared for in the same way is considered to be outdated. The nurses who choose to care for geriatric patients know how to care for this population. Promoting geriatric nursing as a distinct discipline allows nursing care to be managed and treated not merely tolerated[4].

Nursing the elderly may occur in various settings such as acute care, long-term care, assisted living, residential housing, clinics, physician offices and the patient's home. Regardless of the setting the geriatric nurse chooses, their expertise is invaluable to their patients and colleagues. Just as nurses who choose to care for pediatric, obstetric or surgical patients, the geriatric nurse takes pride in the specialized caring of the elderly patient. This includes all factors which impact on the patient, such as family involvement, housing, finances and much more.

CHALLENGES FACING NURSING

Just when health care has begun to recognize the significance and importance of specialized geriatric nurses, it is faced with another pressing challenge. This new challenge is an acute nursing shortage. This is indicated by the dwindling enrolment of students into nursing schools as well as the aging professional nurse who is retiring. The nursing shortage of the late 1980s has prepared us somewhat for this upcoming nursing shortage, that is already noted.

As the population ages, so does the average age of the nurse. The National Sample Survey as summarized by the American Nurses Association indicates that nursing, the largest of the health professions, is also the fastest aging occupation in the USA[5]. The aging of the nurse population is becoming an issue of great concern. In 1996 the average age of all nurses was 44.3 years and, for working nurses, 42.3 years. By 2000, two-thirds of working nurses were expected to be over 40 years old[6]. (Figure 1).

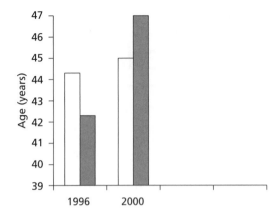

Figure 1   Age and nursing in the USA. White bars, average age of nurses; shaded bars, working age of nurses

Nursing schools have been down in enrolments and there have been indaquate replacements for the retiring nurse, who has spent a lifetime caring for others. Attempts by the nursing profession have been made, such as marketing to students in high schools and colleges and presenting a motivating curriculum which may entice this new generation. The aging nurse population is an issue of great concern and is expected to have the greatest impact over the next 10 years, as nurses decrease their workforce participation.

The World Health Organization warns that a growing shortage of nurses and midwives is jeopardizing health care in many countries due to poor pay and conditions and limited career prospects. We believe that Third World countries will suffer most without competent nurses, since these are being recruited to work in industrialized countries.

We must take aggressive steps now to help prevent a major world wide crisis. Such actions would include improved salaries and working conditions, and recognizing the profession as a much needed and important member of the health-care team.

Nursing has gone beyond backrubs and bedbaths to a new age, where geriatric nurses are essential team players who take responsibility for the care of the elderly patient. The shortage will be an additional burden in the future, but it will not change the need to care for a population that is increasing in numbers each day.

THE GERIATRIC ENVIRONMENT

As we begin to focus on the care of this aging population, concentration needs to be on the environment and its impact on the quality of life. Environmental issues influencing how and where a person lives plays a critical role in the overall care of an older person. There are many different environmental opportunities available to the geriatric patient today. The place where a patient, family or significant other elects to receive care may include a hospital, long-term care setting, assisted living facility, day care facility or the patient's own home.

Regardless of the setting, the environment is a major safety concern. We had the opportunity to participate in the development of a geriatric program including the development of an acute care geriatric in-patient unit. 'Our geriatrics program was planned by a multidisciplinary task force led by a recently appointed medical chief of geriatrics and included other physicians and administrators of the medical center's strategic planning, operations, patient care and nursing departments. We were determined to create a seamless continuum of care'[7].

With the assistance of an interior decorator, we were able to develop a unit specifically designed for the person who has diminished vision, arthritis, dementia, unsteady gait and/or a tendency to fall. Although this unit was created for an acute care facility, many of the environmental modalities and features can be adapted to any area including the patient's own home. The rooms included orientation devices, such as calendars and clocks. As a nurse or other staff member entered the room, they would utilize the calendar and clock to continuously orient the patient to time, place and date. This especially became useful when the patient

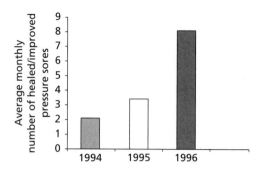

Figure 2 Improvement and healing of pressure sores in an acute care geriatric unit

confused day and night hours. A feature which proved successful was telephones with large dialing numbers, easy handle grips and amplifier ear pieces. These phones became essential for the patient with diminished vision and hearing. Patients were able to stay in touch with their families while in an unfamiliar setting.

Recommendations were made for selecting colors which promote a calm and soothing environment such as light blue, peach, or light pink. If curtains and borders are placed in a room, they should be of a simple pattern. Busy patterns tend to be confusing for the demented patient and may only agitate their behavior.

Pressure relief mattresses are a must if the population is prone to skin problems such as bed sores. These mattresses assist in preventing bed sores from developing and are known to improve the stage of the sore and promote healing. Regardless of what mattress or bed is used for the geriatric patient, nothing replaces proper skin care and turning, positioning and nutrition to decrease the incidence of serious skin breakdowns.

Figure 2 illustrates the improvement and healing of pressure sores from the skin-care practices utilized on our in-patient geriatric unit.

Bathrooms and showers are areas of concern in ensuring proper bathing and toileting. The shower must have a tub chair and a

Table 1   Geriatric design

Item	Specifics
Calendars	single-dated with large numbers
Clocks	large bold numbers
Telephone	large push-button numbers, amplifier earpiece, easy handle grip
Color schemes	soft pastel colors
Beds	pressure-relief mattresses, bed exit sensors
Bathroom/showers	tub chair, hand held shower head, safety rails, handicapped accessible
Activity room	dining, music, arts and crafts
Chairs	rocking chairs, appropriate height and hand grips
Corridor handrails/banisters	rounded
Flooring	simple pattern, no clutter or scatter rugs
Lighting	glare free

hand-held shower head that the caregiver can utilize easily, and the room must be handicapped accessible.

Another aspect for improved quality of life is the importance of socialization and recreational activities. In an institutional setting, a day room may be designated for this purpose. It can be utilized for family and patient visits, communal dining and recreational activities such as watching movies, listening to piano music, playing bingo, playing memory games or planting. This area can be staffed with volunteers. The desk area surrounding the nursing station must be patient friendly. Often the desk is too high for most patients who are either sitting in a wheelchair or who have diminished stature. A recommendation is to create a wheelchair alcove so a person may observe people and activities at the desk rather than the wall of the desk.

It is also very important to accommodate the geriatric patient at home. Almost all of these devices or modalities may be used in the home. Orientation devices such as clocks and calendars are easily obtainable, bathrooms can be modified, and special beds and mattresses are also available. Rooms can be pleasantly painted in soothing colors to promote a calm environment (see Table 1).

Safety is always an important consideration when the environment is evaluated, whether in the home, out-patient setting or institutional setting. Some simple measures include

the evaluation of the chair that the patient utilizes. Chairs need to be of a comfortable height and also have easy-to-grip arm rests. The chairs which we found most comforting for the older population are rocking chairs. These chairs are very soothing to the elderly as they rock and rest, sometimes falling asleep. Beds also must be evaluated for safety. The height of the bed must be appropriate for a frail elderly person to get in and out of easily. Side rails may need to be utilized if the elderly person is restless or agitated. Another device which can be helpful to patients and families is a bed alarm system. Most of these devices include a bed sensor, which is placed in the middle of the mattress under the bed linens. This sensor is connected to a remote sensor box located at the top or bottom of the bed. When the person's body weight is not sensed by the strip, the alarm sounds. This indicates that the person has shifted to the edge of the bed and may be in danger of falling. These devices are very helpful in managing the confused and agitated person both in an institutional setting as well as at home.

Proper handrails are essential for this population. In the institutional setting, rounded handrails are preferred over the traditional flattened handrails. Arthritic hands are able to grasp a round rail better that a flat rail. At home, banisters should be installed for assistance in walking and climbing stairs.

Flooring is another important aspect of the environment that is often overlooked. Floors with multiple designs overwhelm and may cause depth perception difficulties in the older adult. For example, a tiled floor with a border along the edge may cause the patient to walk in the middle of the floor rather than at the sides, where a handrail may be held for support. The border is visualized as a step down and may contribute to an increase in falls. Smaller designs in the center of a floor will deter the patient from walking in the middle of the hallway and guide them to the handrails. At home, special note needs to be made regarding scatter rugs and waxed floors, both of which are not recommended. The floors at home need to be assessed before use and should be free of clutter.

Lighting is the final safety concern to be discussed. It is suggested that lighting be glare free and not too bright. When lights are bright, the elderly tend to squint and look down, away from the light source. Poorly lit areas are also a hazard. Both of these may result in falls and potential injuries. These measures were implemented in our unit. Although over the years the patients were older and sicker, there was no significant increase in falls in our in-patient geriatric unit.

DISCHARGE PLANNING AND FINAL LIVING ARRANGEMENTS

Continuing with our thoughts on the quality of life of the elderly, the greatest concern is the decision making and planning of the final living arrangement. As nurses, we begin this process immediately upon meeting our patient, either in a hospital setting or at home. We begin by asking pertinent questions such as: Is there family involvement? Is the home safe? Can the person manage on their own? Who will shop and clean? How will they get to their physician appointments? Managing the discharge plan is a unique nursing role in our ultimate caring for the patient. We must focus on the patient as a whole, not

as a symptom or a disease entity. When the older adult presents at the hospital or in the home, they often feel alone and have a sense that their world as they know it is falling apart. We as nurses must assure them that we will assist them in making the appropriate plans to meet their needs. In order to do this, it is essential that nurses be an integral member of the health-care team caring for this person. Each discipline caring for this patient has important information that must be shared, to produce a complete picture. The ultimate goal is to utilize this data to determine a safe environment, so that the patient will return to a life style similar to that before the illness.

Home is always the preferred choice for discharge. If the patient is able to return to the familiar surroundings of their home, this is a bonus. At times, the plan must include visits from a home care nurse, physical therapist or social worker. Supplies may also be needed, such as a hospital bed, walker, cane, handrails, and a wheelchair. The older individual may benefit from a temporary arrangement of living with an adult child until they can return to a self-sufficient activity schedule. This may cause some concerns and additional burdens in the family unit. In many parts of the world, it is customary for the care of the elderly to be the responsibility of the extended family. Care management is a concept which is receiving wide international recognition, particularly in Great Britain and Germany. It focuses on optimizing out-patient nursing care which consists of four key elements. These are: need-oriented nursing, continuity of care, assisting family members in providing care and health promotion[8].

An assisted living facility is another alternative for discharge. This can be a solution which provides the best of both worlds. The elderly person usually purchases an apartment in a facility whose mission is the care of the elderly population. In this type of housing, the person has the independence of living alone, but may also utilize the services of the facility such as meals, activities for socialization, medical support when needed, and also cleaning and laundry needs. Several geriatric subjects find this type of living arrangement appealing. However, the drawback is that financial assistance is usually not available. Many elderly do not have the financial means to live in an assisted living facility.

The skilled nursing facility is also referred to as a 'nursing home'. In the USA these facilities were developed in abundance, in order to care for the increased number of elderly. These facilities have attempted to become more 'home-like' than in the past, when they were 'institution-like'. Many of those admitted to nursing homes require skilled nursing care. These are often people who have multi-system and complex medical conditions as well as Alzheimer's disease. These facilities are staffed with professional nurses and nurses aides.

In recent years skilled nursing facilities have broadened their scope of services to include both sub-acute care and rehabilitation placement. Patients may go to a skilled nursing facility for a short period of time, usually 1 month, to receive care which is not acute enough for a hospital but too complex to render at home. An example of this is someone who has undergone hip replacement surgery and requires rehabilitation to walk and return to maximum functioning capacity. This type of 'short-term' placement is usually arranged after hospitalization.

Consideration to place a loved one in a skilled nursing facility often takes special consideration from the health-care team and the family. Guilt and shame often accompany the decision to place an elderly family member. This is often the result of the inability to care for the person at home, either due to the complexities of the medical problems or other family, personal or financial responsibilities. When a decision is made to place a loved one in a skilled nursing facility, often the geriatric nurse facilitates in the decision making process.

END-OF-LIFE CARE

So far we have discussed care of the elderly in various settings and also issues which may influence that care. One aspect of geriatric care that is often overlooked is 'end-of-life care' with the emphasis on decision making, advanced directives, legalities and pain management. While most people state that they would like to die at home, only 23% actually do[9]. Often the elderly do not plan for their end-of-life care by executing an advanced directive. In many cases, the absence of an advanced directive is influenced by cultural norms and belief[9]. In the USA, discussing and obtaining advanced directives is a more accepted practice. The discussion of an advanced directive is mandated in certain states upon admission to a hospital or health-care setting. In the USA and other Western countries, where self determination or autonomy is regarded as a basic right and informed consent an essential element of responsible health care, the idea of withholding from patients the information needed to make informed end-of-life treatment decisions is viewed by many as inexcusable[10]. Many other countries do not hold the same beliefs. Some family members believe that discussing the medical condition or possible outcome of their elders places a burden on the patient, and they may not wish to live any longer. As nurses and health-care professionals, we must be able to adapt and understand the various cultural and religious differences of the patients we care for. The lesson to be learned is that we, as health-care providers, need to be culturally sensitive when we approach end-of-life discussions with our elderly patients. Non-Hispanic White patients were more likely to refuse intubation and continuance of life-sustaining treatment, in case of dementia, than Hispanic or African-American patients. Among Asian and Pacific Island cultures, the interaction of Buddhism, Confucianism and Christianity support filial piety[10]. To protect the elder, the family assumes the decision-making role[10].

Where feasible, it is important for nurses to speak with family members and encourage open communication in understanding the geriatric patient's wishes. It is ideal for this to take place prior to the patient becoming gravely ill. This would be the opportune time for nurses to advocate the appointment of a health-care proxy. This health-care proxy would be the designated person, who is involved in the patient's care, to make health-related decisions when the patient is no longer able.

If a patient decides to appoint a health-care proxy, and documentation is completed, nurses must educate both the patient and the proxy regarding where it should be kept. It is best not to secure it in a place where it will be difficult to be retrieved when needed. Emphasis should be placed on the importance of having both the patient and the proxy keep a copy of the advanced directive with them at all times. Often during the crisis of a sudden illness, the advanced directive is forgotten and can jeopardize the wishes of the patient being followed.

The *New York Times* has stated that there are many reasons that the documents, known collectively as advanced directives, can fail: people lose or forget them; Living Wills are too vague to interpret; relatives disagree about what the patient wanted; hospital staff members mistakenly fear prosecution for stopping life support; or doctors overrule the family and refuse to stop treatment[11].

Although advocacy for elder autonomy is important, special consideration may limit the older adult's ability to act autonomously. These circumstances include internal and external constraints. Internal constraints focus more on when the older adult becomes either physically or mentally incapacitated. External constraints arise when the autonomous actions on the part of the person are limited as a result of being institutionalized, or changes in formal support systems[12].

Regardless of the setting in which we care for the elderly person, it is the nurse as the primary caregiver who has the opportunity to discuss three key issues:

(1) Have they thought about their end-of-life care?

(2) Have they discussed and shared it with the family?

(3) Have they completed the appropriate papers to ensure their wishes are followed?

These papers can include a health-care proxy, a Living Will (which will be used as a guide to their treatment plan), and a power of attorney (this legally appoints someone to oversee their assets). It is the nursing professional who is the advocate for ensuring that the patient's end-of-life wishes are respected. We must also remember the enormous responsibilities placed on family and loved ones who are appointed to carry out the patient's wishes, particularly if they are caring for them at home. As nursing professionals, our role includes caring for all aspects of the patient, which includes the family.

Finally, we focus on pain management. Pain management has become a major theme in health care today, and this is especially true in the elderly, as it relates to quality of life and end-of-life care. Most often the pain experienced by the elderly is musculoskeletal pain due to arthritis or other processes associated with the aging process. This may not appear to be of significant seriousness. However, this chronic pain grossly impacts on the geriatric person's ability to perform activities of daily living.

International research findings indicate that there is a gap between pain management practices. It has been shown that practices that utilize nursing to assist in formalizing their program have proved beneficial[13].

In order to effectively treat pain, we must first know its severity. There are various tools that can assist the nurse and caregiver in assessing pain. Although these tools appear simple, proper assessment of pain is a difficult task. Most pain studies exclude cognitively impaired elderly patients entirely; therefore, few data are available to guide health-care practitioners in selecting effective and appropriate assessment strategies for them[14]. Once we have determined the severity of pain the patient is experiencing, the next step is often the most difficult and challenging. Because they are more likely to need analgesics for chronic pain and take more medications for both acute and chronic conditions, elderly patients are more likely to suffer from adverse effects of drugs and drug interactions[15]. Treating pain appropriately in the elderly is both an art and a science. Extended use of aspirin and non-steroidal anti-inflammatory drugs may harm the geriatric patient, since these drugs have been noted to contribute to gastrointestinal disease, and kidney and liver dysfunction. Since these medications can easily be purchased over the counter at any pharmacy or market, nurses and physicians must educate the elderly about potential side-effects and drug–drug interactions, and instruct the patient on other available pain relief alternatives. If a more potent medication is prescribed for pain relief, the caregiver must alert the family to the possibility to the medicine causing dizziness, which may lead to falls and injury. Patient education and family teaching is essential.

Complementary and alternative medicine may be an option for pain relief, particularly for the elderly. These include a broad range of treatments such as chiropractic, acupuncture, massage therapy, homeopathy, nutrition, and natureopathy[16]. These therapies have proved to be successful in managing pain, and can be a favorable and safe alternative for the geriatric age group.

Our final thoughts are that caregivers should attempt to utilize all available measures to keep the patient as free of pain as possible, in order to maintain quality and dignity at the end of life[17].

CONCLUSION

If we choose to care for the aging population, we have the responsibility to be knowledgeable about the aspects which make them unique. We also must understand that we are first and foremost advocates for our patients. Their treatment and care must be managed in a way that promotes well-being with positive outcomes in their life. We all play a major role in assuring that the latter part of people's lives are fulfilling. Nursing must work collaboratively with other professions in seeking to achieve these outcomes. The future health care of the elderly population depends on the recruitment and retention of new professionals who have a deep commitment and respect for what they can learn from the life experiences of the people they care for.

Nursing in the millennium is much more than bedbaths, backrubs, thermometers and starched white uniforms. It is a profession with advanced skills and knowledge in treating and caring for the patient's body, mind and spirit.

References

1. Ervin S. Fourteen forecasts for an aging society. *Futurist* 2000;34:24–8
2. Brunner LS, Suddarth DS. Medical–surgical nursing. In Intenzo D, Ewan H, eds. *The Lippincott Manual of Nursing Practice*, 4th edn. Philadelphia: JB Lippincott, 1986:3–16
3. Cayne BS, Lechner DE, eds. *The New Webster's Comprehensive Dictionary of the English Language*. New York: Lexicon Publications, 1990:690
4. Fulmer T, Abraham IL. Rethinking geriatric nursing. In James M, Morrison KN, eds. *The

Nursing Clinics of North America. Philadelphia: WB Saunders, 1998:387–93

5. Johnson AE. National sample survey of registered nurses. *Health Resources and Services Administration* (on-line), 2000. *http://bhpr. hrsa.gov//dn/survnote.htm*

6. Gregg M. The new realities in the nurse supply. *The U.S. Nursing Shortage* (on-line), 1997. *http://www.hrlive.com/reports/ rnshortage.html*

7. Dharmarajan TS, Lifrieri R, Gerstner LS. Launching a geriatric unit. *Health Progress* 1998;79:46–51

8. Schaeffer D. Care management: scientific thoughts on a current topic. *Pflege* 2000; 13:17–26

9. Caralis PV, Davis B, Wright K, *et al.* The influence of ethnicity and race on attitudes toward advance directives, life-prolonging treatments and euthanasia. *J Clin Ethics* 1993;4:155–65

10. Mitty E. Ethnicity and end of life decision making. *Reflect Nurse Leadership* 2001; 29–31

11. Grady D. At life's end, many patients are denied peaceful passing. *New York Times* 2000:1–A13

12. Castellucci DT. Issues for nurses regarding elder autonomy. In McDaniel C, ed. *The Nursing Clinics of North America.* Philadelphia: WB Saunders, 1998:265–73

13. Muller-Mundt G, Brinkhoff P, Schaeffer D. Pain management and nursing care – results of a review of the literature. *Pflege* 2000; 13:325–38

14. Wynne CF, Ling SM, Remsburg R. Comparison of pain assessment instrument in cognitively intact and cognitively impaired nursing home residents. *Geriatr Nurs* 2000;21:20–3

15. Miller CA. Advising older adults about pain remedies. *Geriatr Nurs* 2000;21:55–57

16. Thompson E. The alternative model. *Modern Healthcare* 2000;30:26–34

17. O'Donohoe JA. End of life care and catholic ethics. *Health Progress* 2000;81: 46–8

21 Falls

Suzanne D. Fields, MD

INTRODUCTION

In the geriatric literature, by definition, a fall is an event that leads to the conscious subject coming to rest inadvertently on the ground.[1] Some falls occur during hazardous activity; these falls could happen to people of any age. Other falls, especially in frail elder subjects, occur during routine daily activities, and are the subject of geriatric investigation and research.

Approximately 35–40% of community-dwelling elderly fall each year; 10–15% of falls are associated with major injury, including fractures, joint dislocations, burns, broken dentures, hematomas, lacerations, brain injuries and contusions[1,2]. The incidence of fall-related hip fractures is estimated at 25 000/year. Injuries are more likely to occur if the faller lands on a hard surface or if the fall involves the stairs. The more frequent the falls, the greater the risk of sustaining a serious injury and the more likely that placement may be required in a skilled nursing facility[3]. Although death is not a frequent consequence of falls, unintentional injuries are the fifth leading cause of death in older adults. Complications caused by falls (e.g. hip fractures and subsequent thromboembolism, head trauma and subsequent brain injury) are the leading cause of injury-related death in seniors. Many patients over 80 with poor balance and gait are unable to get up from a fall without assistance. Long lies can lead to pressure sores, hypothermia, dehydration and pneumonia, requiring hospitalization as well as fear of falling again, functional decline and social isolation[4].

RISK FACTORS

Epidemiological studies have revealed that certain community-dwelling elderly patients are at higher risk of falling. Advanced age, history of previous falls, cognitive impairment or confusion, use of psychotropic medication, impairments in gait and balance, poor vision, including decreased binocular vision and a loss of edge-contrast sensitivity, 'dizziness', and medical co-morbidity with certain diseases (e.g. arthritis) are predisposing factors[5,6]. Tinetti and colleagues found that among community-dwelling elderly the percentage of persons falling increased from 8% for those with no risk factor to 78% for those with four or more risk factors[5]. Many patients who fall do so repeatedly.

Among nursing home residents, approximately half fall each year and 9% of fallers sustain serious injury[1]. Rates of falling are also higher for hospitalized elderly, where rates of 1.2–7.4/1000 patient-days for older adults have been reported[7]. Patients who fall in the hospital have longer lengths of hospital stay and higher mortality rates than those who do not fall[7]. In a quality assurance analysis we performed at a 500-bed tertiary care teaching hospital, the mortality rate for fallers was over three times that of non-fallers, and the average length of stay was 7.5 times that of non-fallers. We found that 17% of falls resulted in a significant injury. Patients with neurologic and psychiatric diseases had higher rates of falls than patients with other diagnoses (unpublished data). Several investigators have sought to identify patients at high risk for falls, so that fall prevention programs could be instituted to targeted individuals. British researchers, using a case–control technique, developed and evaluated an evidence-based risk assessment tool (STRATIFY) to predict which elderly in-patients would fall. The instrument relies on nursing assessments and identifies patients who have had previous falls, are agitated, are visually impaired, are in need of frequent toileting or who have transfer and mobility scores of 3 or 4 (obtained by combining the transfer and mobility sections of the Barthel Index) as those most likely to fall in the hospital. The instrument, scored 0–5, has a sensitivity and specificity of 93% and 88%, respectively[8]. Other studies have shown that medical co-morbidity and confusion are independent risk factors for falls in hospitalized adults[7].

ETIOLOGY AND PATHOPHYSIOLOGY

Falls are rarely due to a single, isolated process or event; rather, there are intrinsic and environmental factors that are contributory. This fact has clinical implications because data suggest that decreasing even one contributing factor will diminish the risk of future falls[9,10]. Intrinsic factors include physiologic changes of aging and diseases that increase in prevalence with aging as well as the medications used to treat those diseases. Muscle weakness, gait impairment, balance disorders, dizziness or vertigo and postprandial or orthostatic hypotension are common etiologies among the frail elderly. Carotid sinus syndrome is a frequently overlooked cause of recurrent falls and syncope.

Postural control depends on proprioception in the lower limbs, visual contrast sensitivity and depth perception, reaction time and body sway. Changes in depth perception, binocular visual acuity and contrast discrimination were shown in a recent study to predispose elderly patients in the community to fall[6]. As humans age, they tend to have greater glare intolerance and lose the ability to accommodate at night. Diminished proprioception may result from peripheral neuropathy, cervical spondylosis or central nervous system (CNS) diseases.

Gait disorders in the elderly may be secondary to:

(1) Specific CNS diseases, such as Parkinson's disease, normal pressure hydrocephalus, or Lewy body dementia;

(2) Neuromuscular diseases that affect muscle strength (e.g. myopathies), joint strength or mobility (e.g. arthritis);

(3) Foot disorders (bunions, calluses, hammer toes);

(4) Medications with extrapyramidal, cognitive or orthostatic side-effects.

Any cardiovascular condition that results in diminished cerebral perfusion or oxygenation may impair postural stability. Sedative–hypnotic medications, especially long-acting benzodiazepines, have been associated with falls, as have antidepressants. Excessive alcohol consumption may further contribute to the problem. Some risk factors are modifiable (e.g. muscle weakness, medication side-effect, or orthostatic hypotension), whereas others are not (e.g. blindness due to senile macular degeneration, hemiplegia from an old stroke).

Acute medical conditions may also predispose the elderly to falls. In point of fact, the fall may be the presenting sign in acute infections, myocardial infarction, or other serious conditions in frail elderly patients. In more active seniors, environment-related causes are paramount. Clutter, loose rugs, poorly fitting shoes, dim lighting and slippery surfaces may all be contributory.

Accidental falls often result from an inability to compensate for such common environmental hazards. In their sixties and early seventies, people who fall extend their arms and wrists to break the fall by a righting reflex. The result is often a Colles wrist fracture. As people grow older, they lose this ability and a hip fracture ensues.

CLINICAL EVALUATION

For fear of losing their independence, the elderly tend to underreport falls in the out-patient setting. As a result, clinicians may need to question patients specifically about the problem. Often the history can provide clues to the etiology. Here, prevention is key – trying to eliminate risk factors or contributing factors for falls so as to prevent future occurrences. An evidence-based guideline by the American Geriatrics Society (AGS), British Geriatrics Society and American Academy of Orthopedic Surgeons Panel on Falls Prevention[10] provides insight into the proper evaluation and management of falls in older patients. The AGS panel recommends that primary care clinicians perform a brief screen to identify patients at risk. For patients with a history of a single fall, the panel advises checking for a gait or balance problem. With an experience of multiple falls, patients should undergo a complete falls assessment and multifactorial intervention program as appropriate. In the acute situation, where a health provider is called to evaluate a patient for a fall, the approach is somewhat different. Serious injury needs to be ruled out, underlying acute illness excluded and an etiology for the fall sought. Preventive measures can be subsequently instituted (see below) to avert further falling.

History

A simple pneumonic device to recall the key components to a successful falls history is SPLAT: **S**ymptoms, **P**rior falls, **L**ocation of the fall, **A**ctivity during the fall and **T**ime of day the fall occurred. The key is to seek patterns or clues for ascertaining the cause of the fall. For example, do falls always occur after a meal? In this case, postprandial orthostatic hypotension may be operative. Do the falls occur at night? Here, poor lighting may be causative.

In the hospital setting or in the emergency room, questions to ask companions include:

(1) Was the fall witnessed?

(2) Is there an obvious injury, particularly head injury?

(3) Is there currently a change in level of consciousness?

(4) Was there transient loss of consciousness before or after the fall?

(5) Was the patient on anticoagulation or antiepileptic seizure medications at the time of the fall?

(6) What other medication, particularly sedative–hypnotics, does the patient take? (review prescribed and over-the-counter medications).

One then obtains a brief history from the patient, assuming there is no underlying dementia. Ascertain whether the patient is aware of the event, associated symptoms experienced, activities prior to the fall (e.g. coughing, micturating, straining at stool), presence of pain and a history of prior falls. A focused chart review is performed to determine the reason for admission, to obtain relevant history (particularly history of arrhythmias, seizures, autonomic neuropathy and 'sundowning' or night-time confusion) and to review the medication list and most recent laboratory studies.

Physical examination

In the acute setting, the first step in evaluation is to check whether the patient appears alert, groggy or confused, comfortable or in

Table 1 Abnormal gait patterns seen in the elderly. Adapted from reference 14

Type abnormal gait	Manifestations	Example
Sensory ataxic	wide-based; patients lift feet high and uncertainly; eyes are fixed to ground; gait worse in dark	pernicious anemia
Hemiplegic	leg is extended at knee and circumducted at the hip; toes scrape the floor; decreased arm swing	stroke
Parkinsonian	short steps; shuffling feet; stooped trunk; decreased or absent arm swing; retropulsion; hypokinesis; festination	Parkinson's disease
Apraxic	magnetic or glue-footed gait; inability to initiate gait; very clumsy; shuffling may be present; +/−incontinence and memory loss	normal pressure hydrocephalus; other subcortical dementias
Waddling	wide-based, swaying gait	degenerative joint disease; Proximal muscle weakness
Cerebellar ataxic	wide-based, reeling, very unsteady gait	cerebellar stroke; cerebellar degeneration

pain and stable or critically ill. If on anticoagulation, exclude head injury, because such patients require an emergency cranial computed tomography (CT) scan and reversal of anticoagulation. The physical examination needs to assess the extent of injury and focus on relevant organ systems for clues to the etiology of the fall. To exclude serious injury, the following signs should be noted: orthostatic vital signs, pupil size and reaction, examination of the tongue for teeth marks or hematomas, a careful examination of the head, spine and ribs for ecchymoses or localized tenderness, passive range of motion of all four limbs for pain, a complete neurologic examination to exclude new asymmetry and an assessment of level of consciousness by the Glasgow Coma Scale. To help determine the etiology of falls, the physical examination should include: a cardiovascular examination (to exclude arrhythmias and significant murmurs); an examination of the neck for full range of movement and carotid bruits; an examination of joints, feet, vision and proprioception; and a check for cogwheel rigidity, tremors and focal weakness. Probably the most important part of the physical examination is an assessment of mobility, gait and balance. One can use the 'Get up and Go'

test[11], the Functional Reach Test[12], or the Tinetti Gait and Balance Maneuvers[13] to determine functional performance in these areas. In the first assessment, the subject is asked to rise from a standard armchair, walk 3 m across the room, turn around, walk back to the chair and sit down. This sequence of activities can be graded (1, normal to 5, severely abnormal) or can be timed. In the Functional Reach Test, a leveled yardstick is secured to a wall at the height of the acromion. The patient stands so that the shoulders are perpendicular to the yardstick, makes a fist, and extends the arm forward as far as possible without taking a step or losing balance. The total reach is measured along the yardstick and recorded. In the Tinetti Gait and Balance Assessment, one asks the patient to rise from and sit in a chair, walk down a hallway, turn 360°, bend down to pick up an object from the floor, and withstand a sternal nudge. These maneuvers mimic daily activities. While the patient walks, the clinician observes whether the individual requires any assistance with transfer or ambulation. There are characteristic abnormal gait patterns to be noted (Table 1)[14]: sensory ataxic, cerebellar ataxic, Parkinsonian, hemiplegic, apraxic, waddling and steppage[15].

Vital Signs: BP_____ P_____ R_____ T_____ (ORTHOSTATIC CHANGES?)

Level of Pain (0-10 scale) _____

Present Level of Consciousness:

unresponsive [   ] responsive to pain [   ] drowsy [   ] awake [   ]

Injury: No [   ] Yes [   ] if yes, location _____

Brief Description of Event:

_____

_____

_____

Prevention Plan

Start or resume Fall Prevention Protocol

_____

Signature_____ Date _____

Figure 1   Post-fall evaluation progress note – nursing focus

By observing any difficulties, one can co-ordinate a rehabilitation plan. For example, if the patient has trouble transferring from a chair, then transfer training or adative equipment such as a raised toilet seat may be prescribed to help overcome the difficulty[9,13]. All patients with abnormal gait deserve a thorough physical therapy and/or occupational therapy assessment.

Special tests

Laboratory evaluation should be directed by the findings on the history and physical examination. Cardiac monitoring has a low yield in evaluating falls unless syncope is involved. CNS imaging is indicated if the neurologic examination is abnormal or the history is suggestive. Upright carotid sinus massage or tilt testing may be useful for patients with amnesia for loss of consciousness and a history of recurrent unexplained falls with syncope.

MANAGEMENT, INCLUDING PREVENTION

Figures 1 and 2 provide examples of progress notes for nurses and physicians to consider using as a guide for evaluation of patients who fall in the hospital setting. Here, management focuses on treatment of predisposing illnesses and complicating injuries, and targeting patients for intervention programs to prevent future falls. Provisional diagnoses can be multifactorial (e.g. diabetes-induced nocturia, night-time sedation, bedrails that preclude ambulation to the bathroom). Staff education is key. Psychotropic medications should be reduced or eliminated. Call buttons should be readily available for patients. High-risk individuals should be moved closer to the nursing station for more careful observation. At least one bedrail should be kept down at all times to prevent patients from climbing over the rails and falling from a greater height. Early rehabilitation and assisted

Chart Review:

Reason for Admission:_____

FALL WITNESSED? Yes [   ] No [   ]

LOSS OF CONSCIOUSNESS? No [   ] Yes, before fall [   ] Yes, after fall [   ]

ANTICOAGULANTS? Yes [   ] No [   ]; SEIZURE MEDICATION? Yes [   ] No [   ]

Present Level of Consciousness:

Unresponsive [   ] Responsive to pain [   ] Drowsy [   ] Confused [   ] Awake and alert [   ]

Physical Examination:

Impression:

Serious Injury? Yes___ No___

Differential For Etiology:

Treatment Plan: as per order sheet

Signature/Title:_____ ID#_____ Date/Time_____

Figure 2   Post-fall evaluation progress note – medical focus

ambulation can prevent the deconditioning that too often accompanies hospitalization.

In the out-patient setting, management of falls should entail identifying those factors amenable to intervention, and correcting the problems, wherever possible. Eliminating medication with extrapyramidal side-effects, treating underlying medical conditions, changing drug regimens that cause orthostatic hypotension, prescribing support hose for orthostatic hypotensive patients, and making sure patients wear proper footwear and have updated eyeglass prescriptions are some of the simple measures clinicians can take to treat conditions predisposing to falls. Patients with impaired vision should be referred to an ophthalmologist and/or optometrist, and those with abnormal gait should be further evaluated. Adaptive equipment, including ambulation aids (walkers, canes), raised toilet seats, grab bars and shower seats need consideration.

Counseling is provided regarding measures to prevent falls, including rising slowly to change position, 'fall-proofing' the home, minimizing potentially dangerous over-the-counter medications and limiting alcohol ingestion. Advice is offered to rectify hazardous situations, such as loose rugs, electric cords in walkways and poor lighting. Suggestions are made to add fluorescent tape to the last step on a stairway and handrails and traction tape on the entire stairway, and install grab bars in the bathroom. The AGS website has a Patient Education Forum on Fall and Balance Problems, as well as a Patients' Guide to Preventing Falls[16]. The National Institute of Aging has created an Age Page on Falls Prevention[17]. Older adults who live at home should be referred to a monitoring company, so that in the event they fall and cannot get up, a button on their wrist or neck can be accessible to call for assistance. Exercise and balance training are also beneficial.

Tai Chi C'uan, an oriental dance form that promotes balance, has shown promise as a therapeutic modality in falls prevention in preliminary studies. Finally, patients who fall should be evaluated for underlying osteoporosis and considered for treatment if found to have low bone density.

For long-term care patients, comprehensive assessment, staff education, assistive devices and reduction in number of medications have led to decreased rates of falls[10]. Nursing homes have experimented with bed alarms and low-lying beds as well as hip guards. Hip protectors do not prevent falls, but randomized trials support the use of these devices for the prevention of hip fractures in high-risk individuals[18].

RESTRAINTS

A restraint is any manual method or physical or mechanical device that restricts freedom of movement or normal access to one's body. Restraints are *not* the solution to falls; in fact, restraints have serious drawbacks and can contribute to injuries.

There are many reasons clinicians order restraints: to preclude an unsteady patient from getting out of bed, from pulling out intravenous lines or feeding tubes, from wandering, or from injuring one's self, other patients or the staff. Restraints may be mechanical or psychopharmacologic. Mechanical restraints include the obvious – waist belts, chest vests, mittens and bedrails – but also include geri chairs and wheelchairs. There are other 'mobility restrictors' in the hospital setting: intravenous catheter lines, Foley or condom catheters and nasogastric tubes. In fact, the presence of monitoring and support devices predicts the use of mechanical restraints in the acute hospital setting, as do an abnormal mental status examination, a history of dementia and advanced age. A registered nurse may initiate restraints based on appropriate assessment of the patient in the acute setting in an emergency situation. However, a physician must see and evaluate the patient within 24 h to authenticate a verbal order. The restraint must be renewed by a physician every 24 h, and the patient must be observed frequently and carefully monitored while the restraint is in place[19].

Alternatives to restraint use should always be considered[20]. For example, heparin locks rather than intravenous tubing can be ordered to allow for easier mobilization. Foley catheters can often be replaced by bedside commodes and frequent toileting. Paper strips across the doorway and recreational therapy programs can help prevent wandering in hospitalized patients with dementia. Further studies need to be done to assess the effects of these interventions as well as the removal of restraints on risk of falls and serious injuries.

SUMMARY

Falls in the elderly are often multifactorial in origin and require a multidisciplinary approach to prevention and treatment.

References

1. King MB, Tinetti ME. Falls in community-dwelling older persons. *J Am Geriatr Soc* 1995;43:1146–54
2. Rothschild JM, Bates DW, Leape LL. Preventable medical injuries in older patients. *Arch Intern Med* 2000;160:2717–24
3. Tinetti ME, Doucette JT, Claus EB. The contribution of predisposing and situational risk factors to serious fall injuries. *J Am Geriatr Soc* 1995;43:1207–13
4. Tinetti ME, Wen-Liang Liu, Claus EB. Predictors and prognosis of inability to get up after falls among elder persons. *J Am Med Assoc* 1993;269:65–70
5. Tinetti ME, Speechley M, Ginter SF. Risk factors for falls among elderly persons living

in the community. *N Engl J Med* 1988; 319:1701–7

6. Lord SR, Dayhew J. Visual risk factors for falls in older people. *J Am Geriatr Soc* 2001;49:508–15

7. Bates D, Pruess K, Souney P, Platt R. Serious falls in hospitalized patients: correlates and resource utilization. *Am J Med* 1995;99:137–43

8. Oliver D, Britton M, Seed P, *et al.* Development and evaluation of evidence based risk assessment tool (STRATIFY) to predict which elderly inpatients will fall: case–control and cohort studies. *Br Med J* 1997;315:1049–53

9. Tinetti ME, Baker DI, McAvay G, *et al.* A multifactorial intervention to reduce the risk of falling among elderly people living in the community. *N Engl J Med* 1994;331: 821–7

10. American Geriatrics Society, British Geriatrics Society, and American Academy of Orthopaedic Surgeons Panel on Falls Prevention. Guideline for the prevention of falls in older persons. *J Am Geriatr Soc* 2001;49:664–72

11. Mathias S, Nayak USI, Isaacs B. Balance in elderly patients: the 'Get-up and Go' test. *Arch Phys Med Rehabil* 1986;67:387–9

12. Duncan PW, Weiner DK, Chandler J, Studenski S. Functional reach: a new clinical measure of balance. *J Gerontol* 1990;45:M192–7

13. Tinetti ME. Performance-oriented assessment of mobility problems in elderly patients. *J Am Geriatr Soc* 1986;34:119–26

14. Bernat JL, Vincent FM. Tests of coordination, gait, and reflexes. *Diagnosis* 1987; April:61–72

15. Sudarsky L. Geriatrics: gait disorders in the elderly. *N Engl J Med* 1990;322:1441–6

16. Rubenstein LZ. The patient education forum: falls and balance problems. www.healthinaging.org/public-education/pef/falls-and-balance-problems. July 1, 2001 www.american geriatrics.org/education/fallsprevention.pdf. AGS, New York 2002

17. National Institute on Aging. *Preventing Falls and Fractures.* In *Bound for Good Health – A Collection of Age Pages.* Washington, DC: US Department of Health and Human Services, 1991

18. Kannus P, Parkkari J, Niemi S, *et al.* Prevention of hip fracture in elderly people with use of a hip protector. *N Engl J Med* 2000;343:1506–13

19. Marks W. Physical restraints in the practice of medicine. Current concepts. *Arch Intern Med* 1992;152:2203–6

20. Brungardt GS. Patient restraints: new guidelines for a less restrictive approach. *Geriatrics* 1994;49:43–4, 47–50

22 Syncope in older adults

Jerry O. Ciocon, MD, FACP, AGSF, FACA, and
Daisy G. Ciocon, PhD, ARNP

Syncope is a sudden transient loss of consciousness with loss of postural tone and with spontaneous recovery not requiring any resuscitation[1]. Syncope causes significant morbidity and mortality in older adults. Approximately 3% of emergency department visits and 5% of hospital admissions are due to syncope. About 80% of these patients are 65 years or older[2]. The annual incidence of syncope in institutionalized elderly persons is 6%, and 30% of these have recurrences[3]. Recurrent syncope in this population is associated with accelerated functional decline.

PATHOPHYSIOLOGY OF SYNCOPE

Syncope generally results from a transient reduction in oxygen and nutrient (glucose) delivery to the brain. Cerebral blood flow and oxygen-carrying capacity of the blood are the major determinants of brain function that allows wakefulness. For example, an older person with anemia or pulmonary ventilation–perfusion mismatch (as seen with pneumonia or pulmonary embolism) will have inadequate cerebral oxygenation, especially as other disease processes may coexist[4] (Table 1). Certain medications, especially when given after heavy meals, can cause relative hypotension and compromise cerebral blood flow, leading to syncope (Table 2).

Age-related changes and syncope

Cardiovascular system

Blood vessels typically elongate and dilate, and the inner lining thickens with aging

Table 1 Causes of syncope

Hypertension
Hypotension
Reflex syncope or situational stress
   cough syncope
   micturition or defecation syncope
Cardiac disease
   myocardial ischemia
   valvular heart disease (especially aortic stenosis)
   arrhythmias
Neurologic disorders
   Shy–Drager syndrome
   cerebrovascular disease
Medications
   diuretics
   antihypertensives
   drug that predisposes to arrhythmias
   psychoactive drugs
Other disorders
   anemia, especially acute
   psychogenic (panic disorder, pain, depression, somatization)
   pulmonary embolism
   endocrine dysfunction
   electrolyte imbalance
   carotid sinus syncope
   dissecting aneurysm

(Table 3). They progressively stiffen, and thus make compensatory responses to stress less efficient. Arterial vessel stiffening produces high afterload pressures against which the heart must pump, leading to hypertrophy of the cardiac myocytes and thickening of the heart muscles, with higher oxygen demands[5]. Ventricular stiffening is another consequence of myocyte hypertrophy, and could lower preload volume. A low preload can be worsened by states that cause vasodilatation (e.g. sepsis, heat stroke, vasovagal response, heavy

Table 2 Drugs that predispose to syncope when administered with heavy meals

Nitrates
Diuretics
Antihypertensive medications
   β-blockers
   calcium blockers
   ACE-inhibitors
   clonidine
   hydralazine
   α-blockers

ACE, angiotensin converting enzyme

Table 3 Age-related changes and predisposition to syncope

Vascular stiffening
Impaired baroreflex
Impaired thirst response mechanism
Suppressed renin–angiotensin system
Impaired renal concentration ability
Diminished ventricular compliance
Impaired thermoregulation
Renal sodium wasting

meals) and a sudden change in body position (lying to standing).

Autonomic nervous system

Plasma norepinephrine levels increase with age, probably secondary to a norepinephrine spillover from the sympathetic nerve terminals and a reduction of norepinephrine clearance. The β-adrenergic response to these catecholamines is blunted with aging. Consequently, baroreflex sensitivity is also reduced[6]. In some instances, a diminished parasympathetic response to various stimuli can be protective against vagally mediated reduction in heart rate and blood pressure that cause vasovagal syncope. Thus, vasovagal syncope is less common in the very old as compared to the young. However, it is frequently considered the cause, if no other obvious etiology is found.

Homeostasis and body volume

Aging is associated with sodium wasting. Plasma levels of renin and aldosterone fall, while there is an increase in atrial natriuretic peptide. Thus, sodium conservation is not efficient. Thirst is impaired in response to hypovolemia and may contribute to orthostatic hypotension and syncope. This may be additive to other causes of dehydration in older adults, including decreased oral intake of fluids and use of medications (that promote fluid loss or lower blood pressure,

e.g. diuretics and antihypertensives). Preload volume is critical to maintain ventricular filling in the stiff senescent heart. Blood pooling or third spacing of fluid can dramatically reduce preload volume, leading to syncope[7].

Disorders that contribute to syncope

Older adults have an average of three chronic diseases, and many of these may contribute to syncope (Table 1). Hypertension is noted in over 30% of adults aged 75 years or older, resulting from age-related vascular stiffening. Hypertension contributes to reduced baroreflexsensitivity and shifts the threshold for cerebral autoregulation to higher blood pressure levels[8]. This is due to stiffening of the cerebral blood vessel with chronic hypertension. Consequently, cerebral blood flow may begin to fall at higher blood pressure levels, leading to cerebral ischemia and syncope. Longstanding hypertension also increases afterload resistance in the heart, promoting myocardial hypertrophy, which contributes to ischemia and decreased cardiac output due to systolic or diastolic filling dysfunction. Orthostatic hypotension, defined as a fall of systolic blood pressure of 20 mmHg or greater and/or diastolic drop of 10 mmHg upon standing, is common among older adults with chronic uncontrolled hypertension[9]. Postprandial hypotension (20 mmHg or greater decline in systolic blood pressure within 90 min after a meal) occurs in about a third of the frail older persons in the nursing home setting and is believed to cause 8–50%

of syncopal episodes[10]. Splanchnic blood pooling due to vasoactive gastrointestinal peptides is believed to be the main pathophysiologic mechanism of postprandial hypotension. Reflex syncope is commonly caused by vasovagal states, micturition, defecation, cough and/or carotid sinus hypersensitivity[11]. Vasovagal or neurally mediated syncope occurs during intense sympathetic stimulation, and the venous return is reduced in the upright position. This must be differentiated from seizures and complete heart block (Stokes–Adam attacks). The valsalva maneuver is commonly performed during micturition, defecation, lifting heavy objects and coughing. These activities reduce blood flow to the heart and trigger cardioinhibitory reflexes, lowering heart rate and blood pressure. Carotid sinus hypersensitivity is demonstrated by a sinus slowing of $> 50\%$, cardiac asystole of 3 s and/or a decline in systolic blood pressure of ≥ 50 mmHg during carotid sinus massage[12]. This is observed in 10% of older persons, especially males and those with hypertension and ischemic heart disease. Approximately 20% of this group may develop syncope. Drugs that suppresses the sinus node, e.g. β-blockers, calcium channel blockers, digitalis and methyldopa, can predispose to carotid sinus hypersensitivity[13].

Cardiac diseases account for about 34% of syncope (Table 1). Myocardial ischemia or infarction may produce syncope as a consequence of reduced cardiac output, arrhythmias or vagal reflex response[1]. Aortic stenosis or severe forms of aortic sclerosis occurs in about 75% of older adults, and 6% of these are critical[14]. Syncope occurs in about 25% of these patients with exertion, exercise or sudden exposure to hot temperature, e.g. a sauna or Jacuzzi bath, from vasodilatation. Hypertrophic obstructive cardiomyopathy may present with syncope both at rest and with exertion[15]. Ventricular arrhythmia is associated with syncope. Other forms of arrhythmia, e.g. supraventricular, ventricular or bradyarrhythmias, also lead to

a decrease in cardiac output and subsequent syncope[16]. Unfortunately, telemetry data and Holter monitor information are rarely diagnostic for the etiology of syncope. Most studies show poor correlation between syncope and symptoms of palpitation, dizziness and specific cardiac arrhythmias, making the diagnosis difficult.

Neurological conditions (Table 1) affecting the autonomic nervous system can cause vasodilatation and syncope[17]. Diabetes mellitus, tabes dorsalis, amyloidosis, porphyria, alcoholism and spinal cord injuries can disrupt the pathways of the peripheral autonomic nervous system and contribute to syncope. Low levels of serum norepinephrine might provide a clue for this disorder. A more common condition involving multiple system atrophy including the corticospinal, extrapyramidal and cerebellar systems is the Shy–Drager syndrome[18]. Here, the supine plasma norepinephrine levels fail to increase normally on standing, and clinically the syndrome manifests as orthostatic hypotension with parkinsonian features (e.g. joint stiffness or difficulty walking). Other symptoms include fatigue, reduced or excessive sweating, constipation, urinary retention and visual disturbances. Cerebrovascular diseases due to ischemia of the posterior circulation may present with syncope, usually accompanied by one or more of the following: diplopia, vertigo, dysarthria and hemiparesis[19].

Syncope rarely results from severe anemia, pulmonary embolism and certain endocrine conditions (Table 1). Anemia in an older person is usually associated with other chronic diseases; the combination of predisposing factors may cause a decrease in cerebral blood flow. A sudden drop in hematocrit, rather than chronic anemia, is the more common cause of syncope. Pulmonary embolism particularly in postoperative patients may be an overlooked cause. Diabetes mellitus can cause autonomic neuropathy, orthostatic hypotension and subsequent syncope. Uncontrolled diabetes can also cause osmotic

Table 4 Factors in history and examination that may suggest the basis of syncope

History
    onset of symptoms
    offset of symptoms
    associated activities
    previous episodes
    availability of witness to corroborate
    precipitating factors
Medications, including timing of administration
Postural blood pressure
Heart rate and rhythm, including changes with maneuvers
Valvular heart murmurs
Carotid bruits
Fundoscopy
Hemoccult stool examination

diuresis and dehydration. Tightly controlled diabetes mellitus leads to hypoglycemia and to syncope, with recovery. Addison's disease, chronic adrenal suppression from chronic steroid use and hypopituitatism can cause hypoglycemia, hypovolemia and syncope[20].

AN APPROACH TO THE EVALUATION OF SYNCOPE

A detailed chronological sequence of events prior to the occurrence of syncope may provide the diagnosis in 50% of cases and should include details such as precipitating factors, associated symptoms and review of medications (Table 4).

Quick onset and rapid offset or resolution of syncope are observed with cardiac bases such as arrhythmias, or myocardial ischemia. A slow onset and slow offset are commonly seen in vasovagal syncope or with a seizure disorder. Precipitating events often provide clues for the cause[19]. These include cough, emotional stress, neck turning, postural change, meal ingestion and administration of medications. All medications, whether regularly taken or newly prescribed, including over-the-counter medications, should be reviewed and determined as a possible basis[9,19]. Timing of the administration of the medications can have a bearing. In a nursing

home setting, syncope has been observed when antihypertensive drugs, vasodilators or diuretics given immediately after a meal result in postural hypotension. Syncope became less frequent when these medications were given at least 2 h after a meal. Syncope occurring after change from the supine to the upright position may commonly be due to postural hypotension and could be reproduced during examination. The proper manner to check for orthostatic hypotension is measuring the blood pressure after 5 min of supine position and after 1 and 3 min of standing[9]. A drop of blood pressure of more than 20 mmHg systolic and/or 10 mmHg diastolic is a significant finding. Cardiopulmonary examination should focus on arrhythmias and valvular disease, especially aortic stenosis[4,5]. Raising both legs while the patient is supine can increase the venous return and cause the murmur from hypertrophic cardiomyopathy to sound softer. Carotid artery bruits may reveal a possibility of cerebrovascular disease[12]. A delayed carotid upstroke may be observed with significant aortic stenosis[14]. However, this finding may alter with aging, as stiffening of the arteries is common without significant carotid artery disease. Fundoscopic examination may reveal longstanding and poorly controlled hypertension, diabetes mellitus or increase in intracranial pressure. Stools for occult blood may explain the anemia, which may be the basis.

Laboratory and other diagnostic tests may provide clues for the etiology, especially when directed by specific symptoms or clinical presentation (Table 5). An electrocardiogram may suggest myocardial ischemia, infarction and arrhythmias. Multifocal and frequent atrial and ventricular arrhythmias are indications to perform prolonged cardiac monitoring, for example with the Holter monitor and the event monitor. Electrophysiologic studies are indicated if an arrhythmia is identified and further analysis of the arrhythmia will provide guidelines for antiarrhythmic

Table 5 Diagnostic tests for suspected conditions that may cause syncope

Diagnostic test	Suspected condition
ECG	Ischemia or arrhythmia
Stress test	Ischemia or indolent arrhythmia
Echocardiogram	Heart murmur, especially aortic stenosis
Holter or event monitor	Suspected arrhythmias with abnormal ECG
Carotid ultrasound	TIA or presence of carotid bruits
CBC	Pallor, presence of anemia
BUN, creatinine, electrolytes	Dehydration, orthostatic hypotension
Tilt table	Postural syncope
EEG	Seizure suspected from history
Head radiologic imaging	Focal neurologic deficits, head injury

ECG, electrocardiogram; CBC, complete blood count;
BUN, blood urea nitrogen; EEG, electroencephalogram;
TIA, transient ischemic attack

Table 6 Management of orthostatic hypotension

Identify the cause
Non-drug management
  meals
  position
  exercises
  stockings
Drug management
  mineralocorticoids
  midodrine
When related to meals
  alterations in diet
  review drug regimen and timing (relating to meals)

therapy[21]. Non-inducible arrhythmias during an electrophysiologic study predict a low risk for sudden death and low likelihood for malignant ventricular arrhythmias[22].

Stress test may indicate the presence of myocardial ischemia and its severity. Any significant murmurs, especially aortic stenosis, should be evaluated with an echocardiogram. Carotid bruits and clinical findings compatible with cerebral ischemia are addressed by performing a carotid ultrasound examination. The presence of pallor in the conjunctiva, palms and skin folds may be clues for the presence of anemia and should be confirmed with a complete blood count. When orthostatic hypotension is noted, examining the axilla for evidence of poor skin turgor and assessing renal function and electrolytes will support the clinical impression of dehydration. Tilt testing is occasionally helpful to detect vasovagal syncope and is useful in evaluating relatively healthy older adults without structural heart disease, with recurrent syncope. The yield for positive tilt test in older adults is about 37%[23]. If seizure is suspected, an electroencephalogram is helpful. Use of special devices such as an insertable loop recorder may provide long-term monitoring capability to demonstrate seizures as the basis[24]. When there are neurologic deficits such as slurred speech, drooped mouth, or hemiparesis, brain imaging using computerized tomography or magnetic resonance imaging is an appropriate test. Syncope related to trauma or head injury with normal cardiac evaluation and normal electrocardiogram warrants immediate brain imaging to exclude serious and often fatal disorders such as subdural hemorrhage or intracerebral bleeding[25]. However, in older persons, brain imaging often demonstrates abnormalities that may not have any relevance to syncope. Orthostatic hypotension when identified may be corrected to decrease the occurrence of syncope. Proper exercise, correct positioning, gradual change in position, e.g. from supine to standing position, use of pressure stockings, certain medications that can expand vascular volume (Florinef®), increasing sodium content of the diet and timing of medication administration are some ways to correct orthostasis (Table 6). An alpha stimulant, midodrine, has demonstrated benefit in symptomatic orthostatic hypotension.

In conclusion, the approach to syncope should be initiated by the sequence of events, abnormal physical examination findings and performing relevant laboratory tests. Further evaluation should be guided by clues obtained during the comprehensive assessment. Therapy should be focused on the findings believed to be the main cause of syncope.

References

1. Kapoor WN. Syncope in older persons. *J Am Geriatr Soc* 1994;42:426–31
2. Day SC, Cook EF, Funkenstein H. Evaluation and outcome of emergency room patients with transient loss of consciousness. *Am J Med* 1982;75:15–20
3. Lipsitz L, Wei JY, Rowe JW. Syncope in an elderly institutionalized population: prevalence, incidence and associated risk. *Q J Med* 1985;55:45–50
4. McIntosh HD. Cardiac causes of syncope in the elderly. *Cardiology* 1986;3:51–7
5. Wei JY. Age and the cardiovascular system. *N Engl J Med* 1992;327:1735–41
6. Lakatta EG. Catecholamines and cardiovascular function in aging. *Endocrinol Metab Clin North Am* 1987;16:877–82
7. Harizi RC, Bianco LA, Alpert JS. Diastolic function of the heart in clinical cardiology. *Arch Intern Med* 1988;148:99–105
8. Gribbin B, Pickering TG, Sleight P. Effect of age and high blood pressure on baroreflex sensitivity in man. *Circ Res* 1971;29: 424–32
9. Lipsitz LA. Orthostasis hypertension in the elderly. *N Engl J Med* 1989;321:952–62
10. Lipsitz LA, Fullerton KJ. Postprandial blood pressure reduction in healthy elderly. *J Am Geriatr Soc* 1986;34:267–75
11. Waxman MB, Cameron DA, Wald RW. Role of ventricular vagal afferents in the vasovagal reaction. *J Am Coll Cardiol* 1993;21: 1138–45
12. Morely CA, Sutton R. Carotid sinus syncope. *Int J Cardiol* 1984;6:287–93
13. Brignole M, Menozzi C, Gaggioli G, *et al.* Effects of long term vasodilator therapy in patients with carotid sinus hypersensitivity. *Am Heart J* 1998;136:264–8
14. Aronow WS, Kronzon I. Prevalence and severity of valvular aortic stenosis determined by Doppler echocardiography and its association with echocardiographic and electrocardiographic left ventricular hypertrophy and physical signs of aortic stenosis in elderly patients. *Am J Cardiol* 1991;67: 876–82
15. Petrin TJ, Travel ME. Idiopathic hypertrophic subaortic stenosis as observed in a large community hospital: relation to age and history of hypertension. *J Am Geriatr Soc* 1979;27:43–51
16. Camm AJ, Evans KE, Ward DE. The rhythm of the heart in active elderly subjects. *Am Heart J* 1989;99:598–604
17. Robertson RM, Medina E, Shad N, *et al.* Neural mediated syncope: pathophysiology and implications for treatment. *Am J Med Sci* 1999;317:102–9
18. Mosqueda-Garcia R, Furlan R, Fernandez-Violante R, *et al.* Sympathetic and baroreceptor reflex function in neurally mediated syncope evoked by tilt. *J Clin Invest* 1997; 99:2736–44
19. Abe H, Kohshi K, Kuroiwa A. Possible involvement of cerebral hypoperfusion as trigger of neurally-mediated vasovagal syncope. *Pacing Clin Electrophysiol* 1998;21: 613–16
20. Clark CT, Resenblatt R, Somberg JC. Neurocardiogenic syncope with Addison's disease. *Am J Ther* 2000;7:328–31
21. Luria DM, Shen WK. Syncope in the elderly: new trends in diagnostic approach

and nonpharmacological management. *Am J Geriatr Cardiol* 2001;10:91–96

22. Link MS, Kim KM, Hormoud MK, *et al.* Long term outcome of patients with syncope associated with coronary artery disease and a nondiagnostic electrophysiological evaluation. *Am J Cardiol* 1999;83: 1134–7

23. Bloomfield D, Maurer M, Bigger JT Jr. Effects of age on outcome of tilt-table testing. *Am J Cardiol* 1999;83:1055–8

24. Simpson CS, Barlow MA, Krahn AD, *et al.* Recurrent seizure diagnosed by the insertable loop recorder. *J Intervent Cardiac Electrophysiol* 2000;4:475–9

25. Morrison JE, Wisner DH, Ramos L. Syncope-related trauma: rationale and yield of diagnostic studies. *J Trauma Injury Infect Crit Care* 1999;46:707–10

23 Wound care

Robert A. Norman, DO, MPH, and Megan Bock, PA

Wound incidence varies depending on the study, but reports indicate that 10% of hospitalized patients and 20% of nursing home patients suffer from pressure ulcers. Chronic wounds account for at least $1 billion per year in the USA and $7 billion per year worldwide in health care costs[1]. The cost to heal a single pressure ulcer can range between $400 and $40 000.

It is important for a medical practitioner to understand the assessment and management of wounds.

The first step in mastering wound management is assessment and evaluation of the wound; in other words, performing an accurate history and physical examination (Table 1). 'Unfortunately many clinicians are quick to attribute the cause of delayed healing to untreated hypertension, one of the most common causes of chronic leg wounds ... A thorough wound examination combined with relevant historical information will help determine the most appropriate treatment, as well as ensure the best possible clinical outcome for the patient'[2]. For instance, in neuropathic ulcers it is common for the patient to have a history of numbness, burning, paresthesias and pain. Upon physical examination, one would find a deep ulcer over a site where pressure is commonly applied such as the heel. A condensed callus usually surrounds the ulcer. On the other hand, a patient presenting with a venous ulcer customarily has throbbing pain and swelling in the legs. These symptoms are often worse at night and/or when the patient is mobile, standing, or sitting without the leg elevated. More often than not the patient will have some alleviation of symptoms when the leg is elevated. 'Most venous ulcers are located in the so called gaiter area, from 2.5 cm below the malleoli to the point at which calf muscles become prominent posteriorly'[3]. Other symptoms that may be found upon physical examination include varicose veins, lower leg edema, pigmentation eczema and fibrosis.

Patients with arterial ulcers are generally over the age of 45 years. Their medical history may be significant for intermittent claudication, severe ulcer pain and limb pain at rest. The patient may state that the pain is intensified when the limb is elevated. Physical examination may reveal absent or weak peripheral pulses, perpetuated capillary refill time, pallor on limb elevation, rubor, loss of hair, shiny atrophic dry skin and thickened nails.

WOUND PATHOLOGY

The practitioner must distinguish whether one is dealing with an acute or a chronic wound. A chronic wound is defined as a loss in tissue integrity produced by insult or injury that is of extended duration or frequent recurrence. An acute wound is one in which simple medical or surgical intervention produces a resolution. Superficial wounds, where only the epidermis or dermis is injured (partial thickness wound), may heal rapidly via the process of re-epithelialization. Epithelial cells migrate toward one another from

Table 1   Arterial, venous and neuropathic ulcers: differences in history and physical examination

Arterial ulcer	Venous ulcer	Neuropathic ulcer
Ordinarily > age 45 years	Presents with throbbing pain and swelling in the legs, worse at night or when using the limb	History of numbness, burning, paresthesia, pain
Medical history may include intermittent claudication, severe ulcer pain, & limb pain at rest		Physical examination reveals ulcer over site of pressure
Pain may be increased when limb elevated	Physical examination may reveal varicose veins, lower leg edema, pigmentation, eczema and fibrosis	Condensed callus often seen around ulcer
Physical examination shows absent or weak peripheral pulse, delayed capillary refill time, redness, loss of hair on limbs, whiteness on elevation of limb, shiny and dry skin, thickened nails		

the edges of the wound, from the hair follicles, sebaceous glands and sweat glands and eventually close the wound.

With an acute wound it is important to realize that the body begins to quickly heal itself. Within minutes to hours, changes are noticed at the cellular level. The physiology can be divided into three different overlapping phases, namely inflammation, fibroplasia and maturation.

'Perhaps, one analogy would be that wound healing, at least for acute wounds, is like a symphony of several movements. While each movement has its own theme, there are overlaps and indeed a return to previous themes throughout the musical composition'[4]. In other words, phases do not occur individually but rather in rapid sequence as follows.

Within the first 6 h   Neutrophils arrive at the site of the wound, although they do not accumulate in significant numbers in wound healing. A deficiency of neutrophils (neutropenia) will not intervene with healing.

24 h   Neutrophils reach a peak in population. Meanwhile, the initiation of epidermal healing relies on the epidermal cell migration that occurs within the first 24 h.

48 h   With low oxygen and high lactate levels fibroblasts begin to occupy the wound.

A fibroblast is 'Any cell or corpuscle from which connective tissue is developed; it produces collagen, elastin, and reticular protein fibers'.[5] The fibroblasts are responsible for wound contraction. Epidermal healing is dependent on epidermal cell migration, which has now peaked. The rate of re-epithelialization depends on how moist the wound is kept. The more moist the wound, the quicker the epidermal healing.

72 h   The neutrophils begin to disappear.

1 week   Wound contraction begins.

If the wound is properly cared for, the healing time will depend on the size of the wound. The larger and deeper the wound, the longer it takes to heal. If the wound arises from cryosurgery or chemical cautery, it will heal slower than a surgical wound produced by a scalpel. Healing time depends on whether the wound is 'full' thickness or 'partial' thickness. With full thickness wounds, the epidermis and dermis are missing and the wound itself lies beneath the hair follicles and sweat ducts. Full-thickness wounds heal by contraction, granulation tissue formation and re-epithelization. Partial-thickness wounds involve destruction of the epidermis and part of the dermis. Shave excisions, curretage and chemical peels are examples of partial-thickness wounds. These types heal rapidly through re-epithelialization with possibly minor contraction[6].

Chronic wounds often result from surgical procedures, traumatic insults, or metabolic, infectious or neoplastic disorders. Pressure ulcers, diabetic ulcers, lower leg ulcers, vascular ulcers, postoperative open wounds and enterocutaneous fistulae are frequently occurring chronic wounds.

Non-healing wounds generally occur in older individuals with multi-system problems, poor medical care and inadequate health habits. Chronic wounds often arise as a result of diabetes, cancer, liver, renal or gastrointestinal illness.

Radiation trauma victims, transplant patients and burn patients often suffer chronic wounds. Therapy with medications such as steroids can render a person prone to wounds. Obesity, smoking, poor nutrition and immobility can delay wound repair.

Pressure ulcers often occur due to limited mobility and confining physical structures such as wheelchairs and bed rails. With elimination of pressure, and availability of good blood supply and adequate nutrition, the pressure lesions will generally heal.

Given the many factors that predispose our patients to chronic wound development, it is crucial for any physician or caregiver to carefully assess patients and work on preventive strategies such as weight control, smoking cessation, proper nutrition and appropriate prescribing.

STAGING OF PRESSURE ULCERS

Pressure ulcer staging is important in wound evaluation and treatment. The Agency for Health Care Policy and Research (AHCPR) defines pressure ulcers as localized areas of tissue necrosis that can develop when soft tissue is compressed between a bony prominence and an external surface for a period of time. Their guidelines for staging pressure ulcers[7] are as follows:

(1) *Stage I*: Non-blanchable erythema of intact skin. This is the heralding lesion of skin ulceration.

(2) *Stage II*: Partial thickness skin loss involving epidermis and/or dermis. The ulcer is superficial and presents as an abrasion, blister or shallow crater.

(3) *Stage III*: Full thickness skin loss involving damage or necrosis of subcutaneous tissue that may extend to but not through underlying fascia. The ulcer is seen as a deep crater with or without undermining of adjacent tissue.

(4) *Stage IV*: Full thickness skin loss with extensive destruction, tissue necrosis, or damage to muscle, bone or supporting structures. Undermining and sinus tracts may be found.

Along with a comprehensive history and physical examination, certain tests may be used to confirm the diagnosis. The Trendelenburg test may help diagnose a venous ulcer; this is achieved by lifting the patient's leg above the level of the heart until the veins are drained. The leg is then slowly lowered. Venous distention suggests incompetent valves and a venous basis for the ulcer. Another test for venous ulcers is the Perthes' test. Incompetent deep circulation is suggested if there is a change in the superficial circulation after tying a tourniquet above the knee, and asking the patient to ambulate. Color duplex, air plethysmography and photoplethysmography also help determine whether an ulcer is venous. The ankle brachial index (ABI) is useful in diagnosing arterial ulcers. Arteriography may be used to identify an arterial cause.

DEBRIDEMENT

One technique that should be mastered by health-care providers who take care of wounds is debridement. Proper debridement is crucial in all chronic wounds. Wound debridement may be autolytic, chemical, mechanical, surgical or biologic.

The most effortless and customary type of debridement is autolytic. Autolytic debridement is the use of a synthetic dressing over an ulcer that allows self-digestion through the action of enzymes normally present in the wound fluid. This is not indicated for infected ulcers. It is important to compare a moist with a dry environment. Sustaining a moist environment for the wound expedites wound healing by as much as 50% compared to a dry environment caused by air exposure[8]. Wounds that are not covered become dry, making it difficult for re-epithelialization to occur, because a crust forms over the wound. Non-occluded moist autolytic debridement entails a considerable amount of time and labor[9]. A moist, occluded wound encourages autolytic debridement for both acute and chronic wounds; it yields painless debridement, advocates formation of granulation tissue and minimizes persistent pain and tenderness[10].

Chemical debridement, also known as enzymatic debridement, is achieved through the use of proteolytic enzymes. Enzymatic debridement, utilizing topical debriding agents for devitalized tissues, is considered when the patient cannot tolerate surgery and for non-infected ulcers. Proteolytic enzymes have been used for centuries; it is believed that 500 years ago, Christopher Columbus used proteolytic enzymes from pineapple to treat the wounds of his warriors[11]. Currently, fibrinolysin–DNAse is one of the therapeutic combinations used for chemical debridement, marketed as a combination agent, Elase®. Collagenase is another available proteolyic enzyme. It is obtained from *Clostridium histolyticum*. Several clinical trials of collagenase have reported rapid cleansing and enhanced removal of necrotic debris[12]. Finally, there is a combination of papain and urea that is available for chemical debridement. Papain, which is derived from papaya, is useful because it is active in a wide pH range.

Chemical debridement utilizes pH-sensitive agents; when the wound environment changes the agents may become inactivated. The agents are also deactivated by heavy metals, present in numerous topical agents used in wound management.

Although mechanical debridement may be painful and does not differentiate between viable and non-viable tissues, it is useful. Mechanical debridement physically removes debris from the wound in an expeditious manner. Methods of mechanical debridement include dextranomers, hydrotherapy, irrigation and wet-to-dry dressings. Surgical or sharp debridement is the quickest method of mechanical debridement; it involves the expulsion of necrotic areas with surgical instruments. It requires a skilled practitioner and anesthesia. Caution is advised if the patient has a bleeding disorder.

The wet-to-dry dressing method of mechanical debridement involves placing dampened gauze on the wound and allowing it to dry. The dried dressing, in which necrotic debris has become embedded, is removed. Removal of the dressing can be agonizing. Wet-to-dry dressings should not be used on clean granulating wounds, because it can disturb the granulation tissue and new epithelium[13]. Hydrotherapy and irrigation should not be used on clean wounds either. They are best for wounds with heavy exudate. Hydrotherapy is performed by using a whirlpool; irrigation can be accomplished by using syringes or angiocatheters. Dextranomer is manufactured as dry spherical beads and is placed in the wound bed to absorb exudate, bacteria and other debris.

Biological or maggot therapy may also be used for wound debridement. Several studies have indicated that maggot therapy may be effective. One study showed that maggot therapy was able to heal wounds infected with *Staphylococcus aureus* and methicillin-resistant *S.aureus*[14]. Extremities set for amputation have been salvaged with maggot therapy[15]. By applying a chiffon dressing the young sterile maggot larvae encounter the precise area to be debrided[16].

Knowledge of wound dressing is imperative. Dressings act as a barricade protecting the wound. It is useful to know the type of dressing and the reason for use. Dressings include alginates, collagen dressing, films, foams, hydrocolloids, hydrogels, hydrofibers, hydropolymers and superabsorbents[17], all moisture-retentive dressings.

Alginates are derived from seaweed and are composed of calcium alginate. Alginates can be packed into deep wounds and are suitable for wounds with thick exudate. Collagen dressings, good for wounds with moderate exudate, are obtained from cowhide.

Films are thin, adhesive sheets that are penetrable to oxygen and water and impenetrable to bacteria and other fluids. Films, frequently made of polyurethane, make a good secondary dressing, and may be used for minor lacerations, on top of sutures, superficial surgical wounds or minor burns. For an acute wound that has been sutured, films are very useful.

Foams are useful for infected wounds and for wounds with moderate to thick exudate. Foam dressings are fabricated from microporous polyurethane. Hydrocolloids are useful in ulcers, abrasions and postoperative wounds. Hydrogels are beneficial in blisters and wounds caused from chemical peels. Hydrofibers may be packed into wounds or wounds prone to bleeding.

Table 2 lists the advantages and disadvantages of various dressings. Based on data from several sources[17–23], the dressing–wound combinations shown in Table 3 may be considered, depending on the nature of the wound.

After debridement, the wound should be appropriately handled. Following debridement of a diabetic ulcer, crutches or a wheelchair helps keep the patient off their foot completely. This may minimize the need for a limb amputation[24].

Herbal supplements are available to aid in the wound healing process. Supplements such as goldenseal, St John's wort, calendula and goto kola have been claimed to show benefits, not all of which are confirmed by research data.

CLINICAL CARE

Certain therapies or combinations work best for each patient. The following are considerations:

(1) Saline irrigation provides a safe and appropriate cleansing method for most pressure ulcers. Avoid use of agents toxic to wound tissue such as povidone iodine, iodophor, sodium hypochlorite solution, hydrogen peroxide or acetic acid.

(2) Debride any necrotic tissue observed during wound assessment if appropriate. Debride wounds only if the removal of the necrotic tissue speeds up the healing process. Curetting of the borders of the lesions often stimulates increased granulation and wound healing. All infected ulcers should be debrided more rapidly. Consider pain control and prepare the patient. The most rapid method of removing areas of thick, adherent eschar and devitalized tissue is with sharp debridement, generally utilizing sterile surgical scissors[4].

(3) All stage II, III and IV ulcers are bacteria-colonized, which can be minimized through effective wound cleansing and debridement. Swab cultures detect only surface colonization and are not recommended. Needle aspiration or biopsy can be used when a culture is needed. Consider a biopsy to rule out malignancy for any chronic ulcer that does not heal by conventional measures. Consider a 2-week trial of topical antibiotics (triple antibiotic, silver sulfadiazene) if a clean ulcer does not heal or continues to have exudate despite optimal care for 2–4 weeks. Systemic antibiotics are appropriate for patients with bacteremia, sepsis, advancing cellulitis or osteomyelitis.

(4) Aggressive care is warranted with pronounced edema, vascular compromise, gangrene and diabetes. Consider a consult with a vascular surgeon. Conservative measures such as support stockings,

Table 2   The advantages and disadvantages of various wound dressings

Dressing type	Advantages	Disadvantages
Alginate	increased hemostatic characteristics increased fluid collection	risk of drying the wound must be used with other dressing may cause bad odor
Collagen	creates matrix for cell migration	must be used with other dressing may cause erythema
Film	does not require frequent dressing change see-through dressing	may peel away new skin leakage may occur
Foam	shapes to wound good for bony prominence	risk of drying out wound
Hydrocolloid	decreases pain able to remain in water	may cause bad odor may have leakage
Hydrofiber	has more absorption than alginates	risk of drying out wound
Hydrogel	fills dead space cooling effect	poor absorption must be used with other dressing
Hydropolymer	no odor no second dressing needed conforms to wound	may increase wound size

Table 3   Useful combinations of dressings based on wound type

Chronic wound type	Dressing type
Severe exudative	aglinate, foam, or hydrofiber
Moderate exudative	hydrocolloid or foam
Mild exudative	hydrogel or hydrocolloid
Dry and/or necrotic	hydrogel or collagen
Malodorous	charcoal or metro-gel

elevation of legs and so-called 'bunny boots' or other devices may be used for protection whenever indicated. Beware of 'soggy socks syndrome', brought on by keeping the socks on for too long, resulting in maceration and skin breakdown. This contributes to fungal infections as well as foul-smelling feet, and leads to further infection and ulcers. Change the socks (and other clothing) frequently and make sure the socks and shoes fit comfortably. Consider physical therapy consults for patients with contractures. Podiatrists should be utilized for routine care and maintenance of the feet, especially for diabetics.

(5) Assure adequate nutrition. Assess nutrition in an ongoing manner including regular monitoring of intake, weights and appropriate laboratory parameters. Assess anorexia, including possible etiologies such as undiagnosed medical illness, medications, depression or other psychological problems, sensory losses, or swallowing difficulties. Nutritional status can deteriorate rapidly in those who are marginally nourished to begin with. Minimize days of low nutrition status and if prolonged consider alternative forms of nutritional support. Utilize supplements as needed. Ensure an adequate mealtime environment. Provide adequate assistance with meals including the use of adaptive devices. Minimize restrictive diets.

(6) Avoid prolonged bedrest and its adverse effects as much as possible. Minimize the use of restraints; they fail to 'protect' patients and may lead to all the complications of immobility. Involve rehabilitation specialists in occupational and physical therapy early to prevent contractures. Protect against the adverse effects of external forces such as pressure, friction and shear. Utilize proper positioning techniques and repositioning schedules. Elevating the head of the bed is

NORMAN SCALE SKIN CARE ASSESSMENT FORM (copyright 2001 Dr. Robert A. Norman)									
	Dates								
MENTAL STATUS & SENSORY PERCEPTION (score) (Orientation & ability to respond to pressure)									
1 Oriented and cooperative, no sensory impairment 2 Slightly limited (responds to verbal commands) 3 Disoriented or confused, unable to communicate and very limited (responds to painful stimuli) 4 Stuporous, lethargic, or sedated, completely limited sensory perception (unresponsive)	Comments:								
MOBILITY STATUS (score) (Ability to change and control body position)									
1 Full (can turn self) with no limitations	Comments:								
2 Slightly limited (frequent/slight changes)									
3 Limited or restrained: has contractures									
4 Immobile, insensate									
MOISTURE, BOWEL AND BLADDER STATUS (score)									
1 Fully continent, rarely moist 2 Occasionally moist and incontinent of urine, feces (Extra change q day) 3 Very moist (linen/diaper/pad changed q shift) 4 Constantly moist (moisture detected each time moved–Totally incontinent of urine and feces)	Comments:								
SKIN INTEGRITY & FRICTION TEAR (score)									
1 Good turgor with no apparent problem (well hydrated, elasticity WNL for age) maintains good position 2 Potential problem–poor turgor (increased fragility, history of skin breakdown, moves feebly/some sliding) 3 Probable problem (history of ulcers, skin tears, severe purpura, severe sun damage, or moderate to severe stasis dermatitis) 4 Problem (constant friction, existing skin ulcers/lesions)	Comments:								
Resident Name: _____ Admission NO._____									

Figure 1   Form used for wound-care assessment

NORMAN SCALE SKIN CARE ASSESSMENT FORM Dates										
ACTIVITY STATUS (SCORE)										
(Ability to change and control body position) 1 Full (can turn self) with no limitations 2 Slightly limited (Frequent/slight changes) 3 Very limited (restrained, has contractures or infrequent changes) 4 Completely immobile, insensate (requires assistance to move)	Comments:									
NUTRITIONAL/FLUID STATUS (SCORE)										
(Usual food intake & lab parameters) 1 Excellent with IBW, at or above 3.5 serum albumin, BUN and Creat WNL, eats well, spoon fed or self fed, over 90% acceptance 2 Adequate (>1/2 meal, 4 servings protein, Tube/TPN feeding 150% acceptance routinely, above or below IBW, albumin, BUN & creat WNL) 3 Probably adequate (< 3 servings protein, 1/2 meal & BUN/CREAT altered or edema present, above or below IBW, albumin at or below 3.5 gm/dl) 4 Very Poor (Never completes meal with less than 50% acceptance routinely/npo or liquids > 5 days, above or below IBW with albumin at or below 3.5gm/dl, BUN/CREAT altered)	Comments:									
PREDISPOSING MEDICAL PROBLEMS (SCORE) **AND INFLUENCING HEALTH FACTORS:**										
(score (1) for each present) (Severe neurodermatitis, age > 75, recent nicotine abuse of more than 10 pack years, Low pre-albumin, transferrin, hemoglobin, or zinc; infection, edema, temperature elevation, dehydration COPD, ASCVD, PVD, diabetes, liver or renal disease cancer, motor or sensory deficits, osteomyelitis, depression, use of steroids, antipsychotics, anticoagulants) (1) One present (2) Two present (3) Three present (4) Four or more present										
TOTAL SCORE										
10 or under-minimal risk 11–13 low risk 14–15 moderate risk 16 or > high risk comprehensive staff training in wound prevention and care – subtract (5) five points support surface (bed) for wound prevention (and wheelchair if needed) – subtract (5) five points	Comments:									
NURSES INITIALS										
PAGE 2 Resident Name: _____ Admission NO. _____										

Figure 1   *Continued*

conducive to shearing forces; prevent shear injuries by utilizing lifting devices to move patients. Friction injuries may be reduced by the use of lubricants, protective dressings or films, and protective padding.

(7) Evaluate and manage bowel and/or bladder incontinence.

(8) There are several pitfalls to the staging system. Erythema (stage I ulcer) may be missed in dark-skinned individuals; the only signs may be warmth, induration and edema. Ulcers beneath devices such as casts used for orthopedics may not be easily detected. An eschar-covered ulcer cannot be staged, unless debridement is performed. Pressure ulcers do not progress in orderly fashion from stage I to IV, nor do they heal in the opposite order [25].

(9) The occurrence of bacteremia is often underestimated; bacteremia frequently occurs during debridement. Endocarditis prophylaxis should be utilized when appropriate. Osteomyelitis should be excluded, but is often difficult[26]; helpful measures include white blood cell counts, plain radiographs, sedimentation rate and magnetic resonance imaging. Tetanus has been associated with pressure ulcers; immunization against tetanus appears a reasonable measure.

(10) Pain control is important, particularly around the time of debridement, a painful process. A pain rating scale is ideal, but hard to utilize in demented persons. Analgesia is best offered prior to debridement and dressing changes; likewise, occlusive dressings and proper positioning can help minimize pain[25].

(11) Several adjunctive therapies are available including use of hyperbaric oxygen, infra red, ultraviolet and low-energy laser treatments, gold, growth factors, and systemic agents. Most are of unproven benefit. It appears that electrotherapy is one form of adjunctive therapy with some benefit[27].

WOUND CARE IN LONG-TERM CARE FACILITIES

High-risk populations include: quadriplegics, critical care patients, the elderly (especially those with femoral fractures), persons with terminal cancer end-stage renal, liver or heart disease, diabetics and the immunosuppressed. Other risk factors include immobility, poor nutritional status, incontinence and altered level of consciousness.

One of the authors (R.A.N.) has spent years caring for patients in nursing homes. A wound care scale has been designed for wound care prevention and training of the nursing home staff (Figure 1).

Debilitating skin diseases including ulcers in long-term care facilities cause avoidable pain and suffering. In addition, they place an additional burden on low budgets. Although most long-term care administrators and staff recognize the need for improved prevention and management of wounds, they lack the necessary time for these efforts. A systematic approach using risk assessment tools will be effective to reduce the incidence of pressure ulcers and other wounds in the nursing home.

Several scales are available for assessment and prevention of ulcers. Aside from the scale described by the author, the Norton Score and the Braden Scale are recognized instruments used to identify risk for pressure ulcers. The Braden Scale evaluates sensory perception, skin moisture, activity, mobility, nutrition and friction/shear, while the Norton Score assesses physical status, mentation, activity, mobility and incontinence. Scores below 16 for the Braden Scale and 12 for Norton Score suggest a high risk for pressure ulcers[25]. However, inadequate pressure relief and poor recognition by staff are at the very core of pressure ulcer problems. Therefore, an 'interactive' component to the risk assessment tool has been incorporated that includes 'bonus points' (improved score) for those facilities that maintain adequate surface support and staff training.

Wound care is an ever-changing process. Managing wounds does not have to be a complicated procedure if the practitioner is up to date and aware of the choices.

References

1. Margolis, Bilker, Santanna, Baumgarten. Venous leg ulcer: incidence and prevalence in the elderly. *J Am Acad Dermatol* 2002; 46:381–6
2. Cuzzell J. Wound management and evaluation. *Dermatol Nurs* 2000;12:413–14
3. Bello Y, Phillips T. Chronic leg ulcers: types and treatment. *Hosp Pract* 2000;101–6
4. Falanga V. Overview of chronic wounds and recent advances. *Dermatol Ther* 1999; 9:7–17
5. Thomas, Clayton, *et al.*, eds. *Taber's Cyclopedic Medical Dictionary*. Philadelphia: FA Davis, 1997
6. Habif T. *Clinical Dermatology*, 3rd edn. St Louis: Mosby, 1996
7. Panel for the Prediction and Prevention of Pressure Ulcers in Adults. *Pressure Ulcers in Adults: Prediction and Prevention*. Clinical Practice Guideline, Number 3, AHCPR Publication No. 92-0047. Rockville, MD: Agency for Health Care Policy and Research, Public Health Service, US Department of Health and Human Services, 1992
8. Geronemus, Robins. The effect of two new dressings on epidermal wound healing. *J Dermatol Surg Oncol* 1982;8:850–2
9. Woodley DT, Chen JD, Kim JP, *et al.* Re-epithelialization; human keratinocyte locomotion. *Dermatol Clin* 1993;11:642–6
10. Eaglstein W, Falanga V. Chronic wounds. *Surg Clin North Am Wound Healing* 1997;77:689–700
11. Bicherstaff. Hidden powers of the pineapple. *New Sci* 1988;118:46–8
12. Falabella A. Debridement and management of exudative wounds. *Dermatol Ther* 1999;9:36–43
13. Hulten. Dressings for surgical wounds. *Am J Surg* 1994;167:521–4
14. Wolff, Hansson. Larval therapy for a leg ulcer with methicillin-resistant *Staphylococcus aureus*. *Acta Derm Venereol* 1999;79:320–1
15. Mumcuoglu KY, Ingber A, Gilead L, *et al.* Maggot therapy for the treatment of intractable wounds. *Int J Dermatol* 1999; 38:623–7
16. Sherman, Tran, Sullivan. Maggot treatment for venous stasis ulcers. *Arch Dermatol* 1996;132:254–6
17. Bello Y, Phillips T. The practical aspects of dressing therapy. *Dermatol Ther* 1999;9: 66–77
18. Choucair, Phillips. A review of wound healing and dressing materials. *Wounds* 1996;8: 165–72
19. Krasner D. Agency for Health Care Policy and Research Clinical Practice Guidelines, Number 15. Treatment of pressure ulcers: a pragmatist's critique for wound care providers. *Ostomy Wound Manage* 1995; 41:97S–101S
20. Falanga V, *et al.*, eds. *Text Atlas of Wound Management*. London: Martin Dunitz, 2000
21. Ovington LG. The well dressed wound: an overview of dressing types. *Wounds* 1998; A:1A–11A
22. Paquette D, Falanga V. Leg ulcers. *Clin Geriatr Med* 2002;18:80–1
23. Reiber GE, Boyko EJ, Smith DG. Lower extremity foot ulcers and amputations in diabetes. *Diabetes in America*, 2nd edn. Bethesda, MD: National Institutes of Health, 1995;95–1468
24. Kennedy, Tritch. Debridement. In *Chronic Wound Care*, 2nd edn. Wayne, PA: Health Management Publications, 1997
25. Dharmarajan TS, Ugalino JT. Pressure ulcers: clinical features and management. *Hosp Physic* 2002;38:64–71
26. Thomas DR. Prevention and treatment of pressure ulcers: what works? what doesn't? *Cleveland Clin J Med* 2001;68:710–22
27. Frantz RA. Adjuvant therapy for ulcer care. *Clin Geriatr Med* 1997;13:553–64

24 Sleep disorders

T.S. Dharmarajan, MD, FACP, AGSF, *and*
Anna Skokowska-Lebelt, MD

INTRODUCTION

Sleep disorders are common in older adults. Some of these are a result of alteration of the sleep cycle with the aging process, but often times, insomnia is the result of various medical disorders, the use of medications, circadian rhythm changes and/or environmental factors. Insomnia is a common sleep disorder characterized by difficulty in falling asleep or maintaining sleep, with a prevalence ranging from 4 to 70%. While only a few seek help from the physician, many suffer from serious daytime consequences and a decrease in the quality of life; there is also an associated increase in health-care costs[1-4].

NORMAL SLEEP

The normal 'sleep cycle' is characterized by two distinct states recorded by the electroencephalogram (EEG). They are the non-rapid eye movement (NREM) sleep characterized by four stages, and the rapid eye movement (REM) sleep, in which dreams occur. The stages can be differentiated by characteristic EEG changes[5]. The EEG in relaxed, awake persons, with the eyes closed, records alpha waves that are regular, 8-12 cycles/s, low-voltage activity. As one falls asleep, the alpha waves disappear and one enters the NREM stages of sleep. Stages 1 and 2 are the lightest sleep, with low-voltage activity of 3-7 cycles/s, lasting only a few minutes, followed by stages 3 and 4, known as delta sleep or slow-wave sleep, based on the presence of high-amplitude delta waves. Stages 3 and 4 provide the deepest sleep or restorative sleep. NREM is often referred to as 'quiet sleep' because of its 'peaceful' body state with regular respiration, slightly slower blood pressure, infrequent body movements and diminished muscle tone[5-7]. Disturbances in stages 3 and 4 may result in enuresis, somnambulism, nightmares or night terrors.

REM sleep (also called 'paradoxical sleep') is characterized by desynchronized brain activity with increased oxygen consumption, increased heart and respiratory rate, higher blood pressure, sexual arousals and near total skeletal muscle paralysis. Dreams occur in this stage; when fully awake one is usually able to recollect the dream. The REM cycle repeats every 90-100 min with the first episode shorter, at about 10 min, increasing to 40 min as the night progresses[5]. At the same time, deep sleep stages shorten and disappear toward the morning hours. Typically NREM takes up approximately 75% of the sleep cycle, with REM responsible for the remaining 25%. The whole sequence is repeated several times each night[5,6,8,9] (Table 1).

Sleep needs vary substantially from person to person and may be genetically determined. Average sleep time is 7-8 h, but is nevertheless considered normal between 4 and 10 h. Normal sleep requirements are determined on the basis of feeling rested or tired upon

Table 1 Normal sleep physiology. From references 5, 6, 8 and 9

	Non-REM sleep	REM sleep
Alertness	asleep	asleep
Body movement	infrequent, involuntary	inhibited
Eye movement	slow rolling or absent	rapid, abrupt movements
Muscle tone	decreased, not atonic	decreased to absent
Memory/dreaming	dull, non-recalled	vivid, bizarre, recalled if awakened
EEG	varies with stage	desynchronized
EMG	variable	activity absent (atonia)

REM, rapid eye movement; EEG, electroencephalogram; EMG, electromyogram

waking up and the ability to function well during the day[5,10,11].

SLEEP ALTERATIONS WITH AGE

Sleep requirements are not appreciably altered with age. Sleep needs decrease somewhat with aging, but more importantly there are alterations in the pattern of sleep. Sleep *latency*, i.e. the time taken to fall asleep, increases with age; the elderly often experience awakenings (microarousals) during sleep. There are also fewer body movements while asleep, with longer immobility periods. Total actual sleep time is diminished despite longer time spent in bed, indicating that sleep *efficiency* is diminished. A change in posture preference from the prone to the right-sided position has been described. Stage 1 sleep increases, stage 2 remains variable making sleep lighter and the deep (restorative) sleep may be diminished or non-existent. REM sleep is preserved; although the number of REM episodes may increase, total REM time is decreased[12-15].

Older adults experience wakeful episodes toward morning hours, which contribute to a feeling of inadequate sleep. In reality, the healthy older adult should not experience increased daytime drowsiness; however, sleep disturbances contribute to less satisfaction with sleep, more fatigue and frequent naps during the day[6,14-16] (Table 2).

SLEEP DISORDERS, OTHER THAN INSOMNIA

Sleep disorders include disorders of initiating and maintaining sleep, most importantly insomnia, disorders of excessive somnolence, disorders of sleep–wake cycle and parasomnias. The major emphasis in this chapter is on insomnia, which follows a brief discussion of the other sleep disorders.

Narcolepsy

Narcolepsy is a leading cause of excessive daytime sleepiness of unknown etiology, sometimes familial, often associated with cataplexy (sudden loss of muscle tone) and other sleep phenomena such as sleep paralysis and hallucinations. Most patients experience disrupted sleep at night and frequent awakenings. Management of narcolepsy includes non-pharmacological measures (see insomnia) and pharmacological treatment with stimulants, tricyclic agents or short-acting benzodiazepines, depending on symptoms[17].

Obstructive sleep apnea

This is a common disorder seen in older adults, characterized by apneic episodes from complete or partial airway obstruction. The condition is often associated with other medical problems such as obesity, hypertension, heart disease, stroke or hypothyroidism.

Table 2 Sleep changes with age. From references 6, 11, 12, 14, and 16

Sleep is lighter, with an increase in stage 1
Longer sleep latency
Increased sleep fragmentation with microarousals through the night
Reduction of slow-wave sleep (stages 3 and 4)
Changes in sleep architecture (REM episodes increase, but total REM decreases)
Sleep efficiency is decreased
Total sleep time is decreased despite longer time spent in bed
Increased desire for napping during the day
Tendency to depart to bed early with early morning awakenings

REM, rapid eye movement

Patients usually present with snoring and cessation of breathing that leads to hypoxia caused by reduced respiratory effort for more then 10 s. Hypoxia and hypercapnia lead to frequent brief arousals with morning headaches, drowsiness, mood disturbances and decline in functioning. History and physical examination is helpful, with definitive diagnosis by polysomnography.

Management includes recommendations for weight loss, but more helpful is nasal continuous positive airway pressure or bilevel positive airway pressure administered during sleep at night[18].

Restless legs syndrome

Restless legs syndrome (RLS) is a sensory motor disorder increasing in prevalence with age. It is characterized by an uncontrollable urge to move the legs with parasthesias, with worsening at the end of the day. Discomfort is described as a pulling or burning sensation deep in the muscles, relieved by activity, such as moving, kicking or walking. While the cause is unknown, it may be associated with iron deficiency anemia, vitamin B_{12} deficiency, thyroid disorders, uremia or peripheral neuropathy[19]. Treatment is symptomatic, including warm baths or soaks for the legs and regular exercises. If no relief is obtained,

pharmacologic measures include dopaminergic agonists (levodopa–carbidopa), benzodiazepines, gabapentin and opiates.

Periodic limb movement disorder

Periodic limb movement disorder (PLMD), also called 'nocturnal myoclonus', is an idiopathic condition that may accompany RLS or can occur independently. The disorder is characterized by sudden rhythmic leg kicks with ankle dorsiflexion, flaring of toes and painful muscle cramps that force the patient to move the legs every 20–40 s. These movements cause brief arousal from sleep, but may also occur during wakeful periods. PLMD is confirmed by polysomnography. Treatment is similar to that for RLS and includes dopamine agonists and clonazepam[19].

Parasomnias

Parasomnias are abnormal sleep behaviors that occur during NREM sleep and include sleepwalking, talking, nightmares, sleep seizures, enuresis, headache, arrhythmias, angina and asthma. Parasomnias occur at any age and can cause serious injuries or health consequences in older individuals. The concern is regarding the abnormal behavior rather than the impact on the quality of sleep itself[20].

Disorders of the sleep–wake cycle

Disorders of the sleep–wake cycle include jet lag, insomnia related to work hours or irregular sleep–wake schedules, and advanced sleep phase syndrome; these are generally less applicable to the elderly. The circadian rhythm that regulates sleep/wakefulness and physiological body functions is under control of the suprachiasmatic nucleus located in the hypothalamus. This rhythm is influenced by the environment and can be desynchronized with aging. Usually there is an advance in the sleep–wake cycle with age; the 'biological clock' turns off earlier in the evening and turns on sooner than desired in the morning. The result is sleepiness in the evening hours and earlier morning awakenings, noticed even in healthy older people, and referred to as advanced sleep phase syndrome (ASPS). Treatment of ASPS includes exposure to bright light in the evening for at least 2 h. A suggestion is early morning use of melatonin to extend duration of the 'dark phase' and improve sleep efficiency[6,8,21].

Rapid eye movement sleep behavior disorder

REM sleep behavior disorder mostly affects older adults of both genders; half the cases are associated with Parkinson's disease, narcolepsy or stroke. The characteristic feature is a behavior disorder wherein the patient acts out violent, intense, vivid dreams, with preserved memory of the events. Diagnosis is by polysomnography and neurological evaluation. Treatment is bedtime use of benzodiazepines, especially clonazepam, and a safe sleeping environment[22,23] (Table 3).

INSOMNIA

Definition

Insomnia, as defined by DSM-IV criteria, is difficulty in falling asleep and/or maintaining sleep, resulting in sleep that is non-restorative or non-refreshing, despite an adequate opportunity to sleep. The sleep is insufficient in quality or quantity, with the number of hours required for sleep generally a personal perception[24]. Insomnia can be divided into three subtypes; these may occur individually or in combination[7]:

(1) Sleep-onset insomnia associated with increase in sleep latency;

(2) Middle insomnia with excessive middle of the night wakefulness;

(3) Terminal insomnia resulting in early morning awakening.

Another classification of insomnia is based on the length of time it persists. Insomnia can be acute (short-term), lasting days to weeks, or chronic (persistent), lasting months to years. Short-term insomnia is usually a reaction to stressful situations in life, such as illness, hospitalization, death of a close one, unfamiliar environment, retirement or work-related, or bereavement. Causes of chronic insomnia include chronic medical disease, psychiatric illness and medications[8,11,25].

Causes

Disease processes

It is worth emphasizing that age, by itself, is not a significant predictive factor for insomnia. Co-existence of other factors, in addition to aging and biological rhythm changes, often predispose to sleeping difficulties[26].

Insomnia is usually a symptom that masks a medical or behavioral disorder, or a consequence of a disease process and/or its treatment. Increased sleep arousals and early morning awakenings may be symptoms of anxiety, panic attacks or depression. Reasons for secondary insomnia include inability to sleep because of dyspnea (heart failure, chronic obstructive lung disease), pain (osteoarthritis, metastasis), nocturia, prostatism, hyperglycemia, renal failure, peripheral neuropathy, thyroid disease and gastroesophageal reflux disease, amongst others[7,21]. Parkinson's disease and Alzheimer's disease are well known associations, as is also the presence of delirium in the sick older patient[15]. Mental disorders should not be overlooked in the elderly; examples include depression and anxiety[26]. Hormone imbalance at menopause is another well-recognized cause of insomnia, with benefits from hormone replacement therapy. Finally, the use of medications prescribed for an illness, and the often unrecognized use by the

Table 3 Sleep disorders. From references 8, 11–13, 17, 18, 20 and 22

Sleep disorder	Definition	Symptoms	Diagnosis	Treatment
Narcolepsy	excessive daytime sleepiness for at least 3 months	'Sleep attacks' cataplexy or hallucination at beginning or end of sleep	clinical polysomnography MSLT	scheduled naps stimulants methylphenidate
Idiopathic hypersomnia	excessive sleepiness for at least 1 month on a daily basis	prolonged sleepiness during day or night despite adequate sleep	history: familial normal sleep structure, normal sleep study.	stimulants (amphetamines) non-sedating SSRI e.g.fluoxetine, paroxetine, serraline
Obstructive sleep apnea	repeated cessation or reduction of breathing	loud snoring arousals from sleep hypoxemia day-time sleepiness	polysomnography	CPAP weight loss surgery trazadone dopaminergic agents benzodiazepines opiates gabapentin
Restless legs syndrome (RLS)	uncomfortable sensation with urge to move legs relieved by leg movement	motor restlessness during wake delayed sleep onset	history	
Periodic limb movement disorder	idiopathic or associated with RLS	legs jerks during sleep with brief arousals daytime sleepiness	polysomnography	dopaminergic agents clonazepam gabapentin propoxyphene
REM behavior disorder	REM sleep parasomnia with loss of muscle atonia	agitation, violent behavior during sleep	history polysomnography	clonazepam

REM, rapid eye movement; MSLT, Multiple Sleep Latency Test; CPAP, continuous positive airway pressure

patient of over-the-counter (non-prescribed) and topical drugs, may be the basis. Therefore, in the evaluation of insomnia, it is essential to review the medication regimen[27].

Alcohol, caffeine and nicotine

One should enquire about alcohol consumption, since it is often used to promote sleep. In fact, while alcohol facilitates sleep onset from sedation and psychomotor slowing, its eventual adverse effects result in wakefulness and early morning awakening.

Caffeine and nicotine are commonly consumed stimulants associated with sleep disorders. Caffeine is present not only in coffee but also abundantly in chocolate and many popular soft drinks. It is never too late to quit smoking, especially for the older adult who has insomnia[24,28]. Prolonged nicotine intake in any form (smoking, chewing or perhaps second-hand smoke) can affect healthy sleep (Table 4)[29,30].

Environmental factors

Environmental factors associated with insomnia include excessive noise, bright lighting, unsuitable room temperature, uncomfortable beds and inadequate sunlight exposure during the day. These may cause difficulty in

Table 4 Common causes of insomnia*. From references 6–8, 13, 24, 25, 29 and 30

Medical illness
Acute or chronic pain
  arthritis
  osteomalacia
  metastases
Cardiovascular disease
  angina
  congestive heart failure
  arrhythmia
Pulmonary disease
  asthma
  chronic obstructive pulmonary disease
Gastrointestinal disease
  gastroesophageal reflux disease
  peptic ulcer disease
  diarrhea
Genitourinary
  prostatism
  incontinence
  polyuria
Neuropsychiatric
  dementia
  Parkinson's disease
  delirium
  movement disorders
  depression
Endocrine
  diabetes mellitus
  thyroid diseases
  menopause

Sleep–wake cycle disorders
  jet-lag, shift work-related
  delayed sleep phase
  advanced sleep phase syndrome

*Medications**
  alcohol
  bronchodilators
  corticosteroids
  antihypertensive agents
  H_2 receptor blockers
  anticonvulsants
  stimulating antidepressants
  thyroid supplements
  decongestants
  anticholinergics

*List is for illustration, not all-inclusive

falling asleep or maintaining sleep, particularly in the hospital and nursing home settings[8,21].

Behavioral factors

Behavioral factors that negatively impact on sleep include sedentary lifestyle, daytime naps, irregular sleep hours, departing to bed early, consumption of heavy or late meals, and long hours in bed for non-sleep activities such as reading or watching television[21].

Consequences

Insomnia adversely impacts on quality of life. Restorative sleep is essential for emotional and physical health as well as overall well-being. Sleep interruptions may impair next day functioning, causing fatigue, irritability, agitation or drowsiness and contribute to poor job performance, loss of work hours and absenteeism[1,4,26]. Individuals with insomnia are at risk for psychiatric illness, especially depression or alcoholism. Sleep loss and the consequent use of sedative hypnotics may lead to falls and increased risk of automobile and job-related accidents. In those with dementia, sleep disturbances may lead to nursing home placement[7]. Less recognized is the increase in global health-care cost.

Evaluation

Evaluation of sleep disorders includes a focused history regarding sleep habits, medical and psychiatric disorders, besides a review of medications and the use of alcohol, caffeine and nicotine. Clues can be obtained from the patient, bed partner or, in the case of the cognitively impaired, the caregiver. Most patients do not come forward with sleep-related complaints during regular office visits[3]. A complete physical examination is the next important step in diagnosis. Simple bedside observation provides information regarding breathing patterns, apneic episodes, wheezing or abnormal body movements. Identification of fever, upper airway disease, neurologic disorders or conditions that cause pain, dyspnea or discomfort during sleep deserves consideration[29–31].

Laboratory tests help identify secondary causes that are contributory; such testing should be individualized and include complete blood count, full chemistries, thyroid function tests, B_{12} and folate levels, electrocardiogram and chest X-rays. Based on results of the initial evaluation, additional tests may be indicated.

Polysomnography is considered the 'gold standard' test for sleep evaluation. It simultaneously records different physiologic parameters during sleep, such as EEG, electro-oculography (EOG), chin electromyography (EMG), nasal and oral air flow, pulse oximetry and electrocardiogram in correlation with chest and abdominal movements. Polysomnography requires sleep laboratory settings and incurs a cost, and is therefore not recommended for routine evaluation of insomnia. However, there are situations where this test is helpful; these include excessive daytime sleepiness, insomnia unresponsive to usual therapy, movement disorders, obstructive sleep apnea and insomnia of extreme magnitude[7]. Other tests include the Multiple Sleep Latency Test (MSLT), which assesses the length of time to fall asleep, objectively confirmed by EEG. Actigraphy, a recently developed method, records body movements during the sleep–wake cycle with a small, portable device worn on the wrist; it is cheaper, and results correlate with those of polysomnography[10].

Management

Successful management of insomnia improves sleep time, quality of sleep and 'function' during the day. The decision on type of treatment depends on duration of insomnia-related manifestations. Broadly, measures could be divided into lifestyle modifications and pharmacotherapy.

Modification of behavior with implementation of good sleep habits, proper timing of exercise regimens, stimulus control therapy in the bedroom environment, relaxation techniques, cognitive therapy and revision of the medication regimen help develop a better pattern of sleep. Collectively these fall under the term 'sleep hygiene'. The methods can

be used alone, or in combination, and must be individualized[4,11].

Acute insomnia that is caused by bereavement or a new unfamiliar environment, or is triggered by stress, justifies the short-term use of hypnotic medications, in addition to sleep hygiene recommendations. Chronic, persistent insomnia requires more complex strategies to pursue relief, depending on the cause. Here, treatment of primary psychiatric or medical disorders may reduce sleep problems. Behavioral therapy is the mainstay in management of chronic insomnia, with drug therapy playing a secondary role.

Lifestyle modification

Non-pharmacologic measures to modify lifestyle are preferred in treating chronic insomnia in older adults and are generally tried first, although they are more time-consuming and the results not dramatic (Table 5)[32].

The first step is a review of all medications (prescribed and over-the-counter) with discontinuation of potentially offending drugs. Sometimes, it may be necessary to revise the regimen or pick alternatives that have less influence on sleep[6]. The next step is the need to counsel on sleep hygiene, regarding behaviors that promote better sleep. These habits include regular sleep hours, avoidance of daytime naps, limiting time spent in bed without sleeping, setting pre-bed routines and relaxation techniques to help alleviate tension and cognitive arousal. Making the bedroom environment quiet and comfortable is helpful. Physical activities such as exercise should be regular, not strenuous, and not performed within 4–6 h prior to sleep. Exposure to sunlight should be avoided in late hours. Dietary habits with avoidance of heavy meals, excessive fluids, caffeine and alcohol prior to sleep are beneficial[15,28,33]. With sleep hygiene nearly half the individuals using hypnotic drugs may be able to stop their medications, reduce sleep latency and expand duration of sleep by 30–45 min. The techniques are also cost-effective[6,13,15].

Table 5 Insomnia: lifestyle modifications. From references 6–8, 15, 16, 21 and 32–4

Behavioral method	Activity
Sleep hygiene	get up and go to bed at regular hours
	limit alcohol use, never to promote sleep
	avoid stimulants (caffeine, nicotine) close to bed time
	keep bedroom quiet and comfortable
	avoid heavy meals and fluids at bedtime
	establish pre-bed relaxing routines
	avoid hot shower just before bed time
	exercise regularly, not just prior to sleep
	avoid strenuous exercise
	do not watch the clock constantly
	ensure room lighting is not bright
	music, if used, should be relaxing
Stimulus control	use bedroom only for sleep and sex
	go to bed only when sleepy
	leave the bed if unable to fall asleep
	avoid daytime naps
	establish regular wake time
Relaxation therapy	deep muscle relaxation
	cognitive relaxation (meditation)
	biofeedback
	yoga
Light therapy	possibly beneficial, controversial

Behavioral therapies

Behavioral therapies help correct maladaptive sleep habits, and attempt to change an individual's attitude toward sleep requirements and master the ability to relax. The two main forms of behavioral therapy are stimulus control and sleep restriction. Stimulus control includes instructions on sleep-promoting activities at bedtime and methods to minimize sleep disruptive behavior in the appropriate bedroom environment. Many principles of behavioral therapy, such as regular sleep hours, setting bedtime routines and avoidance of daytime napping, are also included under sleep hygiene. Sleep restriction therapy attempts to reduce the extensive amount of time spent in bed as compared to the real sleep time. In this technique, a subject is allowed to stay in bed only for that amount of time actually spent in sleep[32–35].

In addition, mastering relaxation skills can alleviate somatic and cognitive arousal. Techniques includes abdominal breathing, muscle relaxation, meditation, yoga and even hypnosis. These methods usually require help, encouragement and feedback from a professional trainer or psychologist.

Behavioral therapy is safe and effective, and provides long-term results[25,36].

Light therapy

Light therapy is another method that may be helpful in restoring the biological sleep–wake cycle in insomnia. Exposure to bright light (1000–4000 Lux) during evening hours was found to be beneficial in advanced sleep phase syndrome to allow individuals to fall asleep later, and improve sleep quality, daytime functioning and well-being. This method is particularly useful in cognitively impaired adults in nursing home settings[15,37]. Recently, a study demonstrated no improvement in the quality of sleep following light exposure, although a phase shift was achieved[34].

Table 6 Hypnotics: principles of prescribing in the elderly. From references 8 and 37

The lowest effective dose should be used

Intermittent dosing is recommended (2–3 times per week)

Hypnotics are used for short time periods (3–4 weeks)

Gradual discontinuation recommended to avoid rebound insomnia

Short-acting agents are preferred (to minimize daytime sedation)

Be alert to adverse drug effects

Attempt to revise regimen periodically

Pharmacologic treatment

Medication use in older patients with insomnia has to be individualized and applied only when other measures fail. Nevertheless, in practice, hypnotics are common therapy for insomnia. Approximately one-half of all patients with sleep disorders are treated with medications[28].

In most situations, selective benzodiazepine receptor agonists and benzodiazepines are currently the hypnotic agents of choice. In the elderly, sleep medications have to be used with caution, bearing in mind the age-related alterations in pharmacokinetics and dynamics; included are increased volume of distribution due to increased fat/water ratio, reduced phase-1 hepatic metabolism, increased central nervous system sensitivity, concomitant polypharmacy and presence of co-morbid conditions. The result is a higher susceptibility to adverse drug effects. The principles of appropriate prescribing of hypnotics are listed in Table 6[8,38–41].

Preferred therapies Hypnotic agents most commonly prescribed for insomnia include the newer class of benzodiazepine receptor agonists and some benzodiazepines. They have replaced older hypnotics in the treatment of transient insomnia and are approved for short-term therapy.

Benzodiazepine receptor agonists include zolpidem and zaleplon; their chemical structure does not resemble that of benzodiazepines, but the action is on the benzodiazepine receptor, facilitating action of γ-aminobutyric acid (GABA), the predominant inhibitory neurotransmitter in the brain. Selective binding to the ω_1-benzodiazepine receptor complex improves safety, results in fewer side-effects and less tolerance, with no rebound insomnia[7,39,42].

Both zolpidem and zaleplon have short duration of action. Zolpidem has a half-life of 2.5 h and can be used immediately before bedtime. It reduces sleep latency and increases sleep duration. Zaleplon has an even shorter half-life (1 h), and is suitable not only at bedtime but also for night awakenings. No psychomotor impairment or loss of memory has been shown. Benzodiazepine receptor agonists are considered safer for older adults, but caution should always be used with hepatic disease, or with concomitant administration of other drugs that depress the central nervous system. Contraindications include sleep apnea and alcoholism[39].

Benzodiazepines have a long history of use. They are hypnotic agents that bind nonselectively to all benzodiazepine receptors, allowing suppression of neural excitation by opening the chloride channel in response to GABA. They induce sleep onset, decrease nocturnal awakening and increase total sleep time, with a subjective feeling of improved sleep quality. However, they also alter the normal sleep pattern by increasing light sleep and reducing slow-wave and REM sleep[38].

Different benzodiazepines have variable myorelaxant, anxiolytic and anticonvulsant properties. The effects vary and are influenced by absorption, lipophilic properties, rate of hepatic metabolism, presence of active metabolites, elimination rate and receptor binding affinity. Side-effects are dose related, calling for the lowest possible dose to be used. Benzodiazepines may be classified into long acting (half-life above 20 h), intermediate acting (half-life about 10 h) and short acting (half-life less than 6 h)

Table 7 Hypnotics: dosage and half-life. From references 8, 11, 15, 25 and 38

	Geriatric dose (mg)	Half-life (h)
Short-acting agents		
Triazolam (Halcion)	0.125	1.5–5
Zolpidem (Ambien)	5	1.5–4.5
Zaleplon (Sonata)	5	1
Intermediate-acting agents		
Temazepam (Restoril)	7.5	3–25
Lorazepam (Ativan)	0.25–1	8–24
Estazolam (ProSom)	0.5–1	8–24
Oxazepam (Serax)	10–15	3–6
Alprazolam (Xanax)	0.25	8–24
*Long-acting agents**		
Clonazepam (Klonopin)	0.25–1	20–60
Chlordiazepoxide (Librium)	20	5–15
Diazepam (Valium)	5	30–60
Flurazepam (Dalmane)	15	36–120

*Preferably avoided in older individuals

(Table 7). Benzodiazepines with a short half-life are used for sleep-onset insomnia, but may cause retrograde amnesia and/or rebound insomnia. Short-acting agents are generally preferred in the elderly. Agents with an intermediate half-life are helpful in sleep onset and maintenance, and for early morning awakenings. Long-acting agents have a higher incidence of adverse effects and can contribute to falls, hip fracture, daytime sedation, confusion and automobile accidents; they are best avoided in the elderly[29,38,43].

The Food and Drug Administration (FDA) has approved benzodiazepines for bedtime use, for only up to 4 continuous weeks. In general, dosages in older adults should be half of those used for younger individuals, to minimize side-effects.

Therapies generally not recommended
Pharmacotherapeutic options for insomnia treatment include many drugs in prescription form or over-the-counter 'sleeping aids'. Many are no longer recommended because of undesired side-effects. These older agents include barbiturates and barbiturate-like drugs (chloral hydrate, meprobamate and glutethimide); they are associated with low therapeutic index, high risk of tolerance and addiction, besides drug interactions and risk of death in case of overdose.

Sedative antidepressants (amitriptyline, doxepin, trazodone, nefazodone, mirtazapine) are helpful in patients with insomnia who suffer from depression. These agents have a variety of side-effects, including anticholinergic effects, residual sedation, cardiac dysrythmias, orthostatic hypotension, sexual dysfunction, priapism (trazodone), worsening of leg movement disorders and alterations in sleep cycle (REM sleep suppression). Side-effects and potential for overdose limit their use in the majority of patients without depression[8,39,40].

Antihistamines with sedative properties such as diphenhydramine (Benadryl®) and doxylamine (Unisom®) are easily available without prescription as over-the-counter sleeping aids, advertised for temporary relief of insomnia. They have minimal sleep-inducing effects, but can cause residual drowsiness. Use of antihistamines can be dangerous for older adults because of their anticholinergic properties[8,11,36] (Table 8).

Table 8 Hypnotics, preferably avoided in the elderly. From references 7, 8, 15, 38 and 40

Drug	Side-effects
Chloral hydrate	gastrointestinal irritation, nausea, vomiting unpleasant taste and smell delirium, lightheadedness, seizure, ataxia nightmares hepatic and renal toxicity (may be fatal)

Barbiturates
  pentobarbital
  phenobarbital
  secobarbital
	low therapeutic index
	rapid tolerance
	residual sedation, nightmares
	potential for abuse and dependence
	highly lethal with overdose

Antihistamines
  diphenhydramine
  doxylamine
  hydroxyzine
	minimal effect on sleep induction
	daytime drowsiness
	anticholinergic effects (dry mouth, urinary
	  retention, cognitive impairment, orthostatic
	  hypotension, blurred vision)

Sedating antidepressants
  amitriptyline
  trazodone
	anticholinergic effects
	sexual dysfunction
	cardiac toxicity (arrhythmias)
	worsening of restless legs syndrome

Long-acting benzodiazepines
  clonazepam
  flurazepam
  diazepam
	residual daytime drowsiness
	anterograde amnesia
	impaired psychomotor functions
	impaired cognition
	falls
	worsening of sleep apnea

Melatonin	vasoconstriction (avoid in coronary heart disease) sexual dysfunction
Valerian root	may cause hepatotoxicity

Alternatives Melatonin is a hormone secreted by the pineal gland; its release is triggered by darkness and it is suppressed by light. The hormone levels are reduced in the elderly. Melatonin may regulate the circadian rhythm and it is believed that administration may help restore natural sleep drive and improve the quality of sleep in some[28,44]. Use of melatonin, however, is not necessarily safe for everybody; it has vasoconstrictive properties that contraindicates its use in coronary heart disease[7].

Additional alternatives for treatment of insomnia include herbal remedies such as kava and valerian root, and an amino acid, tryptophan (converted to serotonin in the body); these supplements are not under control or approval of the FDA. Tryptophan is believed to be a weak natural hypnotic agent that may improve sleep by reducing sleep latency and nocturnal awakenings. The supplements are generally not recommended in view of potential harm; e.g. a contaminated tryptophan batch was the cause of eosinophilia–myalgia syndrome[7,28].

CONCLUSION

Treatment of insomnia is often difficult. Results can be achieved with a judicious combination of non-pharmacologic measures, with or without short-term, intermittent use of selective hypnotics. An attempt to elucidate an etiology for the sleep disturbance should be made, especially if the insomnia is of recent onset. In our out-patient geriatric clinic, less than 3% of adults ranging from 60 to over 100 years have required the use of pharmacotherapy.

References

1. Leger D. Public health and insomnia: economic impact. *Sleep* 2000;23(Suppl. 3): 69–76
2. Chevalier H, Los F, Boichut D, *et al*. Evaluation of severe insomnia in the general population: results of European multinational survey. *J Psychopharmacol* 1999;13 (Suppl. 1):S21–4
3. Zammit GK. Introduction. In Roberts WO, ed. *Insomnia: Treatment Options for the 21st Century. A Special Report*. Minneapolis, MN: McGraw-Hill Healthcare Information Group, 2000:3–4
4. McCall WV. Pharmacologic treatment of insomnia in the older patient. *Ann Longterm Care* 2000;8:59–63
5. Kaplan HI, Sadock BJ, Grebb JA. Normal sleep and sleep disorders. In Kaplan HI, Sadock BJ, eds. *Kaplan and Sadock's Synopsis of Psychiatry*, 7th edn. Baltimore: Williams & Wilkins, 1994:699–716
6. Haponik EF, McCall WV. Sleep problems. In Hazzard WR, Blass JP, Ettinger WH Jr, Halter JB, Ouslander JG, eds. *Principles of Geriatric Medicine and Gerontology*, 4th edn. New York: McGraw-Hill, 1998: 1413–27
7. Roberts WO, ed. *A Practical Guide to Insomnia*. Minneapolis, MN: McGraw-Hill Healthcare Information, 1999:5–77
8. Uy S. Evaluation and treatment of insomnia in primary care. *Fam Pract Recertification* 2001;23:37–56
9. Ancoli-Israel S, Kripke DF. Sleep and aging. In Duthie EH Jr, Katz PR, eds. *Practice of Geriatrics*, 3rd edn. Philadelphia: Saunders, 1998:237–43
10. Attarian HP. Helping patients who say they cannot sleep. Postgrad Med 2000;107: 127–42
11. Meyer TJ. Evaluation and management of insomnia. *Hosp Pract* 1998;Dec 15:75–86
12. Alessi CA. Sleep problems. In Cobbs EL, Duthie EH Jr, Murphy JB, eds. *Geriatrics Review Syllabus*, 5th edn. New York: Blackwell Publishing, 2002:209–18
13. Neubauer DN. Sleep problems in the elderly. *Am Fam Physician* 1999;59: 2551–8
14. Webb WB. Age-related changes in sleep. Sleep disorders in the elderly. *Clin Geriatr Med* 1989;5:275–87
15. Asplund R. Sleep disorders in the elderly. *Drugs Aging* 1999;14:91–103
16. Ancoli-Israel S. Insomnia in the elderly: a review for the primary care practitioner. *Sleep* 2000;23(Suppl. 1):23–30
17. Bassetti C, Aldrich S. Narcolepsy. *Neurol Clin* 1996;14:545–71
18. Chervin RD, Guilleminault C. Obstructive sleep apnea and related disorders. *Neurol Clin* 1996;14:583–609
19. Trenkwalter C, Walters AS, Henning W. Periodic limb movement and restless legs syndrome. *Neurol Clin* 1996;14:629–51
20. Mahowald MW, Schenck CH. NREM sleep parasomnias. *Neurol Clin* 1996;14:675–97
21. Martin J, Shochat T, Ancoli-Israel S. Assessment and treatment of sleep disturbances in older adults. *Clin Psychol Rev* 2000;20:783–805
22. Schenck CH, Mahowald MW. Parasomnias. *Postgrad Med* 2000;107:145–56
23. Schenck CH, Mahowald MW. REM sleep parasomnias. *Neurol Clin* 1996;14: 697–737
24. Doghramji PP. Detection of insomnia in primary care. *J Clin Psychiatry* 2001;62 (Suppl. 10):18–26
25. Schneider DL. Insomnia: safe and effective therapy for sleep problems in the older patient. *Geriatrics* 2002;57:24–35
26. Ohayon MM, Zulley J, Guilleminault C, *et al*. How age and daytime activities are

related to insomnia in the general population: consequences for older people. *J Am Geriatr Soc* 2001;49:360–6

27. McCrae CS, Lichstein K. Managing insomnia in long-term care. *Ann Long-Term Care* 2002;10:38–43

28. Vitiello M. Effective treatment for age-related sleep disturbances. *Geriatrics* 1999;54:47–52

29. Woodward M. Insomnia in the elderly. *Aust Fam Physician* 1999;28:653–8

30. Katz DA, McHorney CA. Clinical correlates of insomnia in patients with chronic illness. *Arch Intern Med* 1998;158:1099–106

31. Zammit GK. Redefining a good night's sleep. In Roberts WO, ed. *Insomnia: Treatment Options for the 21st Century. A Special Report*. Minneapolis, MN: McGraw-Hill Healthcare Information Group, 2000: 33–40

32. Morin CM, Mimeault VM, Gagne A. Nonpharmacological treatment of late-life insomnia. *J Psychosom Res* 1999;46:103–16

33. Simon RD. Tailoring the treatment of insomnia to the individual patient. In Roberts WO, ed. *Insomnia: Treatment Options for the 21st Century. A Special Report*. Minneapolis, MN: McGraw-Hill Healthcare Information Group, 2000:41–54

34. Suhner AG, Murphy PJ, Campbell CS. Failure of timed bright light exposure to alleviate age-related sleep maintenance insomnia. *J Am Geriatr Soc* 2002;50:617–23

35. Kupfer DJ, Reynolds CF III. Management of insomnia. *N Engl J Med* 1997;336:341–6

36. Hauri P, Esther MS. Insomnia. *Mayo Clin Proc* 1990;65:869–82

37. Ancoli-Israel S, Martin JL, Kripke DF, *et al*. Effect of light treatment on sleep and circadian rhythms in demented nursing home patients. *J Am Geriatr Soc* 2002;50:282–9

38. Mitler MM. Nonselective and selective benzodiazepine receptor agonist – where are we today? *Sleep* 2000:23:39–47

39. Scharf MB. Evaluation of next-day functioning and residual sedation in healthy subjects: zaleplon vs. flurazepam. In Roberts WO, ed. *Insomnia: Treatment Options for the 21st Century. A Special Report*. Minneapolis, MN: McGraw-Hill Healthcare Information Group, 2000:25–32

40. Roth T. Overview of insomnia for the primary care physician. In Roberts WO, ed. *Insomnia: Treatment Options for the 21st Century. A Special Report*. Minneapolis, MN: McGraw-Hill Healthcare Information Group, 2000:5–13

41. Holbrook AM, Crowther R, Lotter A, *et al*. The role of benzodiazepines in the treatment of insomnia. *J Am Geriatr Soc* 2001; 49:824–6

42. Hedner J, Yaeche R, Emilien G, *et al*. Zaleplon shortens subjective sleep latency and improves subjective sleep quality in elderly patients with insomnia. *Int J Geriatr Psychiatry* 2000;15:704–12

43. Vignola A, Lamoureaux C, Bastien CH, Morin CM. Effects of chronic insomnia and use of benzodiazepines on daytime performance in older adults. *J Gerontol* 2000; 55B:54–62

44. Brzezinski A. Melatonin in humans. *N Engl J Med* 1997;336:186–94

25 Urinary incontinence

T.S. Dharmarajan, MD, FACP, AGSF, *Wilson P. Pais,* MD, *and Robin O. Russell,* MD

INTRODUCTION

Urinary incontinence (UI) is common and much more than an annoying problem; in older adults it markedly affects the quality of life of both patient and caregiver. Brocklehurst characterizes UI as a geriatric giant, along with the syndromes of altered mental status, falls and immobility[1]. The prevalence of UI increases with age and is more common in females[2]. In the community, the prevalence is 15% in men, and 30% in women, and in institutions the number rises to 60%[2]. UI may coexist with fecal incontinence. It is a heterogeneous condition with varying severity, ranging from rare episodes of small quantities of urine loss to completely uncontrolled voiding. The cost of managing UI is astronomical. Direct costs in the USA exceed $10 billion annually. This does not include indirect expenses such as those relating to socioeconomic issues[3]. Even though UI is not life threatening, the physical, psychological, social and occupational well-being of the patient as well as the caregiver are adversely affected[4]. UI can result in depression, anxiety, emotional stress and sexual dysfunction[5]. Individuals with UI are a increased risk of developing urinary tract infections, skin breakdown or rashes and falls[6]. Often, the health- care provider may be unaware of the presence of a patient's incontinence[7,8]. Frustration and embarrassment prevent the individual from discussing the condition with the physician. A Japanese study reported that 81% of patients with UI did not seek help for this symptom[9]. UI is treatable in the majority of cases and curable in many.

Incontinence is also common in middle-aged women, the risk increasing with a history of vaginal deliveries, delay in attaining continence in childhood, and obesity[10]. UI is approached by multiple disciplines and may be perceived differently by each. To the geriatrician, it may be perceived as functional impairment; to the urologist, as lower urinary tract dysfunction; the psychiatrist may focus on depression; and the gynecologist sees it as a female problem[11]. From an optimistic viewpoint, the primary physician can successfully manage two-thirds of cases of UI with few instruments in the office[1].

PHYSIOLOGY OF THE URINARY TRACT

Incontinence is the norm at birth. Continence requires several areas of intact function including the urinary tract, neurological system, cognitive function, intact mobility, motivation and an appropriate environment. Incontinence may result from disruption of any of the above. The lower urinary tract consists of three components: the detrusor, the internal sphincter and the external sphincter. The detrusor is the smooth muscle of the bladder and serves as the storage site

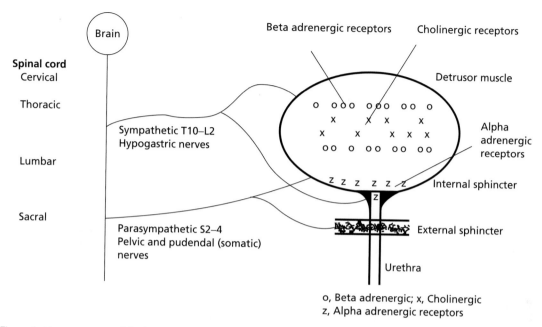

Figure 1 Neuroanatomy of the lower urinary tract

for urine. The internal sphincter consists of smooth muscle, is under involuntary control and is part of the proximal urethra; more precisely, it is a continuation of the bladder muscle and not a distinct entity. The external sphincter is composed of striated muscle and is under voluntary control; it is located in the distal and periurethral area and is particularly well defined in men[2,5]. In addition, compressive forces of urethral musculature, mucosa and submucosal tissue help prevent urinary leakage; this is termed urethral coaptation, a mechanism dependent on estrogen[5]. With estrogen deficiency mucosal coaptation is lost, with consequent lowering of urethral resistance.

Micturition is co-ordinated by the autonomic (sympathetic and parasympathetic) and somatic nervous systems. The sympathetic pathway emanates from spinal cord segments T10 to L2 as the presacral or hypogastric nerves; stimulation contributes to relaxation of the detrusor via β-adrenergic receptors (predominantly in the body of the bladder) and contraction of the internal sphincter via α-adrenergic receptors (predominantly in the

bladder neck). Inhibition of the sympathetic pathway produces the opposite effect. The parasympathetic (cholinergic) pathway originates from the S2–S4 segments as the pelvic nerves. Stimulation causes contraction of the bladder. In addition the somatic pathway, from S2 to S4 via the pudendal nerve, innervates the external sphincter, allowing voluntary contraction of the sphincter[2,5].

The central pathway for micturition has not been precisely delineated. It is believed that a higher central nervous system control located in the cerebellum, basal ganglia and frontal lobe oversees micturition. A pontine micturition center helps co-ordinate sphincter and bladder function. The cerebral cortex apparently has an inhibitory influence, while the brainstem has a facilitatory influence[2,5]. In the central nervous system, the parietal lobes and thalamus receive detrusor afferent stimuli; while the frontal lobes inhibit voiding, the pontine center coordinates these stimuli into the appropriate social act of voiding. Further, voluntary contraction of the pelvic floor musculature can also overcome the parasympathetic tone. When bladder

Table 1 Requirements for continence. From reference 12

Environment
Availability of toilet/urinals
Absence of iatrogenic barriers (e.g. restraints)

Mentation and function
Intact cognition: recognize needs for toileting
Motivation to remain dry
Mobility to reach the toilet

Bladder storage
Accommodate adequate volume at a low pressure
Normal detrusor function
Intact internal and external sphincter function

Bladder emptying
Effective detrusor contraction
Lack of obstruction
Co-ordinated relaxation of sphincters

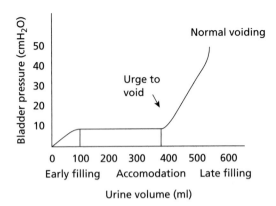

Figure 2 Bladder volume–pressure relationships

volume has reached capacity and circumstances are favorable, micturition occurs by a decrease in the sympathetic and somatic tone, along with a concomitant rise in parasympathetic tone carrying cholinergically mediated impulses to enable bladder contraction (Figure 1 and Table 1[12]). Disruption of the above pathways by any mechanism including medications and disease can result in incontinence[13].

Normal bladder capacity varies among individuals and ranges from 300 to 600 ml. See Figure 2 for bladder pressure–volume relationships. As the bladder fills there is little change in pressure: parasympathetic pathways are inhibited and the bladder remains relaxed. Stimulation of the sympathetic pathways keeps the internal sphincter closed. With normal bladder function, filling occurs at a pressure of 15 cm H_2O or less[2]. The first urge to void occurs at a bladder volume of 150–350 ml; subsequently the pressure rises with increasing urinary volume, and contractions occur[2,5]. Once the bladder is distended, cortical inhibitory control is withdrawn and parasympathetic-mediated contraction along with simultaneous sphincter relaxation lead to voiding. When urination is initiated, bladder pressure overcomes urethral resistance, resulting in micturition. In any case, if this

happens when it is not desired, the result is incontinence. For example, increase in intra-abdominal pressure due to sneezing or coughing may exceed urethral resistance and result in urinary leakage. The above is a simplified description of a complex process, the details of which are still not absolutely clear.

Normally the post-void bladder volume is only a few milliliters. It is measured either by bladder catheterization after micturition, or preferably by ultrasound. A volume above 200 ml is abnormal. Intermediate volumes of 50–200 ml need individualized evaluation[2,13].

AGING AND THE URINARY TRACT

UI is not a normal consequence of the aging process; age-related changes, however, may predispose to incontinence. Aging is associated with a decline in bladder capacity, an increase in involuntary bladder contractions, lower vesical volumes, but higher residual urine volume[14]. Widespread detrusor muscle degradation may be seen on muscle biopsy. The normal urine flow rate is 10–12 ml/second or more. In men an enlarged prostate is a common cause of decreased urine flow rate and nocturia. In women a decline in urethral and bladder outlet resistance is often attributed to lack of estrogen and/or prior injury to the pelvic floor sustained during childbirth, even decades earlier. Estrogen deprivation can cause atrophic vaginitis and

Table 2 Acute (transient) incontinence

Cognition or mood abnormalities
Delirium
Depression

Physical limitations
Restraints
Impaired mobility

Drug adverse effects
See Table 3

Excessive urine production
Excess fluid intake (e.g. water, beer, coffee, etc.)
Volume overload (e.g. congestive heart failure, edema)
Renal insufficiency
Hypokalemia
Hypercalcemia

Endocrine causes
Hyperglycemia
Hypercalcemia
Diabetes insipidus

Miscellaneous
Urinary tract infection
Stool impaction
Atrophic vaginitis

Table 3 Drug adverse effects causing urinary incontinence

Drug class	Example
Diuretics	furosemide
Sedative hypnotics	diazepam
Anticholinergics	diphenhydramine
Antidepressants	amitriptyline
Antipsychotics	haloperidol
Narcotic analgesics	morphine
α-Adrenergic blockers	terazosin
α-Adrenergic agonists	pseudoephedrine
Calcium channel blockers	nifedipine
Caffeine	coffee
Alcohol	beer

List not complete; represents select examples for illustration purpose

urethritis, predisposing to loss of mucosal coaptation, diminished urethral resistance and incontinence. It is now established that the urethra is estrogen sensitive and carries receptors for estrogen[15]. Urethral components such as mucosa, connective tissue, vascularity and smooth muscle cells are influenced by estrogen[15].

With age the ability of the kidneys to handle salt and water is impaired[16]. Altered hormonal status exists with antidiuretic hormone and atrial natriuretic peptide, resulting in inappropriate or untimely delivery of urine to an already compromised bladder. Nocturia and polyuria may result.

DEFINITIONS AND CLASSIFICATION

UI may be defined as the involuntary loss of urine in quantity or frequency sufficient to cause a social and/or hygienic problem[4]. Older adults who have bothersome symptoms such as urgency, frequency, nocturia and occasional unintentional urine loss, requiring lifestyle modification including social isolation and/or need for pads or liners, may not consider themselves incontinent. The health-care provider needs to recognize and identify such patients with the goal of improving the quality of life.

While several classifications are available, the simplest is a broad division into acute (transient) and chronic (persistent) incontinence. Chronic incontinence is further subdivided: urge, stress, overflow and functional incontinence. The subdivisions of chronic incontinence are not necessarily distinct entities, but may overlap or coexist (mixed incontinence). Each type of incontinence may arise from several causes.

Acute (transient) and reversible causes

Acute (transient) incontinence is of recent onset, is usually related to an acute illness or a medication, and subsides when the precipitating factors no longer exist[17]. The causes are listed in Tables 2 and 3. Thus, in acute incontinence a search for an etiology is indicated and treatment is focused on treating the causes. For example, disimpaction for fecal impaction, antibiotics for urinary tract infection, estrogen cream for atrophic vaginitis, and the treatment of hyperglycemia,

Table 4   Chronic (persistent) incontinence

Stress incontinence
Pelvic floor weakness (e.g. prolapse, cystocele)
Internal sphincter weakness

Urge incontinence
Detrusor hyperrefelxia (neurological causes)
　　cerebrovascular accident
　　Alzheimer's disease
　　parkinsonism
　　multiple sclerosis
　　cervical myelopathy
　　detrusor–sphincter dysynergia
Detrusor instability (non-neurological causes)
　　bladder stones
　　foreign body in bladder
　　vesical neoplasm
　　urethral diverticula
　　enlarged prostate
　　infection
　　radiation injury
　　drugs (e.g. cyclophosphamide)

Overflow incontinence
Outlet obstruction (eg.: enlarged prostate, stricture, gynecologic causes)
Abnormal bladder contractility (eg. diabetes mellitus, spinal cord injury)

Functional incontinence
Advanced dementia
Immobility
Depression

Mixed incontinence
A combination of above, commonly stress/urge

Table 5   Diagnostic evaluation for urinary incontinence

History and physical examination
History from both patient and caregiver
Voiding diary
Review of medications (current, past, prescribed and over the counter)
Prior surgery history
Special attention to neurologic and genitourinary systems

Tests
Urine analysis with microscopy
Post-void residual estimation (sonographic or straight catheter)
Blood chemistries
Complete blood count

Special tests when indicated
Urine culture
Renal, bladder and prostate ultrasound
Stress test/cough test
Urodynamics (simple or complex cystometry)

Referral to specialist when indicated
Urology
Gynecology
Neurology

hypercalcemia and delirium will all lead to resolution[2,17]. Urinary catheter use should be minimized. The use of reusable or disposable adult diapers, pads or liners is not ideal, but preferable to catheter use.

Chronic (persistent) incontinence

This exists when acute and reversible causes have been treated or ruled out and incontinence still persists (see Table 4 for causes). Established incontinence should be evaluated with a detailed history, physical examination, urinalysis and post-void residual determination (Table 5). This evaluation will suffice for most types of incontinence, and meet the following objectives:

(1) Identification of reversibility;

(2) Need for further diagnostic testing;

(3) Need for referral to specialist (e.g. urologist);

(4) Development of a management plan.

The types of chronic (persistent) incontinence include urge, stress, overflow, mixed and functional incontinence.

Urge incontinence

This is the most common form of incontinence in adults over the age of 75 years. It is also known as an 'overactive bladder', and is usually caused by abnormal detrusor contractions. It is characterized by an abrupt and strong desire to void[18]. The feeling is sudden, with several known precipitating factors, including, among others, the sound of rushing water (e.g. flushing a toilet or opening a tap), stroking the inner thighs or even the thought of voiding. Voiding may occur before reaching the bathroom. The bladder escapes normal cerebral inhibition and contracts despite contrary wishes. The disorder 'detrusor hyperactivity with impaired contractility' (DHIC) is self-explanatory: it denotes an excessively active detrusor but with weak and ineffective contractions, resulting in incomplete bladder emptying and increased residual volume[2]. Detrusor overactivity can be detrusor hyperreflexia (resulting from neurologic disease), detrusor instability (resulting from non-neurologic causes), and detrusor sphincter dyssynergia (lack of co-ordination between detrusor and external sphincter, usually associated with spinal cord disease)[5] (see Table 4 for causes).

Stress incontinence

This is the most common cause of incontinence in women below the age of 75. It is characterized by loss of urine as a result of the sudden increase in intra-abdominal pressure associated with activities such as coughing, sneezing, laughing or lifting weights[18]. Stress incontinence occurs when intravesical pressure (intra-abdominal pressure is a part of intravesical pressure) exceeds urethral resistance. The conditions that predispose to stress incontinence include pregnancy, vaginal delivery, trauma due to gynecologic or urologic surgery, chronic cough and estrogen deficiency. The amount of urine loss may vary and can occur with change in body position or routine activities. Although uncommon in men, it can occur following prostate surgery or radiation injury[5].

Overflow incontinence

This is the most common form of incontinence in older men; it occurs when the bladder cannot empty normally as a result of obstruction or a neurogenic bladder[18]. Distension of the bladder results, with subsequent loss of urine through overflow. It is often difficult to differentiate from stress and urge incontinence by history. Symptoms vary and include urgency, frequency, hesitancy, nocturia, dribbling, a feeling of incomplete voiding and narrowing of the urinary stream[18]. It is commonly associated with diabetes mellitus, spinal cord trauma, prostate hyperplasia or malignancy, urethral stricture, uterine prolapse, cystocele or rectocele[2,5].

Mixed incontinence

Symptoms of both urge and stress incontinence may be present in mixed incontinence, although other forms can coexist[18]. In mixed incontinence both detrusor overactivity and an incompetent internal sphincter are present. When there is doubt, urodynamic testing may help differentiate the predominant pathology[17].

Functional incontinence

This condition presents with a normal lower urinary tract and normal control mechanisms, but external conditions or cognitive impairment may lead to incontinence. Recognizing the barriers to continence is imperative. For example, use of restraints, pain, impaired mobility, lack of toilet access or presence of dementia can lead to incontinence. Still, it should be kept in mind that, in older adults, the lower urinary tract may not be completely intact, and its ability to compensate for and to withstand stress may be diminished.

EVALUATION

UI is often underreported by the patient and is frequently not adequately evaluated by the health-care provider[19]. Incontinence may be perceived differently by each individual. As revealed by a large national survey of community dwellers, many older adults believed that incontinence is a problem of 'old age' and that the doctor or nurse would be of no help at all in alleviating the problem[20,21]. The situation is worse in many nursing homes,

Table 6   Relevant terminology

Urgency
Intense desire to void, with or without urine loss

Precipitancy
Abrupt sensation of imminent urination, with or without urine loss

Frequency
More than seven diurnal voidings

Nocturia
Two or more nocturnal voidings

Hesitancy
Delay in initiation of micturition

Polyuria
Excessive 24 h urine production

Dysuria
Painful urination, urethral location

Intermittency
Involuntary interruption of the urinary stream

Post-void dribbling
Post-micturition involuntary release of urine

Strangury
Pain of trigonal origin, occurring post-micturition

as physicians visiting such institutions provide 'superficial care', and management is provided by nurse's aides who have limited training[22].

History

It is important that the history of UI be elicited, as the patient typically shies away from the problem. Inquiries about incontinence should be routinely made even in unsuspected cases. Questions should be open-ended to enable better patient self-expression[23]. Typical questions would include: 'do you have any trouble with urination?' or 'do you have any trouble with the bladder or holding urine?' If the patient responds with a 'no', follow-up with questions such as 'did you ever lose control of urine, at any time, even in a small quantity?' or 'do you ever wear a protective pad or undergarment when you go out?'[23]. It is important that the patient understands the questions; privacy should be respected. Similar

questions may be indicated on follow-up visits. The smell of urine may sometimes prompt a discussion. It is equally important to assure the patient that incontinence is a common problem and is treatable. If the patient is demented and has no insight, the caregiver may be interrogated for help. The word 'accident' may be best avoided, as it may connote a 'terrible' problem.

The physician's approach should vary based on the acuity and reversibility of the event. Information should include the duration and characteristics of incontinence such as whether urine loss occurs with coughing, laughing and sneezing, or a failed attempt to reach the rest room in time[24]. The amount of urine loss, the number of incontinent episodes, urinary frequency during day and night, nocturia and associated symptoms suggestive of infection such as fever, burning and pain during micturition are important. Current medical problems, medication review, including prescription and over-the-counter medications, both current and past, deserve importance as adverse drug reactions and polypharmacy resulting in UI are common in older adults[25]. The history should include questions about urgency, frequency, nocturia, polyuria, dysuria and hesitancy (Table 6). Any symptoms such as voiding difficulty, a weak or thin urinary stream, difficulty in initiating micturition and straining to void must be elicited. Predisposing conditions such as pelvic or lower abdominal surgery, childbirth, trauma, or chronic lung disease with or without cough must be identified. A voiding diary along with a record of fluid intake is helpful in characterizing the incontinence and in monitoring progress. The use of protective pads or liners or other similar remedies should be noted.

Physical examination

The physical examination should focus on genital, rectal, abdominal and relevant sensory evaluation, focused neurologic, cardiovascular and respiratory system assessment, particularly for evidence of cerebral or spinal cord disease, e.g. prior cerebrovascular accident, Parkinson's disease, dementia, multiple sclerosis, normal pressure hydrocephalus and spinal cord involvement. Supraspinal neurologic lesions have a lower risk of urologic complications than spinal cord lesions[26]. An assessment of mobility, mental status and cognitive function is essential, as is the estimation of patient motivation and desire to regain continence. Therapy for UI may not be effective in the presence of profound depression, unless the depression is also addressed and treated. Women should have a pelvic examination to exclude uterine prolapse, rectocele, cystocele or atrophic vaginitis. Abdominal examination as well as rectal examination should be performed to test rectal sensation, evaluate prostate size and exclude fecal impaction[23]. The perianal area should be checked for sensation; mild stroking will elicit contraction of the anal sphincter, the 'anal wink reflex' (S4–5). Bulbocavernosus reflexes test the integrity of S4–5. Absence usually denotes injury to the involved nerve roots; however, in older adults this is not necessarily pathologic[27]. A provocative stress test/cough test to detect stress incontinence can be performed in an office setting by asking the patient to cough in a standing position with a full bladder. If urine loss is observed, the test is positive and correlates with stress incontinence[13].

Investigations

Urinalysis should be performed on a clean-catch urine or a clean-catheterized urine specimen, the latter in frail older adults when it is difficult to get a good specimen[28]; seek evidence of infection, hematuria and glycosuria. The presence of hematuria warrants investigation to exclude neoplasia.

A post-void residual (PVR) urine volume determination can be achieved by the use of ultrasound or by catheterization. Effort must be made to obtain the PVR as soon as voiding is complete, as urinary flow into the bladder is continuous. A PVR volume of 50 ml or less is considered normal and over 200 ml is considered abnormal[2,5]. Values in between must be interpreted with care, and require clinical assessment. In practice, volume estimates in the same patient are inconsistent, because several variables determine the eventual volume. An imaging study of the urologic system, such as a sonogram (or a CAT scan) should be considered when the residual volume is high, in order to exclude hydronephrosis[2,5]. PVR volume determination is a helpful tool in management of UI as well, allowing estimation of efficacy of the treatment regimen.

It is essential to be aware that several common medical conditions associated with UI need to be considered when deciding the choice of investigations. Examples include neurological disorders (cerebrovascular diseases, dementia, Parkinson's disease, delirium, spinal cord disorders, normal pressure hydrocephalus), metabolic/endocrine disorders (diabetes mellitus, hypercalcemia), nutritional causes (vitamin B12 deficiency), infections (herpes zoster, cystitis, neurosyphilis), cardiovascular disease (congestive heart failure), pulmonary disorders (cough), and psychiatric disorders (psychosis, alcoholism), among others[18].

In addition to measuring blood urea nitrogen, serum creatinine, serum electrolytes, basic chemistries and complete blood count, other tests may be requested, e.g. screening for diabetes mellitus, estimation of hypercalciuria and excluding renal failure when polyuria is present. Urodynamic evaluation may range from simple 'eyeball urodynamics' (simple cystometrics) to sophisticated (complex cystometrics: multichannel electrical, pressure, flow and video recordings). The latter study is relatively expensive, needs specialized equipment and trained personnel, demands time and is invasive[26]. Cystometry is a graphic representation of intravesical pressure as a function of bladder volume. It is

Table 7 Indications for referral to specialist

Hematuria without obvious explanation
Failure of medical treatment
Difficulty in catheterization
Suspected stricture or obstruction
Excessive post-void residual
Hydronephrosis
Prostate enlargement or suspected prostate cancer
Cystocele, rectocele, uterine prolapse
Recurrent urinary tract infections
Bladder stones
Recent surgery
Radiation injury
Diagnosis not apparent

useful in the evaluation or assessment of bladder function in the presence of urge incontinence or a neurogenic bladder[26]. A cystogram is the radiological visualization of the lower urinary tract during bladder filling, using water or carbon dioxide. If voiding is also studied, it is referred to as a voiding cystourethrogram[26]. Urine flow rate measurement may help in assessing bladder outlet obstruction or impaired detrusor contractility[26]. A peak flow rate of 12 ml or more per second without straining for voids of over 150 to 200 ml excludes obstruction as the basis[18]. Sphincter electromyography can give information on the integrity of innervation and the function of muscles, and in assessing the co-ordination between the detrusor and the external sphincter[13,26]. Even though these tests are precise and aid in diagnosis, they are generally not needed in the evaluation and management of incontinence. Specialist referral may be indicated when the diagnosis is doubtful or when pathology needs to be corrected in order to preserve function (Table 7).

MANAGEMENT

One should consider the patient as a whole, rather than targeting incontinence alone. Cure may rarely be possible, but comfort and satisfaction to the patient and caregiver can almost always be provided. The categories of treatments available are non-pharmacologic, pharmacologic and surgical. The patient should be made aware of all treatment options, and offered the least invasive, most effective regimen with the fewest side-effects. Most of the time a combination of behavior and pharmacologic treatments gives good results.

Non-pharmacologic treatment

Several behavioral interventions targeted at the patient and caregiver are helpful in the management of incontinence. Patient-dependent interventions require intact cognition, motivation and mobility; caregiver-dependent interventions also demand motivation. Non-pharmacologic treatments include pelvic muscle exercises, biofeedback, bladder training, scheduled toileting, prompted voiding, habit training and behavior strategies. Maintaining a bladder diary helps determine the success or failure of a given regimen.

Pelvic muscle (Kegel) exercises

This is a popular technique used for stress incontinence, but it is also useful in urge and mixed stress–urge incontinence. Kegel exercises are frequently not well understood and are inappropriately practiced by the patient, due to a lack of knowledge on the part of the health-care provider. In 1940 Kegel rediscovered the technique with an initial goal of restoring perineal muscle strength after childbirth[29]. The technique involves repetitive contractions of the pelvic floor musculature. The exercise can be taught by asking the patient to initiate micturition and to interrupt the urine flow initially while sitting on the toilet; subsequently the process may be simulated in settings outside the bathroom. In women the exercise may be taught by asking the patient to squeeze the examiner's finger during vaginal examination. It is important that the correct technique is practiced and reinforced to ensure that the appropriate muscles are contracted. Each contraction is held while counting to three and then relaxed while counting to the same number. The patient should work up to 10–15 repeats for each exercise, up to thrice daily. Results are noticed only after several weeks. Once learnt, the exercise can be performed several times a day while standing, sitting or lying down, preferably using all three positions daily for best results. The exercise increases urethral resistance by augmenting periurethral muscle tone and inhibiting reflex bladder contractions[29]. Kegel exercises are an effective modality and benefits are enhanced when they are combined with biofeedback[30].

Biofeedback, not a treatment by itself, is a semi-invasive procedure, using auditory and/or visual feedback to the patient on the use of pelvic floor musculature[30]. Vaginal and rectal pressure probes and electromyography are used to train and provide feedback to the patient regarding muscle contractions[30]. Although useful, it is expensive, and is not always available, neither is it required, although it may be useful in individual cases. Electrical stimulation and vaginal cones have also been used for this purpose.

Bladder training

Intact cognition, co-operation and compliance are essential components of this approach. The patient is encouraged to follow an expanding voiding schedule. One is trained to void following a clock schedule, rather than the subjective urge to void. An initial interval of 2 h between voidings is gradually increased on a weekly basis to 3 h or more over 1–2 months. This technique is especially useful for urge incontinence[2,5]. Bladder training can also be combined with pelvic muscle exercise.

Bladder retraining is also of help following temporary indwelling catheterization for an acute illness[2]. Catheters must always be removed as soon as circumstances permit. A voiding schedule is initiated upon awakening: every 2 h during the day and then every 4 h after going to bed. A voiding diary is kept and PVR measurements are recorded to monitor the progress. If incontinence persists following catheter removal, it must be further investigated to find and treat the causes. Motivated and trained staff or caregivers are essential components for success[31].

Scheduled toileting, habit training, and prompted voiding

These techniques are useful in cognitively impaired individuals who are unable to co-operate and are not adequately motivated. The aim is preventing incontinence, rather than at attempting to achieve continence. As they are caregiver dependent, motivation and commitment on the part of the caregiver are essential.

Scheduled toileting consists of directing the patient to the toilet and encouraging voiding at regular intervals, irrespective of the expressed desire of the patient[2]. This is enforced at 2-hourly intervals during the day and at 4-hourly intervals at night. Habit training is scheduled toileting which has been modified to coincide with the patient's incontinent episodes. The schedule is adjusted to patient habits, such as eating and drinking[28]. For example, the patient is encouraged to void following meals or consumption of liquids.

Prompted voiding involves focusing the patient's attention on the bladder, and asking the patient to void every few hours; if appropriate, social reinforcement of the behavior and a reward for remaining dry are offered[2]. Prompted voiding appears successful for daytime incontinence, particularly in long-term care facilities. Nursing staff can reduce the severity of incontinence in about 75% of patients; adequate staffing is required and may prove cost effective[32].

Behavior strategies

Used in conjunction with other techniques, these strategies are useful and effective.

Table 8   Pharmacotherapy of urinary incontinence (UI)

Drug and dosage	Action	Indication	Contraindication	Adverse effects/ disadvantages
Oxybutynin Ditropan IR 2.5–5 mg bid or tid Ditropan XL 5–30 mg/day	anti-cholinergic	urge, mixed, with urge predominant	overflow or obstructive UI, glaucoma, unstable cardiac status	xerostomia, blurred vision, constipation, delirium, urinary retention
Tolterodine Detrol IR 1–2 mg bid Detrol LA 2–4 mg/day	anti-cholinergic	urge, mixed, with urge predominant	overflow or obstructive UI and glaucoma. Interacts with CYP 3A4. Decrease dose with erythromycin, ketoconazole, etc. and hepatic/renal insufficiency	xerostomia, blurred vision, constipation, delirium, urinary retention
Imipramine (Tofranil) 25 mg tid, max 150 mg/day	anti-cholinergic and α-adrenergic agonist	stress, mixed urge and stress	overflow or obstructive UI, recent MI, cardiac comorbidity	postural hypotension, cardiac conduction defects, xerostomia, blurred vision, constipation, delirium, urinary retention
Pseudoephedrine (Sudafed) 30 mg tid max 180 mg/day	α-adrenergic agonist	stress	overflow or obstructive UI	headache, tachycardia, hypertension
Terazosin (Hytrin) 1–5 mg qhs Doxazosin (Cardura) 1–4 mg qhs Prazosin (Minipress) 1–2 mg tid	post synaptic α-adrenergic antagonist	outflow obstruction from BPH	stress incontinence	dizziness, drowsiness, light headedness, syncope, postural hypotension
Tamsulosin (Flomax) 0.4–0.8 mg qd	selective α_1-adrenergic antagonist	outflow obstruction from BPH	stress incontinence	less postural hypotension than other α-adrenergic antagonists
Finasteride (Proscar) 5 mg qd	5 α-reductase inhibitor	outflow obstruction from BPH	caution with hepatic insufficiency	obtain baseline PSA, decreases PSA by 50% in both BPH and CA. 6–12 months needed to see benefit
Estrogens oral/topical/ vaginal ring	increases periurethral blood flow, mucosal coaptation	stress, urge UI associated with atrophic vaginitis	pregnancy, endometrial and breast cancer	DVT/PE, gall bladder disease, malignancy of breast and uterus
Bethanecol (Urecholine) 10–50 mg po tid–qid or 2.5–5 mg sc tid–qid	cholinergic	overflow incontinence with atonic bladder, in absence of outflow obstruction	outlet obstruction	drowsiness, fainting, bradycardia, hypotension, diarrhea, bronchospasm

After any drug is initiated or added, follow for changes in incontinence pattern and adverse events. BPH, benign prostatic hyperplasia; CYP, cytochrome P450; MI, myocardial infarction; PSA, prostate-specific antigen; CA, cancer; DVT/PE, deep vein thrombosis/pulmonary embolism

Compliance is the key to success[28]. The following is an example of a behavioral strategy used for urge incontinence. When the patient has the urge to void, ask the patient to control the urge and relax. Attempt to shift the mind's focus from the bladder to a distraction, for example TV, music or conversation, and have the patient contract the pelvic floor muscles a few times. When the urge resolves, the patient should slowly go to the bathroom and void. A behavioral strategy for nocturia and night-time incontinence includes an early dinner with fluid restriction after dinner. Eliminate coffee, colas and alcohol in the evening. Leg elevation with the administration of diuretics in the early afternoon will provide post-diuretic volume contraction that decreases urine formation at night. Ensure that voiding occurs prior to going to bed[28]. Lack of adverse effects, low cost and safety of behavioral interventions make them a first-line treatment. Although the techniques are promising, conclusive data based on studies are lacking[33].

Pharmacologic management

Several drugs now available are useful either alone or in combination with behavioral interventions; they are especially effective in the management of urge and stress incontinence (Table 8).

Anticholinergic agents

The most important stimulus for bladder contraction is acetylcholine-induced stimulation of postganglionic parasympathetic receptors in the detrusor[34]. Atropine or atropine-like substances are known to diminish bladder contractions of any cause. Partial inhibition of detrusor activity results in a significant decline in involuntary contractions and consequent improvement in symptomatology[34]. An increase in bladder volume and maximal bladder capacity also results[35]. It is also possible that inhibiting drugs can increase residual urine volume or cause urinary retention[35]. It is conceivable that the use of anticholinergic agents might result in impaired cognition or in diminishing effects of cholinergic drugs (e.g. donepezil and rivastigmine, used in Alzheimer's disease). Data on this kind of drug–drug or drug–disease interaction are presently lacking. Contraindications to the use of anticholinergic agents include narrow-angle glaucoma and unstable cardiovascular disease. Adverse effects include constipation, urinary retention, delirium and dry mouth (xerostomia)[36]. The last symptom is the most common basis for discontinuing therapy.

Oxybutinin chloride (Ditropan®) A popular drug that has stood the test of time, this is a tertiary amine with anticholinergic, smooth muscle relaxant and local anesthetic activity. Oxybutinin reduces frequency, nocturia and incontinence[36]. Side-effects are clearly greater with the short-acting (immediate release) preparations, and are largely minimized by the long-acting (extended release) preparations. The most common side-effects include blurring of vision, xerostomia, dry skin, nausea, constipation and impaired cognition[35]. The usual dosage is 2.5–5 mg two to four times a day. A liquid formulation is available. Extended release formulations are administered in a dose of 5–30 mg once a day[18].

Tolterodine tartrate (Detrol®) This is a new tertiary amine, comparable in efficacy to oxybutinin, with similar adverse effects. It improves symptoms of urgency, frequency and detrusor overactivity. An increase in bladder capacity is observed[35]. Xerostomia is again the most predominant adverse effect leading to discontinuation of therapy. Available in short-acting preparations with the dose 1–2 mg twice daily; for long-acting preparations the dose is 2–4 mg daily[18]. The latter is associated with fewer adverse effects.

Imipramine (Tofranil®) This is a tertiary amine, tricyclic antidepressant used in the treatment of UI[34]. It has anticholinergic and α-adrenergic agonistic properties, in addition to central nervous system and direct muscle relaxant properties[34]. Imipramine diminishes detrusor hyperactivity and increases bladder outlet resistance[35]. Theoretically, it is effective for stress, urge and mixed incontinence. Adverse effects are common and include xerostomia, nausea, constipation, insomnia and agitation. Cardiac arrythmias and central nervous system effects such as confusion are encountered more often in older adults[34]. Other tricyclics in this class include desipramine, doxepin and nortriptyline.

α-Adrenergic agonists

These drugs are used for stress incontinence, because they increase the smooth muscle tone of the bladder neck and urethra, where there is a predominance of α-adrenergic receptors[34]. Examples include phenylpropanolamine and pseudoephedrine; while they cause improvement in symptomatology, adverse effects relate to cardiovascular and cerebrovascular morbidity[35]. The Food and Drug Administration (FDA) has recommended voluntary withdrawal of phenylpropanolamine (PPA).

α-Adrenergic antagonists

These drugs decrease urethral resistance and relax the smooth muscle cells of the internal sphincter by postsynaptic α_1 blockade[36]. α_1-Blockers are useful in the presence of obstruction caused by benign prostatic hyperplasia (BPH). Drugs available in this class include doxazosin, terazosin and prazosin; they serve as antihypertensives in addition to playing a beneficial role at the bladder neck. Adverse effects include orthostatic hypotension, syncope and dizziness. Tamsulosin, in the same class, is an exception, in that it is claimed to be free of antihypertensive properties[36].

Estrogens

These maintain mucosal coaptation and urethral integrity, and increase the sensitivity of α-adrenergic receptors of the bladder neck and urethra[34]. With estrogen use, statistically significant improvement has been observed in combined urge and stress incontinence. The combination of an estrogen and an α-adrenergic agonist produces synergy[35]. Adverse effects include postmenopausal bleeding, sodium and water retention, thromboembolism, malignancy and cardiac events.

Antiandrogens

Finasteride, a 5α-reductase inhibitor, decreases prostate size and may cause improvement in prostatic obstruction-related overflow incontinence[36]. Adverse effects include impotence, diminished libido and gynecomastia. A baseline prostate-specific antigen (PSA) level prior to starting therapy, should be obtained, as PSA levels decline with the use of finasteride. The maximum drug effect takes time[36].

Cholinergics

Although cholinergic agents have been advocated in the treatment of overflow incontinence from detrusor underactivity (e.g. diabetic neurogenic bladder), they are generally ineffective and their use results in unacceptable side-effects (e.g. diarrhea)[36]. The prototype drug is bethanechol.

Role of surgery

Surgery is considered when medical management fails and symptoms are bothersome. Disadvantages include cost, development of new symptoms and/or failure to meet expectations. Urodynamic and other studies are essential and should confirm the diagnosis prior to surgery. Surgical decisions are individualized based on co-morbidity, life expectancy and quality of life. The following are some commonly performed procedures[37,38].

Retropubic suspensions

Known as Marshall–Marchetti–Krantz or Bruch procedures, sutures are placed in the pubocervical fascia around the urethra and urethrovesical junction, and secured to structures in the bony pelvis. They can be performed by a laparoscopic approach, and are used in stress incontinence[37].

Sling procedure

This is the preferred procedure for women with stress incontinence with intrinsic sphincter deficiency and hypermobility. Artificial material or a tissue flap is placed at the bladder neck and attached to rectus fascia above the level of the pubic bone. The procedure provides support to the bladder and prevents descent of the urethrovesical junction following a rise in intra-abdominal pressure[38].

Needle suspensions

Known as Peyrera, Raz, Stamey and Gittes procedures, sutures are placed on either side of the urethrovesical junction and anchored to the rectus abdominus fascia. They are less extensive, and use a combined transabdominal and transvaginal approach[37].

Artificial sphincters

Artificial sphincters are mechanical cuffs placed around the urethrovesical junction, and self inflated or deflated to restore continence. They are preferred for male incontinence. The complication rate is high[37,38].

Collagen injections

Periurethral collagen injections have been tried with limited success in women with intrinsic urethral weakness, but repeated injections are needed. The procedure is performed under local anesthesia and involves injection of collagen into the bladder neck just below the urothelium[38,39].

Nerve stimulation therapy

Nerve stimulation is used for urge incontinence and works as a pacemaker for the bladder. The technique stimulates nerves that modulate voiding. A temporary external device is used to test for efficacy before permanent implantation[38].

Prostate surgery

In men, surgery is typically indicated for outflow obstruction due to prostate enlargement, urinary retention with or without evidence of hydronephrosis, or recurrent infections. Popular surgical procedures include transurethral resection, transurethral incision and simple prostatectomy.

Incontinence garments

These take the form of absorbent liners, pads or shields and are also referred to as adult diapers; sometimes these are improvised at home using tissue paper. Although commonly used and misunderstood as the solution, they are not truly a treatment for incontinence[40]. While they are not first-line measures, they help maintain dignity and comfort, and protect clothing, bedding and floors[40]. Absorbent garments can be disposable or washable and are composed of cotton or synthetic/semisynthetic absorbent fibers or cellulose gel. Allergies, skin irritation and adverse events may be anticipated accordingly. Nevertheless, they should be used in conjunction with other treatment modalities. Additionally, absorbent pads incur cost over time and involve social, hygienic and disposal concerns.

Diapers are commonly overutilized in nursing homes with little attempt to evaluate the UI in the first place. While diapers protect against leakage and provide staff more control with time, they also entail time to be checked and changed. Although debatable, a recent study suggested that disposable diapers were cheaper than the cloth type, with better skin conditions associated with the former[41].

Catheters and catheter care

These are generally not the preferred choice in the long-term management of incontinence, as they do not cure. Sometimes, catheter use

Table 9 Urinary catheter care

Indwelling catheter
Closed system with gravity drainage
Change drainage system using clean, not necessarily
    sterile, technique
Anchor the hard tubing of the catheter to the thigh or
    abdomen with tape, to prevent trauma and fecal soiling
Do not use antibiotics routinely
Do not culture routinely
Treat only symptomatic infection
If recurrent infections occur, consider anatomical
    evaluation
If catheter obstruction occurs, consider increasing
    fluid intake
Avoid using antiseptics to clean catheter insertion site

Intermittent catheterization
Educate and train the patient or caregiver
Use clean, not necessarily sterile, technique

---

is unavoidable[42]. Catheters may be broadly classified as external catheters (e.g. condom catheter), chronic indwelling catheters (e.g. Foley's catheter, suprapubic catheter) and intermittent straight catheters[42]. Appropriate indications for chronic catheterization are urinary retention that cannot be managed medically or surgically, the presence of non-healing pressure ulcers and skin wounds (in order to prevent soiling and to promote healing), and in terminally ill or severely impaired patients (in order to reduce discomfort and suffering). Patient and caregiver preferences influence decision making. Complications from catheter use include infection, local irritation and hematuria. The use of indwelling urethral catheters, even with meticulous hygiene, is associated with bacteriuria at a rate of 3–10% per day; at 1 month, bacteriuria is almost universal[42]. Asymptomatic bacteriuria associated with catheter use in the absence of evidence of infection seldom requires antimicrobial therapy; routine cultures and prophylactic antibiotics are not indicated in this setting[2]. Intermittent catheterization is safe and effective, and can be performed by a trained patient or caregiver 2–4 times daily; for this purpose the catheter should be clean but need not be sterile. It

appears that the incidence of bacteriuria with intermittent catheters is lower when compared to chronic indwelling catheters[42]. Routine catheter care is outlined in Table 9.

The decision to use catheters must be with the knowledge that their utility can result in disease; although there are numerous benefits, catheters are the dominant risk factor associated with hospital acquired urosepsis, the most common nosocomial infection in the US[43]. Catheters are widely and inappropriately used; between 16 and 25% of hospitalized patients in the US have an indwelling urinary catheter[43], partly from ignorance of published recommendations. Often physicians are unaware or forget about the presence of the urinary catheter[43]. Medical and nursing home staff need to be educated about the adverse effects and familiarized with the appropriate use of catheters and non-catheter strategies. Effective 'stop orders' and quality control audits for catheters are recommended[43]. Contrary to common opinions, the use of condom catheters (Texas catheters) in men, also places the resident at higher risk of infection[41].

INCONTINENCE IN THE LONG-TERM CARE SETTING

Management of incontinence in heterogenous nursing home residents is not easy, dealing with the burden of disease, economics and personnel constraints[44]. More than half the incontinent residents have dementia; mobility and functional impairments are additional features. A work-up is warranted in all residents to determine if UI is reversible and therefore treatable; management must be realistic, based on the resident's potential. Prompted voiding and scheduled toileting schedules are effective in reducing incontinence episodes even in the cognitively impaired[41,44]. As an adjunct, pharmacologic management is helpful with the use of bladder relaxants and tricyclic antidepressants, with combined therapy yielding even better results. Attention to bowel regimens to minimize constipation, instituting daily exercises (like walking), limiting use of caffeine to certain hours, ensuring availability of urinals, limiting use of restraints and medication adjustment are all helpful measures. The final choice of diagnostic and therapeutic interventions should be individualized[44]. Incontinence products such as diapers, pads, specialized beds and drainage systems represent a multibillion dollar business and are usually not reimbursable by insurance[45]. Indirect costs of incontinence in the nursing home relating to UI include comorbid conditions relating to incontinence (such as depression, skin breakdown, infections, falls, etc.), and are hard to estimate[45]. Proper completion of the Minimum Data Set (MDS) aids the nursing home staff to collect data for a resident care plan; incontinence is incorporated into the calculation of the Resource Utilization Group scores to help determine services for UI and reimbursement[45].

TREATMENT OF INCONTINENCE: SUMMARY

Treatments discussed in earlier sections are summarized below by type of incontinence.

Urge incontinence

Anticholinergic agents are the drugs of choice for urge incontinence. Oxybutynin and tolterodine are good choices, the development of side-effects being the main limitation. While the OBJECT (Overactive Bladder: Judging Effective Control and Treatment) study suggested that extended-release oxybutinin was more effective than tolterodine as seen from incontinence episodes, adverse events were similar with both drugs[46]. In another study, extended-release tolterodine was shown to be effective, safe and well tolerated for overactive bladder, irrespective of age[47]. Treatment of overactive bladder with once daily extended-release

tolterodine and oxybutinin in the ACET (Antimuscuranic Clinical Effectiveness Trial) study suggested that tolterodine was associated with greater efficacy and tolerability[48]. Overall, the two antimuscarinic, anticholinergic extended-release drugs appear effective. The principal anticholinergic side-effect of immediate-release oxybutinin is dry mouth, probably due to a metabolite; when dry mouth did occur with tolterodine, it was less intense than with oxybutinin. Tolterodine may be more selective, inhibiting the receptors in the bladder more than in the salivary glands[49]. Urinary retention may develop if outflow obstruction co-exists. Checking the post-void residual during therapy may be appropriate, especially if incontinence worsens after initial improvement or if hyperkalemia develops. Patients with Alzheimer's disease should be monitored for anticholinergic delirium. Other, less effective, agents include propantheline and calcium channel blockers. Estrogens may help in the presence of atrophic vaginitis. Trials are underway for the intravesical use of capsaicin and resiniferatoxin[50]. Capsaicin, the active ingredient in chili peppers, is a neurotoxin that inactivates afferent C fibers from the bladder. Its use is based on the fact that stimulation of these C fibers cause voiding[50]. Resiniferatoxin is a potent capsaicin-like substance. Non-pharmacologic measures should be combined with drug therapy.

Stress incontinence

Behavioral therapy with a focus on pelvic floor (Kegel) exercises should be the first step, and is effective in up to two-thirds of patients; several weeks are needed for benefits to be appreciated. α-Adrenergic agonists and estrogens are effective, the former via an increase in internal sphincter tone. These drugs are useful in mild-to-moderate stress incontinence, where there is no major anatomical problem with the urinary tract, and in the absence of contraindications (e.g. coronary artery disease, uncontrolled hypertension). Tricyclic antidepressants (e.g. imipramine, desipramine, nortriptyline) are helpful through a combination of anticholinergic effects on the bladder and α-adrenergic activity at the internal sphincter; their use is limited by anticholinergic side-effects and orthostasis. Drug therapy should be augmented by behavioral techniques. Estrogens in hormone replacement therapy doses have no effect on incontinence; however, they are effective when used in conjunction with α-adrenergic agonists[5]. Estrogens can be used locally in the form of vaginal cream or as rings.

Overflow incontinence

α-Adrenergic antagonists can be tried for bladder outlet obstruction from benign prostatic hyperplasia (e.g. terazosin, doxazosin, prazosin and tamsulosin). Intermittent catheterization is an option for acute retention and when drug therapy has failed. Surgical correction may be necessary for the enlarged prostate, urethral stricture or gynecologic disorders.

Mixed incontinence

Treatment is focused on the major or more bothersome component. A combination of drugs can be used. Imipramine is the single drug possessing both anticholinergic and α-adrenergic agonistic properties. Non-pharmacologic treatment must be part of the regimen.

Functional incontinence

One needs to focus on correcting the factors that limit the patient's ability to remain continent. For example, the release of restraints, the relief of pain or the provision of a bedside commode may solve the problem.

References

1. Brocklehurst JC. Urinary incontinence in old age: helping the general practitioner to make a diagnosis. *Gerontology* 1990;36:3–7

2. Kawas CH. Alzheimer's disease. In Hazzard WR, Blass JP, Ettinger WH Jr, Halter JB, Ouslander JG, eds. *Principles of Geriatric Medicine and Gerontology*, 4th edn. New York: McGraw-Hill, 1999:1595–614

3. Hu T-W. Impact of urinary incontinence on healthcare costs. *J Am Geriatr Soc* 1990;38: 292–5

4. Wyman JF, Harkins SW, Fantl JA. Psychosocial impact of urinary incontinence in the community-dwelling population. *J Am Geriatr Soc* 1990;38:282–8

5. Brandeis GH, Resnick NM. Urinary incontinence. In Duthie EH Jr, Katz PR, eds. *Practice of Geriatrics*, 3rd edn. Philadelphia: WB Saunders, 1998:189–98

6. Rowe JW, Besdine RW, Ford AB, *et al.* Urinary incontinence in adults. National Institutes of Health Consensus Development Conference. *J Am Geriatr Soc* 1990;38:265–72

7. Busby-Whitehead J, Johnson TM. Urinary incontinence. *Clin Geriatr Med* 1998;14: 285–96

8. Brocklehurst JC. Professional and public education about incontinence. The British experience. *J Am Geriatr Soc* 1990;38: 384–6

9. Koyama W, Koyanagi A, Mihara S. Prevalence and conditions of urinary incontinence among the elderly. *Meth Inform Med* 1998;37:151–5

10. Kuh D, Cardozo L, Hardy R. Urinary incontinence in middle aged women: childhood enuresis and other lifetime risk factors in a British prospective cohort. *J Epidemiol Community Health* 1999;53:453–8

11. Resnick NM, Ouslander JG. Urinary incontinence – where do we stand and where do we go from here? *J Am Geriatr Soc* 1990; 38:263–4

12. Williams ME, Gaylord SA. Role of functional assessment in the evaluation of urinary incontinence. *J Am Geriatr Soc* 1990;38:296–9

13. Diokno AC. Diagnostic categories of incontinence and the role of urodynamic testing. *J Am Geriatr Soc* 1990;38:300–5

14. Resnick NM. Initial evaluation of the incontinent patient. *J Am Geriatr Soc* 1990;38: 311–16

15. Cardozo L. Role of estrogens in the treatment of female urinary incontinence. *J Am Geriatr Soc* 1990;38:326–8

16. Dharmarajan TS, Ugalino JT. The aging process. In Dreger D, Krumm B, eds. *Hospital Physician Geriatric Medicine Board Review Manual*. Wayne, PA: Turner White Communications, 2000;1:1–12

17. Resnick NM. Voiding dysfunction and urinary incontinence. In Cassel CK, Riesenberg DE, Sorensen LB, Walsh JR, eds. *Geriatric Medicine*, 2nd edn. New York: Springer-Verlag, 1990:501–18

18. DuBeau CE. Urinary incontinence. *Clin Geriatr* 2001;9:31–47

19. Herzog AR, Fultz NH. Prevalence and incidence of urinary incontinence in community-dwelling populations. *J Am Geriatr Soc* 1990; 38:273–81

20. Jeter KF, Wagner DB. Incontinence in the American home. *J Am Geriatr Soc* 1990; 38:379–83

21. Mitteness LS. Knowledge and beliefs about urinary incontinence in adulthood and old age. *J Am Geriatr Soc* 1990;38:374–8

22. Ouslander JG. Urinary incontinence in nursing homes. *J Am Geriatr Soc* 1990; 38:281–91

23. McCormick KA, Diokno A, Colling J, *et al*. *Urinary Incontinence in Adults: Quick Reference Guide for Clinicians*. AHCPR Publication. No. 92-0041. Rockville, MD: Agency for Health Care Policy and Research, Public Health Services, US Department of Health and Human Services, 1992:232–59

24. Ouslander JG. Incontinence management in long-term care. *Ann Long-term Care* 2000;8:35–41

25. Dharmarajan TS, Tota R. Appropriate use of medications in older adults. *Family Practice Recertif* 2000,22:29–38

26. Blaivas JG. Diagnostic evaluation of incontinence in patients with neurologic disease. *J Am Geriatr Soc* 1990;38:306–10

27. Resnick NM. Noninvasive diagnosis of the patient with complex incontinence. *Gerontology* 1990;36:8–18

28. Ouslander JG, Schnelle JF. Incontinence in the nursing home. *Ann Intern Med* 1995; 122:438–48

29. Wells TJ. Pelvic (floor) muscle exercise. *J Am Geriatr Soc* 1990;38:333–7

30. Burns PA, Pranikoff K, Nochajski T, *et al*. Treatment of stress incontinence with pelvic floor exercises and biofeedback. *J Am Geriatr Soc* 1990;38:341–4

31. Engel BT, Burgio LD, McCormick KA, *et al*. Behavioral treatment of incontinence in the long-term care setting. *J Am Geriatr Soc* 1990;38:361–3

32. Schnelle JF. Treatment of urinary incontinence in nursing home patients by prompted voiding. *J Am Geriatr Soc* 1990; 38:356–60

33. Fantl JA, Wyman JF, Harkins SW, *et al*. Bladder training in the management of lower urinary tract dysfunction in women. *J Am Geriatr Soc* 1990;38:329–32

34. Wein AJ. Pharmacologic treatment of incontinence. *J Am Geriatr Soc* 1990;38: 317–25

35. Thuroff JW, Chartier-Kastler E, Corcus J, *et al*. Medical treatment and medical side effects in urinary incontinence in the elderly. *World J Urol* 1998;16:S48–61

36. Lackner TE. Pharmacologic management of urinary incontinence. *Ann long-term Care* 2000;8:29–37

37. Retzky SS, Rogers RM. Urinary incontinence in women. In Erdelyi-Brown M, Bean KJ, eds. *Clinical Symposia*. Summit, NJ: Ciba-Geigy, 1995;47:1–32

38. Butler RN, Maby JI, Montella JM, *et al*. Urinary incontinence: when to refer for procedural therapies. *Geriatrics* 1999;54: 49–56

39. Gulligan PJ, Heit M. Urinary incontinence in women: evaluation and management. *Am Family Physician* 2000;62:2433–44

40. Brink CA. Absorbent pads, garments, and management strategies. *J Am Geriatr Soc* 1990;38:368–73

41. Johnson T. Nonpharmacological treatments for urinary incontinence in long-term care

residents. *J Am Med Dir Assoc* 2002;3:(Suppl):S25–S30

42. Warren JW. Urine-collection devices for use in adults with urinary incontinence. *J Am Geriatr Soc* 1990;38:364–7

43. Saint S, Lipsky BA, Goold SD. Indwelling urinary catheters: a one-point restraint? *Ann Intern Med* 2002;137:125–7

44. Tannenbaum C, Lepage C. Practical management of urinary incontinence in the long-term care setting. *Ann Long Term Care: Clin Care Aging* 2002;10:26–34

45. Prochoda KP. Medical director's review of urinary incontinence in long-term care. *J Am Med Dir Assoc* 2002;3:(Suppl)S11–S15

46. Appell RA, Sand P, Dmochowski R, *et al.* Prospective randomized controlled trial of extended-release oxybutinin chloride and tolterodine tartarate in the treatment of overactive bladder: results of the OBJECT study. *Mayo Clinic Proc* 2001;76:358–63

47. Zinner NR, Mattiasson A, Stanton SL. Efficacy, safety and tolerability of extended-release once daily tolterodine treatment for overactive bladder in older versus younger patients. *J Am Geriatr Soc* 2002;50:799-807

48. Sussman D, Garely A. Treatment of overactive bladder with once-daily extended-release tolterodine or oxybutinin: the Antimuscarinic Clinical Effectiveness Trial (ACET). *Curr Med Res Opin* 2002;18:177–84

49. Appell RA. The newer antimuscaranic drugs: bladder control with less dry mouth. *Cleveland Clin J Med* 2002;69:761–9

50. Elliot DS, Lightner DJ, Blute ML, *et al.* Medical management of overactive bladder. *Mayo Clin Proc* 2001;76:353–5

26 Osteoporosis and osteomalacia

T.S. Dharmarajan, MD, FACP, AGSF, and Joey T. Ugalino, MD

INTRODUCTION

Of the musculoskeletal disorders in older adults, osteoporosis and osteomalacia are particularly common, and are associated with enormous morbidity from complications. Importantly, the primary health-care provider can play a significant role in the prevention and treatment of these disorders.

BONE PHYSIOLOGY AND AGING

The bone is a dynamic unit, undergoing changes throughout life. At the cellular level, bone remodeling occurs in discrete microscopic loci called basic multicellular units[1] or bone-remodeling units[2]. The greater the number of units, the faster the rate of remodeling.

During bone remodeling, each unit undergoes a four-phase cycle (initiation, resorption, reversal and formation). In the initiation phase, cells that line inactive bone are altered by local or systemic factors. During resorption, these lining cells are replaced by osteoclasts that specialize in removing bone and creating cavities or lacunae on the bone surface. A short period of reversal ensues, followed by the formation phase during which specialized cells or osteoblasts fill the cavity with unmineralized bone (osteoid). The duration of each cycle is approximately 200 days; bone resorption and formation take approximately 3 and 21 weeks, respectively, to complete[1].

Bone has two components: organic and inorganic. Organic bone, also referred to as osteoid, is a matrix of collagenous (mostly type I) and non-collagenous proteins produced by osteoblasts. Inorganic bone contains the mineral hydroxyapatite, derived from calcium phosphate deposited on osteoid during the process of mineralization[3].

Bones may be cortical (compact) or trabecular (cancellous). Cortical bone comprises the cortex of most bones and the outer layer of long bones, and accounts for 75% of the skeletal mass. Trabecular bone is located in the central bone and is composed of a honeycomb-like lattice of intersecting bone plates; it is highly metabolic, has increased turnover rates and has greater susceptibility to fracture[4].

Bone remodeling and mineralization are affected by several regulators, mainly parathyroid hormone (PTH), vitamin D, calcitonin and sex hormones. PTH, secreted by the parathyroid glands, increases osteoclastic activity, reabsorption of urine calcium and renal conversion of inactive vitamin D to the active metabolite. Vitamin D enhances intestinal calcium and phosphorus absorption[5]. Together, PTH and vitamin D act synergistically to maintain serum calcium concentration at the expense of bone resorption. Calcitonin, from the parafollicular cells of the thyroid, inhibits bone resorption by a direct effect on osteoclasts. Estrogen

Table 1   A comparison of osteoporosis and osteomalacia. From reference 6

	Osteoporosis	Osteomalacia
Age of onset	older adults	children and older adults
Etiology	estrogen deficiency, age-related changes, secondary causes	deficiency of vitamin D, calcium, or phosphorus
Pathology	preserved mineral-to-matrix ratio	decreased mineral-to-matrix ratio
Bone volume	decreased	normal or slightly decreased
Clinical presentation	asymptomatic, bony pain, fractures, kyphosis	proximal muscle weakness and tenderness, bony pain, fractures
Diagnostic evaluation		
calcium and phosphorus	normal	normal or decreased
alkaline phosphatase	normal	normal or increased
25-hydroxyvitamin D assay	normal	low
radiology	osteopenia, fracture	osteopenia, fracture
bone densitometry	BMD at 2.5 SD below mean for young adults	variable
Definitive diagnosis	bone mineral densitometry	bone biopsy

BMD, bone mineral density

receptors are present in osteoblasts; the hormone has a negative impact on the secretion of factors (e.g. interleukin 1, macrophage colony-stimulating factor and tumor necrosis factor α) that activate osteoclastic activity[5].

From fetal age, bone grows and reaches maturity in the thirties[3]. Thereafter, an imbalance in bone remodeling leads to progressive bone loss. Imbalance may occur when: osteoclasts create an excessively deep cavity; osteoblasts fail to refill a normal resorption cavity; or both events occur[2]. Failure of bone mineralization after remodeling causes accumulation of osteoid. Osteoporosis and osteomalacia are two different disorders of bone (Table 1).

OSTEOPOROSIS

Osteoporosis is a 'systemic skeletal disease characterized by low bone mass and microarchitectural deterioration with consequent increase in bone fragility and susceptibility to fracture'[5–7]. In the clinical setting, as recommended by the World Health Organization, osteoporosis is objectively diagnosed when the measured bone mineral density (BMD) is 2.5 standard deviations or less below the mean peak value in young, same-sex adults[8].

In Europe, Japan and the USA alone, about 75 million people are afflicted with osteoporosis[7]. As the global population ages, the prevalence is expected to increase. The significance of osteoporosis lies in the consequences, notably fractures. In the USA, more than 1.5 million fractures occur annually[9]. Hip fractures are associated with increased mortality in the elderly, with 20% of women and 40% of men dying within a year. Half the survivors fail to regain their pre-morbid ambulatory status, while 40% eventually require placement in long-term care facilities[10]. Further, the quality of life diminishes, as patients harbor feelings of fear (of falls), anxiety and depression[11]. The impact on health-care cost is staggering. Presently, treatment of osteoporotic hip fractures in the USA costs $20 billion annually, projected to reach $62 billion by 2020[10].

Although osteoporosis is preventable and easily treated, awareness amongst patients and health-care providers remains low globally. It appears that the vast majority of individuals at risk do not receive preventive measures or treatment for subsequent fractures[1].

Classification

Bone growth starts *in utero* and peaks by the third decade of life. Henceforth, bone loss ensues, about 1% annually in women and around 0.7% in men. After menopause, bone

Table 2 Classification of osteoporosis

Primary
(a) Type I or postmenopausal
(b) Type II or age-related/senile

Secondary
(a) Medications: glucocorticoids, heparin, loop diuretics, gonadotropin releasing hormone agonists, phenytoin
(b) Hyperparathyroidism, hyperthyroidism, hypogonadism, Cushing's disease
(c) Malabsorption
(d) Metastatic bone disease, multiple myeloma
(e) Rheumatoid arthritis
(f) Chronic renal failure

Table 3 Risk factors for osteoporosis

Non-modifiable
Advanced age
Female gender
Family history
Race – Caucasian and Asian
Thin body frame

Modifiable
Excessive ingestion of coffee, protein or alcohol
Inadequate exposure to sunlight
Insufficient exercise
Malnutrition (poor calcium and vitamin D intake)
Premature menopause, nulliparity
Smoking
Secondary causes (see Table 2)

loss is accelerated in women, reaching rates up to 5% per year for 5 to 15 years[12]. During this period, significant bone loss occurs.

The etiology of osteoporosis may be primary or secondary (Table 2). Primary bone loss from estrogen deficiency is referred to as type I or postmenopausal osteoporosis and mainly affects trabecular bone. Bone loss from aging is known as type II or age-related (senile) osteoporosis and affects both trabecular and cortical components. Secondary osteoporosis arises in the presence of additional risk factors (e.g. medications, thyroid disease, multiple myeloma and many others)[13].

The vertebrae, which contain a significant amount of trabecular bone, are mainly affected in type I osteoporosis. Femoral bone, relatively more cortical, is mainly involved in type II osteoporosis. Hence, vertebral fractures are encountered in postmenopausal women, while hip fractures occur with increasing frequency in older adults[13].

Risk factors

A discussion of risk factors causative in osteoporosis requires emphasis. Modification of correctable risk factors throughout life (starting from childhood) enables individuals to reach the genetically determined peak bone mineral density by middle age and limit the amount and rate of bone loss in subsequent years. Several risk factors have been associated with osteoporosis (Table 3).

Women with late menarche and/or early menopause are at increased risk[11]. Amenorrhea in young women, as seen with excessive athletic activity or emotional stress, could lead to lower peak BMD and increased bone loss[14].

Caucasians and Asians have lower BMD compared to African-Americans. Lifetime risk of hip fracture above age 50 is higher in Caucasian women (17%) compared to Caucasian men (6%) in the USA. Worldwide the risk varies more in women than in men[15]. A family history of osteoporosis is a risk factor; maternal history of hip fracture was associated with lower BMD and a two-fold increase in fracture risk[16]. Studies have shown that all types of fracture appear to increase in those with low bone density. There is a 50–100% higher likelihood of a fracture in those with a prior fracture[15].

Increased coffee intake (two cups per day) has been associated with decreased bone density; the effect is negated with ingestion of a glass of milk[17]. High dietary protein and sodium leads to increased urinary calcium loss[18]; again, the negative effect on bone density is minimized with adequate calcium intake[11].

Besides associated malnutrition and liver disease, alcohol directly inhibits osteoblast function and decreases levels of 25-hydroxy-vitamin D and 1,25-dihydroxyvitamin D through induction of the cytochrome P450 system[19].

Exercise, through mechanical load, stimulates bone formation[14]. In addition, improved muscular strength, co-ordination and balance lessen the risk of falls and subsequent fracture[20]. Exercise, particularly resistance and high-impact types, leads to a higher peak BMD by middle age and a slower decline in bone density in later life[11].

Medications are well recognized to impact on bone density; thus, a review of all prescribed and over-the-counter medications is important. While furosemide promotes urinary calcium loss, thiazides improve calcium balance through urinary reabsorption[8]. Anticonvulsants (e.g. phenytoin, barbiturates) via induction of the hepatic cytochrome P450 enzyme system enhance the hepatic metabolism of 25-hydroxyvitamin D. When doses of thyroxine are excessive, bone resorption can result[19]. Longstanding heparin is associated with osteoporosis. Glucocorticoid-induced bone loss is well recognized and will be discussed separately.

Of the modifiable risk factors, smoking is common and correctable. Nicotine decreases intestinal calcium absorption[21] and is associated with earlier menopause and lower spine bone density[13].

When evaluating women for osteoporosis, the following five risk factors suggest a tendency for subsequent fractures from osteoporosis: age, race, history of smoking, glucocorticoid use and previous fracture after age 45 or 50. These risk factors not only predict fracture but help in decision making regarding screening for osteoporosis[22].

Presentation

Osteoporosis may be a silent disease, often asymptomatic until a complication occurs. Vertebral fractures may be painless, the presence often discovered incidentally on radiographs. Kyphosis ('dowager's hump'), scoliosis and loss of height suggest the presence of fractures. Pain following a vertebral fracture may last weeks to a few months.

Persistent pain beyond this period suggests another basis. There is often no correlation between symptoms and radiological features[8].

In severe kyphosis, the anterior–posterior diameter of the chest increases. The descent of the rib cage onto the pelvic rim causes local discomfort, leading to protrusion of the abdomen, decreased pulmonary volumes (restrictive lung disease), and reflux esophagitis[13].

Non-vertebral fractures are usually symptomatic. Pain from hip fracture is felt in the inguinal area; external rotation and shortening of the involved leg is recognized on evaluation[23]. Colles' fracture (distal radius) is painful and associated with 'dinner-fork wrist' deformity. While distal radial fracture is common in younger adults, hip fracture occurs in older individuals who are unable to break a fall with an outstretched hand (due to poor reflexes)[13].

Diagnosis

The diagnosis of osteoporosis entails a thorough history and physical examination. Risk factors for osteoporosis and falls must be recognized, including an assessment of gait and balance.

Routine laboratory tests are a good beginning; these should include serum calcium, phosphorus and alkaline phosphatase (Table 4). Most parameters are normal, unlike in osteomalacia (Table 1). Additional tests help evaluate for secondary causes. A high 24-h urinary calcium value (over 4 mg calcium/kg body weight) suggests idiopathic hypercalciuria, while a low level may indicate vitamin D deficiency[13].

When fracture is suspected, radiographs are helpful. Repeat films, computed tomography (CT) scan, magnetic resonance imaging (MRI), and isotope bone scans are helpful to evaluate persistent pain[23]. While radiographs detect fractures, they are not effective for screening; when osteopenia is detected on X-rays, 30% of the bone density has already been lost[8]. Incidental

Table 4 Diagnosis of osteoporosis

Laboratory tests (routine)
Complete blood count, calcium, phosphorus, alkaline phosphatase
Renal function tests

Additional tests (individualized)
24-h urine creatinine and calcium
Parathyroid hormone assay
Liver function tests
Thyroid function tests
Serum testosterone and cortisol assays
Serum and urine protein electrophoresis

Radiology
Plain radiographs for fracture
Dual-energy X-ray absorptiometry
Quantitative ultrasound
Quantitative computed tomography
When indicated (e.g. pain, fracture): computed tomography, magnetic resonance imaging, isotope bone scan

Biochemical markers (primarily for research)
Bone formation
   osteocalcin, bone alkaline phosphatase, carboxy-terminal end of type 1 procollagen
Bone resorption
   pyridinoline, deoxypyridinoline, N- and C-telopeptides of collagen crosslinks

Table 5 National Osteoporosis Foundation: indications for bone densitometry. From references 5 and 24

(1) Estrogen-deficient women at clinical risk of osteoporosis based on history and evaluation (to enable decision for or against treatment)
(2) Radiographic evidence of osteopenia, osteoporosis or fracture
(3) Chronic glucocorticoid therapy (at least 7.5 mg prednisone or equivalent per day for more than 3 months)
(4) Primary hyperparathyroidism
(5) Monitoring response to osteoporosis therapy
(6) Female over 65 years and postmenopausal women below 65 years who have at least one additional risk factor

findings of anterior wedging, flattening and 'codfish' (biconcave) vertebrae suggest severe osteoporosis[13].

Bone densitometry

Individuals at risk for osteoporosis should be considered for bone densitometry; it is most useful in aiding decisions for or against treatment (Table 5). Based on guidelines from the World Health Organization, osteopenia is present when the BMD is between 1 and 2.5 standard deviations (T score of –1 to –2.5) below the mean of young, normal adults; osteoporosis is present when the T score is less than –2.5. On the other hand, the Z score compares the BMD to sex -and age-matched controls[8].

The gold standard for bone densitometry is dual-energy X-ray absorptiometry (DEXA). The test is well accepted for its non-invasiveness, low radiation exposure (less than a standard radiograph), and high sensitivity and specificity[13]. In the presence of osteoarthritis, aortic calcification or compression fractures in the lumbar spine area, vertebral DEXA may yield erroneous values; measurement of the proximal femur is preferred in such settings[8].

Quantitative ultrasound, an alternative to DEXA, measures bone density in the heel, fingers, tibia and patella. It is inexpensive, is easy to perform, and entails no radiation. However, it is currently less sensitive than DEXA[7,13]. Quantitative CT may be used when the above modalities are unavailable. It has limited patient acceptability and higher radiation exposure[7].

Bone markers, indicative of osteoblastic or osteoclastic activity, are largely used for research purposes and for monitoring treatment response[7].

Non-pharmacologic management

Prevention is the primary goal in management and helps avert complications. At present, lifestyle modifications and antiresorptive medications are the core of management.

Lifestyle modifications should begin early in life to achieve the highest peak bone density by middle age (Table 6). Modifiable risk factors should be identified and corrective measures offered. Excessive alcohol and

Table 6 Non-pharmacologic measures of osteoporosis

Ensure adequate intake of calcium and vitamin D
  Calcium (preferred as diet over supplement)
    1000 mg/day for premenopausal women and
    postmenopausal women on estrogen replacement
    1500 mg/day for postmenopausal women (not on
    estrogen) and older men
  Vitamin D
    400–800 IU/day
    multivitamins (contain 400 IU per dose)
Avoid excessive use of coffee and alcohol
Regular weight-bearing exercises
Fall prevention measures
Periodic medication review
Counseling for smoking cessation

Table 7 Calcium supplementation. From references 10, 23, 25 and 27

Dietary calcium (the preferred source)
A serving of milk, yogurt or 1.5 oz cheddar cheese
  contains approximately 300 mg of calcium
Calcium absorption from spinach is poor (complexed
  with oxalate)
If lactose-intolerant, lactose-reduced or lactose-free dairy
  products are alternatives

Calcium preparations
Available as carbonate, phosphate, acetate, citrate,
  lactate and gluconate
Variable elemental calcium per gram of compound
Bioavailability varies with preparation and
  gastric acidity
Enhanced solubility may occur if taken with meals
Consider divided doses of supplements for optimal
  absorption
Calcium carbonate has the highest elemental calcium
  content per gram and is the least expensive

coffee consumption may be curtailed. Assistance may be offered in smoking cessation. Encourage weight-bearing exercises most days a week for both young and older adults. When possible, recognize and correct risk factors for falls. Hip protectors in compliant older individuals help reduce the risk of hip fracture following falls by 60%[24].

Ensure an adequate intake of calcium. Barring contraindications, older men and postmenopausal women over the age of 65 not on hormone replacement therapy (HRT) should receive 1500 mg of calcium per day. For all other women (including those on HRT), at least 1000 mg/day of calcium is recommended[23]. Adequate calcium intake increases the peak bone density, which may reduce the incidence of fracture.

Calcium in the form of diet is preferred over supplements, as the latter is associated with bloating (gas) and constipation[10] (Table 7). A serving of milk, yogurt or cheese contains approximately 300 mg of calcium. The average diet of an older adult contains only 400–800 mg of elemental calcium; for the 50% of older adults unable to meet their daily calcium requirement[11], supplementation may be the solution.

Calcium supplements are mostly available as carbonate, gluconate and citrate. Calcium carbonate contains the highest amount of elemental calcium per gram and is the least expensive. Bioavailability is greater when taken with food. In cases of achlorhydria, calcium citrate may be preferred[25]. To maximize absorption, calcium should be given in split doses of 500 mg or less; calcium is contraindicated in hypercalcemia, hypercalciuria and hyperparathyroidism[23].

Vitamin D deficiency is not uncommon, especially in the frail elderly who are homebound or institutionalized. Decreased dietary intake of vitamin D (coupled with decreased skin production) impairs calcium absorption in the intestine. The recommended daily allowance of vitamin D is 400–800 IU[13]. A dose of multivitamin per day generally supplies 400 IU of vitamin D. Milk is fortified with vitamin D in the USA.

Pharmacologic management

Drugs for the management of osteoporosis may either inhibit bone resorption or promote formation. Currently, all of the available drugs have antiresorptive properties (Table 8). However, some of the medications that stimulate bone formation are currently undergoing clinical trials.

Table 8 Pharmacologic management of osteoporosis. From references 5, 7, 13, 23

Estrogen replacement therapy
Estrogen preparations
    conjugated estrogen 0.3–0.625 mg/day
    micronized estradiol 0.5 mg/day
    transdermal estrogen (cyclic twice weekly or continuous)
Conjugated estrogen with medroxyprogesterone
    continuous: estrogen 0.625 mg/progesterone 2.5 mg
        on days 1–28
    cyclic: estrogen 0.625 mg on days 1–28, progesterone
        5 mg on days 14–28

Bisphosphonates
Etidronate, cyclical: 400 mg/day for 2 weeks, off for
    11 weeks
Alendronate sodium
    prevention: 5 mg/day or 35 mg weekly dose
    treatment: 10 mg/day or 70 mg weekly dose
Risedronate 5 mg/day for prevention and treatment or
    35 mg weekly dose

Selective estrogen receptor modulator
Raloxifene HCl 60 mg/day for prevention

Calcitonin
Calcitonin injectable 100 IU sc every 3 days for treatment
Calcitonin-salmon 200 IU/day (1 spray) alternate nares
    for treatment

Future considerations
Anti-estrogen agents
Calcitriol
Growth hormone
Newer bisphosphonates
Parathyroid hormone
Sodium fluoride
Thiazide diuretics

Hormone replacement therapy

In postmenopausal women, HRT with estrogen increases the bone density by as much as 15% (after 3 years) and may reduce the risk of hip and spine fractures by as much as 50% (after 7 years)[23]; however, additional studies are needed to evaluate reduction in fractures. Though the greatest benefit is achieved when HRT is started within 5 years of menopause[7], effects are also observed when taken even after age 60[26]. In addition, estrogen ameliorates postmenopausal (e.g. hot flashes) and genitourinary (atrophic vaginitis, incontinence) symptoms and favorably alters the lipid profile[13]. The efficacy of low-dose estrogen (conjugated equine estrogen 0.3 mg/day) and transdermal estrogen on bone density has been demonstrated as well[24].

Estrogen replacement therapy is associated with increased risk of uterine and breast malignancy. A regimen of estrogen and progesterone (continuous or cyclic) eliminates the risk of uterine cancer; with cyclic progesterone, withdrawal bleeding may be unacceptable to several[13]. Regular mammograms should be considered for breast cancer screening. Other risks associated with HRT include venous thromboembolism[27] and cholelithiasis.

When estrogen replacement therapy is discontinued, the rate of bone loss increases to the rate in women never started on estrogen[23]. In practice, the majority have discontinued estrogen within 7 years of treatment initiation[24].

Current information derived from the Women's Health Initiative (WHI) study indicate that the use of estrogen and progestin was associated with fewer vertebral and nonvertebral fractures, consistent with observed data. However, also noticed was an absolute increase in risk of cardiac events, strokes, pulmonary embolism and breast cancer. The results suggest that the benefits of postmenopausal estrogen and progestin therapy in osteoporosis must be weighed against the risks of vascular disease and cancer. Thus, use has to be individualized, following detailed discussions on the pros and cons of hormonal therapy and available alternatives[28].

In men with diagnosed hypogonadism, intramuscular depo-testosterone or transdermal testosterone preparations may be considered. Chronic oral testosterone therapy is associated with hepatic tumors[29]. Caution should be exercised in prescribing testosterone for those with prostatic disease or malignancy.

The use of natural estrogens (e.g. phytoestrogens) has not shown significant reduction in the risk of fracture in humans, although results of animal studies have been encouraging[11].

Selective estrogen receptor modulator

Raloxifene HCl increases bone density by 2–2.4% over 2 years of therapy[30] and decreases the risk of vertebral fracture in postmenopausal women[31]. While the risk of thromboembolism remains, the risk of breast cancer is reduced by 76% over 3 years of therapy[31,32]. Neither is there an elevated risk of uterine cancer. While raloxifene lowers levels of total cholesterol and low-density lipoproteins, it does not affect high-density lipoproteins and triglycerides[30]. As hot flushes are a side-effect, raloxifene will not help postmenopausal symptoms. For prevention, the drug is administered at 60 mg per day.

Bisphosphonates

These are synthetic analogs of pyrophosphate and have antiresorptive action from strong affinity for hydroxyapatite. Available forms include etidronate, alendronate and risedronate.

The first bisphosphonate available was etidronate. In the past, its use on a continuous basis resulted in failure of bone mineralization (osteomalacia). With intermittent therapy (400 mg/day for 2 weeks followed by 11 weeks of calcium 500 mg/day), an increase in lumbar and femoral BMD was observed with a decreased risk of vertebral fracture in 3 years[7]. It is given on an empty stomach with avoidance of food and beverages 2 h before and after each dose[29].

Alendronate increased the lumbar spine and femoral neck BMD by 8.8% and 5.9%, respectively, in 3 years[33]; it also decreased the rate of new vertebral and non-vertebral fractures[34]. The bioavailability of alendronate is less than 1%. Absorption is further reduced when taken with meals or fluids other than plain water; even mineral water affects absorption. Elimination is entirely renal; it is contraindicated in renal failure[35]. Common side-effects include gastrointestinal symptoms (nausea, dyspepsia, esophagitis, mucosal ulceration, constipation, diarrhea) and musculoskeletal

pain. Absolute contraindications include esophageal abnormalities (e.g. strictures, achalasia), inability to maintain upright posture after taking the medicine, and hypocalcemia[7,13,35]. Gastroesophageal reflux disease is a relative contraindication[7,23].

Education of individuals on proper administration of alendronate will ensure maximum absorption and minimize side-effects. The drug should be taken alone first thing in the morning with 8 oz (240 ml) of water; it is essential that food, beverages or other medications be avoided, and an upright position be maintained for at least 30 minutes after alendronate ingestion[13]. Alendronate is available in a daily dose of 5 mg for prevention and 10 mg for treatment of osteoporosis. The recently released preparations of once-weekly doses of 35 mg for prevention and 70 mg for treatment have been shown to be therapeutically equivalent to the daily dosing with no increase in adverse side-effects while enhancing compliance. A missed dose can be taken the following day.

Another bisphosphonate used for osteoporosis treatment is risedronate. It is used in daily doses of 5 mg or weekly doses of 35 mg for prevention and treatment. It has been demonstrated to increase lumbar spine, femoral trochanter and femoral neck density in postmenopausal women with at least one vertebral fracture[36]; likewise, the risk of new vertebral and non-vertebral fractures is reduced[24]. Other bisphosphonates, with varying bioavailability, under study for osteoporosis include ibandronate, zoledronate, and clodronate[37].

Calcitonin

Salmon calcitonin has demonstrated a 3% increase in lumbar spine BMD over 2 years of therapy; there is no effect on hip bone density[10,23]. When administered for painful vertebral fractures, a favorable analgesic property has been recognized. However, the benefit for prevention of future vertebral fracture is unclear[10,11,23]. Intranasal salmon calcitonin is administered at 200 IU daily for treatment. Side-effects include nasal irritation, nausea and facial flushing.

Other available forms include calcitonin suppository, which is minimally effective and less tolerable, and injectable calcitonin, which is given subcutaneously or intramuscularly. Aside from the high cost, side-effects include nausea, diarrhea and flushing. With long-term use, neutralizing antibodies develop and render the drug ineffective[7].

Future therapies

Ongoing studies include sodium fluoride, parathyroid hormone, vitamin D metabolites (calcitriol and alfacalcidiol), tibolone, HMG-CoA reductase inhibitors, newer bisphosphonates and selective estrogen receptor modulators (SERMs)[24,37]. In studies, sodium fluoride appears to increase bone density but does not prevent new vertebral fractures[38]. Side-effects include nausea, gastric irritation and stress fractures[7]. In a recent study, subcutaneous parathyroid hormone increased vertebral, femoral and total body BMD and decreased the risk of vertebral and non-vertebral fractures[39]; approval has been received from the US Food and Drug Administration for use in osteoporosis.

Intermittent parathormone injection increase bone strength by new bone formation at periosteal and endosteal surfaces with improvement in cortical and trabecular structure[37]. Recently, statins used in hyperlipidemia have interestingly been associated with substantial reduction in fracture risk not explained purely by the increase in BMD[40].

Glucocorticoid-induced osteoporosis

With the increasing use of steroids for musculoskeletal disorders and pulmonary disease, glucocorticoids have become a recognized cause of secondary (drug-related) osteoporosis. The risk of fracture is dose-dependent, affecting the vertebrae, hip and other non-vertebral areas in decreasing order. Nearly half the patients on chronic glucocorticoids will develop an osteoporotic fracture[41]; 11% will have a vertebral fracture after 1 year of therapy[23]. The rate of bone loss increases, with most loss in the first 6 months of glucocorticoid therapy[23].

Several mechanisms have been proposed for glucocorticoid-induced osteoporosis. Glucocorticoids reduce calcium and phosphate absorption via the intestines, increase calcium loss in the urine and inhibit bone formation through reduction in the function, lifespan and number of osteoblasts. They affect osteoclasts as well, enhancing their number and maturation, leading to greater bone resorption[23,41].

Management of glucocorticoid-induced osteoporosis begins with avoidance of prolonged therapy. When chronic steroid therapy (at least 7.5 mg of prednisone or equivalent for at least 6 months) is anticipated, bone densitometry at baseline and at regular intervals (every 6 months) may be performed to monitor the response to preventive measures[13]. The lowest effective dose of corticosteroids should be used, preferably in topical or inhaled forms whenever possible. Calcium and vitamin D intake should meet the recommended daily allowance. Other measures such as bisphosphonates may be considered as part of the regimen[23].

Osteoporosis in men

Osteoporosis is becoming increasingly recognized as a disorder also affecting men. After the third decade of life, men lose bone at a rate of up to 1% per annum[42]. Most risk factors in women, such as smoking, are also present in men. Secondary causes, such as hypogonadism, glucocorticoid therapy and alcoholism, account for 30–60% of cases[11]. Although fractures may not be as prevalent as in women, one-third of hip fractures and one-fifth of vertebral fractures occur in men[43]. When hypogonadism is suspected, evaluation includes a morning testosterone (abnormal if less than 250 ng/dl), free testosterone and sex hormone binding globulin levels[44]; in confirmed hypogonadism, testosterone therapy is considered in injectable (testosterone enanthate) or patch (transdermal or scrotal) form[13]. Alendronate has been shown to increase spine, hip and total body bone density and prevent vertebral fractures in men[45]. All other life-style measures discussed earlier, relating to alcohol, smoking, calcium and vitamin D intake, are applicable.

The ideal strategy in prevention for osteoporosis is still not clear. We generally resort to use of medications after a fracture (tertiary prevention). Primary prevention targets all postmenopausal women and older adults (both genders) with regards to risk factors, diet, exercise and pharmacotherapy. Screening those with valid risk factors and targeting the individuals with high risk (e.g. low BMD) would be secondary prevention. Eventually, decisions are made based on available resources and evaluation for risk of fracture[46].

OSTEOMALACIA

Osteomalacia is a metabolic bone disease characterized by impaired mineralization of newly formed bone matrix. Unmineralized bone is referred to as osteoid. The true prevalence is unknown, perhaps because of underrecognition of the entity. The most common cause is vitamin D deficiency, which is present in half the older adults in hospitals and homebound community elderly[6].

Vitamin D metabolism

The main sources of vitamin D are dietary and dermal synthesis. With sunlight exposure (ultraviolet B rays), epidermal 7-dehydrocholesterol is converted to cholecalciferol (vitamin D_3) in the skin. Dietary cholecalciferol (vitamin D_3 from animal sources) and ergocalciferol (vitamin D_2 from plant sources) are absorbed in the proximal small intestine[47]. In the circulation, both D_2 and D_3 are bound to a vitamin D-binding protein and hydroxylated in the liver to 25-hydroxyvitamin D (25-OHD). In the kidney, 25-OHD is hydroxylated further to the active metabolite 1,25-dihydroxyvitamin D (1,25-OHD), the stimuli being parathyroid hormone and low serum phosphate. The half-life of 1,25-OHD is only 15 h; serum levels (normal range, N: 20–60 pg/ml) do not necessarily correlate with deficiency. Serum 25-OHD (N: 10–50 ng/ml), with a half-life of 15 days, is a better reflection of the body's vitamin D status[6,48].

Pathophysiology

Age-related physiologic changes predispose the elderly to hypovitaminosis D; these include decreased epidermal concentration of 7-dehydrocholesterol, its less efficient conversion to cholecalciferol, reduction in intestinal absorption of dietary vitamin D with down-regulation of vitamin D receptors and diminished renal synthesis of 1,25-OHD[49,50]. In osteomalacia, the defect lies in the slower mineralization of osteoid, mainly due to deficiencies in vitamin D, calcium or phosphorus.

Vitamin D deficiency is the most common cause of osteomalacia in older adults who are institutionalized or homebound and thus have inadequate sunlight exposure. Sunscreens, windowpane glass and excessive clothing further limit vitamin D production in the skin[51]. Dermal synthesis of vitamin D is also affected by geographical latitude; in the UK, 90% of older adults are said to have decreased vitamin D levels[7]. Diminished sunlight exposure correlates with the lowest vitamin D levels during winter. Heavily pigmented black individuals have lower levels of vitamin D, as melanin competes with 7-dehydrocholesterol for ultraviolet energy[49].

Furthermore, vitamin D deficiency in the geriatric population occurs from inadequate intake (malnutrition) or malabsorption. Malabsorption occurs with impaired fat absorption (pancreatic or biliary disease), gastric surgery, bowel resection or intestinal bypass operations[47]. Lactose intolerance, not uncommon in older subjects, limits consumption of dairy products. Other causes of vitamin D deficiency are end-stage hepatic disease (impaired hydroxylation of vitamin D_2 and D_3) and renal disease (impaired hydroxylation of 25-OHD).

Phosphorus deficiency, yet another cause of osteomalacia, occurs mainly from either gastrointestinal or renal losses. Diarrhea or malabsorption syndromes result in intestinal phosphate loss. Renal phosphate loss occurs in conditions such as renal tubular acidosis, X-linked hypophosphatemia and oncogenic osteomalacia.

Medications may also cause osteomalacia. Anticonvulsants (phenytoin, barbiturates and carbamazepine) increase vitamin D metabolism through activation of the hepatic cytochrome P450 enzymes[6]. Intestinal absorption of phosphate is diminished by excessive use of aluminum antacids, calcium acetate or sucralftate, which act as phosphate binders. Etidronate, if taken continuously for Paget's disease or osteoporosis, impairs bone mineralization. Fluoride stimulates bone formation but inhibits mineralization.

Clinical features and diagnosis

Individuals with osteomalacia commonly complain of diffuse bony pain and generalized fatigue; weakness from type II muscle fiber atrophy may be more pronounced in proximal muscles (e.g. thighs)[50]. Gait abnormality (waddling gait) may be observed as a result of hip pain and thigh weakness. Not uncommonly, fracture is the presenting symptom.

When osteomalacia is suspected, initial laboratory evaluation should include renal and hepatic function tests in addition to serum levels of calcium, phosphorus and alkaline phosphatase. Unlike osteoporosis, alkaline phosphatase is usually elevated (Table 1). Calcium and phosphorus may be low or normal. An assay of 25-OHD, when low, will help confirm the diagnosis. A low 24-h urinary calcium excretion should raise suspicion for vitamin D deficiency. In the presence of renal disease, parathyroid hormone assay may be considered.

Radiographs are non-specific. Pseudofracture or linear cortical lucency (Looser's zone) in the proximal femur (most frequent site), pelvis, ribs and lateral margins of the scapula is suggestive of osteomalacia[23,47]. Bone densitometry gives variable results. Bone biopsy showing unmineralized bone is the definitive diagnostic test. It is unnecessary if the history and laboratory evaluations, including 25-OHD assay, are suggestive of hypovitaminosis D.

Management

The management of osteomalacia requires treatment of the underlying cause. In vitamin D deficiency, an oral dose of 1000 IU/day is prescribed to normalize bone mineralization. Dietary sources of vitamin D include eggs, fish liver oil and chicken liver[6]. In the USA, a quart of milk contains 400 IU of vitamin D; in the UK, margarine is fortified with the vitamin[47]. A regular multivitamin provides approximately 400 IU of vitamin D. Sunlight exposure in institutionalized or homebound elderly for 5–10 min two to three times per week is adequate[6]. In non-compliant individuals, parenteral vitamin D up to 100 000 IU every 6 months is an option[6,50]. Vitamin D and calcium are prescribed long term; precautions include verification for history of nephrolithiasis and need for periodic monitoring of serum calcium level.

Phosphorus deficiency is treated with oral neutral phosphate salts (500 mg three to four times per day); diarrhea is a side-effect.

Dietary sources of phosphorus include dairy products, eggs, meat and cereals[6].

Whenever applicable, medications (e.g. phenytoin, aluminum antacids) that predispose to osteomalacia should be discontinued or replaced. Cyclic etidronate treatment does not cause osteomalacia. In chronic hepatic or renal disease, supplementation with 25-OHD (calcifediol 25–50 μg/day) or 1,25-OHD (calcitriol 0.25–0.5 μg/day), respectively, is recommended[23].

References

1. Baran D. Efficacy and safety of a bisphosphonate dosed once weekly. *Geriatrics* 2001;56:28–32

2. Riggs BL, Melton LJ III. The prevention and treatment of osteoporosis. *N Engl J Med* 1992;327:620–7

3. Kaplan FS. Prevention and management of osteoporosis. *Clin symp* 1995;47:1–32

4. Meier DE. Osteoporosis and other disorders of skeletal aging. In Cassel CK, Cohen HJ, Larson EB, *et al.*, eds. *Geriatric Medicine*, 3rd edn. New York: Springer-Verlag, 1997:411–32

5. Dharmarajan TS, Manalac MM. An understanding of osteoporosis. In: Dreger D, Krumm B, eds. *Hospital Physician: Geriatric Medicine Board Review Manual*. Wayne, Pennsylvania: Turner White Communications, 2000:1:1–12

6. Dharmarajan TS, Ahmed S. Vitamin D deficiency and osteomalacia in older adults. *Family Practice Recertification* 2001;23: 41–50

7. Eastell R. Treatment of postmenopausal osteoporosis. *N Engl J Med* 1998;338: 736–46

8. Ott SM. Osteoporosis and osteomalacia. In Hazzard WR, Blass JP, Ettinger WH, *et al.*, eds. *Principles of Geriatric Medicine and Gerontology*, 4th edn. New York: McGraw-Hill, 1999:1057–84

9. Riggs BL, Melton LJ III. The worldwide problem of osteoporosis: insights afforded by epidemiology. *Bone* 1995;17(suppl): 505–11S

10. Field-Munves E. Evidence-based decisions for the treatment of osteoporosis. *Ann Longterm Care* 2001;9:70–9

11. NIH Consensus Development Panel. Osteoporosis prevention, diagnosis, and therapy. *J Am Med Assoc* 2001;285:785–95

12. Hurley DL, Khosla S. Update on primary osteoporosis. *Mayo Clin Proc* 1997;72: 943–9

13. Dharmarajan TS, Ugalino JT. Current trends in the prevention and treatment of osteoporosis. *Family Practice Recertification* 2000; Special Geriatrics Issue: 17–26

14. Carbon RJ. Exercise, amenorrhea and the skeleton. *Br Med Bull* 1992;48:546–60

15. Cummings SR, Melton III LJ. Epidemiology and outcomes of osteoporotic fractures. *Lancet* 2002;359:1761–7

16. Cummings SR, Nevitt MC, Browner WS, *et al*. Risk factors for hip fracture in white women. Study of Osteoporotic Fractures Research Group. *N Engl J Med* 1995;332: 767–73

17. Barrett-Connor E, Chang JC, Edelstein SL. Coffee-associated osteoporosis offset by daily milk consumption. The Rancho Bernardo Study. *J Am Med Assoc* 1994; 271:280–3

18. Celotti F, Bignamini A. Dietary calcium and mineral/vitamin supplementation: a controversial problem. *J Int Med Res* 1999;27:1–14

19. Bohannon AD, Lyles KW. Drug-induced bone disease. *Clin Geriatr Med* 1994;10: 611–23

20. Lane JM, Nydick M. Osteoporosis: current modes of prevention and treatment. *J Am Acad Orthop Surg* 1999;7:19–31

21. Krall EA, Dawson-Hughes B. Smoking increases bone loss and decreases intestinal

calcium absorption. *J Bone Miner Res* 1999;14:215–20

22. Lyles KW, Colon-Emeric CS. Can we identify women at high risk of osteoporotic fractures? *J Am Geriatr Soc* 2002;50:1161–2

23. Pacala JT. Osteoporosis and osteomalacia. *Clin Geriatr* 2000;8:35–47

24. McGarry KA, Cyr MG. Prevention and bone loss and fractures in postmenopausal osteoporosis. *Clin Geriatr* 2001;9:47–56

25. Morgan SL. Calcium and vitamin D in osteoporosis. In Lane NE, ed. *Rheumatic Disease Clinics of North America*. Philadelphia: WB Saunders, 2001;27:101–30

26. Schneider DL, Barrett-Connor EL, Morton DJ. Timing of postmenopausal estrogen for optimal bone mineral density. The Rancho Bernardo Study. *J Am Med Assoc* 1997; 277:543–7

27. Grady D, Wenger NK, Herrington D, *et al.* Postmenopausal hormone therapy increases risk for venous thromboembolic disease. The Heart and Estrogen/progestin Replacement Study. *Ann Intern Med* 2000; 132:689–96

28. Rossouw JE, Anderson GL, Prentice RL, *et al.* Risks and benefits of estrogen plus progestin in healthy postmenopausal women: principal results from the Women's Health Initiative randomized controlled trial. *JAMA* 2002;288:321–33

29. Zaqqa D, Jackson RD. Diagnosis and treatment of glucocorticoid-induced osteoporosis. *Cleveland Clin J Med* 1999;66:221–30

30. Delmas PD, Bjarnason NH, Mitlak BH, *et al.* Effects of raloxifene on bone mineral density, serum cholesterol concentrations, and uterine endometrium in postmenopausal women. *N Engl J Med* 1997;337: 1641–7

31. Ettinger B, Black DM, Mitlak BH, *et al.* Reduction of vertebral fracture risk in postmenopausal women with osteoporosis treated with raloxifene: results from a 3-year randomized clinical trial. Multiple Outcomes of Raloxifene Evaluation (MORE) Investigators. *J Am Med Assoc* 1999;282: 637–45

32. Cummings SR, Eckert S, Krueger KA, *et al.* The effect of raloxifene on risk of breast cancer in postmenopausal women: results

from the MORE randomized trial. Multiple Outcomes of Raloxifene Evaluation. *J Am Med Assoc* 1999;281:2189–97

33. Liberman UA, Weiss SR, Broll J, *et al.* Effect of oral alendronate on bone mineral density and the incidence of fractures in postmenopausal osteoporosis. *N Engl J Med* 1995;333:1437–43

34. Black DM, Cummings SR, Karpf DB, *et al.* Randomised trial of effect of alendronate on risk of fracture in women with existing vertebral fractures: Fracture Intervention Trial Research Group. *Lancet* 1996;348: 1535–41

35. Ragsdale AB, Barringer TA III, Anastasio GD. Alendronate treatment to prevent osteoporotic fractures. *Arch Fam Med* 1998;7:583–6

36. Harris St, Watts NB, Genant HK, *et al.* Effects of risedronate treatment on vertebral and nonvertebral fractures in women with postmenopausal osteoporosis: a randomized controlled trial. Vertebral efficacy with risedronate therapy (VERT) study group. *J Am Med Assoc* 1999;282:1344–52

37. Delmas PD. Treatment of postmenopausal osteoporosis. *Lancet* 2002;359:2018–26

38. Meunier PJ, Sebert JL, Reginster JY, *et al.* Fluoride salts are no better at preventing new vertebral fractures than calcium–vitamin D in postmenopausal osteoporosis: The FAVO Study. *Osteoporos Int* 1998; 8:4–12

39. Neer RM, Arnaud CD, Zanchetta JR, *et al.* Effect of parathyroid hormone (1–34) on fractures and bone mineral density in postmenopausal women with osteoporosis. *N Engl J Med* 2001;344:1434–41

40. Pasco JA, Kotowicz MA, Henry MJ, *et al.* Statin use, bone mineral density and fracture risk. Geelong Osteoporosis Study. *Arch Intern Med* 2002;162:537–40

41. Lane NE. An update on glucocorticoid-induced osteoporosis. In: Lane NE, ed. *Rheumatic Disease Clinics of North America*. Philadelphia: WB Saunders, 2001; 27:235–53

42. Amin S, Felson DT. Osteoporosis in men. In Lane NE, ed. *Rheumatic Disease Clinics of North America*. Philadelphia: WB Saunders, 2001;27:19–47

43. Eastell R, Boyle IT, Compston J, *et al.* Management of male osteoporosis: report of the UK Consensus Group. *Q J Med* 1998;91:71–92

44. Swan KG, Lobo M, Lane JM, Nydick M. Osteoporosis in men: a serious but under-recognized problem. *J Musculoskeletal Med* 2001;18:310–16

45. Orwoll E, Ettinger M, Weiss S, *et al.* Alendronate for the treatment of osteo-porosis in men. *N Engl J Med* 2000;343: 604–10

46. Sedrine WB, Reginster J. Risk indices and osteoporosis screening: scope and limits. *Mayo Clin Proc* 2002;77:622–3

47. Raisz L, Pilbeam C. Osteomalacia. In Evans JG, Williams TF, eds. *Oxford Textbook of Geriatric Medicine.* New York: Oxford University Press, 1992:411–15

48. Gunby MC, Morley JE. Calcium, vitamin D, and osteopenia. In Morley JE, Glick Z, Rubenstein LZ, eds. *Geriatric Nutrition,* 2nd edn. New York: Raven Press, 1995:107–14

49. Clemens TL, O'Riordan JLH. Vitamin D. In Becker KL, ed. *Principles and Practice of Endrocrinology and Metabolism,* 2nd edn. Philadelphia: JB Lippincott, 1995:483–91

50. Gloth FM III. Impaired vitamin D status in the elderly. In Vellas BJ, Sachet P, Baumgartner RJ, eds. *Facts and Research in Gerontology.* New York: Springer Publishing, 1995:17–22

51. Holick MF. Environmental factors that influence the cutaneous production of vitamin D. *Am J Clin Nutr* 1995; 61(suppl): 638–45S

52. Jennings J, Perkel V, Baylink DJ. Osteo-porosis. In Calkins E, Ford AB, Katz PR, eds. *Practice of Geriatrics,* 2nd edn. Philadelphia: WB Saunders, 1992:363–77

27 Constipation and fecal incontinence

T.S. Dharmarajan, MD, FACP, AGSF, *Ajit J. Kokkat*, MD,
and C.S. Pitchumoni, MD, FACP, FRCP(C), MACG, MPH

INTRODUCTION AND AGE-RELATED CHANGES IN BOWEL FUNCTION

'Constipation' is a general term used by patients to indicate fewer bowel movements, hard stools, painful defecation and feelings of bloating, abdominal discomfort or incomplete elimination. An international committee included these symptoms in an operational definition of chronic functional constipation[1-3] (Table 1). Studies in North America estimate the prevalence of self-reported constipation in community-dwelling older adults to vary between 21 and 40% and between 11 and 22% when the criteria for chronic functional constipation are applied[2,4,5]. Women are more likely to report constipation and use laxatives than men[2]. The prevalence of constipation in long-term care patients is estimated to be around 27.5%. However, the routine use of laxatives was recently reported to be higher at 53.8%, suggesting a potential overuse or an inadequate documentation to justify their use[6]. Constipation accounts for 2.5 million physician visits per year, with almost all visits (85%) leading to prescription of laxatives and significant increase in costs of health care[3]. Fecal incontinence (accidental and involuntary defecation) is more prevalent in the long-term care and hospital settings than in the community[7]. Shame, humiliation and fear of institutionalization are the basis for under-reporting the problem of incontinence in older adults.

Tensile strength of collagen in the colonic wall decreases with aging due to collagen fibrils becoming smaller and more tightly packed. Lack of accommodation of the intra-luminal pressure by less compliant areas of the colonic wall, e.g. site of perforating arteries, results in diverticula formation, especially in the sigmoid and descending colon[8]. The number of neurons in the myenteric plexus is reduced, but colonic transit time is not affected[7-9]. The mass movements and segmental contractions of the colon in older adults are enhanced postprandially, provided these individuals are not bed-bound[10]. Internal sphincter tone and external anal sphincter contractile pressure do not change significantly[10]. The rectum is less distensible, perhaps due to degeneration of rectal wall connective tissue and increased rectal smooth muscle tone[11]. The rectal volume (rectal distension by stool) required to stimulate internal anal sphincter relaxation and external anal sphincter contraction is reduced. The threshold pressure needed to elicit this rectoanal inhibition reflex increases with aging[11].

Table 1 Criteria for diagnosing chronic functional constipation. From references 1–3

A. Presence of two or more of the following symptoms for at least 12 weeks in the preceding year:
   1. straining with ≥ 25% of bowel movements
   2. sense of incomplete evacuation with ≥ 25% of bowel movements
   3. hard or pellet stools with ≥ 25% of bowel movements
   4. manual evacuation maneuvers with ≥ 25% of bowel movements
   5. feeling of anorectal blockage with ≥ 25% of bowel movements
   6. number of bowel movements two or less per week
B. Absence of loose stools and insufficient criteria for irritable bowel syndrome

Table 2 Drugs commonly associated with constipation*. From reference 14

Aluminum hydroxide
Anticholinergics
Anticonvulsants
Antihistamines
Anti-Parkinsonian drugs
Antipsychotics
Bismuth
Calcium channel antagonists
Calcium preparations
Diuretics
Iron salts
Non-steroidal anti-inflammatory drugs
Opioids
Tricyclic antidepressants

* The list is partial and for illustration only

CONSTIPATION

Pathophysiology

Colonic motility consists of segmenting, propagating and high-amplitude contractions. Contents of the colon are mixed by segmenting contractions, propelled over short distances in either the cephalad or caudal direction by propagating contractions and moved over long distances toward the anus by high-amplitude contractions[1]. Constipation with slow transit time is associated with marked slowing of colonic motility; in contrast, constipation-prone irritable bowel syndrome is associated with an increase in segmenting contractions, which hinders transit of stool through the left colon[1]. Immobility and decreased physical activity are linked to reduced colonic motility[12]. The ascending and transverse colon are more compliant than the sigmoid colon, the former functioning as reservoirs of stool while the latter is associated with rapid evacuation. The proximal colon is often lengthened or pendulous in constipated patients with prolonged proximal colon transit time[8].

Pelvic floor dyssynergia, the unconscious contraction of the pelvic floor muscles during defecation, results in increased anal canal pressure preventing passage of stool[1,5,13]. Rectal emptying in women is hampered by pelvic floor weakness. Weakening of the perineal body (fibromuscular structure where the transverse perineal, bulbocavernosus, external sphincter and puborectalis muscles interdigitate) and the rectovaginal fascia may allow the rectal wall to bulge into the vagina with straining, causing a rectocele. The bolus of stool moves into the rectocele and manual pressure on the perineum or posterior vaginal wall is then needed to evacuate the rectum. Attenuation of the levator ani muscles creates 'lateral pockets' in the rectum and increased abdominal pressure is needed to expel the stool. Megarectum (dilatation of the rectum in the elderly with longstanding constipation) reduces defecation forces and diminishes rectal sensation[1]. Anal fissures, perirectal abscesses and hemorrhoids cause voluntary inhibition of defecation due to pain. Altered mental state, e.g. dementia, is well known to be associated with abnormal bowel habits.

A careful review of medications including over-the-counter preparations and nutritional supplements is necessary to exclude drug-related constipation (Table 2). Constipation is listed as an adverse effect of more than 750 brand-name drugs[14]. Diseases associated with chronic constipation include gastrointestinal, metabolic and neuropsychiatric disorders (Table 3).

Table 3 Disorders commonly associated with constipation. From reference 14

Gastrointestinal	Endocrine/Metabolic	Neuropsychiatric
Obstruction	Hypothyroidism	Dementia
Anal fissure	Hypercalcemia	Parkinson's disease
Rectocele	Hypokalemia	Cerebrovascular accident
Diverticulosis	Hypomagnesemia	Depression
Strictures	Diabetes mellitus	Autonomic neuropathy
Amyloidosis	Renal failure	Multiple sclerosis

Evaluation

The importance of the history is to determine whether clinical constipation exists and to detect reversible risk factors. The health provider needs to review appetite, physical activity, sleep pattern, weight changes and diet. It is worth maintaining a 2-week bowel diary listing food intake, frequency of bowel movements, straining at defecation, time spent toileting and character of stools. Although alternating constipation and diarrhea might suggest irritable bowel syndrome, colon cancer must always be ruled out. Alarm symptoms such as blood in stools and weight loss should be looked for. Pain during defecation is common with anal disorders. Physical examination along with rectal and perineal examinations detect fissures, masses, fistulae, hemorrhoids and perirectal abscesses. Useful laboratory studies include complete blood cell counts, electrolytes including calcium and phosphorus, fasting blood glucose, thyroid function tests and fecal occult blood testing[12].

Sigmoidoscopy with double contrast barium enema or colonoscopy can detect malignancy, strictures, megacolon, volvulus and melanosis coli. Stools positive for occult blood warrant colonoscopy as the initial diagnostic procedure. Plain radiographs of the abdomen can suggest stool retention in each of four abdominal quadrants and help monitor results of bowel cleansing (Figure 1). Barium radiographs demonstrate obstructing lesions, colonic dilatation and megarectum. Colonic transit studies utilize radio-opaque markers to measure transit time; persistence of the markers after 3 days is abnormal, and indicates colonic inertia (proximal slowing) if distributed throughout the colon, or anorectal motility disorder (outlet delay) if limited to the rectosigmoid region[1,15,16]. Anorectal manometry measures resting and squeezing pressures of the anal sphincters. Defecography (barium imaging) identifies anatomical problems, e.g. rectoceles, mucosal prolapse and abnormalities in perineal descent during defecation[12,15].

Management

Patient education

Educating the patient about normal bowel habits helps correct misconceptions. A regular time for defecation should be established, utilizing the gastrocolic reflex (Table 4). Exercise, e.g. walking for about 30 min most days each week, is beneficial. Adequate water intake (minimum 1500 ml/day) helps reduce the risk of constipation[12].

Dietary fiber

'Dietary fiber' is a term for dietary substances of plant origin resistant to digestion by small intestinal digestive enzymes, and help increase stool bulk. The term 'dietary fiber' previously referred to plant cell wall components, cellulose and hemicellulose, but currently includes gums, pectins, mucillages and lignin[17]. Bran and raisins are sources of fiber; other natural sources include vegetables such as beans and broccoli and raw fruits

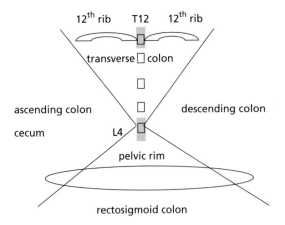

Figure 1 Constipation: use of the plain radiograph of the abdomen. Four lines drawn from the 4th lumbar vertebra to the lateral ends of the 12th ribs and the lateral aspects of the pelvic rim divide the abdominal radiograph into four quadrants; each quadrant represents a segment of the colon: ascending, transverse, descending and rectosigmoid segments. Adapted from reference 16

such as berries[13,18]. Fiber from citrus fruits and legumes encourages colonic bacterial growth, increasing fecal mass[1]. Fiber particle size is important in that larger and coarser particles have a greater laxative effect[1,17].

The calorie-dense, low-fiber diets of the Western world result in a smaller and harder stool mass among healthy individuals (100 g of stool weight/day) compared to people in countries with high-fiber, less calorie-dense diets (> 300 g/day)[17]. Fiber acts by decreasing total gut transit time; it is useful in constipation due to colonic inertia, but has little to no effect in pelvic floor dyssynergia[5]. Colonic bacteria metabolize dietary fiber producing gas, accounting for the adverse effects of fiber such as abdominal bloating and flatulence. A step-up supplementation of fiber starting with 10 g day and titrating gradually to 20–25 g/day enhances patient tolerance[12]. Stressing the need for sufficient water intake to prevent fecal impaction and intestinal obstruction, although essential, may be difficult in elderly patients with cognitive impairment.

Table 4 Using the gastrocolic reflex

Eat an adequate breakfast
Ingest a hot drink, e.g. tea, coffee, warm water or milk
Sit on the toilet for up to 10 min
Use the Valsalva maneuver
Hold the breath after inspiration for 10 s, several times
Avoid distractions such as reading
Do not deny the urge to defecate, if possible
Stop after 10 min, even if no bowel movements have occurred
Make this a daily routine

Stool softeners

Docusates are anionic surfactants that act as stool-wetting and softening agents to help prevent straining during defecation. Adverse effects include loose stools, abdominal cramps and rash. Docusates, available as sodium, potassium or calcium salts, increase intestinal absorption of drugs such as phenolphthalein, mineral oil and quinidine, promoting drug toxicity[19]. Stool softeners in conjunction with dietary and lifestyle changes may help minimize use of laxatives. The daily dose, ranging from 50 to 500 mg, can be given with milk or fruit juice[16,19].

Laxatives

Misconceptions about the normal or desirable frequency of bowel movements, the easy availability of laxatives over the counter and ignorance of the adverse effects of these agents (Table 5) have resulted in their sometimes unwarranted use. Laxatives act in various ways; the classification in this chapter is based on their general mechanisms of action[1,16,19].

Bulk-forming laxatives e.g. psyllium, methylcellulose and calcium polycarbophil bind ions and water in the colonic lumen, resulting in increased fecal mass and water content with rapid colonic transit. Psyllium also binds bile acids, promoting their excretion and consequent reduction of cholesterol in low-density

Table 5 Laxatives: classification, dosage and adverse effects. From references 16 and 19

Laxative class	Dose range	Adverse effects*
Bulk-forming		flatulence, fecal impaction
Psyllium	1 tablespoon or 1 biscuit OD-TID	
Methylcellulose	2–4 tabs OD	
Calcium polycarbophil	1 g OD-QID	
Saline		
Magnesium salts	15–40 ml OD	magnesium toxicity
Sodium phosphate	10–30 ml OD	hypocalcemia, hyperphosphatemia
Osmotic		flatulence, abdominal cramps
Lactulose	15–30 ml OD-QID	
Glycerin	rectal suppository	
Sorbitol	15–30 ml OD-QID	
Polyethylene glycol	8 oz–4 liters OD	
Stimulant		
Phenolphthalein	30–200 mg OD	Stevens–Johnson syndrome, colitis, osteomalacia, protein-losing enteropathy
Bisacodyl	10–15 mg OD	colitis, abdominal cramps
Anthraquinones (senna, cascara)	10–30 mg OD	urine discoloration, nephritis melanosis coli
Castor oil	15–60 ml OD	colic, malabsorption
Mineral oil	15–45 ml OD	lipid pneumonitis, rectal irritation, anal leakage, malabsorption of fat-soluble vitamins and drugs

OD, once daily; TID, three times a day; QID, four times a day
* Electrolyte disturbances and volume depletion could occur to variable extent with any of the above

lipoproteins[19]. Drug interactions may occur, e.g. reduction of intestinal cardiac glycoside and salicylate absorption by cellulose, binding of warfarin by psyllium and decrease in tetracycline absorption due to calcium polycarbophil[19]. Allergic reactions, although rare, may occur to plant gums, while flatulence is common. Ingestion of these agents must be accompanied by adequate water intake to prevent esophageal and intestinal obstruction[19]. In particular, fecal impaction may occur after use of bulk-forming laxatives with insufficient fluid intake in patients who have intestinal stenosis, ulceration or adhesions. Thus it would be prudent to avoid the initiation of fiber as a remedy for constipation in the acutely ill, hospitalized, bed-bound patient.

Saline laxatives e.g. magnesium sulfate (Epsom salt), magnesium hydroxide (milk of magnesia), magnesium citrate and sodium phosphate, exert an osmotic effect to retain water in the colon. Magnesium salts also stimulate cholecystokinin release and thus increase intestinal motility. Toxicity can occur with use in renal failure[19]. Sodium phosphate worsens congestive heart failure or renal disease. Phosphate absorption can lead to hyperphosphatemia and hypocalcemia. Saline laxatives are hypertonic solutions that can result in dehydration if concurrent water intake is insufficient.

Osmotic laxatives e.g. lactulose, glycerin, sorbitol and polyethylene glycol–electrolyte solutions are neither digested nor absorbed in the small intestine and act by their osmotic properties. Bacterial metabolism of lactulose to lactate, acetate and formate in the colon and distal ileum increases the osmotic effect of the laxative, reduces luminal pH, and enhances motility and secretion[19]. Lactulose is also useful to reduce intestinal absorption of ammonia in individuals with hepatic encephalopathy. Glycerin is administered as a rectal suppository and may additionally stimulate rectal contraction. Sorbitol, another osmotic laxative, may be used by itself or as a vehicle to prevent the constipating effect of sodium polystyrene sulfonate (used in the treatment of hyperkalemia). Polyethylene glycol–electrolyte solutions, which are isotonic (isotonicity makes dehydration unlikely), can be used for initial colon cleansing prior to colonoscopy and/or long-term management of constipation. Ingestion of large volumes of these non-absorbable solutions results in efficient removal of solid wastes from the gut; contraindications include intestinal obstruction, perforation and toxic mega-colon. Polyethylene glycol, a metabolically inert polymer resistant to bacterial degradation, is now available as a laxative to treat constipation in ambulatory and long-term care facility patients[14].

Stimulant laxatives e.g. diphenylmethane derivatives (phenolphthalein, bisacodyl) and anthraquinone derivatives (senna, cascara sagrada) stimulate intestinal motility and reduce absorption of water and electrolytes from the colonic lumen. Diphenylmethane derivatives can damage enterocytes, cause colitis and lead to fluid and electrolyte deficits. Additionally, phenolphthalein has been linked to Stevens–Johnson syndrome, osteomalacia, protein-losing enteropathy and fixed drug eruptions[19]. Senna and cascara are prodrugs that are converted to active forms by colonic bacterial activity. Adverse effects of anthraquinone laxatives include urine discoloration; chronic use causes a benign, reversible pigmentation of the colonic mucosa known as melanosis coli[19].

Castor oil has a strong cathartic effect causing copious diarrhea and therefore its use is not recommended. Pancreatic lipases hydrolyze the oil in the small intestine, resulting in accumulation of ricinoleate that reduces fluid and electrolyte absorption and stimulates peristalsis[19]. The evacuation of intestinal contents is so complete that a normal bowel movement may take several days to occur. The purgative action of castor oil damages the intestinal epithelium causing colic, dehydration, electrolyte abnormalities and malabsorption.

Mineral oil penetrates and softens the feces, reducing water absorption from the colon. Adverse effects include lipid pneumonitis, anal leakage of oil, rectal irritation and malabsorption of fat-soluble vitamins (such as vitamin D) and medications; thus risk outweighs benefit[19].

In general, laxative use should be infrequent; the lowest effective dose should be administered and therapy discontinued promptly after constipation resolves. Contraindications to laxative use include cramps, colic, undiagnosed abdominal pain and acute abdomen[19]. The delay in onset of normal bowel movements after thorough intestinal evacuation (for medical procedures) may at times be erroneously labeled as 'constipation' by patients, prompting laxative abuse. Bowel habits could eventually become so abnormal (cathartic colon) that the subject relies on daily laxative use for a bowel movement. Habitual use can lead to irritable bowel syndrome, secondary aldosteronism from volume depletion, hypoalbuminemia from protein-losing enteropathy and osteomalacia from loss of vitamin D and calcium in the stool[19]. Laxatives are often excessively prescribed without a clear diagnosis of constipation in the long-term care facility either to 'prevent' constipation or as part of a standing order. Saline and stimulant laxatives are the most commonly prescribed agents for constipation in nursing homes in addition to stool softeners[6].

Enemas

Enemas distend and lavage the colon, stimulating bowel movements. Tap water enemas are relatively safe; other preparations include soap suds, mineral oil and phosphate enemas[7]. Complications such as perforation, mucosal injury and rectal ischemia occur rarely. Hyperphosphatemia, hypocalcemia and metabolic acidosis are complications of therapy with phosphate enemas; predisposing factors include dehydration, renal disease and aging[20]. Kayexalate (sodium polystyrene sulfonate) administered for treatment of hyperkalemia with sorbitol enemas, can cause colonic ulceration if cleansing tap water enemas are not administered subsequently.

Prokinetic agents

Gastric motility is stimulated by cholinergic neurons, inhibited generally by adrenergic neurons and modulated by the enteric nervous system via neurotransmitters, e.g. dopamine and serotonin[19]. Agonists of 5-HT$_4$ and motilin receptors and antagonists of D$_2$ and 5-HT$_3$ receptors stimulate gastric motility.

Metoclopromide accelerates gastric emptying and transit of intestinal contents up to the ileocecal valve; it has little effect on colonic motility[19]. The mechanism of action, although not fully understood, may be via dopamine receptor antagonism and promotion of acetylcholine release from myenteric neurons. Adverse effects may be extrapyramidal symptoms, hyperprolactinemia, anxiety, drowsiness and depression. Cisapride lacks dopamine antagonist activity. Unlike metoclopromide, it increases colonic motility. Drug interactions with cisapride resulting in fatal arrhythmias have curtailed its use. Domperidone (not available in the USA), a D$_2$ receptor antagonist with poor central nervous system penetration, decreases small intestinal transit time, but colonic motility remains unchanged. Adverse effects of domperidone include headaches and hyperprolactinemia. Prucalopride, a 5-HT$_4$ agonist, accelerates colonic transit in patients with functional constipation and is awaiting phase III trials[21]. Motilin initiates the intestinal interdigestive myoelectric complex and stimulates gastric postprandial contractions[19]. This may explain the prokinetic effect of erythromycin, which acts as an agonist at motilin receptors in the antrum and duodenum.

Surgical therapy

Subtotal colectomy with ileorectal anastomosis is performed only if medical therapy has failed to correct chronic severe incapacitating constipation, provided anorectal function is normal and intestinal pseudo-obstruction is absent[1]. Surgical complications include persistent abdominal pain, postoperative infections, diarrhea and small intestinal obstruction. Rectocele repair may improve constipation in elderly women.

Biofeedback

The modality is used for pelvic dyssynergia. Patients watch sphincter activity or pressure recordings and attempt to modify the inappropriate contraction of pelvic muscles during defecation through trial and error.[1] This technique is time-consuming and performed on an out-patient basis.

Complications

Complications from constipation frequently occur in older adults (Table 6). While fecal impaction is a common, nagging problem to patient and provider, other complications such as arrhythmias, syncope, transient ischemic attacks and cardiac ischemia are rare[22]. Longstanding constipation often results in laxative abuse. A discussion on fecal impaction and sigmoid volvulus follows.

Table 6 Complications of constipation[22]

Fecal impaction
Rectal prolapse
Hemorrhoids
Megacolon
Megarectum
Sigmoid volvulus
Cecal perforation
Arrhythmias
Cardiac ischemia
Syncope
Transient ischemic attacks

Fecal impaction

Fecal impaction usually occurs in the rectosigmoid colon. Symptoms may be misleading; they include anorexia, nausea, vomiting, spurious diarrhea (watery stool forced around the hard fecal ball), fecal incontinence, urinary frequency and/or incontinence, colonic ulceration with occult blood in stools and abdominal pain[7]. Digital rectal examination reveals the fecal mass unless impaction is proximal. In these patients, there is a need for greater rectal dilatation to stimulate defecation[7]. Management of distal fecal impaction involves manual disimpaction; proximal impaction requires enemas and laxatives. After resolution of fecal impaction, appropriate dietary modification and laxative regimens must be initiated to prevent recurrence. Regimens are individualized to suit patient preferences.

Sigmoid volvulus

Volvulus usually occurs in bed-bound, institutionalized elderly with chronic constipation[13]. Abdominal distension and cramps result. Plain radiograph of the abdomen is helpful in diagnosis. Passage of a flexible endoscope reduces the loop, failing which surgery is needed. Without treatment, the intestinal blood supply becomes compromised with subsequent fatal outcome.

FECAL INCONTINENCE

Pathophysiology

Various physiologic safeguards ensure continence; interference with any of these mechanisms can result in fecal incontinence. Voluntary contraction of the external anal sphincter allows enough time for the rectum to adapt and accommodate the feces. Contraction of the internal anal sphincter is involuntary, and the resting tone is important for constant anal closure; relaxation occurs with rectal dilatation. Action of the puborectalis muscle causes the anal canal to form an acute angle with the rectum, creating a posterior rectal pouch which accommodates more feces without increasing anal canal pressure[23]. Intra-abdominal pressure pushes the anterior rectal wall on to the upper end of the anal canal, occluding the lumen (so-called anorectal flap valve). Further, increased rectal pressure from stools lifts the anterior rectal wall and opens the valve, facilitating downward movement of feces. The perineal body bolsters the deficient anterior portion of the puborectalis. The descending colon acts as a storage for formed stools. The rich nerve supply of the lower half of the anal canal differentiates between solid stool, flatus and liquid stool and signals external sphincter contraction. Anal contour is important for complete closure of the anal canal. Cognition plays an essential role in ensuring continence. Disease processes adversely affecting any of the above factors may result in fecal incontinence (Table 7).

Evaluation

A focused history on diarrhea, constipation, perianal surgery and perineal trauma in addition to a detailed obstetric history are essential[24]. Inspection of the perianal region is indicated for scars, fistulas, external hemorrhoids and fissures. The patient is asked to bear down to detect rectal prolapse and external sphincter contraction is verified

Table 7 Causes of fecal incontinence. From references 23 and 24

Factor	Disease process
Internal anal sphincter	trauma
	anal surgery
	spinal cord lesions
	neuropathy (diabetes)
	neoplasm
	Crohn's disease
External anal sphincter	trauma
	anorectal surgery
	neoplasm
	rectal prolapse
Puborectalis and perineal body	trauma
	obstetric or gynecologic injury
Rectal sensation	impaired mental status
	diabetes mellitus
	peripheral neuropathy
	spinal cord lesions
Rectal distensibility	radiation proctitis
	inflammatory bowel disease
	rectal ischemia

during digital rectal examination. Fecal impaction must be excluded.

Anoscopy, sigmoidoscopy or colonoscopy detects scars, neoplasms and inflammatory lesions. Anorectal manometry measures the resting anal canal pressure and the maximal squeeze pressure (highest anal pressure produced during efforts to contract the external anal sphincter)[11,24]. Balloon inflation evaluates rectal compliance and sensation. Anal endosonography defines the anal sphincter anatomy prior to surgical repair. Pudendal nerve conduction is measured before sphincter repair, because the pudendal nerve innervates the external anal sphincter[24]. Defecography images the anorectal area using barium and detects rectal intussusception or prolapse; the test is of questionable benefit.

Management

Medical

Sphincter exercises benefit patients who are cognitively intact and have a functioning external sphincter. The patient contracts the sphincter while slowly counting to five in the supine posture, repetitively for 5 min, and performs this exercise 3–4 times/day. Low-residue diet may be helpful. Constipation is treated to avoid impaction with subsequent incontinence. Diarrhea should prompt investigation for the cause. Patients with spinal cord lesions, poor sphincter function and no rectal sensation benefit from regular use of enemas[24].

Surgical

Failure of medical therapy or existence of a correctable cause, e.g. obstetric trauma, favors the surgical approach. Surgery focuses on repairing the sphincters and perineal body – either direct sphincter repair or anterior sphincter repair with perineorrhaphy. Neoanal sphincters (creation of a sphincter using gracilis or gluteus muscle) and implantation of artificial sphincters are technically difficult procedures performed only in select centers[24]. Fecal diversion with either colostomy or ileostomy is an option.

Electrostimulation

Short-term stimulation of sacral nerves by electrodes implanted in the sacral foramen prevents incontinence; long-term benefit is not clear[24]. Electrostimulation is useful in those not candidates for sphincter repair.

Biofeedback

Often subjects have difficulty understanding instructions to contract their external anal sphincter and may mistakenly contract their abdominal or buttock muscles, especially after anal surgery. In such situations, an intra-anal electrode and electromyometer records sphincter contractions, enabling the patient to determine initiation and strength of sphincter contractions with conscious effort.

SUMMARY

Constipation is a frequent complaint in older adults. The role of the physician is to remove offending drugs, if any, and evaluate for underlying disorders. The US Preventive Services Task Force has recently published recommendations on screening options for colonoscopy, sigmoidoscopy, fecal occult blood testing and barium enema[25]. Colonoscopy is a useful screening and diagnostic test[26], particularly in older adults with altered bowel habits. While several pharmacologic remedies are available, dietary modification and patient education should be the primary approaches and are preferable to drug therapy. Laxatives, stool softeners and enemas, along with the administration (staffing) expenses, add substantially to the cost of chronic constipation care in nursing homes[27]. Fecal incontinence, common in the frail elderly, is an often neglected problem and a basis for social morbidity leading to institutionalization[28].

References

1. Wald A. Constipation. *Med Clin North Am* 2000;84:1231–46
2. Pare P, Ferrazzi S, Thompson WG, *et al.* An epidemiological survey of constipation in Canada: definitions, rates, demographics, and predictors of health care seeking. *Am J Gastroenterol* 2001;96:3130–7
3. Locke GR, Pemberton JH, Phillips SF. American Gastroenterological Association medical position statement: guidelines on constipation. *Gastroenterology* 2000;119:1761–78
4. Talley JN, Fleming KC, Evans JM, *et al.* Constipation in an elderly community: a study of prevalence and potential risk factors. *Am J Gastroenterol* 1996;91:19–25
5. Cheskin LJ, Kamal N, Crowell MD, *et al.* Mechanisms of constipation in older persons and effects of fiber compared with placebo. *J Am Geriatr Soc* 1995;43:666–9
6. Phillips C, Polakoff D, Maue SK. Assessment of constipation management in long-term care patients. *J Am Med Dir Assoc* 2001;2:149–54
7. De Lillo AR, Rose S. Functional bowel disorders in the geriatric patient: constipation, fecal impaction and fecal incontinence. *Am J Gastroenterol* 2000;95:901–5
8. Camilleri M, Lee JS, Viramontes B, *et al.* Insights into the pathophysiology and mechanisms of constipation, irritable bowel syndrome and diverticulosis in older people. *J Am Geriatr Soc* 2000;48:1142–50
9. Meier R, Beglinger C, Dederding JP, *et al.* Influence of age, gender, hormonal status and smoking habits on colonic transit time. *Neurogastroenterol Motil* 1995;7:235–8
10. Dharmarajan TS, Pitchumoni CS, Kokkat AJ. The aging gut. *Practical Gastroenterol* 2001;25:15–27
11. Akervall S, Nordgren S, Fasth S, *et al.* The effects of age, gender and parity on rectoanal functions in adults. *Scand J Gastroenterol* 1990;25:1247–56
12. Wilson JA. Constipation in the elderly. *Clin Geriatr Med* 1999;15:499–510

13. Abyad A, Mourad F. Constipation: common-sense care of the older patient. *Geriatrics* 1996;51:28–36

14. DiPalma AM, DiPalma JA. New perspectives on constipation – a clinician's viewpoint. *Practical Gastroenterol* 1999;23:20–41

15. Jaffe PE. Constipation. In Greene LH, Johnston WP, Lemche D, eds. *Decision Making in Medicine: An Algorithmic Approach*, 2nd edn. St Louis: Mosby, 1998:188–9

16. Harari D. Constipation in the elderly. In Hazzard WR, Blass JP, Ettinger WH Jr, *et al.*, eds. *Principles of Geriatric Medicine and Gerontology*, 4th edn. New York: McGraw-Hill, 1999:1491–505

17. McRorie J, Kesler J, Bishop L, *et al.* Effects of wheat bran and olestra on objective measures of stool and subjective reports of GI symptoms. *Am J Gastroenterol* 2000;95:1244-52

18. Johanson JF, Lafferty J. Epidemiology of fecal incontinence: the silent affliction. *Am J Gastroenterol* 1996;91:33–6

19. Brunton LL. Agents affecting gastrointestinal water flux and motility; emesis and antiemetics; bile acids and pancreatic enzymes. In Hardman JG, Limbird LE, *et al.*, eds. *Goodman and Gilman's The Pharmacologic Basis of Therapeutics*, 9th edn. New York: McGraw-Hill 1996:917–36

20. Kirschbaum B. The acidosis of exogenous phosphate intoxication. *Arch Intern Med* 1998;158:405-8

21. Camilleri M. Management of the irritable bowel syndrome. *Gastroenterology* 2001;120:652–8

22. Quirk DM, Friedman LS. Approach to gastrointestinal problems in the elderly. In Yamada T, Alpers DH, Laine L, *et al.*, eds. *Textbook of Gastroenterology*, 3rd edn. Philadelphia: Lippincott Williams and Wilkins, 1999:1015–33

23. MacLeod JH. Continence and incontinence. In *A Method of Proctology*. Hagerstown: Harper and Row, 1979:85–92

24. Soffer EE, Hull T. Fecal incontinence: a practical approach to evaluation and treatment. *Am J Gastroenterol* 2000;95:1873–80

25. Berg AO, Allan JD, Frame PS, *et al.* Screening for colorectal cancer: recommendations and rationale. US Preventive Services Task Force. *Ann Intern Med* 2002;137:129–31

26. Arce DA, Ermocilla CA, Costa H. Evaluation of constipation. *Am Fam Physician* 2002;65:2283–90

27. Pekmezaris R, Aversa L, Wolf-Klein G, *et al.* The cost of chronic constipation. *J Am Med Dir Assoc* 2002;3:224–8

28. Whitehead WE. Fecal incontinence: a neglected area of gastroenterology. *Gastroenterology* 2002;122:5

28 Thermoregulation and aging

T.S. Dharmarajan, MD, FACP, AGSF, and May Luz F. Bullecer, MD

INTRODUCTION

Several physiologic changes occur with age; impaired thermal regulation is one of them[1]. The presence of multiple chronic illnesses, along with the use of numerous medications, predispose the elderly to temperature dysregulation. This vulnerability to hyperthermia and/or hypothermia in the geriatric population leads to increased morbidity and mortality.

PHYSIOLOGY OF TEMPERATURE REGULATION

Temperature regulation comprises an interplay of body metabolism, the neuroendocrine system and the hypothalamus[2,3]. The normal internal temperature in adults ranges from 96.8 to 99.5°F (36–37.5°C); in the elderly, oral readings range from 96.4 to 98.2°F (35.7–36.7°C) and rectal readings from 98.2 to 98.9°F (36.7–37°C). This narrow range of temperature is maintained by a fine-tuned equilibrium between heat produced, heat conserved and heat lost. Heat production depends on basal metabolic processes: muscle activity such as shivering, which increases heat production two-to five-fold[1]; and the effects of hormones (such as thyroxine and catecholamines). Heat conservation is attained through the insulating effects of skin, subcutaneous fat and muscle, as well as vasoconstriction[4]. The mechanisms of heat transfer to the environment are mainly through radiation (electromagnetic transfer of energy), conduction (direct heat transfer to adjacent cooler areas), convection (heat transfer through air currents) and evaporation (dissipation of heat through conversion of sweat to water vapor)[1,3]. The skin is endowed with 'cold' and 'warm' receptors; these peripheral thermoreceptors transmit impulses to the central receptors integrated in the preoptic area of the anterior and posterior hypothalamus. As the core temperature increases, skin vasodilatation, sweating, decreased heat production and behavior modification (moving to a cooler environment, removal of clothing, decreasing activity level) follow. A decrease in core temperature causes vasoconstriction, piloerection, increased heat production, and again alteration in behavior (transfer to a warmer environment, adding more clothing, increase in activity level).

It should be recognized that, in the geriatric age group, cognitive impairment and physical limitation in mobility may interfere with the behavioral response. Further, with aging there is reduced ability to perceive cold or heat, and defective heat generation, conservation and loss. In addition, the ability to preserve volume status is impaired. Renal concentrating and diluting functions are subnormal, interfering with the ability to conserve or excrete water. Likewise, the ability of the kidneys to conserve or excrete a sodium load is impaired with aging[5,6]. Obese older subjects have a higher risk for hyperthermia due to reduced dermal blood flow, lower sweat gland mass and a greater layer of adipose tissue for insulation[7] (Table 1).

Table 1 Age-related factors that impair temperature regulation. From references 1, 3 and 11

Reduction of the ability to sense warmth and cold
Defective heat generation
   diminished basal metabolism
   less efficient shivering response
Defective heat retention and loss
   impaired skin vasodilatory and vasoconstrictive
     response
   blunted heart rate and cardiac output response
     to exercise
   reduced sweat gland function
   decreased subcutaneous fat
Impaired maintenance of volume status
   decreased response to thirst
   reduced renal concentrating and diluting capacity
   impaired renal ability to conserve and excrete sodium
Alteration in pharmacokinetics and dynamics

Table 2 Causes of thermoregulatory disorders in the elderly. From references 1, 3, 9–11, 15–17

Hyperthermia
Environmental (heat exposure), e.g. prickly heat, heat
   edema, heat syncope, non-exertional heat stroke
Diseases, e.g. thyrotoxic crisis, pheochromocytoma,
   pontine hemorrhage
Drugs
   drug-induced hyperthermia, e.g. antihistamines,
     anticholinergics, diuretics, β-agonists
   neuroleptic malignant syndrome, e.g. phenothiazines,
     butyrophenones, tricyclic antidepressants,
     metoclopramide, fluoxetine, clozapine
   serotonin syndrome, e.g. selective serotonin reuptake
     inhibitors, buspirone, meperidine, trazodone,
     selegiline, phenelzine, levodopa
   malignant hyperthermia e.g. halothane,
     succinylcholine

Hypothermia
Environmental (cold exposure)
Secondary
   sepsis
   drugs, e.g. sedatives, alcohol, clonidine,
     phenothiazines, opioids, hypoglycemic agents,
     lithium, cyclic antidepressants
   metabolic abnormalities, e.g. hypothyroidism,
     hypoglycemia, hypoadrenalism, malnutrition
   hypothalamic lesions
   renal and hepatic failure
   exfoliative skin lesions and burns

HYPERTHERMIA

Hyperthermia is defined as 'an elevation of body temperature above the hypothalamic set point due to insufficient heat dissipation or excessive heat production'[8]. Fever is 'temperature elevation due to an increase in hypothalamic set point as a result of stimulation by pyrogenic cytokines'[8,9]. The causes of hyperthermia include exposure to environmental heat, several diseases (e.g. thyrotoxic crisis, pheochromocytoma) and drugs (Table 2).

Causes and clinical manifestations

Environmental heat-related illnesses usually occur during the summer months; however, excessive use of indoor heat during winter may also be contributory. Prickly heat, heat edema, heat tetany, heat cramps, heat syncope, heat exhaustion and heat stroke are all manifestations of heat illness[1]. In particular, the elderly are predisposed to: prickly heat, characterized by pruritic papulovesicular skin lesions; heat edema, pitting in nature involving the hands and feet, resulting from prolonged exposure to heat; heat syncope, a type of vasovagal syncope from arteriolar vasodilatation without reflex tachycardia, resulting from prolonged standing in a warm environment and worsened by the use of β-blockers and calcium channel blockers; and non-exertional/classic heat stroke, occurring in those who have concomitant chronic medical conditions that inhibit appropriate thermoregulation and physical limitations that prevent moving away from a warm environment. The presence of mental status changes and hyperthermia (temperature greater than 105°F (40.5°C) characterizes heat stroke[1,9–11].

Several diseases predispose to hyperthermia in older subjects. The mechanisms for hyperthermia in thyrotoxic crisis are not well understood, but may be related to the release of bound hormones resulting in increased metabolic activity[12]. This syndrome is typified by delirium, temperature of 105°F or higher, tachycardia, restlessness and hypotension. Pheochromocytomas, tumors that produce, store and release catecholamines, occur in all ages but are more common in the young. In the presence of paroxysms of hypertensive crisis, tachycardia and apprehension occur[13], along with catecholamine release, increased metabolic activity and hyperthermia[1,3]. Pontine hemorrhage is a well-known cause of hyperthermia. Infections, both bacterial and viral syndromes, should always be considered and excluded.

Several medications predispose older subjects to thermoregulatory disorders[14]. These conditions may be primarily drug related or secondary to genetic predilection. A description of drug-induced hyperthermia with an emphasis on neuroleptic malignant syndrome, serotonin syndrome and malignant hyperthermia follows.

Drug-induced hyperthermia

This may occur with the use of antihistamines, tricyclic antidepressants and anticholinergic agents, by inhibiting sweat production through their effects on the parasympathetic nervous system. Diuretics decrease intravascular volume, predisposing to dehydration with impairment of heat loss and sweating. β-Agonists and thyroid hormones stimulate metabolism and heat production, while β-blockers modify cardiac response to stress, affecting temperature regulation[3,15]. As older subjects are typically on several medications, hyperthermia as a drug-induced adverse effect should be borne in mind.

Neuroleptic malignant syndrome

This occurs in all ages with a mortality rate of 10–20%[4,14,15]. Neuroleptic malignant syndrome is an idiosyncratic adverse drug reaction. The exact mechanism is not well understood, but it is believed to result from dopaminergic blockade in the basal ganglia and hypothalamus[16]. Initiation of antipsychotic neuroleptic agents or sudden withdrawal of dopamine agonists (levodopa) for the treatment of Parkinson's disease may precipitate the syndrome. Manifestations include hyperthermia, delirium and muscle rigidity, with consequent rhabdomyolysis and autonomic dysfunction occurring from a few days to several weeks after the initiation of antipsychotic agents. Thus, neuroleptic malignant syndrome is a differential diagnosis in geriatric subjects with delirium and hyperthermia[14]. Dopamine agonists are helpful in the management.

Serotonin syndrome

This results from increased stimulation of the central nervous system (CNS) 5-hydroxytryptamine 1_A receptors with manifestations that may be difficult to differentiate from neuroleptic malignant syndrome[16,17] (Table 3). The use of selective serotonin reuptake inhibitors has led to its increased incidence. Symptoms may occur within minutes to a few hours after the inciting drug is administered. Hyperthermia, muscle rigidity and altered mental status are also noted, but are less pronounced than with neuroleptic malignant syndrome[17]. While features overlap, muscle rigidity and rhabdomyolysis are more pronounced with neuroleptic malignant syndrome, and myoclonus is rarer. Serotonin antagonists may be of help.

Malignant hyperthermia

This is a genetic disorder, mostly autosomal dominant, due to a mutation of the calcium channel receptor in the sarcoplasmic reticulum of skeletal muscle. Exposure to halothane or succinylcholine causes uncontrolled calcium efflux, manifested as tetany, resulting in increased skeletal muscle metabolism and heat production.

Diagnosis

A thorough history, review of prescribed and over-the-counter medications, and physical

Table 3 A comparison between serotonin syndrome (SS) and neuroleptic malignant syndrome (NMS). From references 14 and 17

	SS	NMS
Receptor involved	5-hydroxytryptamine$_{1A}$ stimulation	dopamine blockade
Onset of manifestations	abrupt (minutes to hours)	gradual (days to weeks)
Hyperthermia	common	observed
Autonomic instability	observed	common
Delirium	observed	common
Muscle rigidity	seldom	common
Rhabdomyolysis	seldom	common
Myoclonus	observed (lower extremities)	seldom
Exaggerated DTR	observed	seldom
Leukocytosis	seldom	common
Therapeutic agents	serotonin antagonists may help	dopamine agonists

DTR, deep tendon reflexes; common, ~ 90%; observed, ~ 50%; seldom, < 20%

examination aid in diagnosis. For those with cognitive impairment, the caregiver's role is important, to obtain the relevant history such as housing conditions (especially ventilation, air conditioning), concomitant chronic medical illness and medications. Physical evaluation may reveal hyperthermia, autonomic instability (including labile blood pressure, tachycardia, arrhythmias), altered mentation ranging from confusion to coma, and muscle rigidity. An underlying infectious etiology should be meticulously looked for.

Initial laboratory studies must include complete blood count for leukocytosis, especially in the presence of infection, and thrombocytopenia for possible consumptive coagulopathy (accompanied by elevated prothrombin time and activated partial thromboplastin time). Electrolytes, blood urea nitrogen, creatinine and liver function tests should be obtained. Creatine phosphokinase and urinalysis will help determine the presence of rhabdomyolysis. Chest X-ray will aid in excluding a pneumonic process. Thyroid function tests will exclude thyroid crises, and drug screening will help to exclude drug toxicity. Computed tomography of the brain and lumbar puncture are relevant when underlying CNS etiology is suspected[10]. The combination of exposure to heat, hyperthermia and CNS dysfunction points to heat stroke, while the use of medications may suggest a drug-related etiology.

Management

Stabilization of the airway, breathing and circulation with simultaneous rapid cooling to decrease the temperature to 102°F (38.8°C) within the hour of presentation is acceptable[10,18]. Cooling measures include removal of the clothing, and application of ice packs applied to the scalp, axilla, neck and groin[19]. However, the best method is by evaporation and convection, with the use of water spray mists and large fans blowing over the subject[1]. The use of iced peritoneal lavage is invasive and technically difficult[1,3,10].

Treatment of neuroleptic malignant syndrome includes withdrawal of the offending medication, and use of dopaminergic agonists, e.g. bromocriptine 2.5–7.5 mg every 8 h or amantadine 100–300 mg daily in divided doses (adjust for renal status). Muscle relaxants, e.g. dantrolene 0.8–3 mg/kg every 6 h to a maximum of 10 mg/kg per day, and benzodiazepines (indirectly increase dopamine activity through their action on the basal ganglia and substantia nigra)[20], are found effective. Cooling measures should nevertheless be instituted.

For serotonin syndrome, withdrawal of the causative medications and administration of cyproheptadine, an antiserotonergic agent, in doses of 0.5 mg/kg per day is helpful, aside from the general supportive and cooling measures[17].

Administration of dantrolene may be helpful in malignant hyperthermia, as it inhibits the release of calcium from the sarcoplasmic reticulum[10].

Some general comments are worth remembering. No pharmacological agent appears to enhance cooling by itself; the role of antipyretic therapy is not clear either[21]. There is no data from controlled studies comparing the benefits of the various cooling techniques. These cooling techniques may be classified as external (cold water immersion, cold pack application, cooling blankets) or internal (iced gastric or peritoneal lavage), and work on the principle of conduction. Fans and body cooling units work on the basis of evaporative or convective cooling[21]. Prompt treatment is important as residual brain damage may occur with delay, resulting in high mortality. Institutions must therefore be equipped to measure high temperatures in the range of 40–47°C. Ongoing monitoring is recommended for rhabdomyolysis, renal injury, electrolyte imbalance, respiratory failure, seizures, hypotension and other organ failure[21].

HYPOTHERMIA

Hypothermia is common in the elderly and defined as 'a core body temperature (tympanic, esophageal, rectal or urine) of less than 95°F (35°C)'[1-3]. At this temperature humans lose their capacity to generate sufficient heat to maintain body functions[1]. As the posterior hypothalamus receives signals through the spinothalamic tract and senses the cold temperature of the cerebral blood flow, it acts to increase core heat production within the insulating fat layer and reduces heat transfer. Increased release of catecholamines results in peripheral vasoconstriction, rapid heart and respiratory rates, increase in cardiac output and blood pressure, as well as heat production from muscle contraction[1,4]. The shivering mechanism is preserved in the elderly; however, the latency of shivering is prolonged in response to cold exposure, and a lower peak of muscle contraction is achieved.

Older individuals are predisposed to hypothermia, be it environmental (due to cold exposure) or secondary (the presence of underlying or predisposing factors) (see Table 2). As stated earlier, age-related physiologic changes are a predisposition. A decrease in lean body mass occurs, along with reduction in basal metabolic rate and thermogenesis. Older subjects also have an abnormal vasoconstrictor response to cold, with decreased ability to conserve heat. Secondary debilitating conditions, metabolic abnormalities (hypoglycemia, hypothyroidism, hypoadrenalism and malnutrition), sepsis, hypothalamic lesions, renal failure, hepatic failure, burns, exfoliative skin diseases and several drugs increase the risk[1,3]. The presence of hypothermia should be taken as a possible warning sign for infection; here, failure to treat infection influences outcome.

Drugs are significant contributors to hypothermia. Sedatives and alcohol can impair the sensitivity to cold temperature and interfere with hypothalamic thermoregulatory function[3]. Hypoglycemics reduce the substrate for thermogenesis. Antihypertensives, especially the centrally acting sympatholytic agents (clonidine, reserpine and guanabenz) inhibit reflex vasoconstriction. β-Blockers affect heat production. Phenothiazines inhibit the shivering response[3,4].

Causes and clinical manifestations

In older subjects, subnormal temperatures may be experienced for days or weeks prior to eventual hypothermia. The initial response to hypothermia manifests as increased metabolic rate, heart rate, respiratory rate and blood pressure in addition to vasoconstriction and shivering. As temperature drops further the manifestations are protean. Mild hypothermia (89–95°F; 32–35°C) may present with fatigue, confusion, apathy, lethargy, clumsiness, ataxia and cool skin. Cold stimulates the production of copious bronchial secretions (cold bronchorrhea) and together with inhibition of the cough reflex predisposes to pneumonia. Moderate hypothermia (82–89°F; 27.7–32°C) results in cessation of shivering, stiff muscles, and stupor that may progress to coma. Cardiac output along with heart rate, blood pressure and respiratory rate begin to decline. Oxygen consumption decreases by 50% as temperature reaches 82°F. Arrhythmias are common with prolongation of PR, QRS and QT intervals. Atrial fibrillation and ventricular premature contractions can occur. Severe hypothermia (less than 82°F) increases the risk of ventricular fibrillation markedly. Non-reactive and dilated pupils, absent deep tendon reflexes and diminished response to pain may be noted. At 80°F (26.6°C) oxygen consumption is decreased to 25% and J or Osborn waves (second upward deflection immediately following the S wave) may be seen at the junction of the QRS and ST segment in the electrocardiogram[3,19]. At 65°F (18°C) asystole results and a flat line on the electroencephalogram is observed[3]. Caution should be exercised in pronouncing death in the presence of hypothermia.

Diagnosis

The use of special low-reading thermometers renders the diagnosis of hypothermia possible[1–3]. The core temperature may be measured by using rectal, esophageal, tympanic or freshly voided urine readings. For rectal temperature it is essential that the thermometer probe be inserted to approximately 15 cm in the rectum; rectal temperature is 1°F higher than the oral temperature[1]. An astute observation for the subtle signs of hypothermia helps diagnose mild and moderate cases[1], bearing in mind that hypothermia can occur in any type of weather[2].

In addition to routine tests, laboratory assessment includes examination of the endocrine, hepatic and renal functions. An infectious etiology should be investigated appropriately with a chest X-ray (to exclude pneumonia), blood cultures, urinalysis (urosepsis) and even cerebrospinal fluid evaluation for CNS infections, if suspected. Other tests include electrocardiograms, cardiac enzymes, toxicology screen, coagulation profile and arterial blood gas. Care should be exercised with interpretation of laboratory data, as the patient's status is labile and test results are prone to wide fluctuations. Platelet function and clotting factors are affected, with consequent coagulopathy resembling disseminated intravascular coagulopathy. Hypoxemia results from ventilation perfusion mismatch, left shift of the oxyhemoglobin curve and increased blood viscosity. Metabolic acidosis occurs, due to reduced clearance of lactate and acid by the kidneys. Serum glucose may be elevated, due to diminished secretion of insulin. Both hyperkalemia (from metabolic acidosis) and hypokalemia (from reduced tubular absorption) may result. Elevated cardiac enzymes without ischemic changes in the electrocardiogram may be an artifact or signify subendocardial damage or small transmural infarctions[4].

Management

Like any medical emergency, management of hypothermia should include stabilization of the airway, breathing and circulation. Therapy comprises correction of fluid and electrolyte balance, avoidance of further heat loss, attaining an acceptable core temperature and evaluating for an underlying basis[2,22]. Suspicion for infection warrants the use of

Table 4 Thermoregulatory disorders: preventive measures

General
Educate patients and caregivers on risks and presentation of hyper- and hypothermia
Ensure comfortable indoor temperature
Ensure thermostat and equipment (heating/cooling) in working order
Review medications, revise as appropriate
Identify patients at risk (dementia, limited mobility, poor living conditions)
Provide early assistance to those at risk

Hyperthermia
Ensure adequate fluid intake
Provide adequate ventilation and cooling
Minimize prolonged exposure to direct sunlight during warm weather
Decrease rigorous physical activity in a warm environment
Use appropriate light, loose clothing

Hypothermia
Provide appropriately warmed meals
Avoid leaving the windows open during cold weather
Recommend immediate drying of the body after bathing
Promote physical activities, e.g. exercise program
Use appropriate (multilayered) clothing

empiric antibiotic therapy. In those with mild hypothermia (more than 89°F) and normal cardiac rhythm, removal of wet clothing and passive rewarming with blankets is appropriate and the safest method of treatment. Active external rewarming with the use of electric heated blankets, warm mattresses, submersion in warm tub water and heat lamps are not recommended for use. These methods may cause the return of the sequestered cool blood from the surface to the core, termed an 'after drop'; peripheral vasodilatation may result in hypotension[1,3,4]. Warm, humidified oxygen is simple and provides non-invasive active core rewarming; it is recommended for use in all instances of hypothermia in older subjects[1,2]. Other methods for active core rewarming include: heated intravenous fluids (normal saline) up to 104°F (40°C), bladder and gastric irrigation, mediastinal lavage, extracorporeal circulation, and peritoneal and hemodialysis. In moderate and severe hypothermia, active core rewarming is suggested.

Treatment of the underlying etiology, if known, should be implemented (e.g. thyroid hormone for myxedema, steroids for adrenal insufficiency, glucose for hypoglycemia, antibiotics for infection). Medications should be administered with caution in hypothermia, as drug effects may be erratic, needing frequent alterations in regimen. Following cardiac arrest, cardiopulmonary resuscitation should be continued until the temperature is at least 89°F (31.6°C). The lowest temperature recorded from which successful resuscitation was performed is 58.8°F (14.8°C)[23].

PREVENTIVE MEASURES

Education of the elderly patient and caregiver plays an important role in the prevention of hyperthermia and hypothermia. The need to wear appropriate apparel is emphasized. During summer, light and loose clothing gives comfort, while in winter, layers of warm clothing are recommended. Suitable indoor conditions ought to be maintained by ensuring that the thermostat, air conditioners, fans and heaters are in working condition. Adequate fluid intake is enforced, with consideration for pre-existing medical conditions. Periodic review of the entire drug regimen will help, e.g. indication for diuretics and the need for or restriction of water intake. Hot meals and drinks may be appropriate when the subject is exposed to cold temperatures, whereas cold refreshments are helpful during warm and humid conditions. The elderly are instructed to limit outdoor physical activity during hot weather. The presence of cognitive impairment, limited physical mobility, poor living conditions and inadequate family or caregiver support systems magnify the difficulty in the implementation of preventive measures in general (Table 4).

SUMMARY

Thermoregulatory disorders are more common in the elderly than in the young. Physiologic changes that accompany the aging process predispose the geriatric patient to hyperthermia and hypothermia, especially in the presence of underlying co-morbidity. In particular, physical limitations, cognitive impairment and a variety of medications may play a role. Appropriate use of preventive measures goes a long way in minimizing morbidity and mortality.

The occurrence of hyper- and hypothermia appears to be on the increase. Thermoregulatory failure and impaired stress response in the elderly may be a basis for progression of these disorders and increase in resultant tissue injury. Research in the understanding of cellular and molecular responses to thermal injuries will help achieve better preventive and management strategies in the future[21].

References

1. Harchelroad F. Acute thermoregulatory disorders. *Clin Geriatr Med* 1993;9:621–37
2. Dharmarajan TS, Manalo MG, Manalac MM, Kanagala M. Hypothermia in the nursing home: adverse outcomes in two older men. *J Am Med Dir Assoc* 2002;3: S35–S38
3. Brody GM. Hyperthermia and hypothermia in the elderly. *Clin Geriatr Med* 1994;10: 213–29
4. Hirsch CH. Hypothermia and hyperthermia. In Duthie EH Jr, Katz PR, eds. *Practice of Geriatrics*, 3rd edn. Philadelphia, PA: WB Saunders, 1998:244–55
5. Dharmarajan TS, Ugalino JT. The aging process. In Dreger D, Krumm B, eds. *Hospital Physician Geriatric Board Review Manual*. Wayne, PA: Turner White Communications, 2000;1:12
6. Taffet GE. Age related physiologic changes. In Cobbs EL, Duthie EH Jr, Murphy JB, eds. *Geriatrics Review Syllabus*, 4th edn. Dubuque, Iowa: Kendall/Hunt Publishing, 1999;10–23
7. Bar-Or O, Lundgren H, Buskirk ER. Heat tolerance of exercising obese and lean women. *J Appl Physiol* 1969;26:403–9
8. Gelfand JA, Dinarello CA. Alterations in body temperature. In Fauci AS, Braunwald E, Isselbacher KJ, *et al.*, eds. *Harrison's Principles of Internal Medicine*, 14th edn. New York: McGraw Hill: 1998:84–9
9. Simon HB. Current concepts: hyperthermia. *N Engl J Med* 1993;329:483–7
10. Mechem CC. Severe hyperthermia: heat stroke; neuroleptic malignant syndrome; and malignant hyperthermia. *UpToDate* 2000;8:3
11. Khosla R, Guntupalli KK. Environmental emergencies: heat related illnesses. *Crit Care Clin* 1999;15:251–63
12. Wartofsky L. Diseases of the thyroid. In Fauci A, Braunwald E, Isselbacher, *et al.*, eds. *Harrison's Principles of Internal Medicine*, 14th edn. New York: McGraw Hill, 1998:2013–35
13. Landsberg S, Young J. Pheochromocytoma. In Fauci AS, Braunwald E, Isselbacher KJ,

et al., eds. *Harrison's Principles of Internal Medicine*, 14th edn. New York: McGraw Hill, 1998:2057–60

14. Dharmarajan TS, Bullecer MF, Gorich G. Drug related hyperthermia. *J Am Med Dir Assoc* 2001;2:160–5

15. Chan TC, Evans SD, Clark RF. Drug induced hyperthermia. *Crit Care Clin* 1997;13:785–808

16. Carbone JR. The neuroleptic malignant and serotonin syndromes. *Emerg Med Clin North Am* 2000;18:317–25

17. Mills KC. Serotonin syndrome a clinical update. *Crit Care Clin* 1997;13:763–83

18. Abrass IB. Disorders of temperature regulation. In Hazzard WR, Blass JP, Ettinger WH, *et al.*, eds. *Principles of Geriatric Medicine and Gerontology*, 4th edn. New York: McGraw Hill, 1999:1437–41

19. Cohen R, Moelleken BRW. Disorders due to physical agents. In Tierney LM, McPhee SJ, Papadakis MA, eds. *Current Medical Diagnosis and Treatment*, 38th edn. Stamford, CT: Appleton & Lange, 1999: 1474–94

20. Khaldarov V. Benzodiazepines for treatment of neuroleptic malignant syndrome. *Hosp Physician* 2000;36:51–5

21. Bouchama A, Knochel JP. Heat stroke. *New Engl J Med* 2002;346:1978–88

22. Morgan LW. Hypothermia. In Ham RJ, Sloane PD, Warshaw A, eds. *Primary Care Geriatrics: A Case Based Approach*, 4th edn. St Louis: Mosby, 2002;649–55

23. Matz R. Hypothermia: mechanisms and countermeasures. *Hosp Pract* 1986;21:45

29 Dementia

T.S. Dharmarajan, MD, FACP, AGSF, and Joey T. Ugalino, MD

Dementia is characterized by progressive loss of memory and other cognitive domains, affecting an individual's ability to maintain normal social or occupational function. Behavioral problems (e.g. wandering, agitation, delusions, hallucinations) are common accompaniments, increasing caregiver despair, often leading to institutionalization. The causes of dementia are multiple (Table 1), with the most common being Alzheimer's disease (over half), diffuse Lewy body dementia, frontotemporal dementia and vascular dementia[1].

ALZHEIMER'S DEMENTIA

Alzheimer's disease is a progressive neurodegenerative disorder seen in older adults; it is the most common cause of dementia in the elderly and the underlying disorder in over 50% of individuals with significant memory loss[2]. The disease was named after Alois Alzheimer, a German neurologist who cared for Augusta D, hospitalized from 1901 to 1906 for intolerable paranoid delusions, confusion, agitation and aggressive behavior[3]. Following the patient's death, Dr Alzheimer

Table 1 Etiology of dementia in older adults: common causes

Cause	Examples
Degenerative disorders	Alzheimer's disease frontotemporal dementia Lewy body dementia Pick's disease Parkinson's disease
Vascular dementia	large or small vessel disease vasculitis
Metabolic and endocrine	hypothyroidism, hyperthyroidism uremic encephalopathy hepatic encephalopathy vitamin deficiency (B_{12}, folic acid, nicotinic acid)
Infection based	neurosyphilis Jakob–Creutzfeldt disease HIV dementia
Toxin related	alcohol (Korsakoff's psychosis, Wernicke's syndrome) heavy metals medication toxicity
Miscellaneous	post-traumatic encephalopathy intracranial tumor normal pressure hydrocephalus subdural hematoma anoxic encephalopathy

discovered clumps (subsequently identified as senile plaques) and knots (later termed neurofibrillary tangles) in the brain biopsy, findings now considered anatomical hall-marks of the disease.

In the USA, about 4 million people suffer from Alzheimer's disease, impacting on health care to the tune of more than $65 billion annually in the 1990s[4]. The number is expected to increase as the population ages. The prevalence of the disease increases exponentially with age; the risk of developing Alzheimer's disease doubles every 5 years between 65 and 85 years of age, with approximately half the people at age 85 afflicted with the disease[5].

Classification of Alzheimer's disease

Based on the age when symptoms are evident, individuals may be termed to have early-onset or late-onset Alzheimer's disease; the former occurs in 5–10% of cases while the latter accounts for the rest[2].

Familial Alzheimer's disease manifests early, usually between the ages of 30 and 60 years. Nearly 50% have inherited mutations in one of several genes: amyloid precursor protein (APP) gene on chromosome 21, presenilin 1 gene on chromosome 14 and presenilin 2 gene on chromosome 1[2]. APP gene mutation leads to formation of β-amyloid (the core substance in neuritic plaques); affected individuals are rare worldwide. Likewise, cases of presenilin 2 gene mutation are rare (seen in some German families), while mutation of the presenilin 1 gene is common. All mutations are transmitted as an autosomal dominant trait disorder.

More common than familial Alzheimer's disease is late-onset Alzheimer's disease with symptoms of dementia manifesting after age 65. In some cases, a susceptibility gene has been identified. Apolipoprotein E (APOE) is a cholesterol-carrier protein usually found in very low-density lipoprotein (VLDL), high-density lipoprotein (HDL) and chylomicrons. The APOE gene is located on chromosome 19 and has three alleles: $\epsilon 2$, $\epsilon 3$, and $\epsilon 4$. While the risk of acquiring Alzheimer's disease is increased in individuals with at least one APOE $\epsilon 4$ allele, the $\epsilon 2$ allele is considered to be protective and $\epsilon 3$ appears to be the most common inherited allele. APOE $\epsilon 4$ is not invariably associated with Alzheimer's disease; many carriers do not get the disease.

The National Institute of Neurological and Communicative Disorders and Stroke and the Alzheimer's Disease and Related Disorders Association (NINCDS-ADRDA) criteria for clinical diagnosis classifies Alzheimer's disease into three categories: possible – typical clinical presentation with the presence of additional systemic or brain disorder known to cause dementia but not considered the primary cause; probable – typical clinical presentation with no other identifiable causes of dementia; and definite – typical clinical presentation with tissue confirmation through brain biopsy[6]. Other classifications exist (e.g. the American Psychiatric Association's DSM-IV, the World Health Organization's ICD-9); these basically share the same criteria[2].

Pathophysiology

Acetylcholine is a neurotransmitter that links the hippocampus to the cerebral cortex. Through the action of an enzyme, acetyltransferase, acetylcholine is formed from choline and acetyl CoA, is released from vesicles in the pre-synaptic neuron and binds to post-synaptic receptors. Thereafter, cholinesterase enzymes break down acetylcholine into acetate and choline. The two forms of cholinesterases are acetylcholinesterase (predominant in the brain) and butyrylcholinesterase (predominant in the periphery).

The primary deficit in Alzheimer's disease is impairment of the cholinergic system in the brain, particularly those areas involved in learning and memory[7]. The level of choline acetyltransferase, responsible for the synthesis of acetylcholine, is decreased by 58–90% in the hippocampus and neocortex. In addition, a degeneration of cholinergic neurons occurs in the basal forebrain[8,9]. Thus, a progressive decrease in acetylcholine production occurs. Other neurotransmitters (e.g. norepinephrine, glutamate and corticotropin releasing factor) may also be involved in cognitive dysfunction[2].

The hallmark anatomical findings in Alzheimer's disease are the neuritic plaques and neurofibrillary tangles typically concentrated in the cortex and limbic system[2]. Neuritic plaques are rich in β-amyloid peptides that accumulate outside the neuron from abnormal processing of glycoprotein APPs. Neurofibrillary tangles, on the other hand, result when the neuronal cytoskeleton collapses because of unstable microtubules.

While it is not clear as to how the disease results, it is evident that tangles develop inside the neurons and plaques outside the brain cells; whether they occur in sequence or together is uncertain. The relation of tau to β-amyloid is not resolved. Secretases make proteins called β-amyloid (excessively in Alzheimer's disease), being snipped off a larger, so-called APP. These plaques enlarge and get denser, triggering reactions to kill other cells. Tau is a molecule that maintains microtubules to support the cell structure, resembling a railroad track; chemical change (hyperphosphorylation) causes an alteration in the tau molecules, such that the 'railroad ties' ('railway sleepers') begin to get twisted, resulting in a tangle and cell death.

Risk factors

Several risk factors have been associated with Alzheimer's disease (Table 2). The risk of acquiring the disease increases exponentially with advancing age. Women are afflicted more with the disease partly due to their longer life expectancy. Higher education may have a protective effect, perhaps on the basis of enhanced cognitive reserve. An inherited mutation in some genes (APP, presenilin 1 and presenilin 2) may lead to early-onset

Table 2 Risk factors for Alzheimer's dementia

Increasing age
Female gender
Level of education
Genetic
  apolipoprotein ε4 (chromosome 19)
  amyloid precursor protein gene (chromosome 21)
  presenilin 1 gene (chromosome 14)
  presenilin 2 gene (chromosome 1)
Head trauma
Toxins

dementia. A family history of Alzheimer's disease or inheritance of the apolipoprotein ε4 allele(s) increases the risk of developing dementia. Head trauma may be a risk factor only in individuals with an APO ε4 allele[6]. An elevated plasma homocysteine level has recently been described as an independent risk factor for dementia[10]. Homocysteine levels rise with age and increase the risk of Alzheimer's disease or other dementia; the mechanism appears to be oxidative vascular injury resulting in a prothrombotic state and development of atherosclerosis[11]. Thyroid disease has been considered a risk; estrogen and non-steroidal auti-inflammatory drugs (NSAIDs) are discussed under adjuvant therapy.

Clinical course

The duration of Alzheimer's disease is 3–20 years, with a mean of 8–10 years[12]. Frequently, the clinical feature that brings an older adult to the doctor is short-term memory loss or forgetfulness. Still later, a progressive decline in cognition and function is observed. In the early stages, aside from recent memory loss, the individual may encounter difficulties in managing finances, word finding and learning directions in new places. In the next stage, remote memory is also affected. Relatives and friends are now considered strangers. The individual does not recognize familiar surroundings and may

Table 3   Diagnostic criteria for dementia of the Alzheimer's type. From reference 13

A. The development of multiple cognitive deficits manifested by both

    (1) memory impairment (impairment of the ability to learn new information or to recall previously learned information)

    (2) one (or more) of the following cognitive disturbances:

        (a) aphasia (language disturbance)

        (b) apraxia (impaired ability to carry out motor activities despite intact motor function)

        (c) agnosia (failure to recognize or identify objects despite intact sensory function)

        (d) disturbance in executive functioning (i.e. planning, organizing, sequencing, abstracting)

B. The cognitive deficits in Criteria A1 and A2 each cause significant impairment in social or occupational functioning and represent a significant decline from a previous level of functioning.

C. The course is characterized by gradual onset and continuing cognitive decline.

D. The cognitive deficits in Criteria A1 and A2 are not due to any of the following:

    (1) other central nervous system conditions that cause progressive deficits in memory and cognition (e.g. cerebrovascular disease, Parkinson's disease, Huntington's disease, subdural hematoma, normal pressure hydrocephalus, brain tumor)

    (2) systemic conditions that are known to cause dementia (e.g. hypothyroidism, vitamin B_{12} or folic acid deficiency, niacin deficiency, hypercalcemia, neurosyphilis, HIV infection)

    (3) substance-induced conditions

E. The deficits do not occur exclusively during the course of a delirium

F. The disturbance is not better accounted for by another Axis I disorder (e.g. Major Depressive Disorder, Schizophrenia)

Reprinted with permission from the Diagnostic and Statistical Manual of Mental Disorders. Copyright 1994 American Psychiatric Association

get lost; wandering is often a troublesome feature, particularly to the caregiver. Speech deteriorates as aphasia worsens, with the vocabulary becoming sparser. Judgement becomes impaired. In the late stages, the individual develops complete dependence for activities of daily living (ADL) and is unable to provide basic self-care. The patient is incapable of feeding and eventually may not swallow food placed in the mouth. The individual eventually becomes bedridden and develops urinary and bowel incontinence. The vocabulary is now only a few words with echolalia and palilalia apparent in some. The causes of death are usually complications from restricted mobility such as aspiration pneumonia, urinary tract infection or pressure ulcers, often associated with malnutrition[6].

Behavioral problems are common in all stages of the disease and are often the triggering points in institutionalization, compounded by increased caregiver burden. Wandering, sleep/wake disorders, agitation, aggressive behavior, delusions (usually paranoia) and hallucinations are some of the behavioral disorders seen.

Evaluation

A clinical diagnosis of Alzheimer's dementia can be made reliably following evaluation (Table 3)[13]. Alzheimer's disease is no longer a diagnosis of exclusion. A focused history and physical examination is the initial step when an older adult presents with memory loss. The objective is to delineate any risk factor or etiology for memory impairment, and offer remedial measures. It is best to interview the older adult and the caregiver separately, if possible. Any information obtained from the affected individual requires corroboration by the family or caregiver. Eventually, both patient and caregiver may be interviewed together to discuss management.

It is important to characterize the memory loss, establish the presence of dementia based on set diagnostic guidelines and consider differential diagnoses. The presence of aphasia (disturbance in language), apraxia (impaired ability to perform motor activities despite intact motor function), agnosia (inability to recognize or identify objects despite intact sensory function) or impaired executive functioning (e.g. abstraction, organization) associated with social and occupational dysfunction is suggestive of dementia. Family medical history is relevant in familial cases of dementia.

Basic ADL are skills essential for personal care and include transferring, toileting, bathing, grooming, dressing and feeding. Instrumental ADL (IADL) represent interaction with one's environment; examples include handling finances (e.g. writing checks), traveling, shopping, cooking, making telephone calls and performing household chores. Functional capabilities of older individuals are followed on a regular basis. In dementia, the ability to perform IADL is lost initially; with disease progression, the ability to provide basic self-care (ADL) is lost as well.

The physical examination must include a complete neurological evaluation. Focal neurological findings, carotid bruits, cogwheel rigidity, or gait abnormality (shuffling or wide-based) may indicate vascular dementia, Parkinson's disease, or normal pressure hydrocephalus. Muscle fasciculation and myoclonus suggest Creutzfeldt–Jakob disease. Screening tests for cognition may be utilized (e.g. the Mini-Mental Status examination (MMSE), the mini-Cog test and the clock drawing test (CDT)). A discussion on these tools follows.

Initial laboratory tests help to exclude causes of dementia other than Alzheimer's disease. Complete blood count, blood chemistries, thyroid function tests, folic acid and vitamin B_{12} levels, and serological tests for syphilis comprise the basic tests. Additionally, Lyme titer, HIV testing[14], antinuclear antibodies and others may be requested on a selected basis. Erythrocyte sedimentation rate is helpful when vasculitis is suspected.

Even in the absence of focal neurologic signs, it may be prudent to include a neuroimaging study in addition to the initial diagnostic tests to detect any potentially treatable cause of dementia (e.g. hydrocephalus, subdural hematoma, brain tumor). If intracranial pathology is suspected (e.g. stroke, hydrocephalus), an initial computerized tomography (CT) scan or magnetic resonance imaging (MRI) of the head is necessary. Positron emission tomography (PET) scanning, used in some centers, is based on glucose metabolism in the brain and is an ancillary test. In general, neuroimaging is not diagnostic in Alzheimer's disease, but sequential studies over time may help correlate with the clinical diagnosis.

Routine genetic testing for apolipoprotein E alleles is not recommended at this time, as inheritance of either the $\epsilon2$ or $\epsilon4$ allele does not ensure protection from or predict the development of Alzheimer's disease, respectively. Genetic testing for mutations involving the APP, presenilin 1 and presenilin 2 genes is expensive and limited to patients with a strong family history of early-onset dementia. Genetic testing may not provide enough information to justify the cost and social impact. There is presently no consensus on appropriate selection of individuals for testing.

Electroencephalogram (EEG) and lumbar puncture are performed as indicated on an individualized basis. The EEG may be helpful in cases of suspected seizure or Creutzfeldt–Jakob disease[15] and a lumbar puncture for cerebrovascular fluid pressure and analysis in normal pressure hydrocephalus and neurosyphilis.

A simplified approach to the evaluation of dementia is presented in Table 4.

Tests for cognition

Several screening instruments for dementia are available for use in the initial and periodic evaluation of patients presenting with memory loss and cognitive dysfunction.

The Alzheimer disease assessment scale – cognitive subscale

The Alzheimer Disease Assessment Scale – Cognitive Subscale (ADAS-COg) is a standard

Table 4 Evaluation of dementia

History
Conduct separate interviews with patient and
    caregiver
Search for risk factors for dementia
Elicit family history of dementia, if applicable
Evaluate patient's functional status (ADL and IADL)
Review medications and diet

Physical examination
Complete neurological examination
Use screening tests for cognition and mood

Diagnostic tests*
Laboratory
    complete blood cell count, thyroid function tests,
    folic acid and vitamin B_{12} levels, electrolytes,
    serologic test for syphilis, renal and hepatic function
    tests
Neuroimaging
    CT or MRI of the brain
Additional tests
    electroencephalogram, lumbar puncture (for
    cerebrospinal fluid pressure and analysis), HIV
    screening, erythrocyte sedimentation rate, PET or
    SPECT imaging, apolipoprotein E genotyping

*Selection of tests is individualized

neuropsychological test and consists of 11
items that assess memory, language, orientation, reasoning and praxis. The maximum
score is 70 points[16]. The higher the score, the
more severe the cognitive impairment.

The Mini-Mental Status Examination

The MMSE is reasonably brief and easy to
administer. It evaluates a person's basic orientation, attention, calculation, memory, language and visuospatial ability[17]. A score of
24 or more (maximum possible score 30) is
considered normal. However, factors such as
educational attainment, visual or hearing
impairment and mood may affect test performance. A near perfect score does not
exclude mild Alzheimer's disease or mild
cognitive impairment, nor does a score below
24 rule in dementia.

Clock Drawing Test

The patient is asked to draw a clock and
place the hands of the clock to show a

particular time (e.g. twenty past ten). This
test evaluates the person's memory, visuospatial skills and executive functioning. A
score of 5 or less suggests dementia[15].

Mini-Cog

A recent study involving the use of the three-
word recall test in addition to the CDT
shows promise as a screening test for dementia. The estimated time to complete this test
was 2 min. However, the test needs to be
validated in different populations[18].

Seven-minute screen

This is a battery of tests with four components: orientation to time; enhanced cued
call using flash cards; CDT; and verbal flu-
ency tests (naming objects in a general category within a minute).

Clinical dementia rating

The clinical dementia rating (CDR) is accomplished in 10–15 min, during which the
patient's memory, orientation, judgement,
problem solving, community affairs, home and
hobbies, and personal care are evaluated[19].

Pharmacotherapy in Alzheimer's disease

The goal of treatment is to manage the symptoms (especially behavioral) and slow the
progression of the disease. General management (including non-pharmacological measures and pharmacological management of
behavioral problems associated with dementia) is discussed in a subsequent section of
this chapter. An early diagnosis and initiation
of treatment for the disease can delay institutionalization[20], allowing time for the individual and family to set things in order (e.g.
Living Will, advance directives) and enjoy
quality life together in preparation for the
future.

The mainstay of treatment for cognitive impairment in Alzheimer's disease is the use of cholinesterase inhibitors. To improve tolerance and minimize adverse reactions, the drugs are given with food, with slow titration of the dose upward to the maximum tolerated dose, to attain maximum benefit. All cholinesterase inhibitors have a definite dose-related response[21-23]. Starting treatment early may slow the progression of the disease. The medications are continued even after institutionalization, as long as they help the individual maintain some function and recognize or communicate with the family and others. In suspected cases of mixed dementia (vascular and Alzheimer's type), the use of a cholinesterase inhibitor is worth a try; data suggest benefit even in vascular dementia[24].

The first drug approved by the United States Food and Drug Administration (FDA) for the treatment of Alzheimer's disease was tacrine in 1993. It reversibly inhibits both acetylcholinesterase (AChE) and butyl-cholinesterase (BuChE), has a terminal elimination half-life of 2–3 h, and is metabolized by the hepatic cytochrome P450 system[21]. Although effective, the use of this drug is no longer favored, because of side-effects and the availability of alternative drugs. Significant asymptomatic hepatotoxity may occur, requiring monitoring of liver function tests on a regular basis. Other gastrointestinal side-effects include nausea, vomiting, abdominal discomfort, diarrhea and anorexia. Frequent dosing several times a day is cumbersome in demented patients and leads to non-compliance. The optimal dose is 120–160 mg/day.

Donepezil is a reversible piperidine-based AChE inhibitor with a terminal elimination half-life of 70 h, allowing once-daily dosing. Metabolism is through the cytochrome P450 system. In contrast to tacrine, donepezil is not hepatotoxic, obviating the need for liver function monitoring. Donepezil is initiated in a dose of 5 mg daily for 4–6 weeks and increased to 10 mg daily to achieve maximum benefit. Side-effects include diarrhea, nausea, vomiting, anorexia, muscle cramps and fatigue[21].

Rivastigmine inhibits both AChE and BuChE. It has an elimination half-life of 1.5 h; inactivation occurs by enzymatic cleavage at the cholinesterase sites rather than at the liver. The initial dose is 1.5 mg twice daily, increasing by 1.5 mg daily every 2–4 weeks. A maximum dose of 6 mg twice a day is recommended for highest efficacy. Side-effects include nausea, vomiting and diarrhea[21].

Galantamine, originally extracted from *Leucoium aestivum*, is now synthesized for commercial use[25]. It has two actions that enhance acetylcholine activity. Aside from reversible and competitive inhibition of AChE, it also amplifies cholinergic nicotinic neurotransmission by modulating nicotinic acetylcholine receptors. Galantamine improves cognitive and global function significantly, irrespective of whether the individual has an APOE ϵ4 allele or not[9,26]. The terminal elimination half-life is 7 h and metabolism is via the hepatic cytochrome P450 system[21]. The drug is started in a dose of 4 mg twice daily for the first 4 weeks, and increased to 8 mg twice daily for a few weeks until the optimum dose is reached of 12 mg twice a day (range 16–32 mg/day). A rapid escalation of the dose results in side-effects, which include gastrointestinal symptoms (nausea, anorexia, diarrhea, vomiting, abdominal pain), weight loss, headache, tremors, dizziness and agitation[9]. Table 5 compares the properties of available cholinesterase inhibitors.

Adjuvant therapies

Several other medications have been studied in relation to their effect on slowing the progression of dementia. Though implicated in the past, no study supports the benefit of nicotine in dementia. Although estrogen has been touted to enhance cognition, recent large double-blinded placebo-controlled studies have not conclusively proved the benefit from estrogen replacement therapy

Table 5 Available cholinesterase inhibitors for Alzheimer's disease. From references 2, 20, 21, 22 and 23

	Tacrine	Donepezil	Rivastigmine	Galantamine
Chemical class	aminoacridine	piperidine	carbamate	alkaloid
Action	non-competitive, reversible inhibitor	non-competitive, reversible inhibitor	non-competitive pseudoirreversible inhibitor	competitive, reversible inhibitor
	non-selective AChE and BuChE inhibitor	selective for central AChE inhibitor	selective for central AChE and BuChE inhibitor	presynaptic nicotinic receptor modulator selective central AChE inhibitor
Dosing	four times daily	once daily	twice daily	twice daily
Daily dose	40–160 mg	5–10 mg	6–12 mg	8–24 mg
Side-effects	nausea, vomiting, diarrhea, anorexia, dizziness, hepatotoxicity	nausea, vomiting, diarrhea, anorexia, muscle cramps, insomnia	nausea, vomiting, diarrhea, anorexia, dizziness, weight loss, sweating	nausea, vomiting, diarrhea, anorexia, dizziness, weight loss, sweating

AChE, acetylcholinesterase; BuChE, butylcholinesterase

claimed by earlier epidemiologic studies[27,28]. The decreased incidence of dementia in people on chronic NSAIDs[29] emphasizes the possible role of inflammation in the brain in Alzheimer's disease. However, NSAIDs are not recommended for management of Alzheimer's disease, partly due to their side-effect profile involving other body systems. Likewise, whether cyclo-oxygenase-2 inhibitors will make safer alternatives needs further study. *Ginkgo biloba* has been propagated to have a beneficial effect on dementia[30] but has not been consistently observed[31]. The use of antioxidants is based on the theory that free radicals in the brain can cause oxidative damage to tissues and eventual death of neurons. Patients treated with either vitamin E or selegiline for 2 years showed a slight delay in the progression of Alzheimer's disease but without substantial benefit to cognitive dysfunction[32]. Vitamin E in doses of 1000 IU twice a day has been recommended for adjunctive therapy.

Future treatments would be likely to involve a vaccine that would prevent β-amyloid plaque formation on the neuronal surface. The use of stem cells or fibroblasts that produce nerve growth factor is another area that is currently being explored[21].

MILD COGNITIVE IMPAIRMENT

An older adult with complaints of consistent forgetfulness (e.g. forgetting names) not associated with other cognitive dysfunction or interference with work or social function may have 'mild cognitive impairment' (MCI). Synonymous terms used include 'benign senescent forgetfulness' and 'age-associated memory impairment (AAMI)'. Yearly neuropsychological assessment of affected individuals is indicated, since 10–15% of cases with MCI per year may progress to develop Alzheimer's disease, compared to 1–2% for controls[33].

Previously, the term AAMI was used for the gradual decline of memory associated with aging; such individuals over age 50 had a decline in memory but did not suffer from depression or dementia and were generally healthy. The concept proved to be of little use, as it was found that most older adults would fit the diagnosis[34].

VASCULAR DEMENTIA

Vascular dementia accounts for 15–30% of all dementias in the USA but appears more common as the cause in Japan. Risk factors

Table 6 Vascular dementia (formerly multi-infarct dementia). From reference 13

A. The development of multiple cognitive deficits manifested by both

 (1) memory impairment (impaired ability to learn new information or to recall previously learned information)
 (2) one (or more) of the following cognitive disturbances:

   (a) aphasia (language disturbance)
   (b) apraxia (impaired ability to carry out motor activities despite intact motor function)
   (c) agnosia (failure to recognize or identify objects despite intact sensory function)
   (d) disturbance in executive functioning (i.e. planning, organizing, sequencing, abstracting)

B. The cognitive deficits in Criteria A1 and A2 each cause significant impairment in social or occupational functioning and represent a significant decline from a previous level of functioning.
C. Focal neurological signs and symptoms (e.g. exaggeration of deep tendon reflexes, extensor plantar response, pseudobulbar palsy, gait abnormalities, weakness of an extremity) or laboratory evidence indicative of cerebrovascular disease (e.g. multiple infarctions involving cortex and underlying white matter) that are judged to be etiologically related to the disturbance.
D. The deficits do not occur exclusively during the course of a delirium.

Reprinted with permission from the *Diagnostic and Statistical Manual of Mental Disorders*, 4th edn. Copyright 1994 American Psychiatric Association

include hypertension, hyperlipidemia, atrial fibrillation, hyperhomocysteinemia and cerebral amyloid angiopathy. Vascular dementia results from thrombosis, embolism and hemorrhage. Infarcts may be cortical or subcortical; in Binswanger's disease, there may be diffuse involvement of the white matter with lacunar infarcts. Neuroimaging may reveal evidence of vascular disease, with MRI superior to CT for small infarcts. The infarcts may be single or multiple, large or small; based on the location of infarcts, presentation may vary considerably.

Vascular dementia commonly co-exists with Alzheimer's disease[24]. Unlike Alzheimer's disease, deterioration in cognitive ability and function is sudden and stepwise in character and physical examination may reveal focal neurologic findings (Table 6). The Hachinski Ischemic Scale (HIS) helps differentiate Alzheimer's disease from vascular dementia, based on a constellation of features in the latter (abrupt onset, stepwise deterioration, hypertension, focal neurologic signs and symptoms, emotional incontinence and history of strokes). A score of 4 or above suggests vascular dementia.

Treatment includes the use of an antiplatelet agent (e.g. aspirin, clopidogrel or ticlodipine) and adequate management of known risk factors (e.g. hypertension, diabetes mellitus, hyperlipidemia). Adequate long-term control of hypertension has been shown to decrease the onset of cognitive impairment and vascular dementia[35]. Recent data suggest that statins appear to decrease the incidence of cerebrovascular disease; they decrease platelet aggregation and favorably impact on prothrombotic and fibrinolytic processes, independently of their cholesterol-lowering action[36]. As vascular dementia and Alzheimer's disease can co-exist, patients may benefit from a trial of cholinesterase inhibitors[24,37].

DIFFUSE LEWY BODY DEMENTIA

Diffuse Lewy body dementia (DLBD) is characterized by dementia, fluctuating cognition, recurrent hallucinations and Parkinsonian features. Hallucinations are a prominent feature and are more visual than auditory. Parkinsonian features include bradykinesia, tremors and rigidity. Unlike in Parkinson's disease, where Parkinsonian features appear early and dementia is a late feature, in DLBD, Parkinsonian manifestations follow the development of dementia. The pathologic characteristic of this disease entity is the presence of concentric, eosinophilic cytoplasmic inclusions (Lewy bodies) in neurons of the cerebral cortex, substantia nigra, tegmentum, basal forebrain and the dorsal raphe nucleus[38].

DLBD is associated with both dopaminergic and cholinergic deficits. Side-effects limit the dosage of dopaminergic drugs in this disorder. Extrapyramidal side-effects are common with the typical antipsychotics (e.g. haloperidol) and risperidone. Other atypical antipsychotics (e.g. olanzapine, quetiapine) may be used with caution.

FRONTOTEMPORAL DEMENTIA

Like Alzheimer's disease, the onset of frontotemporal dementia is insidious and slowly progressive. However, behavioral changes occur earlier and include sexual disinhibition, hyperorality (excessive eating, smoking and alcohol use) and poor hygiene. Examination may reveal progressive speech deterioration (mutism), rigidity and tremor. Surprisingly, calculation and visuospatial skills remain intact. Atrophy of the frontal and temporal lobes is seen during neuroimaging or postmortem biopsy. EEG may reveal diffuse or frontal-temporal slowing. With single-photon emission CT (SPECT), diminished cerebral perfusion is seen in the anterior hemispheric regions (as opposed to posterior cerebral regions in Alzheimer's disease)[39]. Antipsychotic medications may be used to control the behavioral problems. Pick's disease falls under this category.

REVERSIBLE DEMENTIAS

Several conditions, when diagnosed early and treated adequately, may improve with varying degrees of reversibility. These disorders include depression, endocrine disorders, normal pressure hydrocephalus, medication toxicity and nutritional deficiencies, among others. In some cases where detection of the underlying problem is delayed (e.g. vitamin B_{12} deficiency),

cognitive impairment may persist or only partially improve if timely treatment is not initiated[40,41].

DIFFERENTIAL DIAGNOSIS OF DEMENTIA, DEPRESSION AND DELIRIUM

In addition to delineating an etiology, dementia must be differentiated from depression and delirium; often dementia may co-exist with depression and delirium. Although the prevalence of major depression in community residents appears surprisingly low among older adults (1–2% in women and less than 1% in men), the prevalence of 'minor' or subsyndromal depression approaches 15%[42]. Depressed individuals may appear demented, hence the term 'pseudodementia'. In such situations, the Yesavage Geriatric Depression Scale is a useful screening tool. In some instances, a trial of treatment with antidepressants and psychotherapy may improve cognitive function, and help differentiate the two.

Delirium is common in older adults and associated with increased morbidity and mortality. It is characterized by acute onset, fluctuating mental status, inattention, change in level of consciousness and the presence of one or more etiological medical conditions[43]. Dementia and advanced age are also risk factors clearly associated with delirium. Table 7 offers a comparison between dementia, delirium and depression. The differentiation can be quite difficult at times.

MANAGEMENT

The goals in the management of patients with dementia are to delay the progression of cognitive impairment, increase independence by improving function and enhance quality of life for patient (and caregiver). Depending on the etiology of dementia (as discussed earlier), specific treatment may be available. The following focuses on other aspects of care.

Table 7 Differential diagnosis of cognitive dysfunction

	Dementia	Delirium	Depression
Onset	insidious	acute	acute or chronic
Duration	persistent, often years	hours to weeks	episodic or persistent
Consciousness	awake, co-operative	waxing and waning	usually intact
Memory	impaired, initially recent, later remote	impaired	may be impaired
Psychosis	delusions (usually paranoid); possibly hallucinations	visual, auditory, and tactile hallucinations and delusions	delusions involve worthlessness; paranoid ideation
Reversibility	progressive	potential present	potential present
Evaluation of cognition (e.g. MMSE)	co-operative but erroneous answers	difficulty in focusing (rambles)	uninterested: 'do not know' answers

MMSE, Mini-Mental Status Examination

General management

Management begins when the diagnosis of dementia is initially disclosed to the patient and caregiver. The patient with insight has the legal and moral right to know about the diagnosis. A family meeting may be arranged for this purpose to inform those concerned on future expectations and available options. It is essential to convey the fact that progression of dementia is associated with behavioral disturbances and increasing dependence on caregivers for basic care.

An early diagnosis enables the patient with mild dementia an opportunity to participate actively in care planning and be involved in end-of-life decisions. Preparation of advance directives, Living Will and durable power of attorney should be encouraged at the first opportunity. The patient's preferences on cardiopulmonary resuscitation, life support systems (e.g. mechanical respiration) and feeding tubes must be appropriately documented. Planning regarding institutionalization (e.g. assisted living, nursing homes) and financial issues should involve both patient and family.

Depending on the stage, demented individuals present with common geriatric syndromes such as urinary and fecal incontinence, constipation, visual and hearing impairment, anorexia, sleep disorders and falls. Management of treatable conditions helps improve the patient's quality of life and decrease caregiver stress; each of these is discussed elsewhere in the book.

Management of common behavioral problems

Cognitive and functional dysfunctions are often associated with behavioral changes in demented patients. These include agitation, wandering, psychosis, personality changes, sleep disorders and care resistance. Half the patients in the community with Alzheimer's disease manifest one or more behavioral problems; in long-term care facilities, up to 90% are affected[44]. Understandably, disruptive behavior is a common basis for institutionalization in conjunction with worsening caregiver stress.

The initial step in managing behavioral disturbances is to identify and treat the precipitating cause, if possible (Table 8). New-onset agitation may be the result of an acute medical problem or a medication. Patients with dementia are often unable to express their complaints clearly. In Parkinson's dementia, psychosis can be a result of the use of dopaminergic drugs. Drugs with strong anticholinergic effects (e.g. diphenhydramine, amitriptyline) are best avoided in Alzheimer's dementia. Environmental factors (e.g. loud noise) may contribute to behavioral disturbances. Pain or

Table 8 Non-pharmacological management of dementia

Agitation, aggression, catastrophic reaction
Identify precipitating factor
Reduce overstimulation
Simplify tasks to prevent frustration

Wandering
Provide identification bracelet or anklet
Provide a safe area for wandering (e.g. wander garden)
Install door locks or alarms
Have a recent photograph for the police if patient gets lost
Encourage participation in structured activities to minimize boredom

Delusions, hallucinations
Evaluate for delirium
Do not confront the patient or reinforce
Use distraction tactics
Provide adequate lighting
Avoid situations that contribute to paranoia
Correct sensory impairments, if possible

Sundowning
Avoid sudden environmental changes
Encourage adequate daytime exercise
Provide easy to read clocks and calendars
Encourage familiar environment and caregiver
Provide exposure to light in the afternoon
Have a night-light at bedtime

discomfort from fecal impaction, skin wounds and arthritis, amongst other causes, can contribute to an acute change in behavior. Treatment of the inciting medical problem or withdrawal of the offending medication often leads to resolution of the behavioral disorder. An empirical trial of analgesics may be considered when patients are unable to express themselves. Environmental modification may be helpful in the management.

Catastrophic reaction, agitation and aggression

Catastrophic reactions are verbal, physical or emotional outbursts secondary to patient frustration[45]. Agitation and aggression may be precipitated by events or conditions in the patient's environment. Unfamiliar, new surroundings tend to increase confusion and anxiety. When the demented patient is unable to complete complex tasks, frustration and anger may result.

Identification and correction of precipitant factors (e.g. time, situation, person) should be tried before pharmacologic treatment is initiated. Situations that lead to catastrophic reactions should be avoided. For example, if bathing in the morning is associated with aggressive behavior, leaving the patient alone for a while or giving an afternoon bath may be options. A familiar environment should be maintained, with change introduced only gradually. Easy to read clocks and calendars help maintain orientation to time. Reality orientation questions are helpful but may cause irritation when repetitive. Complex tasks could be broken down into easier tasks to help the patient, depending on the severity of dementia. The choices made available for an activity (e.g. mealtime) should be limited and simplified.

In addition, objects may be removed or rearranged for reasons of safety. To develop familiarity, a long-term (consistent) staff and one-to-one relationship with the patient help development of trust. This is also encouraged at mealtime. A predictable daily routine minimizes confusion and provides the patient with a sense of control. Provision of stimulating activities and an enriched environment (simulating a home environment) leads to decreased agitation and disruptive behavior. Overstimulation (loud radio and TV) can cause agitation[46]. Soothing music and reminiscing (with familiar videotapes and photo albums of families and friends) are preferable alternatives.

Wandering

Wandering is a common behavioral problem seen in a fifth of patients with mild dementia and half of those with severe dementia. Precipitants include relocation, environmental stimuli, boredom, psychosis and agitated depression. Wandering is a risky behavior, as exposure to environmental hazards has the potential for injury.

Patients who wander should have their names and assigned floor location in facilities (or home address) sewed onto their clothing or exhibited in a bracelet, necklace or wallet card[46]. Exit doors may be disguised or fitted with a complex lock[45]. Alarm systems have been used to alert the staff or caregivers of patients who wander.

Provision of a safe area for wanderers to walk around may be helpful. An example is the wander garden[47]. To prevent wandering from boredom, daytime interventions for socialization and structured activity programs can be planned. Restraints are best avoided and used only when all other interventions are unsuccessful.

Psychotic features

Psychotic features (e.g. hallucinations, delusions, illusions) affect a third of individuals with Alzheimer's disease and more than half of those with Lewy body dementia; psychosis characteristically presents before cognitive dysfunction in the latter[48]. A common visual or auditory hallucination is 'communication with deceased family members or friends'. Typical delusions include false beliefs that close ones or strangers are attempting to steal one's belongings or that the spouse is unfaithful. Coexisting sensory impairments (e.g. hearing, visual) increase paranoia.

It is not advisable to confront patients about their delusions. Likewise, situations that contribute to paranoia are best avoided (e.g. talking softly or whispering). Hearing and visual impairments need consideration for evaluation and correction. When psychotic symptoms do not result in violence or agitation, pharmacotherapy is not indicated[45,49]. An antipsychotic medication may be resorted to for the exceptions.

Sundowning

Sundowning is a syndrome characterized by confusion, unexplained restlessness and/or agitation in the late afternoon or night, with relatively calm daytime behavior. The reason for sundowning, a form of delirium, is not clear; it may be a result of sensory deprivation (hearing, vision), new environment or new caregiver, a change in daily structured activities, or an acute, occult medical problem[50]. Exposure to light in the afternoon and a nightlight at bedtime, adequate daytime stimulation, provision of eyeglasses and hearing aids may help. Changes in the environment or activities should be introduced gradually. Familiar objects (e.g. pictures) and presence of close ones (or caregiver) may provide reassurance and calm.

Pharmacotherapy

When behavioral interventions fail, pharmacotherapy is a last resort. Conventional antipsychotic medications (e.g. haloperidol) are effective in controlling aggression and psychosis in dementia. Their use is limited by adverse drug events that include extrapyramidal syndrome (EPS), tardive dyskinesia (TD), orthostatic hypotension, sedation and anticholinergic effects. TD is an iatrogenic disorder seen in individuals on neuroleptics, especially those with baseline alcohol abuse/dependence or subtle movement disorders. In a prospective longitudinal study involving 266 older adults, the cumulative incidence of TD increased from 26% in the first year to 60% in the third year of neuroleptic treatment[51].

Atypical antipsychotic medications, with relatively safer side-effect profile, have replaced earlier neuroleptics as first-line treatment for psychosis and behavioral disorders in the elderly. Their selectivity for the mesolimbic systems (responsible for behavior and memory) rather than the niagrastriatal systems (responsible for movements) lessens the risk for EPS. Examples of medications in this group include risperidone, olanzapine, quetiapine and clozapine.

Risperidone has optimal efficacy and minimal side-effects at a dose of 1 mg/day. Higher doses (2 mg daily) increase the incidence of somnolence, orthostatic hypotension and EPS[52]. Peripheral edema is a common associated side-effect[53,54]. Olanzapine is better than placebo for agitation, psychosis and aggression in doses between 5 and 10 mg/day; at higher doses, sedation, abnormal gait and increased risk of falls are evident. Weight gain is also a side-effect. Quetiapine has affinity for serotonin, dopamine, histamine and adrenergic receptors. The dose is titrated from 25 mg once or twice daily to 100 mg/day. At higher doses, sedation, dizziness, seizure, postural hypotension and EPS have been documented. Lower doses are used in the presence of liver disease, as the drug is extensively metabolized in the liver. Due to possible cataract formation associated with its use, eye evaluation at initiation of treatment and every 6 months thereafter is recommended[55]. Clozapine is not the first-line agent in Alzheimer's disease, due to its potent anticholinergic action; on the other hand, this property makes clozapine a consideration with dopamine-induced psychosis in Parkinson's disease. Other side-effects with clozapine include agranulocytosis, postural hypotension and seizures[48].

Mood stabilizers such as carbamazepine, valproic acid and gabapentin have been evaluated for the treatment of agitation. Initial studies suggest that carbamazepine and divalproex sodium are effective. Both drugs need monitoring of white blood cell counts, hepatic function and drug levels[56].

Caregiver burden

As dementia progresses, the primary caregiver may experience mental and physical fatigue. The majority of caregivers are women, often the spouse, daughter or daughter-in-law[57]. The age of the caregiver is a relevant factor, since many are aging and in the 'older age group'[45]. Watching a close family member deteriorate with progressive physical dependence over time contributes to caregiver stress. Behavioral problems (e.g. aggression, delusion), insomnia and incontinence exacerbate caregiver burden.

Caregivers of patients with dementia are known to have a higher prevalence of medical illness, including but not limited to rheumatological disorders, diabetes mellitus, hypertension, headaches and depression[57]. It is not unusual for them to seek medical attention, at times even from the same health-care provider of the patient. The physician may hence need to provide adequate time for both patient and caregiver to help their illness or burden.

Caring for the family is part of the management of dementia. A list of available community resources (e.g. home care, adult day care services and respite services) or groups (e.g. Alzheimer's Association support group) may be made available to the family and caregiver to ease stress and assist in providing care. Referral to an elder-law attorney and a case manager is an option.

References

1. Bolla LR, Filley CM, Palmer RM. Dementia DDX: office diagnosis of the four major types of dementia. *Geriatrics* 2000;55:34–46
2. Marin DB, Sewell MC, Schlechter A. Alzheimer's disease: accurate and early diagnosis in the primary care setting. *Geriatrics* 2002;57:36–40
3. Schneider LS. Pharmacologic management of behavioral problems in dementia. *Ann Long-term Care* 2000;8:53–5
4. Ernst RL, Hay JW. The US economic and social costs of Alzheimer's disease revisited. *Am J Public Health* 1994;84:1261–4
5. Evans DA, Funkenstein HH, Albert MS, *et al*. Prevalence of Alzheimer's disease in a community population of older persons. *J Am Med Assoc* 1989;262:2551–6
6. Kawas CH. Alzheimer's disease. In Hazzard WR, Blass JP, Ettinger WH, Halter JB, Ouslander JG, eds. *Principles of Geriatric*

Medicine and Gerontology, 4th edn. New York: McGraw-Hill, 1999:1257–69

7. Davis KL. Alzheimer's disease: seeking new ways to preserve brain function. *Geriatrics* 1999;54:42–7

8. Burke JR, Morgenlander JC. Update on Alzheimer's disease. *Postgrad Med* 1999; 106:85–96

9. Raskind MA, Peskind ER, Wessel T, Yuan W, and the Galantamine USA-1 Study Group. Galantamine in AD. *Neurology* 2000;54: 2261–8

10. Seshadri S, Beiser A, Selhub J, *et al.* Plasma homocysteine as a risk factor for dementia and Alzheimer's disease. *N Engl J Med* 2002;346:476–83

11. Loscalzo J. Homocysteine and dementias. *N Engl J Med* 2002;346:466–8

12. Volicer L. Dementia and personality. In Mahoney L, Volicer L, Hurley AC, eds. *Management of Challenging Behaviors in Dementia*. Baltimore: Health Professions Press, 2000:11–28

13. *American Psychiatric Association. Diagnostic and Statistical Manual of Mental Disorders*. 4th edn. Washington, DC: American Psychiatric Association, 1994

14. Small GW, Rabins PV, Barry PP, *et al.* Diagnosis and treatment of Alzheimer disease and related disorders. Consensus statement. *J Am Med Assoc* 1997;278: 1363–71

15. Steffens DC, Morgenlander JC. Initial evaluation of suspected dementia. *Postgrad Med* 1999;106:72–83

16. Rosen WG, Mohs RC, Davis KL. A new rating scale for Alzheimer's disease. *Am J Psychiatry* 1984;141:1356–64

17. Folstein MF, Folstein SE, McHugh PR. 'Mini-mental state.' A practical method for grading the cognitive state of patients for the clinician. *J Psychiatr Res* 1975;12: 189–98

18. Scanlan J, Borson S. The Mini-Cog: receiver operating characteristics with expert and naïve raters. *Int J Geriatr Psychiatry* 2001;16:216–22

19. Morris JC. Clinical dementia rating: a reliable and valid diagnostic and staging measure for dementia of the Alzheimer type. *Int Psychogeriatr* 1997;9(Suppl 1):173–8

20. Gauthier S, Gelinas I, Gauthier L. Functional disability in Alzheimer's disease. *Int Psychogeriatr*, 1997;9(Suppl):163–5

21. Hake AM. Use of cholinesterase inhibitors for treatment of Alzheimer disease. *Cleveland J Med* 2001;68:608–16

22. Sramek JJ, Alexander BD, Cutler NR. Acetylcholinesterase inhibitors for the treatment of Alzheimer's disease. *Ann Long-term Care* 2001;9:15–22

23. Evans RM, Farlow MR. Acetylcholinesterase inhibition in the treatment of Alzheimer's disease. *Grand Rounds Alzheimer's Dis* 2001;1:24–9

24. Zekry D, Hauw J-J, Gold G. Mixed dementia: epidemiology, diagnosis and treatment. *J Am Geriatr Soc* 2002;50: 1431–8

25. Sramek JJ, Pharm D, Alexander BD, Cutler NR. Efficacy of galantamine in the treatment of Alzheimer's disease. *Clin Geriatr* 2001;9:55–60

26. Wilcock GK, Lilienfeld S, Gaens ELS. Efficacy and safety of galantamine in patients with mild to moderate Alzheimer's disease: multicenter randomised controlled trial. *Br Med J* 2000;321:1445–9

27. Mulnard RA, Cotman CW, Kawas C, *et al.* Estrogen replacement therapy for treatment of mild to moderate Alzheimer disease. *J Am Med Assoc* 2000;283: 1007–15

28. Henderson VW, Paganini-Hill A, Miller BL, *et al.* Estrogen for Alzheimer's disease in women: randomized, double-blinded, placebo-controlled trial. *Neurology* 2000; 54:295–301

29. Stewart WF, Kawas C, Corrada M, Metter EJ. Risk of Alzheimer's disease and duration of NSAID use. *Neurology* 1997;48:626–32

30. Le Bars PL, Katz MM, Berman N, *et al.* A placebo-controlled, double-blind, randomized trial of an extract of *Ginkgo biloba* for dementia. *J Am Med Assoc* 1997;278: 1327–32

31. Van Dongen M, Van Rossum E, Kessels A, Sielhorst H, Knipschild P. The efficacy of ginkgo for elderly people with dementia and age-associated memory impairment: new results of a randomized clinical trial. *J Am Geriatr Soc* 2000;48:1183–94

32. Sano M, Ernesto C, Thomas RG, *et al.* A controlled trial of selegiline, alpha-tocopherol, or both as treatment for Alzheimer's disease. *N Engl J Med* 1997; 336:1216–22

33. Ritchie K, Kildea D. Is senile dementia 'age related' or 'aging related'? Evidence from a meta-analysis of dementia prevalence in the oldest old. *Lancet* 1995;346:931–4

34. Shah Y, Tangalos EG, Petersen RC. Mild cognitive impairment. When is it a precursor to Alzheimer's disease? *Geriatrics* 2000;55:62, 65–8

35. Birkenhager WH, Forette F, Seux ML, *et al.* Blood pressure, cognitive functions, and prevention of dementias in older patients with hypertension. *Arch Intern Med* 2001;161:152–6

36. Aronow WS. Rationale for lipid lowering in older patients with or without coronary artery disease. *Geriatrics* 2001;56:22–30

37. Erkinjuntti T, Kurz A, Gauthier S, *et al.* Efficacy of galantamine in probable vascular dementia and Alzheimer's disease combined with cerebrovascular disease: a randomized trial. *Lancet* 2002;359:1283–90

38. Fago JP. Dementia: causes, evaluation, and management. *Hosp Pract* 2001;36:59–69

39. Reichman WE, Cummings JL. Dementia. In Duthie EH Jr, Katz P, eds. *Practice of Geriatrics*, 3rd edn. Philadelphia: WB Saunders, 1998:267–78

40. Dharmarajan TS, Koshy A, Sipalay M, Norkus EP. The need to screen: a case in point. In Herbert V, ed. *Vitamin B12 Deficiency*. London: Royal Society of Medicine Press, 1999:9–13

41. Dharmarajan TS, Norkus EP. Approaches to vitamin B_{12} deficiency. *Postgrad Med* 2001;110:99–106

42. Meyers BS. Depression and other mood disorders. In Cobbs EL, Duthie EH, Murphy JB, eds. *Geriatric Review Syllabus: A Core Curriculum in Geriatric Medicine*, 5th edn. Malden, MA: Blackwell Publishing for the American Geriatrics Society, 2002:219–28

43. Marcantonio ER. Delirium. In Cobbs EL, Duthie EH, Murphy JB, eds. *Geriatric Review Syllabus: A Core Curriculum in Geriatric Medicine*, 5th edn. Malden, MA: Blackwell Publishing for the American Geriatrics Society, 2002:131–9

44. Neugroschl J. Agitation: how to manage behavior disturbances in the older patient with dementia. *Geriatrics* 2002;57:33–7

45. Ham RJ. Confusion, dementia, and delirium. In Ham RJ, Sloane PD, eds. *Primary Care Geriatrics: a Case-based Approach*, 2nd edn. Philadelphia: Mosby-Year Book, 1992:259–311

46. Burnside I. Nursing care. In Jarvik LF, Winograd CH, eds. *Treatment for the Alzheimer Patient: The Long Haul.* New York: Springer, 1988:39–58

47. Detweiler MB, Trinkle DB, Anderson MS. Wander gardens: expanding the dementia treatment environment. *Ann Long-term Care* 2002;10:68–74

48. Morris SK, Jeste DV. Schizophrenia and other psychotic disorders. In Hazzard WR, Blass JP, Ettinger WH, Halter JB, Ouslander JG, eds. *Principles of Geriatric Medicine and Gerontology*, 4th edn. New York: McGraw-Hill, 1999:1341–9

49. Burke JR, Morgenlander JC. Managing common behavioral problems in dementia. *Postgrad Med* 1999;106:131–40

50. Small GW. Dementia. In Cobbs EL, Duthie EH, Murphy JB, eds. *Geriatric Review Syllabus: A Core Curriculum in Geriatric Medicine*, 5th edn. Malden, MA: Blackwell Publishing for the American Geriatrics Society, 2002:117–25

51. Jeste DV, Caligiuri MP, Paulsen JS, *et al.* Risk of tardive dyskinesia in older patients. A prospective longitudinal study of 266 outpatients. *Arch Gen Psychiatry* 1995;52:756–65

52. Katz IR, Jeste DV, Mintzer JE. Comparison of risperidone and placebo for psychosis and behavioral disturbances associated with dementia: a randomized, double-blind trial. *J Clin Psychiatry* 1999;60:107–15

53. Hwang JP, Yang CH, Yu HC, *et al.* The efficacy and safety of risperidone for the treatment of geriatric psychosis. *J Clin Psychopharmacol* 2001;21:583–7

54. Katz IR, Jeste DV, Mintzer JE, *et al.* Comparison of risperidone and placebo for

psychosis and behavioral disturbances associated with dementia: a randomized, double-blind trial. Risperidone Study Group. *J Clin Psychiatry* 1999;60:107–15

55. Madhusoodanan S, Brenner R, Gupta S, Bogunovic O. Quetiapine for elderly patients with psychosis. *Clin Geriatr* 2001; 9:46–56

56. Neugroschi J. Agitation: How to manage behavior disturbances in the older patient with dementia. *Geriatrics* 2002;57:33–7

57. Dunkin JJ, Anderson-Hanley C. Dementia caregiver burden: a review of the literature and guidelines for assessment and intervention. *Neurology* 1998;S1(Suppl 1): S53–60

30 Delirium

T.S. Dharmarajan, MD, FACP, AGSF, *and Dilip Unnikrishnan,* MD

INTRODUCTION

Delirium, also known as acute confusional state, acute brain failure, acute brain syndrome, metabolic encephalopathy or acute toxic psychosis, is a common neuropsychiatric disorder in the geriatric population, with serious immediate and long-term consequences. Because of the wide spectrum of clinical features, the syndrome of delirium is often misdiagnosed as depression, dementia, schizophrenia or other mood disorders, with the disorder missed in up to two-thirds of patients[1-4]. The prevalence of delirium ranges from 10 to 40% of hospital admissions, with an incidence of 25–60% during hospitalization[3,5]. It is roughly estimated that 10–15% of patients in acute medical–surgical wards at any given time have delirium[6,7]. Many causes of delirium are emergent or life threatening, requiring hospitalization for immediate evaluation, treatment and patient safety[8]. Individuals with delirium manifest increased morbidity, prolonged hospitalization and higher rates of institutionalization, all with significant financial implications[3,5,7,9,10]. Several studies have confirmed a higher overall mortality in delirious patients, both during hospitalization and up to a year after discharge.

PATHOGENESIS

While multiple neurotransmitters are probably involved, several models of delirium suggest a derangement in glucose metabolism and resultant cerebral metabolic insufficiency as the probable final mechanism following a variety of insults[1]. Medications with anticholinergic activity are an important cause of delirium, suggesting that impaired cholinergic transmission might play a role in the pathogenesis[4,11,12]. Hypoxia and hypoglycemia may impair the production of acetylcholine. Decline in cholinergic activity correlates with delirium in several states (e.g. following surgery). Structurally, both cortical and subcortical areas of the brain appear to be involved[12]. Relief of delirium-related symptoms by haloperidol, a dopamine blocker, suggests excess dopaminergic activity. In hepatic encephalopathy, increased serotonin and γ-amino butyric acid (GABA) levels have been noted. Elevation of plasma β-endorphins, their disrupted relation to cortisol circadian rhythms and cytokines have been incriminated in the basis[7,13].

RISK FACTORS

Common causes of delirium are summarized in Table 1. In any given individual, multiple interacting factors may be responsible; repeated assessment is thus required to identify predisposing, precipitating and perpetuating factors[3,5,14]. Risk factors, especially in hospitalized patients, include electrolyte disturbances (hyponatremia, hypernatremia, hypokalemia, hypercalcemia), hyperthermia or hypothermia, severity of illness, pre-existing cognitive impairment, sleep deprivation, social isolation, malnutrition and history of

Table 1 Common causes of delirium. From references 1–3, 6, 7, 12, 14, 17, 18, 20 and 24

Infections
Urinary tract, pneumonia, intra-abdominal

Metabolic
Electrolyte abnormalities (sodium, potassium, calcium, magnesium)
Hyper- or hypoglycemia
Hyper- or hypothyroidism
Hypoxia, hypercarbia
Adrenal insufficiency, renal, hepatic or respiratory failure

Medications
Anticholinergics, antihistamines, psychoactive drugs with anticholinergic effects
Sedative hypnotics (benzodiazepines, barbiturates, paraldehyde, chloral hydrate)
Analgesics (opioids, dextropropoxyphene, salicylates)
Cardiovascular (digoxin, clonidine, β-blockers, lidocaine, reserpine)
Steroids, non-steroidal anti-inflammatory drugs (ibuprofen, indomethacin, naproxen)
Intoxication, overdose (alcohol, sedatives)
Withdrawal (drug or alcohol)
H_2-receptor blockers (cimetidine, ranitidine)
Antiparkinson drugs (levodopa, carbidopa, amantidine)
Antidiarrheal drugs (atropine, belladonna)
Theophylline

Other
Cardiac failure, myocardial infarction
Neurologic disease (stroke, post-ictal, raised intracranial pressure)
Fever or hypothermia
Vitamin B_{12} deficiency
Altered volume status, hypotension, shock
Anemia
Pain
Constipation
Unfamiliar environment (e.g. hospital)

The list is illustrative and not necessarily all-inclusive

psychoactive drug use[1,2,7,9,15,16]. A higher incidence of delirium is typically seen following fractures, narcotic or antipsychotic drug use, and with azotemia[1]. Use of three or more medications, physical restraints, bladder catheters and any iatrogenic event can precipitate delirium[1,15]. Advanced age is a risk factor, consequent upon structural brain disease, altered drug kinetics, sensory deprivation (vision, hearing) and co-morbid illnesses[1]. Patients with dementia are clearly at a higher risk for development of delirium, especially in the setting of an unfamiliar environment and limited social interaction.

Medications

Medications are amongst the most common causes of delirium in the hospitalized elderly.

Polypharmacy, in particular, increases the risk. Usual inciting drugs include anticholinergics and sedative–hypnotics[3]. Any patient with an alteration in mentation needs assessment for a recent change in medications and possible drug–drug interactions. In high-risk individuals with dementia or sensory impairment, a single dose of a sedative medication might be enough to cause delirium. A review of prescribed, over-the-counter and topical medications is indicated in the evaluation of delirium. Intoxication with alcohol and withdrawal from alcohol or medications (benzodiazepines, opioids) can result in delirium and necessitates consideration when screening an agitated patient. Meperidine and its active metabolite, normeperidine, accumulate in older adults because of impaired renal function (limiting excretion of parent drug and metabolite) resulting in agitated delirium, tremors and seizures; the medication is best avoided in the elderly[17].

Co-morbid illnesses

Infections, cardiac failure, neurologic illnesses, volume depletion and azotemia are all associated with the development of delirium[11,15]. A search for occult infections is always indicated, since older individuals may not necessarily manifest fever or leukocytosis. In the elderly, delirium may be the only clinical sign of life-threatening states such as acute myocardial infarction, pneumonia, impending respiratory failure or stroke[11,18]. Dementia, depression, visual impairment and abnormal serum sodium concentrations have been found to have a significant association with delirium[15].

Dementia

Pre-existing dementia is a well-recognized risk factor for the development of delirium, contributing up to five times the risk during hospitalization[3]. Individuals with Alzheimer's disease and other neurodegenerative conditions have decreased central cholinergic transmission, and are thus predisposed to anticholinergic medication toxicity. Although the relationship between delirium and future development of dementia is less clear, it appears that some delirious patients do not recover completely and have sustained cognitive impairment many months later.

Postoperative factors

Delirium complicates 15–25% of elective procedures and 25–65% of emergency procedures in older individuals[17,19,20]. Hip surgery appears to be particularly related; here, delirium appears associated with frailty, prior cognitive impairment, poor functional status, nursing home residence and medical co-morbidity. Other risk factors for delirium include male sex, age, stroke, heart disease, depression and treatment with multiple medications[7,20]. In the perioperative phase, urinary retention, urinary and wound infections, fever, hypotension, feeding problems and anemia are known to induce delirium[12,20]. Occurrence of delirium predicts poor functional recovery at 1 and 6 months, and is considered a reliable predictor of outcome following hip fracture[19,20]. Patients undergoing cataract surgery may develop delirium consequent to visual impairment and use of anticholinergic medications[12]. Prolonged surgical procedures and cardiac surgery are well-known associations. Delirium is associated with worsening postoperative functional status, independent of baseline cognition and function; patients with persistent delirium at 1 month had a poorer prognosis than those who had recovered by that time[19].

Environmental factors

Factors resulting in sensory overload or deprivation can cause delirium. Unfamiliar surroundings or alteration in environment, sleep deprivation, noisy instruments (such as in intensive care units) or restraints can precipitate or prolong delirium in a prone individual. Therefore, attention to environmental factors is vital in the prevention and treatment of delirium.

CLINICAL FEATURES

The constellation of clinical features suggesting a diagnosis of delirium include acute onset, altered consciousness, fluctuating course, inability to focus attention and reversibility[1,2,8,14]. In the older adult, the onset could be insidious, with restlessness, sleep disturbances, anxiety or irritability during the prodromal stage[1,8]. Attention, orientation, planning and concentration ability are impaired[6,14]. An alteration in the level of consciousness is important in distinguishing delirium from dementia and other psychiatric disturbances. Symptoms fluctuate during the course of a day and between days, and are sometimes worse at night, resembling

Table 2 Criteria for delirium from the *Diagnostic and Statistical Manual of Mental Disorders*, 4th edn. (DSM-IV)*

(1) Disturbance of consciousness (reduced clarity of awareness of the environment) with reduced ability to focus, sustain or shift attention.
(2) A change in cognition (memory deficit, disorientation, language disturbance) or the development of a perceptual disturbance that is not better accounted for by a pre-existing, established, or evolving dementia.
(3) The disturbance develops over a short period (usually hours to days) and tends to fluctuate during the course of a day.
(4) There is evidence from the history, physical examination, or laboratory findings that the disturbance is caused by the direct physiologic consequences of a general medical condition.

*Washington, DC: American Psychiatric Association Press, 1994. Reprinted with permission. Copyright 2000 American Psychiatric Association

'sundowning' in dementia, often with 'lucid intervals'[1,2]. Impaired immediate and recent memory is common; often patients are amnesic or have patchy memory of the episode after recovery[8]. Inappropriate behavior, persecutory delusions, and visual and auditory hallucinations may be present[1]. The hallucinations may be vivid and frightening; accidents may result.

Occasionally, patients experience sleep abnormalities (reversal of the sleep–wake cycle), psychomotor hyper- or hypoactivity, mood alterations (anxiety, panic, apathy, sadness) and disorganized thought. Sleep is fragmented, night sleep short, with daytime drowsiness and naps. Neurologic examination may reveal constructional apraxia (defects in copying designs or drawing to command, in the absence of motor or sensory deficits), dysgraphia (difficulty in the automatic sequence of writing), dysnomia (inability to name objects in the absence of sensory deficits), tremors, myoclonus, asterixis or alterations in muscle tone. Asking the patient to draw a clock or name common objects serves to screen for apraxia and dysnomia. Those with hypervigilant delirium (intoxication, alcohol withdrawal) manifest features of agitation, while the more common hypersomnolent type presents with lethargy; mixed states also occur[1,4,6,8].

DIAGNOSIS

Maintaining vigilance for the syndrome is vital to diagnosis. Any alteration in mentation with a fluctuating cognitive status, decreased attention or disorientation should be treated as delirium, prompting a history, with information on baseline mentation from family or caregiver, physical examination, review of medications and investigations to uncover any precipitating factors for delirium. Several minor factors could be additive in causing delirium (e.g. hypercalcemia and anemia); these should not be ignored[2]. In the elderly, delirium might be the first sign of a serious underlying illness; for example, urosepsis may present with confusion, in the absence of fever or leukocytosis.

The two commonly used criteria for diagnosis of delirium are the *Diagnostic and Statistical Manual of Mental Disorders*, fourth edition (DSM-IV) criteria (Table 2) and the Confusion Assessment Method (CAM) (Table 3)[10,11]. The CAM as an instrument was adapted from the DSM-III R criteria and provides a simple, validated tool for the detection of delirium; the diagnosis is based on four major clinical features and has a sensitivity of 94–100% and a specificity of 90–95%[3,10]. The Mini Mental Status Examination provides a useful screening tool to assess cognitive status (attention, orientation, apraxia) and serial follow-up of the clinical course[6,7,9], but it was not designed as an ideal tool for delirium. Instruments such as the Delirium Rating Scale, Confusion Rating Scale and Delirium Symptom Interview are available but mostly for research use[6].

Laboratory evaluation should include serum electrolytes, glucose, calcium, and renal and liver function tests[3,7,11,12].

Table 3   The confusion assessment method (CAM) diagnostic algorithm. From reference 10

Feature 1. Acute onset and fluctuating course
This feature is usually obtained from a family member or nurse and is shown by positive responses to the following questions. Is there evidence of an acute change in mental status from the patient's baseline? Did the (abnormal) behavior fluctuate during the day, that is, tend to come and go, or increase and decrease in severity?

Feature 2. Inattention
This feature is shown by a positive response to the following question. Did the patient have difficulty focusing attention, for example, being easily distractible, or having difficulty keeping track of what was being said?

Feature 3. Disorganized thinking
This feature is shown by a positive response to the following question. Was the patient's thinking disorganized or incoherent, such as rambling or irrelevant conversation, unclear or illogical flow of ideas, or unpredictable switching from subject to subject?

Feature 4. Altered level of consciousness
This feature is shown by any answer other than 'alert' to the following question. Overall, how would you rate this patient's level of consciousness? (alert (normal), vigilant (hyperalert), lethargic (drowsy, easily aroused), stupor (difficult to arouse), or coma (unarousable)).

The diagnosis of delirium by CAM requires the presence of features 1 and 2 and either 3 or 4. Reprinted with permission from the *Annals of Internal Medicine*

Evaluation for occult infection should include complete blood count, urine analysis and chest radiographs. Electrocardiogram, oxygen saturation measurement and toxicology screening is undertaken in the appropriate clinical setting. Vitamin B_{12}, drug or ammonia levels, computed tomography (CT) scan or magnetic resonance imaging (MRI) of the brain, electroencephalogram (EEG), cerebrospinal fluid analysis and additional tests may be requested on a select basis[3]. Neuroimaging has a poor yield when there is no focal neurologic deficit, but may be performed when delirium persists without an evident cause[21]. EEG is useful when seizures are the etiology[13]. In delirium, EEG shows diffuse non-paroxysmal δ-wave slowing; some patients with agitation may have low-voltage fast activity[1,2]. The EEG abnormalities are non-specific and not diagnostic by themselves. A normal EEG makes the diagnosis of delirium less likely; the diagnostic sensitivity is about 75%[22].

DIFFERENTIAL DIAGNOSIS

Delirium has to be distinguished from dementia and other psychiatric illnesses such as depression, mood or psychotic disorders; salient features to differentiate delirium from dementia are provided in Table 4[23–25]. Attention to mode of onset, fluctuating course and level of consciousness help make the differentiation. Dementia does not alter attention or consciousness (except in advanced stages), is of slower onset and without the fluctuant nature of delirium[3]. When delirium is superimposed on dementia, especially in the absence of known baseline status, diagnosis may be difficult. Patients with pre-existing psychiatric disorders are prone to delirium from medications, drug abuse or other illnesses[2].

MANAGEMENT

Prevention

Prevention is probably most important in the management of delirium and can reduce the risk by up to 40%[3,5,9]. Individuals with predictors for the development of delirium need to be closely monitored with timely institution of appropriate interventions. Careful attention to medications, minimizing the use of indwelling catheters, promoting mobilization, using frequent cues to maintain orientation, limiting unnecessary environmental stimulation, giving attention to fluid–electrolyte balance, providing adequate pain relief and minimizing use of anticholinergic or sedative medications are

Table 4 Differentiation of delirium from dementia. From references 3, 7, 12, 13, 21 and 23

	Delirium	Dementia
Onset	acute (hours to days)	insidious (months to years)
Duration	days to weeks	months to years
Attention	impaired	normal*
Consciousness	fluctuates	normal*
Memory	impaired (poor attention)	impaired (even when awake, alert)
Speech	incoherent, rambling	coherent*, word-finding difficulty
Hallucinations	prominent feature	often absent
Reversible cause	more likely	less likely
Systemic illness	evident	usually absent
EEG	pronounced, diffuse changes	normal or mild abnormalities

EEG, electroencephalogram
*Except in advanced stages of the disease

helpful[10,12]. Exercise and ambulation limit deconditioning, development of pressure ulcers and pulmonary atelectasis. In the perioperative setting, appropriate management of hypotension, anemia, hypoxemia and infections helps prevent development of delirium[20,25].

Non-pharmacologic measures

Most non-pharmacologic measures aim at reducing sensory deficits, immobility, sleep disturbances and cognitive impairment[12,14]. Simple instructions, strategies to improve orientation, encouraging the participation of family members, involving the patient in decision-making, frequent eye contact and encouraging self-care are helpful. An agitated patient may be moved closer to the nurse's station for closer monitoring. Use of physical (and chemical) restraints should be minimized, as they contribute to immobility, agitation and delirium. The patient is encouraged to use glasses, hearing aids and dentures while in the hospital to maintain adequate sensory input. Non-pharmacologic measures also help treat behavioral disorders and sleep problems, thus lowering the use of psychoactive medications[3]. A discussion with the family explaining the clinical condition will alleviate anxiety and fear. Some useful measures to maintain a therapeutic environment are summarized in Table 5.

Pharmacologic therapy

No ideal drug for treatment of delirium exists; personal preferences often come into play. Therapy needs to balance symptom control and potential adverse effects from the medications. Sedatives and hypnotics can cause further cognitive dysfunction, impair evaluation of mental status and increase the risk of falls. However, at times, medications may be required to control agitation and problem behavior, for patient protection; this indication should be clearly recognized prior to initiating pharmacotherapy. Antipsychotics are often the drugs of choice, except in alcohol/drug withdrawal states when benzodiazepines are preferred[14]. Haloperidol in low dose (0.5–1 mg orally or intramuscularly) offers the advantages of fewer anticholinergic effects, less sedation and hypotension, and flexibility of different routes for administration[3,11,12,17]. Adverse reactions include hypotension, dystonia, anticholinergic and extrapyramidal effects. Higher doses of haloperidol (including the intravenous routes) are used in intensive care; adverse effects include neuroleptic malignant syndrome and QT prolongation with torsade de pointes[21]. Newer antipsychotics such as olanzapine and risperidone, available only in oral forms, are increasingly used, due to less sedation and fewer extrapyramidal side-effects. Amongst the benzodiazepines, lorazepam (0.5–2 mg orally or intramuscularly) has

Table 5   Environmental measures to treat delirium. From references 3, 5, 6, 9, 11 and 14

Maintain orientation (use of clocks, calendars, television, frequent reminders)
Keep familiar objects in the room (photographs)
Use measures to enhance cognition (trivia games)
Involve family members or close friends (supportive contact)
Make appropriate use of sensory aids (glasses, hearing aids, dentures)
Give clear and simple instructions to maintain daily routines
Communicate schedules (with use of an orientation board or center)
Ensure adequate lighting, including at night
Minimize sources of noise, especially at night (equipment, staff)
Limit room and staff changes, utilizing familiar staffing (if possible)
Maintain activity (ambulation, range of movement exercises)
Avoid sleep interruptions; adjust timing of medication administration, monitoring of vital signs
Use relaxation techniques (music, massage)

rapid onset and shorter duration of action, no active metabolites and low risk of accumulation. It should be emphasized that lower doses of medications should generally be used in older individuals, particularly if they are on other medications with potential for drug interactions.

While haloperidol appears to have a history of extensive use, intravenous (or intramuscular) use of droperidol is helpful when rapid effect is required, with monitoring for torsade again recommended. Although the second generation antipsychotics such as risperidone, olanzapine and quetiapine have been used for management of delirium, data from controlled studies confirming their efficacy is pending[25]. In situations where there is cholinergic deficiency, the off-label use of physostigmine salicylate (an anticholinesterase) has been found helpful; the use is associated with several risks especially in the presence of cardiac or pulmonary disease and intestinal ileus[25].

PROGNOSIS

A diagnosis of delirium carries significant morbidity and mortality, the latter perhaps because delirium is part of a terminal illness. Complications such as infections, falls and pressure sores may prolong hospitalization[6,15]. Persistent delirium in the postoperative setting is associated with a poor outcome; rehabilitation measures should be intensified in this group. While delirium can resolve in hours or days when correctable factors are addressed (e.g. hypo- or hypernatremia), many individuals do not return to their prior level of function. Mortality in hospitalized patients with delirium is estimated to range from 10 to 65%[1]. Upon discharge, delirium may persist for some time; in some, the transitional phase may persist for 6 months[11]. Nevertheless, a heightened awareness, coupled with timely institution of measures, can lower its incidence and improve the prognosis.

References

1. Tune LE. Perioperative management of the older adult. In Hazzard WR, Blass JP, Ettinger WH Jr, *et al.*, eds. *Principles of Geriatric Medicine and Gerontology*, 4th edn. New York: McGraw Hill, 1999: 1229–37
2. Caine ED, Grossman H, Lyness JM. Delirium, dementia, and amnestic and other cognitive disorders and mental disorders due to a general medical condition. In Kaplan HI, Sadock BJ, eds. *Comprehensive Textbook of Psychiatry*, 6th edn. Baltimore: Williams & Wilkins, 1995:729–32
3. Inouye SK. Assessment and management of delirium in hospitalized older patients. *Ann Long-term Care* 2000;8:53–9

4. Sandberg O, Gustafson Y, Brannstrom B, Bucht G. Clinical profile of delirium in older patients. *J Am Geriatr Soc* 1999;47:1300–6

5. Inouye SK. Delirium: a barometer for quality of hospital care. *Hosp Pract* 2001;36: 15–16, 18

6. Wise MG, Gray KF. Delirium, dementia, and amnestic disorders. In Hales RE, Yudofsky SC, eds. *Synopsis of Psychiatry*, 1st edn. Washington: American Psychiatric Press, 1996:305–43

7. Murphy BA. Delirium. *Emerg Med Clin North Am* 2000;18:243–52

8. Glick RL, Riba M. Common psychiatric emergencies in the office setting. In Knesper DJ, Riba MB, Schwenk TL, eds. *Primary Care Psychiatry*, 1st edn. Philadelphia: WB Saunders, 1997:45–60

9. Inouye SK, Bogardus ST Jr, Charpentier PA, *et al*. A multicomponent intervention to prevent delirium in hospitalized older patients. *N Engl J Med* 1999;340:669–76

10. Inouye SK, van Dyck CH, Alessi CA, *et al*. Clarifying confusion: the confusion assessment method. A new method for detection of delirium. *Ann Intern Med* 1990;113: 941–8

11. Inouye SK. Delirium and other mental status problems in the older patient. In Goldman L, Bennett JC, eds. *Cecil Texbook of Medicine*, 21st edn. Philadelphia: WB Saunders, 2000:20–2

12. Winawer N. Postoperative delirium. *Med Clin North Am* 2001;85:1229–39

13. Chan D, Brennan NJ. Delirium: making the diagnosis, improving the prognosis. *Geriatrics* 1999;54:28–30, 36, 39–42

14. Meagher DJ. Delirium: optimising management. *Br Med J* 2001;322:144–9

15. Zeleznik J. Effectiveness of interventions to prevent delirium in hospitalized patients: a systemic review. *J Am Geriatr Soc* 2001;49: 1730–2

16. McCusker J, Cole M, Abrahamowicz M, *et al*. Environmental risk factors for delirium in hospitalized older people. *J Am Geriatr Soc* 2001;49:1327–34

17. Frierson RL. Dementia, delirium, and other cognitive disorders. In Tasman A, Kay J, Lieberman JA, eds. *Psychiatry*, 1st edn. Philadelphia: WB Saunders, 1997:892–926

18. Johnson JC, Jayadevappa R, Baccash PD, Taylor L. Nonspecific presentation of pneumonia in hospitalized older people: age effect or dementia? *J Am Geriatr Soc* 2000; 48:1316–20

19. Marcantonio ER, Flacker JM, Michaels M, Resnick NM. Delirium is independently associated with poor functional recovery after hip fracture. *J Am Geriatr Soc* 2000; 48:618–24

20. Edlund A, Lundstrom M, Brannstrom B, *et al*. Delirium before and after operation for femoral neck fracture. *J Am Geriatr Soc* 2001;49:1335–40

21. Marcantonio ER. Delirium. In Cobbs EL, Duthrie EH Jr, Murphy JB, eds. *Geriatric Review Syllabus*, 5th edn. Malden, MA: Blackwell Publishing, 2002:131–8

22. Bair DB. Delirium. In Cobbs EL, Duthie EH Jr, Murphy JB, eds. *Geriatric Review Syllabus*, 4th edn. Dubuque, Iowa: Kendall Hunt Publishing, 1999:111–15

23. Brauer C, Morrison RS, Silberzweig SB, Siu AL. The cause of delirium in patients with hip fracture. *Arch Intern Med* 2000; 160:1856–60

24. Lipowski ZJ. Delirium in the elderly patient. *N Engl J Med* 1989;320:578–82

25. Samuels SC, Evers MM. Delirium: pragmatic guidance for managing a common, confounding and sometimes lethal condition. *Geriatrics* 2002;57:33–8

31 Depression in older adults

Seshagiri Rao Doddi, MD

INTRODUCTION

Symptoms of depression are common in older people[1] and these symptoms contribute to significant psychological and physical distress, physical disability[2] and higher mortality[3]. Depression is underdiagnosed and undertreated by primary care physicians[4]. Most elderly patients receive mental health care in primary care settings and are reluctant to accept referral to mental health specialists. It is essential for primary care providers to acquire knowledge and clinical skills to diagnose and treat depressive disorders in this age group. Diagnosis of depression in the elderly poses a challenge. Some of the contributing factors for difficulty in recognizing depression are listed in Table 1.

DEPRESSION AND AGE-RELATED ALTERATIONS IN THE BRAIN

The monoamine hypothesis attributes depression to decreased availability of neurotransmitters, specifically norepinephrine (noradrenaline) and serotonin, or altered sensitivity of receptors to these neurotransmitters. Selective degeneration of neurons occurs with advancing age, and compensatory dendrites proliferate. Acetylcholine, dopamine and norepinephrine decrease in the central nervous system with advancing age[5]. Monoamine oxidase (MAO), the enzyme involved in the degradation of monoamines, increases. The receptors decrease in number[6] with increased resistance to diffusion of drugs.

These changes may increase the biological vulnerability to depression in older adults. Due to the large reserves, the loss of cerebral function and cognitive decline is minimal in normal aging. The memory decline is normally limited to acquisition and retrieval of new information in secondary memory. Normal age-related changes in the brain do not affect ordinary functions of daily living until the person reaches the late seventies. Depression is not a part of normal aging.

EPIDEMIOLOGY AND RISK FACTORS

Depression is a generic term. It is important to recognize the difference between mood symptoms and mood syndromes (cluster of signs and symptoms with a characteristic course). Two main categories of depressive disorders are major depression and dysthymic disorder. The estimated prevalence for these disorders is lower in older adults compared to the young. In the majority of elderly suffering from depression, the symptoms do not meet the established criteria for these disorders. The prevalence of clinically significant symptoms of depression that need treatment interventions in the geriatric age group is estimated to be much higher, especially in general medical settings and in extended care facilities. Table 2 summarizes the epidemiological data[1,7–9] and Table 3[10–12] summarizes the risk factors for depression in the elderly.

Table 1 Factors contributing to difficulty in recognizing depression in older adults

Misconception that the depressive symptoms are part of normal aging
Reluctance to admit that one is depressed, due to stigma attached to mental disorders
More emphasis on physical symptoms and underreporting of psychiatric symptoms by older individuals. Psychiatric symptoms and emotional distress expressed in somatic terms rather than as depression
Inability to communicate and report, due to hearing or cognitive impairment
Diagnostic criteria for depressive disorders and structured interview schedules not sensitive or suitable for the elderly
Difficulty in distinguishing symptoms due to depression and co-existing medical and neurologic illnesses
Overlap of depressive symptoms with medication-related side-effects (such as anorexia, insomnia, weakness, fatigue)
The dysphoria experienced is often attributed to an understandable response to adversity with the diagnosis of depression missed

Table 2 Prevalence (%) of depression in the older population

Type of setting	Major depression	Depressive symptoms*
Community[1]	1.8	13.5
Primary care[7]	5–10	20
Hospitalized medically ill[8]	10–14	14–25
Long-term care[9]	12	30

*Clinically significant, causing distress and interfering with daily functioning

Table 3 Depression in older adults: risk factors. From references 10–12

Physical disability due to chronic disabling medical illness
History of depression
Death of spouse
Death of close family members or friends
Low socioeconomic status
Poor social support and loss of close social contact
Recent adverse and unexpected life events and situations of severe stresses
Alcohol or other substance abuse including prescription and non-prescription drugs
Cognitive impairment

CLASSIFICATION OF DEPRESSIVE DISORDERS

The relevant categories of depressive disorders, as classified in the *Diagnostic and Statistical Manual*, 4th edition (DSM-IV)[13] include (1) bipolar disorder, depressed or mixed type; (2) major depression (single episode, recurrent, with or without melancholia, with or without psychotic features); (3) dysthymic disorder; and (4) cyclothymic disorder. DSM-IV criteria for a major depressive episode and dysthymia

are summarized in Tables 4 and 5. Criteria for these disorders exclude symptoms due to physical illness, substance use and medications. The categories that are more prevalent in the geriatric age group are complicated bereavement, depressive disorders due to general medical conditions, substance- and medication-induced mood disorders, adjustment disorders with depressed mood, recurrent brief depressive disorders and mixed anxiety–depressive disorders. Some of these subthreshold depressive syndromes are referred to as 'minor depressive disorders'[14].

SUBTYPES AND SPECIFIC CLINICAL PRESENTATIONS

Late-onset major depression

This is a subtype of major depressive syndrome in elderly people who experience their first major depressive episode after age 60. Late-onset depression is associated with a loss of motivation or interest, less frequent family history of mood disorders, fewer bipolar II disorders, more unipolar disorders

Table 4 DSM-IV criteria for major depression. From reference 13

A. Five (or more) of the following symptoms have been present during the same 2-week period and represent a change from previous functioning; at least one is either (1) depressed mood or (2) loss of interest or pleasure.
    Note: Do not include symptoms that are clearly due to a general medical condition, or mood-incongruent delusions or hallucinations.

(1) depressed mood most of the day, nearly every day
(2) markedly diminished interest or pleasure in all, or almost all, activities most of the day, nearly every day
(3) significant weight loss when not dieting or weight gain, or decrease or increase in appetite nearly every day
(4) insomnia or hypersomnia nearly every day
(5) psychomotor agitation or retardation nearly every day (observable by others, not merely subjective feelings of restlessness or being slowed down)
(6) fatigue or loss of energy nearly every day
(7) feelings of worthlessness or excessive or inappropriate guilt (which may be delusional) nearly every day (not merely self reproach or guilt about being sick)
(8) diminished ability to think or concentrate, or indecisiveness, nearly every day
(9) recurrent thoughts of death (not just fear of dying), recurrent suicidal ideation without a specific plan, or a suicide attempt or a specific plan for committing suicide

The symptoms

B. Do not meet criteria for a mixed episode
C. Cause clinically significant distress or impairment in social, occupational, or other important areas of functioning
D. Are not due to the direct physiological effects of a substance or a general medical condition
E. Are not better accounted for by bereavement, i.e. after the loss of a loved one, the symptoms persist for longer than 2 months or are characterized by marked functional impairment, morbid preoccupation with worthlessness, suicidal ideation, psychotic symptoms, or psychomotor retardation

Reprinted with permission from the *Diagnostic and Statistical Manual of Mental Disorders*, Fourth Edition, Text Revision. Copyright 2000, American Psychiatric Association

and more relapses[15,16]. These patients develop a higher rate of dementia on follow-up, greater enlargement of lateral brain ventricles and increased prevalence of white-matter hyperintensities leading to the hypothesis of 'vascular depression'[17–19].

Psychotic depression (delusional depression)

Major depression with psychotic (delusional) symptoms is common in the in-patient geriatric psychiatry setting. The patients are severely depressed, manifest more psychomotor retardation and have a history of psychotic depressive episodes. The types of delusions with psychotic depression are frequently of the somatic and nihilistic type[20]. The response to treatment with antidepressants alone is poor in psychotic depression.

Combinations of antipsychotic and antidepressant medications or electroconvulsive therapy (ECT) are the treatments of choice.

Minor depression

Minor or mild depression[14,21–23] is common in the elderly and causes significant distress and disability. Subthreshold minor depression may present in two ways: first, as a quantitatively minor variant of depression or a depression-like state with fewer symptoms or with less continuity; second, as qualitatively different from major depression with fewer suicidal thoughts or feelings of guilt or worthlessness, while worries about health and weariness of living occur with a similar frequency[21]. Minor depression is not a stable entity and can predict the development of major depression. Minor depression is

Table 5 DSM-IV diagnostic criteria for dysthymic disorder. From reference 13

A. Depressed mood for most of the day, for more days than not, as indicated either by subjective account or observation by others, for at least 2 years. **Note:** In children and adolescents, mood can be irritable and duration must be at least 1 year.

B. Presence, while depressed, of two (or more) of the following:

   (1) poor appetite or overeating
   (2) insomnia or hypersomnia
   (3) low energy or fatigue
   (4) low self-esteem
   (5) poor concentration or difficulty making decisions
   (6) feelings of hopelessness

C. During the 2-year period (1 year for children or adolescents) of the disturbance, the person has never been without the symptoms in Criteria A and B for more than 2 months at a time.

D. No Major Depressive Episode has been present during the first 2 years of the disturbance (1 year for children and adolescents); i.e. the disturbance is not better accounted for by chronic Major Depressive Disorder, or Major Depressive Disorder, In Partial Remission.
   Note: There may have been a previous Major Depressive Episode provided there was a full remission (no significant signs or symptoms for 2 months) before development of the Dysthymic Disorder. In addition, after the initial 2 years (1 year in children or adolescents) of Dysthymic Disorder, there may be superimposed episodes of Major Depressive Disorder, in which case both diagnoses may be given when the criteria are met for a Major Depressive Episode.

E. There has never been a Manic Episode, a Mixed Episode, or a Hypomanic Episode, and criteria have never been met for Cyclothymic Disorder.

F. The disturbance does not occur exclusively during the course of a chronic Psychotic Disorder, such as Schizophrenia or Delusional Disorder.

G. The symptoms are not due to the direct physiological effects of a substance (e.g. a drug of abuse, a medication) or a general medical condition (e.g. hypothyroidism).

H. The symptoms cause clinically significant distress or impairment in social, occupational, or other important areas of functioning.

Reprinted with permission from the *Diagnostic and Statistical Manual of Mental Disorders*, Fourth Edition, Text Revision. Copyright 2000, American Psychiatric Association

roughly twice as common as major depression, with a higher frequency in residential or medical in-patients compared with community-dwelling elderly. There is also a steep increase in people over age 80. Minor depression is associated with significant functional impairment[22,23]. Treatment remains unclear, but in the absence of evidence to the contrary, antidepressant medication and psychotherapeutic interventions, alone or combined, are currently the recommended course of action.

Depression and bereavement

Complicated grief and bereavement-related depression poses another challenge regarding recognition and treatment. Older adults experience multiple losses, leading to grief and bereavement. Symptoms include searching, yearning, preoccupation with thoughts of the deceased, crying, disbelief regarding the death, feeling stunned by the death and lack of acceptance of the death. Complicated grief results in impairment in global functioning, mood, sleep and self-esteem[24]. The prolonged symptoms of complicated grief should be recognized and treated aggressively to prevent morbidity and mortality.

Depression and anxiety

Depression presents most often as anxiety in older people. A high level of co-morbidity exists between anxiety disorders and depressive disorders. The presence of a co-morbid anxiety disorder was associated with poor social functioning and a higher level of somatic symptoms and suicidality[25]. Antidepressants are the primary treatment of choice for anxiety symptoms associated with depression.

DEPRESSION AND GENERAL MEDICAL CONDITIONS

Depression is a common associated symptom of several medical conditions that are frequent in older adults. The following is a partial list.

(1) Dementias: Alzheimer's disease and vascular (post-stroke) dementias;

(2) Post-myocardial infarction (MI);

(3) Neurological disorders: Parkinson's disease, Huntington's disease, multiple sclerosis;

(4) Endocrine disorders: hypothyroidism, hyperthyroidism, hyperparathyroidism, Cushing's disease;

(5) Malignancies: cancer of the head of the pancreas, metastatic bone cancer;

(6) Nutritional: vitamin B_{12} and folate deficiencies;

(7) Autoimmune: systemic lupuserythematosus;

(8) Infections: syphilis, Lyme disease, viral illnesses.

Depression and dementia

Depression and dementia are two common mental illnesses in the geriatric age group. Depression could present as dementia (depressive pseudodementia), and early stages of dementia could present as depression. Co-existing depression and dementia are also common; approximately 50% of demented individuals manifest depressive features of varying intensities.

Depression may be an early manifestation of Alzheimer's disease before cognitive symptoms become apparent. Small left hippocampal size on neuroimaging may be a marker for dementia in depressed patients who have not yet met criteria for a clinical diagnosis of a dementing disorder[26]. Elderly depressed patients with cognitive impairment may experience improvement in specific domains following antidepressant treatment, but may not necessarily reach normal levels of performance, particularly in memory and executive functions. This subgroup of late-life depression is at risk for developing progressive dementia[27]. A therapeutic trial of an antidepressant is warranted whenever the diagnosis is not clear. Treatment could improve the quality of life, even in those with severe dementia.

Post-stroke depression

Clinically significant depression is frequent after ischemic stroke[28] and may influence functional recovery[29] and mortality. Proximity of the lesion to the left frontal pole increases the risk for depression within 2 years following the stroke[30]. Remission of post-stroke depression is associated with improvement in recovery of activities of daily living (ADL)[29].

Medication and substance-induced depression

Alcohol abuse and inappropriate use of prescription drugs, such as benzodiazepines, is not uncommon in the elderly, but is often unrecognized by the health-care providers. Any medication or a substance that causes depressive effects on the central nervous system potentially could contribute to induction of depression in the vulnerable individual[31]. Polypharmacy is common and leads to drug–drug interactions with adverse effects. Anorexia, insomnia, fatigability, restlessness, anxiety and depression are common adverse drug reactions, which may also be symptoms of depressive disorders. The medication may not be the sole perpetrator, but a contributing

Table 6 Drugs known to contribute to development of depression*. From references 31 and 32

Antibacterials	*Cardiovascular drugs*	*Narcotics*
Anti-TB drugs	Amiodarone	Codeine
Cephradine	β-blockers (lipophilic drugs may	Meperidine
Clotrimazole	be more likely)	Morphine
Cotrimoxazole	Atenolol	Methadone
Dapsone	Nadolol	
Griseofulvin	Labetalol	*NSAIDs and analgesics*
Mefloquine	Oxprenolol	Diflunisal
Metronidazole	Timolol	Indomethacin
Piperazine	Acebutol	Nabilone
Primaquine	Pindolol	Nalbuphine
Sulfonamides	Metoprolol	Pentazocine
	Propranolol	Sulindac
Anticonvulsants	Acebutol	Tramadol
Carbamazepine	Nadolol	
Clobazam	Timolol	*Respiratory*
Clonazepam	Clonidine	Aminophylline
Ethosuximide	Diltiazem	Ephedrine
Phenobarbital	Enalapril	Flunisolide
Vigabatrin	Felodipine	Theophylline
	Hydralazine	
Antiparkinsonian drugs	Methyldopa	*Steroids*
Amantadine	Nicardipine	Dexamethasone
Anticholinergics	Nifedipine	Prednisolone
Levodopa	Prazosin	Prednisone
	Procainamide	Stanozolol
Anxiolytics	Quinapril	
Alprazolam	Quinidine	*Miscellaneous*
Bromazepam	Streptokinase	Allopurinol
Clordiazepoxide		Astemizole
Diazepam	*Gastrointestinal*	Cinnarizine
Lorazepam	Cimetidine	Clomiphene
Oxazepam	Metoclopramide	Diphenoxylate
Buspirone	Ranitidine	Disulfiram
	Sulphasalazine	Etretinate
Chemotherapeutic agents for		Fentanyl (transdermal)
cancer	*Hypnotics and sedatives*	Interferon
Interferon-α	Barbiturates	Ondansetron
Mesna	Chloral hydrate	Oral contraceptives
Mithramycin	Flurazepam	Phenylpropanolamine
Plicamycin	Meprobamate	Pravastatin
Tamoxifen		Progestogens
Triamcinolone		Roaccutane
		Simvastatin
		Trimeprazine/alimemazine
		Xylometazoline

*Some of these drugs may not be available in some countries. TB, tuberculosis; NSAIDs, non-steroidal anti-inflammatory drugs

agent for development of depression. Medications known to induce depression are listed in Table 6[31,32]. Management includes discontinuation or altering the offending agent, if feasible. If depressive symptoms persist, treatment with antidepressant medications is warranted.

MORBIDITY AND MORTALITY

Consequences of depression in the elderly include:

(1) Psychological and physical suffering;

(2) Diminution in quality of life;

(3) Physical disability with decline in performance of basic activities of daily living[2,23];

(4) Increased mortality of the aged, even after adjustment for age, number of current diseases, smoking status and gender[3,33,34];

(5) Predisposition for development of cardiovascular illness[35] and this could be a contributing risk factor for cerebrovascular disease[36];

(6) Interference with recovery following medical illness such as stroke[29,37], MI[38,39] and hip fractures;

(7) Increased use of medical resources[40,41];

(8) Decreased immune response;

(9) Increased burden on families and caregivers.

DEPRESSION AND SUICIDE

The majority of older suicide victims suffer from a depressive disorder at the time of death. Old age is a risk factor for suicide; risk is higher in the age group of 65 years and above, and highest in the age group above 85 years of age. Other risk factors include severe medical illness and functional disability; alcohol abuse; white male widowed or divorced older men; a history of a suicide attempt; co-morbid anxiety; and psychotic depression[42]. Older individuals who commit suicide tend to seek physicians for somatic complaints shortly before their death. Suicide assessment should be routinely performed in all patients in the high-risk category, and the clinician should never hesitate to question regarding suicide. Inquiry about suicide begins by questioning about passive death wishes, not uncommon in the elderly. Enquiring should proceed by asking about active suicidal ideas, intentions and plan. Strategies for prevention should include providing a safe environment, involving the family, addressing underlying problems, crisis intervention and treatment of underlying depression.

Psychiatric referral and hospitalization should be considered, based on the severity of suicidal symptoms and associated risk factors.

DIAGNOSIS

A comprehensive history, physical examination and laboratory tests are indicated in depressed patients, prior to initiating treatment. The purpose is to diagnose and identify any underlying medical conditions (e.g. hypothyroidism), establishment of baseline function (e.g. cognitive abilities when dementia coexists with depression) and medical risk factors that may influence choice of treatment.

(1) *History* The history should include information from significant others and primary caregivers. The change in pattern should be more emphasized, rather than getting information for mere presence or absence of various neurovegetative symptoms such as sleep, eating and interest in activities, social behavior, etc. Information should be obtained regarding episodes of depression, history of alcohol and substance use, family history of depression, medical history and all medications (including over the counter), social history including recent psychosocial stressors, major life events, changes in living arrangements and changes in ADL and instrumental activities of daily living (IADL) functions.

(2) *Physical examination* The examination should include neurologic examination and mental status examination for cognition (Mini-Mental Status examination).

(3) *Rating scales* The rating scales are useful for longitudinal follow-up to assess progress or lack of progress with treatment interventions. Commonly used rating scales include the Hamilton Depression Scale[43], the Geriatric Depression Scale[44], and the Beck[45] and Zung[46] self-rating scales.

(4) *Laboratory tests* These include blood counts, hemoglobin, hematocrit and chemistry panel to include glucose, blood urea nitrogen, creatinine, basic liver and cardiac profile, B_{12} and folate levels, thyroid function and screening tests for syphilis, electrocardiogram and chest X-ray. Further evaluation may be individualized based on aforementioned test results.

TREATMENT

The treatment modalities include pharmacotherapy, ECT, psychotherapy and psychosocial interventions. Referral to a psychiatrist is recommended if the depression is resistant to treatment, if depression is associated with psychotic symptoms and if the patient is considered a high suicidal risk.

Pharmacotherapy

General principles of pharmacotherapy in the elderly are as follows:

(1) Assess benefit/risk ratio.

(2) Start low and go slow.

(3) Avoid subtherapeutic doses. Gradually increase to appropriate therapeutic doses, as long as the medication is tolerated without significant side-effects.

(4) Onset of antidepressant effect may take longer in the elderly. An adequate trial should last up to 6–12 weeks at full therapeutic dose of the medication.

Generally, antidepressants display similarity in efficacy; however, effectiveness may be substantially different within different classes of antidepressant medications. The selection of an antidepressant is based on side-effect profiles, drug interaction potential, the patient's prior drug response and effect on other co-morbid medical conditions[47-51].

Table 7 presents the commonly prescribed antidepressants, mechanisms of action, side-effect profile and dosage recommendations for the geriatric age group[49-55].

Tricyclics

The efficacy of tricyclics (TCAs) is well established. TCAs affect multiple neurotransmitters with potential for intolerable side-effects in the elderly. They are also lethal in overdose. Secondary amine TCAs have an advantage over tertiary, especially nortriptyline, with less tendency for orthostatic hypotension. Nortriptyline is shown to have a 'therapeutic window' between plasma levels of 50 and 150 ng/ml; the dose could be adjusted on the basis of blood levels.

Monoamine oxidase inhibitors

Monoamine oxidase inhibitors (MAOIs) are effective in depression and also mixed anxiety depressive conditions, including panic disorders and phobias. In general, they are well tolerated, but orthostatic hypotension could contribute to falls and fractures. Another disadvantage of MAOIs is the need for dietary restrictions and potential for adverse drug interactions leading to fatal hypertensive crisis.

Selective serotonin reuptake inhibitors

Selective serotonin reuptake inhibitors (SSRIs) are well tolerated with fewer side-effects. SSRIs are effective and reasonably safe in elderly depressed patients with co-morbid illness[54]. A number of potential adverse effects are unappreciated by clinicians. These include falls, hyponatremia, weight loss, sexual dysfunction and drug interactions. These potential risks, however, appear to be equally balanced by advantages such as fewer anticholinergic effects, a benign cardiovascular profile, ease of use and safety with overdose[55]. All SSRIs block cytochrome

Table 7 Antidepressants in the elderly. From references 49–55

Name of the medication	Starting dose (mg/day)	Target dose (mg/day)	Mechanism of action	Adverse effects and comments
Tricyclics (TCAs)				
Tertiary amines				
Amitriptyline	10–25	75–150	inhibition of norepinephrine	dryness of mouth, blurred vision,
Clomipramine	10–25	75–150	and serotonin re-uptake	constipation, urinary retention,
Doxepin	10–25	75–150	(therapeutic action), but also	sedation, weight gain, orthostatic
Imipramine	10–25	50–150	block cholinergic receptors,	hypotension, confusion,
Trimipramine	25	50–150	H₁ histaminic and	cardiotoxicity and fatal in overdose.
Secondary amines			α₁-adrenergic receptors	
Desipramine	10–25	50–150	(side-effects)	Nortriptyline therapeutic window
Nortriptyline	10–25	50–100		plasma level 50–150 ng/ml
Protriptyline	5–10	15–20		
Monoamine oxidase inhibitors (MAOIs)				
Phenelzine	15	15–60	inhibition of monoamine	orthostatic hypotension,
Isocarboxazide	20	20–60	oxidase, but also dose-related	insomnia, sexual dysfunction.
Tranylcypromine	20	20–40	α-adrenergic blocking effects	Serious drug–drug and drug–food interactions (hypertensive crisis with foods high in tyramine and sympathomimetic drugs)
Selective serotonin reuptake inhibitors (SSRIs)				
Fluoxetine	10	10–50	selective inhibition of serotonin	headache, dizziness, anxiety,
Fluvoxamine	50	100–300	reuptake with minimal	restlessness, agitation, insomnia,
Paroxetine	10	10–40	impact on other receptors	GI side-effects, sexual dysfunction,
Sertraline	25	50–150		drug–drug interactions due to
Citalopram	10	20–40		inhibition of P450 (except citalopram)
Norepinephrine and dopamine reuptake inhibitors (NDRIs)				
Bupropion			active metabolite of bupropion	GI side-effects, headache, insomnia,
Sustained release	100	150–300	blocks the reuptake of dopamine and norepinephrine reuptake	restlessness, agitation and risk of seizures. No cardiotoxicity and sexual side-effects
Serotonoin-2 antagonist and reuptake inhibitors (SARIs)				
Trazodone	25	75–300	Both are 5-HT₂ antagonists and	trazadone causes very high sedation
Nefazodone	100	100–400	5-HT reuptake inhibitors. In addition, they block α₁-adrenergic receptors and trazadone also blocks histamine receptors	and orthostatic hypotension. Nefazodone causes GI side-effects, agitation, insomnia, dizziness and drug–drug interactions due to inhibition of P450 3A4
Serotonin and norepinephrine reuptake inhibitors (SNRIs)				
Venlafaxine			potent inhibitors of 5-HT and	venlafaxine causes dose-related
Extended release	37.5	75–225	norepinephrine uptake;	elevation in diastolic BP, GI and
Mirtazapine	7.5–15	15–45	weak inhibitors of dopamine reuptake, but mirtazapine also has histaminergic blocking effect	sexual side-effects, and has activating properties. Mirtazapine causes sedation, weight gain, dizziness, dry mouth, constipation and rarely neutropenia and mild transient elevation of liver enzymes.
Duloxetine				Unknown (under development)
Selective norepinephrine reuptake inhibitors (SNRIs)				
Reboxetine	2	4–12	norepinephrine reuptake	not available in USA. Initial reports
			inhibitors without serotonin	indicate no significant side-effects.
Viloxazine	unknown	unknown	reuptake inhibition activity	Unknown (under development)

5-HT, 5-hydroxytryptamine; GI, gastrointestinal; BP, blood pressure

P450, causing interaction with other drugs and altering pharmacokinetics. Differences among SSRIs are not significant in general clinical practice, but in geriatric practice they may be a factor in selection. Fluoxetine has an active metabolite with prolonged half-life (4–16 days), which can be an advantage when weaning the patient off therapy, in that it may reduce the incidence of discontinuation symptoms, but a significant disadvantage if the patient cannot tolerate the drug or experiences an adverse drug–drug interaction. Citalopram and sertraline may have comparatively less effect on cytochrome P450 and be less likely to be involved in significant drug–drug interactions than fluoxetine, fluvoxamine and paroxetine[54].

Mixed reuptake inhibitors

Several newer antidepressant medications have specific inhibitory action on reuptake of two ('dual action') or more neurotransmitters. Venlafaxine is a specific serotonin and norepinephrine reuptake inhibitor (SNRI) with a weak effect on the dopamine receptor. Compared to TCAs, it has minimal anticholinergic, antihistaminergic and antiadrenergic effect. It is shown to have excellent efficacy in mixed anxiety and depressive disorders and in those who respond poorly to SSRIs. In a small number of patients, significant elevation of diastolic blood pressure was reported, but much less with the extended release form.

Bupropion has an active metabolite, which blocks the reuptake of dopamine and norepinephrine. It has no known cardiotoxicity and minimal effect on sexual function. It can cause insomnia and has to be avoided in patients with seizure risk, even though the risk is much less with the sustained-release form.

Mirtazapine has multiple effects including blockade of presynoptic α_2-adrenergic receptors and inhibition of both 5-hydroxytryptamine (5-HT) and norepinephrine reuptake. Mirtazapine also has a histaminergic blocking effect and causes sedation and weight gain. Sedation is marked in the lower dose range.

Psychostimulants

Dextroamphetamine and methylphenadote improve apathy and anergy in patients with advanced cancer and other medical illnesses[56,57]. Psychostimulants have rapid action, minimal side-effects and low risk for addiction in the ill elderly. They could cause anorexia, anxiety, agitation and confusion.

Electroconvulsive therapy

ECT is used increasingly in the older population for major depression, particularly when unresponsive to medications, or not tolerated because of side-effects, or when depression is accompanied by life-threatening complications such as severe weight loss or catatonia, where a rapid definitive response is required. ECT is considered a low-risk procedure that can be successfully administered to ill older adults[58], but is associated with a brief period of increased blood pressure and heart rate, leading to increased myocardial oxygen demand. ECT may cause brief periods of delirium, particularly in the cognitively impaired.

Psychotherapy and psychosocial interventions

Very few controlled studies exist regarding the effectiveness of various forms psychotherapy in the treatment of geriatric depression. There is some evidence to suggest that combined psychotherapy and pharmacotherapy may be more effective than either alone[59,60]. Psychotherapy could be provided in an individual or group format. The psychotherapy formats used in the elderly include the supportive, behavioral, cognitive, interpersonal and psychodynamic. Problem solving and reminiscence are other forms of therapy. In general, an eclectic approach with flexibility and active participation by the therapist are the preferred choices in treating older adults.

Social interventions, environmental management and other concrete services such as a visiting nurse, home care, day care, referral to senior citizen centers, placement in retirement or group homes and psychoeducation to patient and families are other measures that need to be utilized in the treatment of the depressed elderly.

Continuation and maintenance treatment

Relapse and recurrence of major depression and other depressive disorders after initial remission is common. The objective of continuation treatment is to decrease the likelihood of relapse of symptoms during the current episode. For a major depressive episode, the general guidelines are to continue the same dosage of medication for 1 year[60]. Maintenance treatment is aimed at preventing a new episode of depression in vulnerable individuals. Patients who have had three episodes of major depression have a 90% chance of having another episode, and long-term maintenance on antidepressant medication for longer than 3 years is recommended. The number of episodes, time between episodes, severity of the episodes and risk of suicide are some of the factors that need to be considered in deciding the need for maintenance treatment. Maintenance medications are generally of the same type and dosage found effective in the acute phase of treatment.

References

1. Beekman AT, Copeland JR, Prince MJ. Review of community prevalence of depression in later life. *Br J Psychiatry* 1999;174: 307–11
2. Penninx BWJH, Guralnik JM, Ferrucci L, *et al*. Depressive symptoms and physical decline in community-dwelling older persons. *J Am Med Assoc* 1998;279:1720–6
3. Schulz R, Beach SR, Ives DG, *et al*. Association between depression and mortality in older adults: the Cardiovascular Health Study. *Arch Intern Med* 2000;160:1761
4. Katon W, von Korff M, Lin E, *et al*. Adequacy and duration of antidepressant treatment in primary care. *Med Care* 1992; 30:67–76
5. Strong R. Neurochemical changes in the aging human brain: implications for behavioral impairment and neurodegenerative disease. *Geriatrics* 1998;53(Suppl. 1):S9–12
6. Schocken DD, Roth GS. Reduced beta-adrenergic receptor concentration in aging man. *Nature (London)* 1977;26:856–8
7. Schulberg HC, Mulsant B, Schultz R, *et al*. Characteristic and course of major depression in older primary care patients. *Int J Psychiatry Med* 1992;28:421–36
8. Koenig HG, George LK, Peterson BL, *et al*. Depression in medically ill hospitalized older adults: prevalence, characteristics, and course of symptoms according to six diagnostic schemes. *Am J Psychiatry* 1997; 154:1376–83
9. Parmelee PA, Katz IR, Lawton MP. Depression among institutionalized aged: assessment and prevalence estimation. *J Gerontol* 1989;44:M22–9
10. Schoevers RA, Beekman AT, Deeg DJ, *et al*. Risk factors for depression in later life; results of a prospective community based study. *J Affect Disord* 2000;59:127–37
11. Brilman EI, Ormel J. Life events, difficulties and onset of depressive episodes in later life. *Psychol Med* 2001;31:859–69
12. Raccio-Robak N, McErlean MA, Fabacher DA, *et al*. Socioeconomic and health status differences between depressed and nondepressed ED elders. *Am J Emerg Med* 2002;20:71–3
13. American Psychiatric Association *Diagnostic and Statistical Manual of Mental Disorders*, 4th edn. Text Revision. Washington, DC: American Psychiatric Association, 2000:327, 349

14. Tannock C, Katona C. Minor depression in the aged. Concepts, prevalence and optimal management. *Drugs Aging* 1995;6:278–92

15. Heun R, Kockler M, Papassotiropoulos A. Distinction of early- and late-onset depression in the elderly by their lifetime symptomatology. *Int J Geriatr Psychiatry* 2000; 15:1138–42

16. Benzzi F. Late-life chronic depression: a 399-case study in private practice. *Int J Geriatr Psychiatry* 2000;15:1–6

17. Alexapoulos GS, Meyers BS, Young RC, et al. 'Vascular depression' hypothesis. *Arch Gen Psychiatry* 1997;54:915–22

18. Krishnan KR, Hays JC, Blazer DG. MRI-defined vascular depression. *Am J Psychiatry* 1997;154:497–501

19. Nebes RD, Vora IJ, Meltzer CC, et al. Relationship of deep white matter hyperintensities and apolipoprotein E genotype to depressive symptoms in older adults without clinical depression. *Am J Psychiatry* 2001;158:878–84

20. Gournellis R, Lykouras L, Fortos A, et al. Psychotic (delusional) major depression in late life: a clinical study. *Int J Geriatr Psychiatry* 2001;16:1085–91

21. Geiselmann B, Bauer M. Subthreshold depression in the elderly: qualitative or quantitative distinction? *Compr Psychiatry* 2000;41(2 Suppl. 1):32–8

22. Hybels CF, Blazer DG, Pieper CF. Toward a threshold for subthreshold depression: an analysis of correlates of depression by severity of symptoms using data from an elderly community sample. *Gerontologist* 2001;41:357–65

23. Williams JW, Kerber CA, Mulrow CD, et al. Depressive disorders in primary care: prevalence, functional disability, and identification. *J Gen Intern Med* 1995;10:7–12

24. Prigerson HG, Frank E, Kasal SV, et al. Complicated grief and bereavement-related depression as distinct disorders: preliminary empirical validation in elderly bereaved spouses. *Am J Psychiatry* 1995; 152:22–30

25. Lenze EJ, Mulsant BH, Shear MK, et al. Comorbid anxiety disorders in depressed elderly patients. *Am J Psychiatry* 2000; 157:722–8

26. Geerlings MI, Schoevers RA, Beekman AT, et al. Depression and risk of cognitive decline and Alzheimer's disease. Results of two prospective community-based studies in the Netherlands. *Br J Psychiatry* 2000; 176:568–75

27. Butters MA, Becker JT, Nebes RD, et al. Changes in cognitive functioning following treatment of late-life depression. *Am J Psychiatry* 2000;157:1949–54

28. Pohjasvaara T, Leppavuori A, Siira I, et al. Frequency and clinical determinants of poststroke depression. *Stroke* 1998;29: 2311–17

29. Chemerinski E, Robinson RG, Kosier JT. Improved recovery in activities of daily living associated with remission of poststroke depression. *Stroke* 2001;32:113–17

30. Starkstein SE, Robinson RG, Price TR. Comparison of cortical and sub cortical lesion in the production of poststroke mood disorders. *Brain* 1987;110: 1045–59

31. Dhondt T, Derksen P, Hooijer C, et al. Depressogenic medication as an aetiological factor in major depression: an analysis in a clinical population of depressed elderly people. *Int J Geriatr Psychiatry* 1999;14: 875–81

32. Bazire S, Benefield WH Jr. Drug induced psychiatric disorders. In Bazire S, Benefield WH Jr, eds. *Psychotropic Drug Directory*. Oxford, UK: Alden Press, 2001:302–4

33. Takeida K, Nishi M, Miyake H. Mental depression and death in elderly persons. *J Epidemiol* 1997;7:210–13

34. Saz P, Dewey ME. Depression, depressive symptoms and mortality in persons aged 65 and over living in the community: a systematic review of the literature. *Int J Geriatr Psychiatry* 2001;16:622–30

35. Ariyo AA, Haan M, Tangen CM. Depressive symptoms and risks of coronary heart disease and mortality in elderly Americans. Cardiovascular Health Study Collaborative Research Group. *Circulation* 2000;102: 1773–9

36. Krishnan KR. Depression as a contributing factor in cerebrovascular disease. *Am Heart J* 2000;140(4 Suppl.):70–6

37. Gillen R, Tennen H, McKee TE, *et al*. Depressive symptoms and history of depression predict rehabilitation efficiency in stroke patients. *Arch Phys Med Rehabil* 2001;82:1645–9

38. Lesperance F, Frasure-Smith N, Talajic M, *et al*. Five-year risk of cardiac mortality in relation to initial severity and one-year changes in depression symptoms after myocardial infarction. *Circulation* 2002; 105:1049–53

39. Frasure-Smith N, Lesperance F, Talajic M. Depression following MI in patients on 6 month survival. *J Am Med Assoc* 1993;270: 1819–25

40. Luber MP, Meyers BS, Williams-Russo PG, *et al*. Depression and service utilization in elderly primary care patients. *Am J Geriatr Psychiatry* 2001;9:169–76

41. Bula CJ, Wietlisbach V, Burnand B, *et al*. Depressive symptom as a predictor of 6-month outcomes and services utilization in elderly medical inpatients. *Arch Intern Med* 2001;161:2609–15

42. Suffens DC, Blazer DG. Suicide in the elderly. In Jacob DG, ed. *The Harvard Medical School Guide to Suicide Assessment and Intervention*. San Francisco, CA: Jossey-Bass Publishers, 1999:443–62

43. Hamilton M. A rating scale for depression. *J Neurol Neurosurg Psychiatry* 1960;23: 56–62

44. Yesavage JA, Brink TL, Rose TL, *et al*. Development and validation of a geriatric depression screening scale: a preliminary report. *J Psychiatr Res* 1983;17:37–49

45. Beck A, Ward CH, Mendelson M, *et al*. An inventory for measuring depression. *Arch Gen Psychiatry* 1961;4:53–63

46. Zung WWK. A self-rating depression scale. *Arch Gen Psychiatry* 1965;12:371–9

47. Depression Guideline Panel. *Depression in Primary Care: Detection, Diagnosis, and Treatment*. Clinical Practice Guideline Number 5. AHCPR Publication 93-0550. Rockville, MD: US Department of Health and Human Services, Public Health Service, Agency for Health Policy and Research, 1993

48. Lebowitz BD, Pearson JL, Schneider LS, *et al*. Diagnosis and treatment of depression in late life: consensus statement update. *J Am Med Assoc* 1997;278:1186–90

49. Barkin RL, Schwer WA, Barkin SJ. Recognition and management of depression in primary care: a focus on the elderly. A pharmacotherapeutic overview of the selection process among the traditional and new antidepressants. *Am J Ther* 2000;7: 205–26

50. Sable JA, Dunn LB, Zisook S. Late-life depression. How to identify its symptoms and provide effective treatment. *Geriatrics* 2002;57:18–19, 22–3, 26

51. Nelson JC. Diagnosing and treating depression in the elderly. *J Clin Psychiatry* 2001;62(Suppl. 24):18–22

52. Mulrow CD, Williams JW, Chiquette E, *et al*. Efficacy of newer medications for treating depression in primary care patients. *Am J Med* 2000;108:54–64

53. Stahl SM, ed. *Psychopharmacology of Antidepressants*. London, UK: Martin Dunitz, 1997:29–82

54. Solai LK, Mulsant BH, Pollock BG. Selective serotonin reuptake inhibitors for late-life depression: a comparative review. *Drugs Aging* 2001;18:355–68

55. Herrmann N. Use of SSRIs in the elderly: obvious benefits but unappreciated risks. *Can J Clin Pharmacol* 2000;7:91–5

56. Homsi J, Nelson KA, Sarhill N, *et al*. A phase II study of methylphenidate for depression in advanced cancer. *Am J Hosp Palliat Care* 2001;18:403–7

57. Frye CB. Methylphenidate for depression in the elderly, medically ill patient. *Am J Health Syst Pharm* 1997;54:2510–1

58. Rabheru K. The use of electroconvulsive therapy in special patient population. *Can J Psychiatry* 2001;46:710–19

59. Lenze EJ, Dew MA, Mazumdar S, *et al*. Combined pharmacotherapy and psychotherapy as maintenance treatment for late-life depression: effects on social adjustment. *Am J Psychiatry* 2002;159:466–8

60. Alexopoulos GS, Katz IR, Renolds CF III, *et al*. The expert consensus guideline series: pharmacotherapy of depressive disorders in older patients. *Postgrad Med* 2001;(Special Report):1–86

32 Cerebrovascular disease

John T. Hughes, MD

INTRODUCTION

Geriatric neurology deserves greater attention and study as our population ages. The classical history and physical examination are essential in evaluating many geriatric neurologic problems, such as gait disorders, and the neurodegenerative disorders, including dementias, which affect our geriatric population. In assessing the distinction between the features of aging and diseases that affect individuals in their older years, we must recognize norms for expected involution which occur in all people, some with striking penetrance and in others with less obvious features or marked delay. Furthermore, this distinction may be obscured due to superimposition of a variety of diseases upon the aging individual.

ANATOMY AND PHYSIOLOGY

Even the casual lay observer notices the insidious changes that characterize the aged. The slow tentative gait, shorter steps, hunched posture, slowed unreliable reflexes, dependency on banisters to negotiate steps and hypophonic raspy voice are all conscious and unconscious observations that characterize senescence. These observations have a physiologic and anatomic basis. The changes entail time-dependent neurodegeneration involving neuronal loss and death.

Neurodegeneration and effects on bodily and psychological changes have been estimated by biologists. Table 1 shows the estimated losses in function for age 30–80 that have been proposed by Shock[1]. Actual measurements of the effects of aging have also been looked at in terms of brain weights. Brain weight varies widely in the elderly in the seventh and eighth decades and is estimated at 930–1350 g. In those who are neurologically and histologically intact, the loss in brain weight becomes most evident in the seventh, eighth and ninth decades. Male brains are heavier than female brains by 9%, and the reduction in weight is 11% from 19 to 86 years of age. Much of the decrease in weight is related to cerebral and cerebellar cortical neuronal loss. Estimates of approximately 50% of neuronal loss can be seen in cortical layers two and four in the superior temporal gyrus, pyramidal cell layers and in the visual cortex. Smaller losses are seen in the Purkinge cells (25%) and hippocampal neurons (12%). Cholinergic neurons comprising the nucleus basalis of Meynert typically involve a 65% reduction in neurons between 20 and 80 years of age[2]. It is estimated that a threshold below 100 000 cholinergic neurons is strongly associated with Alzheimer's disease. Neuronal loss also occurs in critical subcortical nuclei and spinal cord anterior horn cell pools including the substantia nigra, pars compacta and locus ceruleus. Vestibular nuclei, inferior olives, and fourth, sixth and seventh cranial nuclei show no significant losses with age. It is

Table 1 Physiologic and anatomic deterioration at 80 years of age

	Relative decrease
Brain weight	+
Blood flow to brain	++
Cardiac output at rest	+++
Creatinine clearance	+++
Nerve fiber density	+++
Nerve conduction velocity	+
Number of taste buds	++++
Maximum ventilation volume	++++
Power of hand grip	++++
Maximum work rate	+++
Basal metabolic rate	+
Body water content	+

then easy to see how these cellular changes and neuronal atrophy and death, which occur in 'typical aging', can predispose many patients to characteristic neurodegenerative diseases such as a myriad of dementias, cerebral atherosclerosis and neoplasms, to name a few. Systemic disease may interact with the 'aged brain' and result in acute neurologic syndromes such as delirium and metabolically induced encephalopathies. Quantitative volumetric magnetic resonance imaging (MRI) studies of the brain have been looked at in a cohort of 46 non-demented neurologically normal patients. Mueller and co-workers have found that there are small constant rates of brain atrophy with aging, but interestingly there were stable linear changes without accelerated volume loss in the latest decade of life[3]. The largest decreases in brain volumes were seen in those patients suffering from dementing diseases.

Structural changes in neurons and glial support cells in aging are well documented. Dendritic tree remodeling, alterations in cytoskeletal proteins, accumulation of proteins (such as amyloid) and lipid by-products are common to the aging nervous system. There are common features seen in both aging brains and in brains of patients with such states as Alzheimer's disease. The findings that characterize Alzheimer's disease, including neurofibrillary tangles, neuritic plaques, granulovacuolar degeneration and

Hirano bodies are also commonly found, albeit much lower in numbers, in the medial temporal brain in non-demented patients. It is controversial whether these findings represent the beginning of a superimposed pathologic process. Other cellular changes include increased astrocytic fibrillary subpial intracytoplasmic corpora amylacea, intracytoplasmic inclusions and increased neuropigments such as lipofuscin in nerve and support cells.

There are a variety of non-specific axonal responses to injury which are seen in advancing age and a wide variety of pathologic states. Polymers of protein which act as the neuronal cytoskeleton may accumulate within axons in both aging and pathologic states. In mesial temporal areas, microtubule-associated proteins (MAPs) can be found accumulating in the phosphorylated state (tau protein in axons). Calcium mediates proteolysis and accumulation of MAP-2 is seen in dendrites of aging neurons. Similar but striking changes are seen in major neurodegenerative disorders of Alzheimer's disease, Parkinson's disease and amyotrophic lateral sclerosis. These changes include a marked increase of neurofibrillary tangles composed of tau and MAP proteins and a decrease in neuronal microtubules. Intracellular calcium mediated proteolysis of cytoskeletal protein and accumulation of MAP and phosphorylated protein result in neurofibrillary tangles and focal swelling of axons (spheroids). In Parkinson's disease abnormal accumulation of neurofilaments form the distinguishing Lewy body. Glutamate-mediated calcium influx leads to dendritic degeneration and excitotoxic synaptic injury.

Marked vascular changes occur with aging. At age 80, brain blood flow decreases by an estimated 20–28% and this parallels a decline in the cerebral metabolic rate[4]. There is also an expected increase in cerebrovascular resistance with cerebral atherosclerosis, vessel fibrosis and endothelial involution. Greater reduction in flow is seen in prefrontal areas and cortical regions than subcortical white matter. Even in those patients with preserved blood flow at age above 70, cerebral glucose metabolism is independently reduced[5]. The blood–brain barrier (BBB) becomes less discriminative, and transport functions, such as the transfer of glucose, are diminished.

Amyloid accumulates in advancing brains, and few brains aged 90 years or more are free of these 'senile' plaques, made up of amyloid β-peptide. These insoluble proteins appear in non-demented individuals, although relatively few are present in the brains of mentally intact individuals. This is in contrast with the large number of plaques observed in patients with Alzheimer's disease. Interestingly, there is a predilection for amyloid to accumulate in the learning regions of the brain and those structures serving memory (hippocampus and entorhinal cortices)[6]. It is accepted that amyloid β-protein induces a severe oxidative stress on neurons and eventual cell death. Amyloid β-protein is also deposited extensively in the blood vessels of patients with Alzheimer's disease, rendering the BBB inefficient in transport and vulnerable to vascular occlusion and rupture (amyloid angiopathy).

Many biochemical changes occur in aging cerebral tissues. DNA, RNA and components of myelin diminish with age. Neurotransmitters, including acetylcholine, dopamine, norepinephrine and GABA, all decline in aging. It is speculated that these reductions reflect the neuronal cell reduction in the nucleus basalis of Meynert, and the nuclei of the basal forebrain and substantia nigra[7].

Certain changes occur in the peripheral nervous system and musculature. The effectors of the central nervous system (i.e. muscle fibers) undergo atrophy and cell reduction. This translates into diminished overall power production and endurance. The loss in muscle mass is multifactorial and related to myopathic changes, disuse and denervation due to anterior horn cell loss. There is an expected decrease in nerve conduction velocity and compound muscle action potentials, reflecting muscular atrophy. Sensory nerve action potentials are diminished, and are also indicative of peripheral sensory neuronal loss.

The focus of the physician should not be limited to the diagnosis of medical ailments that the elderly face, but also to assessing functional impairments. It is these functional impairments that are just as threatening to an individual's independence as the most devastating stroke or advanced case of dementia.

CEREBROVASCULAR DISEASE

Epidemiological studies have characterized stroke as a leading cause of morbidity and mortality, with a worldwide incidence of approximately 150 per 100 000. It runs third to coronary disease and cancer in overall mortality figures. Stroke is a disease of middle aged and elderly individuals. The rate of stroke increases with age and rises dramatically in postmenopausal women[8]. The Framingham study shows stroke incidence in men 45–54 years old at 20/100 000, in the 65–74 age group at 90/100 000 and in men over 75 at 176/100 000. Postmenopausal women have stroke rates very similar to those of men over the age of 65. In the USA, nearly 500 000 people suffer from a stroke each year and 175 000 die from stroke yearly. Just as important, showing equal or even greater burden, is the fact that at any one time there are over two million stroke survivors. At least one-half of all neurologic admissions to general hospitals are due to stroke.

The effect of stroke on the individual can be devastating. The sudden loss of neurologic function is unanticipated. Most young and practically all older patients experience dramatic lifestyle changes, may never return to employment and may become dependent for even the simplest activity of daily living.

Emergent diagnostic testing, broadening treatment modalities including endovascular procedures and drugs have catapulted us into an exciting era in the management of patients with acute stroke. Stroke is a heterogeneous entity. Stroke entails damage to the brain or

Table 2   Classification of stroke

Ischemic
Atherosclerotic thrombosis
Embolism (cardiogenic, artery to artery, paradoxical)
Watershed infarction (hypotensive)
Transient ischemic attack
Arteritis (connective tissue, temporal arteritis,
   meningovascular, systemic arteritides, meningitides)
Hypercoagulable conditions
Carotid dissection
Aortic dissection

Hemorrhagic
Parenchymal
   hypertensive
   angiopathy (arteritis, amyloid, mycotic)
   vascular malformations
   trauma
   iatrogenic (anticoagulants)
Subarachnoid
   vascular malformations (arteriovenous
      malformation, berry aneurysm)
   trauma
   iatrogenic (anticoagulants)

---

spinal cord caused by an abnormality of its blood supply. As seen in Table 2, there are two major categories of stroke: ischemia and hemorrhage. Ischemia can be further divided into thrombosis, embolism and decreased systemic perfusion. Hemorrhage can be subdivided into two types: subarachnoid and intracerebral. The overall ratio of infarcts to hemorrhage is about 4 : 1.

Atherothrombotic infarction

Atherothrombotic infarction accounts for 85% of ischemic stroke. Thrombosis is an obstruction of blood flow due to a localized occlusive process within one or more blood vessels. Occlusions may occur due to an alteration in the vessel wall or superimposed clot formation. Most underlying cerebrovascular disease is attributed to the effect of atherosclerosis and hypertension. Hypertension may cause the vascular wall to become infiltrated by hyaline lipid material (known as lipohyalinosis). Vessels affected by lipohyalinosis may undergo narrowing and subsequent thrombosis[9]. Focal vessel wall weakening with formation of Charcot Bouchard microaneurysms may also lead to eventual small vessel rupture with classical subcortical intraparenchymal hemorrhage. There is a tendency for atheromatous plaques to form at branch points or areas of tortuosity in larger extracranial and intracranial vessels. Most frequent areas of involvement include the juncture of the common carotid and internal carotid arteries, the cervical portion of the vertebral artery, the vertebrobasilar junction and the main bifurcation of the middle cerebral artery (MCA). Vessel occlusion occurs secondary to atherosclerotic vessel narrowing and superimposed thrombosis. Platelets play an important role and may adhere to plaque. Platelet clumping serves as a nidus for deposition of fibrin thrombin and clot, important when considering treatment. Less commonly, clots form due to a hypercoagulable state, polycythemia or thrombocytosis.

Embolism

Embolism is due to clots that form elsewhere in the heart or vascular tree and lodge in vessels, shutting off blood flow. 'Red clots' typically form in the heart or in occluded blood vessels in the form of stump emboli (e.g. complete carotid occlusion). These are best treated with heparin and warfarin. 'White clots' are a combination of platelet and fibrin debris which adhere to atherosclerotic surfaces (e.g. the carotid artery or aorta), can dislodge and cause transient ischemic attack (TIA) or stroke. These are best approached with antiplatelet agents. There is clinical utility in correctly classifying the stroke and understanding the pathophysiology for appropriate treatment. In most cases clots fragment from the heart, but intra-arterial sources, such as the carotid sinus and the 'shaggy' aorta, are also likely areas for clot formation. Any vascular territory is prone to embolism; however, emboli that traverse the common carotid artery most often end within the MCA bifurcation[10].

Brain embolism is predominantly from heart disease, and 75% of cardiogenic emboli lodge in the brain[11]. Atrial fibrillation is by far the most common heart condition associated with stroke. Mural thrombi generated by myocardial infarction, valvular disease, cardiac surgery and prosthetic valves are also common cardiogenic sources of emboli.

Decreased systemic perfusion

Decreased systemic perfusion typically causes 'watershed' infarctions. These are found in the border zones between anterior and middle and/or middle and posterior circulations. The common substrate for this type of stroke is systemic hypoperfusion; however, superimposed large vessel extracranial stenosis can make patients prone to watershed infarct. Causes include cardiogenic shock (pump failure or dysrhythmia) and various entities associated with systemic hypotension (arrest, sepsis, acute blood loss). These are usually symmetric, although they can be asymmetric, depending on location and severity of pre-existing atherosclerotic vascular lesions[12].

Transient ischemic attack

TIA is caused by reversible hypoperfusion of various parts of the brain. The average duration of a TIA is 15 min (range 2–20 min) and it may last up to 24 h[13]. Specific symptoms are determined by impaired branch circulation. Even though the clinical examination returns to normal, MRI and positron emission tomography (PET) scanning may demonstrate reversible ischemic changes due to transient hypoperfusion. The underlying pathophysiologic mechanism is usually atherothrombotic. Single transient prolonged episodes are usually due to embolism, whereas repeated episodes of uniform type usually herald an impending small vessel occlusion. The occurrence of a focal TIA is associated with a 23% 5-year cumulative rate

of cerebral infarction. Almost 20% of infarcts that follow TIAs occur within 1 month after the first attack and about 50% within 1 year. Equally important, there is almost as high an incidence rate (21%) for myocardial infarction[14]. The occurrence of a TIA is a predictor of cerebral infarction and myocardial infarction. TIAs may occur in virtually any cerebral artery: anterior or posterior arterial distribution, and in large and small arteries.

Transient monocular blindness (TMB) is usually due to platelet thrombi originating in an atherosclerotic carotid artery or aortic arch, or cholesterol emboli from similar sources. TMB is associated with 13% chance of stroke within 6 years of the event. Nearly 50% of patients have no further attacks. Those patients with normal carotid angiograms have extremely low chances of future stroke, whereas in those patients with carotid stenosis or occlusion, over a third will have an eventual stroke. Patients with TMB before age 45 typically do not suffer strokes[15].

Brainstem TIAs are clinically dissimilar to carotid distribution TIAs. They have a longer duration, are less stereotypic and more likely to end in a completed stroke. The clinical picture is quite diverse, due to the large number of cranial nuclei and long tracts that occupy the brainstem. Vertigo, diplopia, perioral facial numbness, ataxia, hemibody and tetrabody sensory and motor symptoms and clinical signs are the hallmarks of vertebral–basilar insufficiency. When the symptoms and signs occur alone they are much less specific for basilar ischemia; when appearing together they are a signature for brainstem ischemia.

Most cases of TIA are due to vascular stenosis and intimal atherosclerosis with endothelial ulceration. Thrombus formation and embolization of white platelet thrombi is commonly invoked as the underlying pathogenesis for most TIAs. Single transient episodes that are prolonged for more than 1–2 h, and events involving multiple cerebral circulations, suggest embolization from a central source (i.e. heart or great vessels). In contrast, brief 5–15-min episodes in similar vascular distributions are indicative of atherosclerotic mechanisms and thrombosis.

Carotid artery stenosis

Carotid artery stenosis is usually due to atherosclerotic plaque, and the restricted diameter of the internal carotid artery may significantly reduce blood flow to the cerebrum. Carotid artery stenosis may be associated with ipsilateral TIA, stroke and TMB. Carotid atherosclerosis accounts for up to 20% of cases of cerebral stroke[16]. It is clear that in patients with TIAs and carotid stenosis of 50–99%, there is an associated increased risk of stroke[17]. The North American Symptomatic Carotid Endarterectomy Trial (NASCET) showed that patients with *symptomatic severe carotid stenosis* of 70% or more who were medically treated suffered a 26% 2-year ipsilateral stroke rate[18]. The European Carotid Surgery Trial (ECST) showed similar risks of stroke in *symptomatic severe carotid stenosis*. In patients with severe stenosis (> 70%), the overall 3-year ipsilateral stroke or death rate in the surgically treated group was 12.3%, while there was a 21.9% risk of stroke in medically treated patients[19]. The NASCET trial showed that the absolute 5-year stroke reduction in surgically treated patients was 17%. Stroke incidence can be reduced with surgical treatment. The two main strategies employed in the treatment of carotid stenosis are prevention or slowing of the atherosclerotic process and surgical or endovascular interventional techniques. The benefit of carotid endarterectomy in patients with *moderate stenosis* (50–69%) is generally less dramatic, but greatest for men older than 75 years of age, patients with recent stroke and hemispheric transient ischemic attacks. Surgical treatment of *moderate stenosis* in NASCET trials showed an absolute 5-year stroke reduction of 6.5%. Advising surgery is indicated in patients with significant vascular risk factors and a surgeon with acceptable perioperative complication rates (< 3%).

Asymptomatic carotid stenosis is associated with a definite but lower risk for stroke in comparison to *symptomatic carotid stenosis*. The risk of stroke is about 3% per year for asymptomatic stenosis in the range of 60–99%, increasing only minimally with progressive degrees of stenosis. The asymptomatic carotid stenosis treatment trials overall showed a significant, but more modest, absolute stroke risk reduction of 6% at 5 years. The skill of the surgeon takes on particular importance with asymptomatic carotid stenosis, due to the smaller benefit of surgery. A perioperative complication rate greater than 3% would offset any surgical benefit. The decision to perform surgery is dependent on the availability of surgical expertise, and a good surgical candidate with significant vascular risk factors. Carotid endarterectomy should be considered in patients under age 80 with stenosis of more than 60%. The absence of significant other medical problems, life expectancy and patient preferences are factors which help in the decision-making process.

Carotid artery angioplasty and stenting is a relatively new procedure and is an alternative treatment for patients with contraindications to surgery with general anesthesia, postoperative recurrent stenosis, radiation-induced stenosis and distal carotid stenosis beyond surgical reach. Comparative data between endarterectomy and angioplasty with stenting are scant but promising. Several protective devices are currently being studied and will hopefully make this procedure even safer. Angioplasty and stenting is very attractive in geriatric populations due to shortened hospital stays and avoidance of general anesthesia, and is the preferred application for patients with multiple medical problems.

Intracranial hemorrhage

Approximately 10% of strokes are caused by intracranial hemorrhage[20]. Intracranial hemorrhage can be subdivided into two categories: subarachnoid and intracerebral. Subarachnoid hemorrhage has traumatic and non-traumatic causes. Intracerebral or parenchymal bleeding may be located in subcortical basal ganglia and brainstem areas, or cortical/lobar areas.

Primary or hypertensive hemorrhage is the most commonly encountered type of intracerebral bleed. The most common cause is hypertension. Hypertension and atherosclerosis interact to weaken arterial perforators of the MCA, posterior cerebral artery (PCA), and basilar arteries. Lipohyalinosis of small intraparenchymal arteries is the common arterial lesion leading to arterial rupture. Lobar hemorrhages are thought to be non-hypertensive in many cases. Hypertension is present in 72–81% of patients with subcortical basal ganglia/brainstem bleeds. Populations with a high incidence of hypertension, such as African-Americans, Chinese and Japanese, have a higher incidence of intracerebral hemorrhage. There has been a general decline over the past decade in the incidence of intracerebral hemorrhage as a result of improved detection and treatment of hypertension.

Subarachnoid hemorrhage (SAH) is due to leakage of blood from the cerebral vasculature on to the surface of the brain into the subarachnoid spaces and ventricles. SAH is most commonly due to berry aneurysm in the circle of Willis, but arteriovenous malformations, bleeding diathesis or trauma can also be sources. In most series of SAH due to berry aneurysms, approximately 50% of patients remember a 'sentinel' hemorrhage within the preceding 2 weeks. This is actually a warning leak. Aneurysmal rupture is associated with 30% mortality within the first 24 h[21]. Patients typically present with an excruciatingly severe headache with sudden onset. The sudden appearance of symptoms distinguishes this as a serious type of headache. Meningismus may be the only clinical sign on examination.

Non-hypertensive hemorrhages are associated with bleeding diathesis (anticoagulants and trauma), vascular malformation and vasculopathies (primarily amyloid angiopathy). Cerebral amyloid angiopathy (CAA) is associated with deposition of amyloid in small and medium-sized arteries of the cortex and leptomeninges. A staggering 60% of individuals over age 90 have amyloid deposition in their arteries, deserving special mention in the geriatric age group. Due to the predilection for small and medium-sized arteries, hemorrhage is frequently seen in lobar areas. Local subarachnoid bleeding may be seen secondary to leptomeningeal vessel involvement. Although the diagnosis is ultimately left to the pathologist, CAA should be considered in patients with simultaneous or recurrent lobar hemorrhage. A disturbing note is that there is a significant proportion of patients with CAA who may present with transient ischemic attack symptoms prior to major lobar hemorrhages, further complicating management. The mechanism of rupture is due to mere weakening of the vessel wall, or formation of microaneurysms in association with the effects of hypertension. Other events associated with hemorrhage include trauma, neurosurgical procedures, coexistence of granulomatous angiitis, and use of fibrinolytic agents for treatment of myocardial infarction and thrombolitic or embolic stroke. The expected rate of hemorrhage with tissue plasminogen activator (t-PA) in myocardial infarction is approximately 1.5% with t-PA doses of > 100 mg. The hemorrhage rate associated with t-PA use in stroke is 6.3%. Mortality rates are in the range of 44–87%. An additional feature of CAA is its association with clinical dementia in up to 30% of patients. Neuritic plaques are identified in almost 50% of patients.

Stroke-associated seizure

Cerebrovascular disease is responsible for the abrupt rise in incidence of seizures and epilepsy in patients over the age of 60. Early necropsy studies and epidemiologic studies support the hypothesis that there is a definite link between stroke and seizures. The rate of seizures after stroke is estimated as 4–17%[22]. In a study of over 1000 stroke patients, Kilpatrick et al.[23] found an overall seizure rate of 4.4%. Seizures were more common with lobar hemorrhages (15.4%) than with cortical infarcts (7%). Partial seizures were seen in 60% of patients. A third with early seizures also had late seizures. It is clear that cortical insults are most frequently associated with seizures. While they do not occur with pure subcortical lacunar infarcts, subcortical slit hemorrhages may be associated with seizures.

The timing of seizures is bimodal and is similar to the pattern observed in post-traumatic epilepsy. Often seizures occur either within the first 2 weeks or 6–12 months after a stroke. Intracerebral hemorrhage is associated with greater incidence of an early seizure, with 30–70% occurring within the first 48 h.

Simple partial seizures occur in most individuals, and secondary generalized tonic clonic seizures in approximately a third. The observed mortality rate is 20–40% with early seizures. Limb-shaking attacks may be seen in patients with severe carotid stenosis, not to be confused with focal seizures. These events are usually seen in association with severe carotid stenosis and orthostatic blood pressure changes. There may be disinhibition of subcortical motor control mechanisms resulting in this coarse extremity tremor.

The electroencephalogram (EEG) may be helpful in predicting which individuals may experience seizures. Those with periodic lateralizing epileptiform discharges (PLEDs) or focal spikes on EEG have a greater risk of developing post-stroke seizures. All patients with cortical strokes (hemorrhagic or ischemic) are at risk for post-stroke seizures, with larger strokes associated with greater risk.

Post-stroke seizures should be treated aggressively. Some have worsening of neurologic deficits after seizure, and a higher associated in-hospital mortality. An increased risk of aspiration and pneumonia could potentially worsen a stroke. Although the seizure may be simply due to the effects of a cortical infarct or hemorrhage, many factors could account for the emergence of seizure. Metabolic causes (hypo/hyperglycemia, hypocalcemia, hypo/hypernatremia), drugs (antibiotics, psychotropics, baclofen) or hemorrhagic transformation of an infarct may all be contributory. Entities such as cerebral abscess, encephalitis, tumor or subdural hematoma may all be incorrectly diagnosed as stroke. Seizures should be managed in the usual way. The risk of recurrence after the first seizure is 50%. Those with a lone seizure after a stroke may be observed, with recurrence warranting anticonvulsant treatment. Management entails a search for contributing factors. Historical aspects may be helpful in distinguishing between focal onset seizure (partial) vs. a generalized seizure (i.e. drug or alcohol withdrawl). Benzodiazepines such as diazepam or lorazepam are indicated in prolonged generalized seizures or status epilepticus. These are given intravenously to ensure adequate blood levels. The anticonvulsant effect lasts from 10 to 20 min, therefore a long-acting preparation must be given following the benzodiazepine. Phenytoin and phenobarbital are commonly used. Phenytoin is given as an intravenous bolus of 20 mg/kg at a rate of 50 mg/min, with blood pressure monitoring during infusion. Fosphenytoin may be given at the same dosage as phenytoin, but at twice the rate. Phenobarbital may also be used as an additional drug if seizures continue, at a rate of 100 mg/min intravenously up to a total dose of 20 mg/kg. Respiratory depression during the infusion may be handled with intubation and ventilation. Further management is best recommended in an intensive care unit.

Vascular dementia

Dementia due to ischemic cerebrovascular insults is known as vascular dementia. This is the second leading cause of dementia, second to Alzheimer's disease. Strokes may induce cortical or subcortical types of dementia. Subcortical leukoencephalopathy is due to multiple small white matter infarcts[24]. There is a confluence of these infarcts in the watershed (border zone) areas between penetrating cortical and basal ganglionic arteries. Predictive factors for dementia include educational level, stroke severity, dominant hemisphere infarction, old age, large areas of leukoencephalopathy and two or more cortical infarcts, all favoring development of dementia.

MANAGEMENT

The 'best medicine' is prevention. Identification of risk factors is not as glamorous or nearly as exciting as angioplasty and stenting or lysing acute clots in cerebral arteries. Risk factors such as hypertension, heart disease, diabetes mellitus, hypercholesterolemia, smoking and excessive alcohol intake must be identified by primary care physicians and treated.

Treatment is instituted once the symptoms or signs of stroke have begun. It is important to establish the underlying pathophysiologic mechanisms that underlie the neurologic deficit and findings, so the appropriate treatment may be given.

TIAs may affect small or large vessel distributions. The small vessel lacunar TIAs often 'stutter' at onset. Anterior circulation (carotid) lacunar TIAs are best managed with antiplatelet regimens with aspirin (ASA), clopidogrel, or ASA/dipyridamole combination. Slightly better stroke prevention may be seen with the latter two agents, but cost differences are significant. There is no rule for anticoagulation in these small vessel-induced TIAs. It may be difficult to discriminate between small- and large-vessel TIA, therefore admission to the hospital with an expeditious evaluation is warranted in most cases.

Single transient TIA episodes lasting more than an hour and multiple episodes of different pattern suggest embolism. These contrast with brief stereotypic attacks lasting minutes which are usually caused by atherosclerosis and thrombosis. Large-vessel carotid distribution TIAs are often complex, involving many cortical functions including language, spatial orientation, faciobrachial motor and sensory modalities. These are typically embolic from heart to artery or artery to artery sources. Anticoagulation is often employed to prevent recurrence of embolization. Non-valvular artrial fibrillation is best managed with anticoagulation after the age of 60. Other cardiac sources, including acute myocardial infarction with associated mural thrombus, valvular problems including endocarditis and right to left shunting of embolic material, all require specialized evaluation and individualized treatment.

Carotid distribution TIAs or stroke secondary to carotid stenosis of > 50% with hemispheric TIA symptoms should undergo carotid endarterectomy. Patients with retinal TIAs have a better prognosis, but if the evaluation shows a high-grade stenosis of ≥ 70%, then surgery is indicated. Vertebrobasilar insufficiency must be suspected by presenting symptoms and signs. Posterior circulation TIA may indicate an impending basilar artery occlusion which is life threatening in most cases. Long-term anticoagulation appears to be the most viable and effective option for posterior circulation TIA due to basilar narrowing or occlusion.

Ascending aorta atheromatous plaques ('shaggy aorta') are an important source of embolism, and have been reported to account for as many as 38% of emboli in a group of patients with no discernible embolic source[25]. These types of emboli are best treated with standard antiplatelet agents.

Thrombolytic therapy using recombinant t-PA has been effective in restoring circulation in small- and large-vessel stroke[26]. When administered within 3 h of the onset of symptoms, t-PA causes a 30% increase in the number of patients who show little or no neurologic deficit at 3 months and 1 year. t-PA is given in a dose of 0.9 mg/kg, 10% given in a bolus, followed by a 1-h infusion of the remaining dose. A 6% risk of symptomatic hemorrhage is seen. There is a 50% fatality rate in patients who experience hemorrhage. Although the risk of hemorrhage is higher in patients with larger infarction (greater than two-thirds of the hemisphere), the patients who survive have a greater comparative functional recovery than patients who underwent thrombolysis with smaller strokes. Data regarding efficacy and hemorrhage rate is not known for patients over 80 years. Administration of t-PA is reserved for those patients in whom the time of onset of stroke is clear, and following initial evaluation, the infusion is administered under 3 h. The computerized tomography (CT) scan should show no evidence of hemorrhage or significant early stroke findings. Small strokes and very large strokes are normally not treated with t-PA.

Intracerebral hemorrhage poses different challenges and management. Management of intracranial pressure and adequate ventilation are paramount. Most patients are hypertensive immediately after the hemorrhage, with blood pressure management in the acute stage controversial. Most bleeding stops within 1–3 h. Lowering the mean arterial blood pressure too aggressively may compromise cererbral perfusion pressure. Lowering mean arterial blood pressure to less than 110 mmHg helps prevent worsening cerebral edema. Increased intracranial pressure may be life threatening and frequently requires osmotic agents (mannitol) and hyperventilation (Pco_2 in the 23–27-mmHg range) for control. Surgical intervention is appropriate to prevent herniation and may be employed for lobar hemorrhages and basal ganglia hemorrhages. Patients may be saved from herniation and brain death by surgical decompression; however, neurologic functional outcomes remain unchanged. Special mention regarding cerebellar hematomas is warranted. These may claim life quickly due to proximity to the brainstem and development of hydrocephalus from fourth ventricular compression. Most hematomas of 4 cm or greater will require surgical evacuation.

When patients present with TIA or stroke symptoms and signs, an expeditious evaluation and treatment in most cases entails admission to the hospital. Basic laboratory parameters may reveal a hypercoaguable state, coagulopathy or other abnormality, which may cause a state mimicking a stroke (e.g. hypoglycemia, hypercalcemia, etc.). A CT scan is readily available, quick and easy, and does not require as much co-operation as an MRI scan. It is usual that the CT scan within 24 h will not show the clinically presumed stroke, and a repeat scan should be performed to identify the lesion. Non-invasive vascular studies including magnetic resonance angiography (MRA), carotid duplex and transcranial Doppler are now readily available for investigation of the aortic arch, cervical and intracranial vessels. MRI is the preferred modality in evaluating posterior circulation stroke, or when the differential diagnosis includes vascular malformations, or there is any question of tumor or infection (abscess or encephalitis); it is particularly helpful in identifying small lacunar infarcts missed by CT scanning. MRI diffusion weighted images are helpful in determining acute infarcts difficult to discern in patients with multiple strokes or extensive white matter disease.

Depression is common in up to 50% of patients in the year following a stroke[27]. Left hemisphere strokes involving the frontal pole and right hemispheric subcortical strokes are more frequently associated with depression. Common symptoms include insomnia, anhedonia, diminished appetite, poor attention and concentration, and a withdrawn feeling. The depression may interfere with rehabilitative efforts, and is amenable to psychological and psychotropic treatments.

Stroke rehabilitation programs are important in preventing many of the complications of stroke. Conditioning is critical for recovery. Strength can deteriorate 3% per day if conditioning exercises are not implemented. Physical therapy should be started within 48 h of a stroke. Speech and swallowing evaluations are part of initial stroke evaluations and feedings should be withheld for the first 24–48 h until a full speech and swallow evaluation is performed and aspiration risk is assessed. Aspiration pneumonia and ensuing fever are detrimental to the patient. Appropriate positioning is critical in helping prevent cutaneous breakdown. Deep vein thrombosis prophylaxis is initiated upon admission to prevent complications such as pulmonary embolism. Addressing these issues will lessen pain and suffering, help patients deal better with their deficits and hopefully, in some, help them overcome these deficits.

References

1. Shock MW. System integration. In Finch CE, Hayflick L, eds. *Handbook of the Biology of Aging*. New York: Van Nostrand Reinhold, 1977:23–30
2. Davis RL, Robertson DM, eds. *Texbook of Neuropathology*, 3rd edn. Baltimore, MD: Williams and Wilkins, 1997:1064–7
3. Mueller EA, Moore MM, Kerr DC, *et al.* Brain volume preserved in healthy elderly through the eleventh decade. *Neurology* 1998;51:1555
4. Obrist WD. Cerebral ciruclatory changes in normal aging and dementia. In Hoffmeister F, Muller C, eds. *Brain Function in Old Age*. Berlin: Springer-Verlag, 1979:278–87
5. Sokoloff L. Effects of normal aging on cerebral circulation and energy metabolism, In Hoffmeister F, Muller C, eds. *Brain Function in Old Age*. Berlin: Springer-Verlag, 1979:367–80
6. Mattson M. Cellular and neurochemical effect of the aging human brain, In Hazzard W, Blass J, Walter E, *et al.*, eds. *Principles of Geriatric Medicine and Gerontology*. New York: McGraw Hill, 1999:1193–208
7. Decker MW. The effects of aging on the hippocampal and cortical projections of the forebrain cholinergic system. *Brain Res* 1987;434:423–5
8. Wolf PA, Kannel WB, Verter J. Current status of risk factors for stroke. *Neurol Clin* 1983;1:317–43
9. Caplan L. *Caplan's Stroke*, 3rd edn. Boston: Butterworth-Heinemann, 2000:225–31
10. Gacs G, Merer FT, Bodosi M. Balloon catheter as a model of cerebral emboli in humans. *Stroke* 1982;13:39–42
11. Victor M, Ropper A. *Principles of Neurology*, 7th edn. New York: McGraw-Hill, 2001:870–5
12. Mohr JP. Neurological complications of cardiac valvular disease and cardiac surgery including systemic hypotension. In Vinken P, Bruyn G, eds. *Handbook of Clinical Neurology*, vol 38. Amsterdam: North Holland, 1979:143–71
13. Millikan CH, McDowell FH. Treatment of transient ischemic attacks. *Stroke* 1978;9: 299–308
14. Heyman A, Wilkinson WE, Hurwitz BJ, *et al.* Risk of ischemic heart disease in patients with TIA. *Neurology* 1984;34: 626–30
15. Poole CMJ, Ross Russell RW. Mortality and stroke after amaurosis fugax. *J Neurol Neurosurg Psychiatry* 1985;48:902–3
16. Sacco R. Extracranial carotid stenosis. *N Engl J Med* 2001;345:1113–18
17. Grotta JC, Bigelow RH, Hu H, *et al.* The significance of carotid stenosis or ulceration. *Neurology* 1984;34:437–42
18. North American Symptomatic Carotid Endarterectomy Trial Collaborators. Beneficial effect of carotid endarterectomy in symptomatic patients with high-grade carotid stenosis. *N Engl J Med* 1991; 325:445–53
19. European Carotid Surgery Trialists' Collaborative Group. MRC European

Carotid Surgery Trial: interim small results for symptomatic patients with severe (70–99%) or with mild (0–29%) carotid stenosis. *Lancet* 1991;337:1235–43

21. Ingall TJ, Whisnant JP, Wiebers DO, *et al.* Has there been a decline in subarachnoid hemorrhage mortality? *Stroke* 1989;20: 718–24

22. Fisher M, Bogousslavsky J. *Current Review of Cerebrovascular Disease*, 2nd edn. Philadelphia: Current Medicine, 1996: 107–17

23. Kilpatrick CJ, Davis SM, Tress BM, *et al.* Epileptic seizures in acute stroke. *Arch Neurol* 1990;47:157–60

24. Hachinski VC, Potter P, Mersky H. Leukoaraiosis. *Arch Neurol* 1987;44:21–3

25. Amarenco P, Cohen A, Tzourio C, *et al.* Atherosclerotic disease of the aortic arch and the risk of ischemic stroke. *N Engl J Med* 1994;331:1474–82

26. National Institute of Neurological Disorders and Stroke RT-PA Stroke Study Group. Tissue plasminogen activator for acute ischemic stroke. *N Engl J Med* 1995;333:1581–7

27. Robinson RG, Starr LB, Lipsey JR, *et al.* A two-year longitudinal study of post-stroke mood disorders. *J Nerv Ment Dis* 1985;173:21–7

33 Parkinson's disease

John T. Hughes, MD

INTRODUCTION

Parkinson's disease (PD) is a hereditary degenerative disorder affecting over 1 million people in the USA. The disorder is prevalent worldwide, although seen with less propensity in African-Americans (one-quarter as common) and half as common in Asian populations. Most patients with PD are managed by primary care physicians.

PD is named after James Parkinson, who outlined the features of this syndrome in 1817. His *Essay on the Shaking Palsy* predated formal neurologic examinations and placed particular emphasis on tremor and generalized weakness. Charcot added rigidity to the clinical description. The 'classical triad' and signature of PD includes resting tremor, bradykinesia and rigidity. This triad does not include the equally important gait and postural stability problems which also constitute the syndrome. The association of PD with the pathological lesion in the substantia nigra was observed in the early 20th century. Patients with advanced PD demonstrating resting tremor, cogwheel rigidity, bradykinesia, stooped posture with festinating gait and reptilian stare rarely pose a diagnostic challenge. Early PD presenting as a limp or frozen shoulder in a 35-year-old patient may not be as obvious, taking considerably longer for diagnosis. On the other hand, many are erroneously diagnosed with PD, do not respond to the usual pharmacopea and actually have Parkinsonism from one of many non-PD extrapyramidal disorders. Jellinger reported an autopsy series of 500 patients, of which 60–75% Parkinsonian patients actually had PD. Of the remaining, 15% had multisystem degeneration, 6–8% had cerebrovascular disease and 3% were postencephalitic. Isolated cases may be related to toxins, drugs and tumors[1].

The recognition of PD by the physician is devastating for the patient, being labeled with a chronic degenerative disease. Early treatment is effective, with the use of a considerable armamentarium of drugs, and gratifying for the physician and patient. Initial excitement is tempered by stark realization that one is dealing with an inexorably progressive course confounded by neurological, medical and possibly orthopedic complications, all of which will claim life prematurely. The almost miraculous discovery of levodopa (L-dopa) for treatment of PD has not been paralleled with discovery of neurotransmitters for other extrapyramidal disorders. L-Dopa was first given to 'repigment' the substantia nigra. In actuality, this led to an increase in dopamine in the striatum responsible for clinical improvement. Unfortunately, L-dopa embodies the notion that 'the treatment can be worse than the disease', on the basis of numerous motor and neuropsychiatric problems which complicate L-dopa treatment.

ETIOLOGY AND PATHOPHYSIOLOGY

In 1919 Tretiakoff linked PD to the substantia nigra[2]. Lewy first described concentric hyaline cytoplasmic inclusions in the dorsal vagal nucleus and nucleus substantia inominata. Lewy bodies may also be observed in Alzheimer's disease and many Parkinson-plus syndromes; they are not specific, but rather a sensitive marker for PD. Parkinson-plus syndromes are degenerative neurologic disorders with Parkinsonian features associated with other neurologic findings of pyramidal, cortical, oculomotor, cerebellar and autonomic dysfunction. Disorders such as progressive supranuclear palsy, multisystem atrophy, olivopontocerebellar degeneration, corticobasal ganglionic degeneration and Shy–Drager syndrome are included in Parkinson-plus syndromes. Neuronal loss, Lewy bodies and gliosis are noted symmetrically in the substantia nigra, locus ceruleus, dorsal vagal nucleus and nucleus basalis of Meynert. The motor symptoms are due to substantia nigra lesions, whereas the autonomic features are due to pigmented neuronal loss in the intermediolateral column of the spinal cord and other pigmented nuclei of the brainstem. Lesions within the nucleus basalis of Meynert may contribute to the dementia observed in PD. Dopaminergic neurons undergo degeneration in the zona compacta of the substantia nigra, leading to dopamine loss in the striatum (globus pallidus, putamen and caudate). PD begins to manifest when 70–90% of nigral neurons are destroyed.

The etiology of PD is not clear. There may be synergy between genetic constitution, environmental toxic exposure, effects of aging and perhaps infection in the ultimate expression of PD. Nigral cells diminish with age. The normal dopaminergic pool of neurons of approximately 425 000 decreases to 200 000 at age 80[3]. A remarkable Parkinsonian state has been identified where methyl-phenyltetrahydropyridine (MPTP) has been self administered. The MPTP molecule, an analog of meperidine, has great affinity for monoamine oxidase which oxidizes MPTP. Oxidized MPTP binds to melanin pigment and is lethal to dopaminergic neurons, resulting in a Parkinsonian state. This finding has stimulated much research into environmental toxins as a possible etiology for PD. Cycad ingestion in Guam has been strongly linked to Parkinsonism, amyotropic lateral sclerosis (ALS) and PD dementia. Primates given β-n-methylamino-I-alanine, an amino acid from cycad, developed basal ganglia dysfunction.

The genetic influence on development of PD is not clear. There is a lack of concordance of PD in twins. It is still possible that genetic factors may play an important role. Interestingly, positron emission tomography (PET) imagery has shown striatal dysfunction in 75% of asymptomatic twins[4]. This was true for patients developing PD prior to age 50. First-degree relatives of a patient with PD have a two- to five-fold increased risk for the disease. A mutation on chromosome 6 characterized as a deletion, coding for a protein called parkin, has been associated with autosomal recessive juvenile-onset familial PD[5].

Several biochemical abnormalities have been identified in the substantia nigra in PD. There is evidence of increased free radical production and oxidative damage to lipid, protein and DNA. Increased iron content in the substantia nigra may increase oxidative stress. In addition, mitochondrial complex I deficiency in PD substantia nigra has been postulated as decreasing ATP synthesis, increasing free radical production, reducing mitochondrial membrane potential, decreasing cell growth rate and increasing cell death. Inflammatory cytokine production is also noted in the substantia nigra; however, these cytokines are higher in concentration in Huntington's disease and Alzheimer's disease.

CLINICAL FEATURES

PD is the most common extrapyramidal disease affecting the elderly. The usual onset is between 50 and 70 years of age, and seldom before the age of 30, except for some familial case onsets prior to age 30. Tremor is the most common presenting symptom. Many early motor disabilities go unrecognized by

Table 1 Parkinson's disease tremor vs. essential tremor

Feature	Parkinson's disease	Essential tremor
Typical onset	adult/elderly	adolescence/young adulthood
Common presentation	unilateral arm, fingers, tongue, lips, leg, foot	unilateral arm, head, or vocal cords
Progression	over years	over decades
Frequency of tremor	4–5 Hz	6–12 Hz, slowing with age
Tremor presence	at rest	with action
Alcohol effects	no change	suppression
Family history	rare	common (autosomal dominant)
Other neurologic signs	bradykinesia, rigidity, gait problems, masked face	usually none
Tremor type	'Pill rolling' (agonist–antagonist alternately activated)	low-amplitude 'beating' (antagonists are simultaneously activated)
Treatment	L-dopa and others	beta blockers, primidone, topiramate

the patient as the onset is insidious. The masked face, slowness of movement (bradykinesia), resting tremor, stooped posture (simian posture), axial instability, poor righting reflexes, drooling and hypophonic speech are all characteristic signs that present in varying combinations. The diagnosis may become suddenly apparent to a family member or treating physician. Many early changes may be attributed to 'aging' as the gait, coordination and postural changes seen in aging superficially resemble those seen in PD. A common early complaint is that a limb is 'weak'. When tested, the confrontation strength is fine, but the slow-moving and rigid limb is found, and interpreted by the patient as 'weak'. Typically, degenerative neurologic conditions are symmetric in onset. However, PD is one exception (as is ALS), where there is a hemibody presentation. Perhaps counterintuitive, most cases presenting with tremor show greater involvement on one side. The tremor which usually brings the patient to the physician has a frequency of 4–5 cycles/s; it occurs at rest, and diminishes or abates with action. The tremor increases with stress or anxiety; this can be demonstrated by challenging the patient with mental exercises. In contrast to essential or action tremor, Parkinsonian tremor decreases with finger-to-nose testing. Tremor is a 'to and fro'

or pill-rolling movement with high-amplitude motion. Alternate rhythmic excitation of agonist and antagonist muscles differentiates this tremor from others. Essential tremor is quicker (6–12 Hz) and has much smaller excursion (Table 1). It is well known, however, that an action (kinetic) tremor may be found in PD patients; this may be seen in outstretched hands and fingers. Action tremor begins with muscle contraction, while resting tremor dampens or ceases with contraction. In 20–25% of cases there may be only mild intermittent tremor.

Although tremor is a common presenting symptom in up to one-half of patients, immobility and bradykinesia may be the first feature noted by family members. There is a stiffness and slowness of movement, with a diminished arm swing while walking, a frequent finding early in the disease. Frozen shoulder may also be the presenting complaint due to paucity of movement in one arm. Blinking may be markedly decreased from the normal 12–20 blinks to 5–10/min seen in PD. Bradykinesia manifests as infrequency of swallowing, drooling, slow chewing, diminished speed of postural reflexes, tendency to fall and readying movement prior to executing a motor act. These symptoms are frequently interpreted by the patients as 'feeling weak'.

Micrographia is another common phenomenon. The speech becomes hypophonic, muffled and even inaudible. The gait gradually deteriorates and steps become shortened and shuffling. Extra steps are taken when turning. Pivoting is noted while walking and the 'pull test' impaired. Postural challenge with the pull test is a measure of postural stability and righting reflexes. The examiner, while behind, pulls at the shoulders and patients with PD will take small corrective steps, chase their center of gravity backwards and may fall into the examiner's arms. This retropulsion is common in PD and the number of steps may be used as a grading system. The vestibular system is also affected. Using caloric testing and electronystagmography, 31% of patients with PD had reduced responses while 31% had absent reponses. Up to 91% with impaired postural instability had absent or reduced responses[6]. These patients, however, typically do not complain of common vestibular symptoms. There is an interesting subset of patients who may present with isolated postural reflex impairment and fall without loss of consciousness. Extensive cardiac and general medical evaluations are found to be normal. On closer examination, they have historical and other clinical features consistent with PD. They may respond to dopaminergic agents early on; however, pharmacologic treatement for PD is least effective for the gait and postural instability which is often the greatest source of morbidity and mortality in moderate to severe disease[7]. This postural impairment is well known to occur independently of PD in elderly patients. Gait problems probably parallel the decline in dopaminergic mechanisms seen with aging, and are common findings among elderly patients even without PD.

Sensory symptoms occur in about 10% of cases. Complaints include painful sensory feelings (dysesthesia), paresthesia, tightness and stiffness. They are ill-defined and usually do not have associated examination findings.

Dementia is common in PD with estimates of 10–15%, and as high as 30%[8]. This frequency rises dramatically in older patients and is as high as 65% over the age of 80. The deficits are variable and may range from an isolated cognitive deficit to global cortical dysfunction. It may be difficult at times to discern dementia from side-effects of anti-Parkinson drugs including anticholinergics, L-dopa and dopaminergic agents. In addition, these agents may also induce delirium, which may be interpreted as dementia. It has become clear that the severity of PD, particularly the degree of bradykinesia and rigidity, parallels cognitive decline[9]. It is postulated that the reduction of dopamine and associated diminished stimulation of the prefrontal cortex, limbic structures and basal ganglia results in the respective diminished intellectual ability, depression, bradykinesia and rigidity.

Autonomic dysfunction may be associated with PD. The spectrum of clinical difficulties includes orthostatic hypotension, delayed gastric emptying, urinary bladder dysfunction and temperature dysregulation. Orthostatic hypotension may be seen, but this is not commonly associated with PD[10]. Syncope is seen in a minority, and if prominent, other diseases with Parkinsonism should be sought (especially Shy–Drager syndrome and striatonigral degeneration). Treatment with dopaminergic agents may cause postural blood pressure fluctuations.

DIAGNOSIS

The diagnosis of PD is a clinical one. Conventional laboratory studies may help indirectly by identifying other disorders that present with Parkinsonism. Computerized tomography (CT) and magnetic resonance imaging (MRI) scans are usually normal or show mild atrophy or other non-specific changes. They may be helpful in discerning other disease states associated with Parkinsonism (Table 2). PET using 6-[^{18}F]-fluorolevodopa shows reduced uptake of isotope in the striata. This

Table 2 Causes of Parkinsonism

Toxins
MPTP
Methanol
Manganese
Carbon monoxide
Carbon disulfide

Drugs
Neuroleptics
Reserpine
Meperidine
Ethanol
Diltiazem
Lithium
Amiodarone
Alpha-methyldopa
Amphotericin

Neurodegenerative disorders
Multisystem atrophy
Alzheimer's disease
Pick's disease
Progressive supranuclear palsy
Corticobasal ganglionic degeneration
Cruetzfeldt–Jakob disease

Hereditary disorders
Wilson's disease
Huntington's disease

Post-infectious causes
Viral encephalitis
Postencephalitis lethargica

Miscellaneous
Post-traumatic
Multi-infarct state
Brain tumors
Arteriovenous malformations
Hydrocephalus

MPTP, methyl-phenyl-tetrahydropyridine

modality is costly and usually not necessary for diagnosis. It is commonly reserved for research protocols and presurgical assessments for stereotactic functional neurosurgery. Diagnosis in the early stage may take time and repeated observation. The diagnosis may be delayed with just unilateral akinesia or rigidity, and there may be reluctance to diagnose PD without tremor.

Features of aging may masquerade as early PD. A combination of signs of physiologic aging such as decrease in muscle mass, arthritic joints, diminished vestibular performance, isolated postural instability, memory decline and motor frailty may suggest early PD. Asymmetry of findings is more consistent with PD, whereas the aging process is usually symmetrical. Paratonia should not be mistaken for rigidity, and is common in multi-infarct states and degenerative dementias. Parkinson syndromes associated with post-encepahalitic forms of Parkinsonism, toxins and drugs, and other degenerative neurologic disorders need to be excluded if atypical features are seen in the patient. Bradykinesia, rigidity, resting tremor, gait and postural instability are the cardinal features. The presence of resting tremor would make a strong case for PD. Once Parkinsonism is noted, secondary causes should be excluded such as the use of neuroleptic agents, reserpine, lithium and aldomet, and maganese exposure, or carbon monoxide poisoning. One distinguishing feature between PD and drug- or toxin-induced Parkinsonism is that PD usually starts unilaterally, while drug-induced Parkinsonism is bilateral early on. Drug-induced Parkinsonism is common in the elderly. The aging central nervous system associated with diminished dopaminergic function and reserve may predispose individuals to medication-induced motor side-effects. This form of Parkinsonism is more likely to present without tremor. Unusual features such as paralysis of vertical gaze, cerebellar features, pyramidal tract signs, severe dysphonia or prominent autonomic failure would suggest other neurodegenerative disorders.

In the past an arteriopathic (vascular) form of PD was occasionally diagnosed. Pseudobulbar palsy due to a confluence of subcortical white matter and basal ganglia lacunar infarcts is characterized by dementia, emotional incontinence, pyramidal tract signs, dysarthria, dysphagia, hyperactive bulbar reflexes, and paresis of tongue and facial muscles. This syndrome may superficially resemble PD, but closer scrutiny will differentiate the two disorders.

A diagnosis can be made in most patients who are examined closely. Secondary causes for Parkinsonism must be ruled out; the objective criteria of bradykinesia, resting tremor, postural changes and instability, and cogwheel rigidity are variably present. A clinical response to L-dopa helps secure the diagnosis of PD; however, 10% of PD patients are non-responders. Observation over months with repeat examinations may be necessary in less obvious cases.

MANAGEMENT

Non-pharmacologic management

While pharmacologic intervention provides the most dramatic response, non-pharmacologic measures are cornerstones in the management of PD. Sensible and measured educational efforts are important. Although the disease is progressive, subgroups progress at variable rates. Most respond to pharmacologic treatment and there is usually a substantial period when the quality of life with intervention will be satisfying. Comprehensive medical, social and psychologic assessments should be undertaken early. Attention to the patient's emotional state, insomnia, depression, stress level and financial status is helpful. Introduction to PD patients with good functional status can be an asset and allay fears. Patients and family may be directed to their local PD society chapter. Exercise is essential and may slow the secondary effects of tremor, bradykinesia and rigidity. A balanced exercise program includes aerobic training, strengthening and stretching. Adequate nutrition will help maintain muscle mass, strength and overall well-being.

Pharmacologic treatment

This is summarized in Table 3.

Neuroprotective agents

The decision to begin pharmacologic treatment is based on the degree of functional impairment. Anti-Parkinson medication should be employed to return patients to their previous functioning level and is an option in any patient with functional impairment (Table 4). There has been great interest generated in neuroprotective treatments. Clinically, the monoamine oxidase B inhibitor (MAO-B inhibitor) selegiline has undergone extensive study. The capacity of selegiline to block formation of free radicals has led to its use in clinical studies[11]. Selegiline may delay the emergence of disability and progression of signs and symptoms in previously untreated patients. However, it is unclear whether it is the symptomatic effects or prevention of free radicals and neuroprotective effects of selegiline that translate into the delay in functional disability and better neurologic function. Selegiline enhances the dopaminergic effects of L-dopa; however, in the elderly, it may lead to increased dyskinesia and neuropsychiatric side-effects. It should be used cautiously in patients over 60, due to limited efficacy, potential side-effects and cost concerns. Because of the putative neuroprotective properties and enhancement of L-dopa effects, it is commonly employed in the young. Vitamin E in doses of 2000 IU was ineffective in preventing progression of disease. Prevailing theories make vitamin E an attractive and inexpensive therapy, as it has antioxidant properties and is not harmful. Riluzole, an inhibitor of glutamine release, is currently being investigated for neuroprotection in PD. Dopaminergic drugs are also being tested as neuroprotective agents because of their capacity to induce an L-dopa-sparing effect, direct antioxidant effects and inhibition of excitatotoxicity mediated by overacitivity of the subthalamic nucleus[12].

It is appropriate to start treatment with functional impairment, including difficulties in managing activities of living, threatened

Table 3 Pharmacotherapy for Parkinson's disease

Drug	Dosage	Indications	Comments
Selegiline (MAO-B inhibitor)	5 mg twice a day	neuroprotection (?) adjunct to L-dopa provides increased 'on' time decreases motor fluctuations L-dopa sparing	neuropsychiatric complications neuroprotective effects unconfirmed does not stop progression of disease insomnia
L-dopa–carbidopa	10/100 ⎱ 25/100 ⎰ Sinemet® 25/250 ⎰ 25/100 ⎱ Sinemet CR® 20/200 ⎰ (long acting) (carbidopa/L-dopa)	most effective anti-Parkinsonian drug maintains capacity to perform ADL	neuropsychiatric complications motor fluctuations dyskinesia does not treat freezing, postural instability, dementia, autonomic dysfunction oxidant stress: ? accelerates disease by formation of free radicals may cause an acute delirium/hallucinations (non-threatening human images)
Dopamine agonists	bromocriptine 5–40 cabergoline 0.5–5 lisuride 1–2 ropinirole 0.75–24 pramipexole 1.5–4.5 pergolide 0.75–5 (mg/day)	anti-Parkinson properties L-dopa-sparing drug potential neuroprotective effect diminished L-dopa-related adverse motor complications	limited anti-Parkinson effect orthostatic hypotension neuropsychiatric complications somnolence
Anticholinergics	benztropine 0.5–2 mg twice a day trihexiphenidil 0.5 mg twice a day to 2 mg three times a day	alternative drug in those unable to tolerate L-dopa use may delay use of L-dopa in younger patients	high incidence of neuropsychiatric complications delirium, sedation, dry mouth, blurred vision, urinary retention, constipation

(Continued)

Table 3 (Continued)

Drug	Dosage	Indications	Comments
Amantadine	50–100 mg three times a day	acts by releasing dopamine from striatal neurons anticholinergic properties diminishes L-dopa-induced dyskinesia modest anti-Parkinsonian effect spares early use of L-dopa in younger patients	lower extremity swelling confusion anticholinergic symptoms
COMT inhibitors	entacapone 200 mg with each dose of L-dopa–carbidopa up to 8 times/day tolcapone 100 mg three times a day (used rarely, due to side-effects – see comments)	increases availability of L-dopa to the brain increases L-dopa half-life by 75% provides stable plasma L-dopa levels diminishes 'off' time smoother L-dopa plasma levels reduces L-dopa-related side-effects	increases dopaminergic side-effects (especially dyskinesia) diarrhea and hepatic necrosis with tolcapone usage – should be avoided in most cases

COMT, catechol-O-methyl transferase; MAO-B, monoamine oxidase B

Table 4 Principles of therapy in early Parkinson's disease

Non-pharmacologic treatments
Education
Support
  emotional needs
  peer and group support
  referral to Parkinson's disease society and associations
Legal and financial counseling
Exercise, physical and occupational therapy
Nutritional support

Consider neuroprotection
Early use of dopamine agonist (delay use of L-dopa with associated induced oxidant stress and motor
  complications from long-term L-dopa treatment)
Selegiline (avoid after age 60, patients with cognitive impairment and advanced disease due to high incidence
  of neuropsychiatric side-effects and motor-induced problems)
Vitamins C and E (not proven)

Symptomatic treatment (pharmacologic treatment)
Institute with functional disability or threatened loss of employment
Dopamine agonists can be used as a first-line drug in patients less than 70 years old (delays L-dopa
  introduction; however, clinical efficacy is limited up to 3 years and is significantly less potent than L-dopa)
If L-dopa started as first-line treatment, use with a decarboxylase inhibitor (COMT inhibitor)
Sustained release L-dopa compound (Sinemet CR) is preferred (if switching from immediate to sustained release
  formulations, increase sustained release dose by 20–30%)
L-dopa should be started at a low dose (25/100) and slowly titrated using the lowest dose necessary for good
  clinical response (usually 300–500 mg/day in early disease)
L-dopa is best administered on an empty stomach (1 h before meals)
L-dopa dosages > 600 mg/day are avoided due to higher risk of motor complications
In advancing disease, use combination therapy with L-dopa and dopamine agonist, both at lower dosages
L-dopa combined with COMT inhibitor is preferred in any patient with cognitive impairment, regardless of age
Cost considerations must be part of any treatment plan

COMT, catechol-O-methyl transferase

loss of employability and gait disturbance with falling. The decision to treat should consider the nature of Parkinson symptoms which are paramount. Bradykinesia, for example, is more disabling than tremor. Involvement of the dominant hand with tremor, rigidity or bradykinesia would favor early treatment.

Symptomatic treatment

There is no known treatment for neurorescue of the substantia nigra; however, there is an assortment of drugs for symptomatic treatment. Medical therapies are relied upon primarily to control symptoms of PD. Surgical treatments are available as well.

L-Dihydroxyphenylalanine (L-dopa) is clearly the best drug for symptomatic control.

It was introduced in the 1960s and was initially used in an effort to 're-pigment' the substantia nigra. Although the most effective drug, its place in the treatment of PD is evolving. It is fraught with difficult management problems with chronic treatment. Motor fluctuations and dyskinesias, especially in younger patients, limit its usefulness. Ten per cent of the oral dose is eventually delivered to the brain. L-Dopa is converted in the periphery to dopamine which is unable to pass through the blood–brain barrier. Peripheral dopamine is responsible for the side-effects of L-dopa such as nausea, vomiting and hypotension. Therefore, L-dopa is coupled with a decarboxylase inhibitor (carbidopa) in order to prevent the peripheral conversion of L-dopa to dopamine. This diminishes side-effects and allows more

L-dopa to pass through the blood–brain barrier, enhancing its therapeutic effect. At least 75 mg/day of carbidopa is necessary for effective peripheral dopadecarboxylase inhibition. Increased carbidopa dosage above 75 mg/day may reduce bothersome side-effects. This can be given as pure carbidopa (Lodosyn®) or compounded with L-dopa in Sinemet®. Available dosage strengths of carbidopa/L-dopa (Sinemet) include 10/100, 25/100 and 25/250. Sustained release formulations are available as Sinemet CR®, in 25/100 and 50/200 doses.

Most physicians prefer to start with small doses of L-dopa, one-half of a 25/100 Sinemet tablet three times per day. Normally, dosage of L-dopa in the 300–600 range suffices in the early stages. As there is decreased absorption of the sustained release product, the dosage should be increased by 20–30%.

L-Dopa initially controls rigidity, bradykinesia and tremor quite well. Postural instability and gait problems are less responsive to L-dopa, which can ultimately be a major source of morbidity and mortality. L-Dopa is less effective in treating mental changes, dysarthria, dysphagia, sialorrhea and dysautonomia[13]. Progression of disease and motor fluctuations induced by L-dopa are the main reasons for eventual failure of treatment. Progression of disease is associated with diminished numbers of dopaminergic nerve terminals where L-dopa is converted to dopamine. The main problem with L-dopa is development of motor fluctuations including shorter periods of 'on time' requiring higher and more frequent dosing, dyskinesia and the 'on–off' phenomenon. The 'on–off' phenomenon is the abrupt decline in therapeutic drug effect despite an adequate serum level.

Motor fluctuations are curious, with the underlying mechanism not understood. Motor complications in the form of fluctuations and dyskinesias usually occur after 5 years of treatment with L-dopa[14]. Both presynaptic and postsynaptic events induced by abnormal pulsatile stimulation of the dopamine receptors result in dysregulation of genes and proteins in dopaminergic neurons and abnormal firing patterns in the basal ganglion neurons[15]. It is postulated that the normal physiologic state is continuous dopaminergic stimulation. Long-acting L-dopa preparations (Sinemet CR) have become popular. The addition of catechol-O-methyl transferase (COMT) inhibitors increases the availability of L-dopa by diminishing the peripheral metabolism of L-dopa to the inactive 3-O-methyldopa metabolite. By inhibiting aromatic amino acid decarboxylase by carbidopa and inhibiting catechol-O-methyl transferase by COMT inhibitors (such as tolcapone or entacapone), the two main peripheral degradation pathways of L-dopa, there results a marked increase in the availability and more continuous dopaminergic stimulation[16]. This is theoretically desirable, and ongoing studies are investigating whether this strategy will diminish eventual development of motor complications due to L-dopa. Tolcapone (Tasmar®) has a pharmacologic advantage over entacapone (Comtan®) in that it inhibits central nervous system COMT as well. Due to hepatotoxicity (5% of patients) and rare fulminant liver failure, tolcapone is used rarely. Entacapone (200 mg with each dose of L-dopa) increases 'on time', reduces Parkinson disability scores and may allow reduction of L-dopa daily dosage.

Dopaminergic agonists are drugs that directly stimulate dopamine receptors (D_2) in the basal ganglia. The advantage over L-dopa is that they do not require metabolism to an active neurotransmitter, thus bypassing the diminishing pool of nigral neurons. Ergot derivatives such as bromocriptine, pergolide and lisuride and the newer non-ergot dopamine agonists ropinirole and pramipexole may be used to supplement L-dopa. Dopamine agonists have less risk for inducing motor complications and may be associated

Table 5 Principles of therapy in advanced Parkinson's disease

1. Advanced stages of Parkinson's disease will require an assessment for home health services
2. There is a greater potential for interaction between L-dopa and dietary protein in advanced Parkinson's disease
3. Motor complications can be expected in most patients on L-dopa
   motor fluctuations ('on and off', freezing)
   dyskinesia
   short duration response
   strategies:
      COMT inhibitor may help reduce 'off' time and improve motor response
      higher doses of L-dopa in patients without dyskinesia and smaller more frequent doses in patients with dyskinesias may help reduce motor fluctuations and short-duration responders
4. Orthostatic hypotension is treated by first eliminating antihypertensives; increased salt and fluid intake, elevating the head of the bed; fludrocortisone and midodrine are useful
5. Dysphagia may occur in up to 40%, not directly linked to severity of disease. Such things as swallowing evaluation, soft diet, eating during 'on' time and feeding gastrostomy are helpful in the correct setting
6. Behavioral impairment is common and may present as depression, anxiety, panic attacks and agitation
   sustained depression
      counseling
      antidepressants
   agitation (medication induced)
      discontinue non-Parkinson medication, anticholinergics, amantadine, selegiline, dopamine agonists
   anxiety
      counseling
      antidepressants
      anxiolytics
7. Hallucinations and delirium occur spontaneously or may be medication induced; watch closely for medication effects and eliminate in a stepwise fashion. Always exclude acute medical conditions, particularly infection
8. Exercise programs, exercise in groups, and appropriate PT/OT referrals are helpful
9. Surgical therapies including pallidotomy, deep brain stimulation and fetal transplantation therapies are realistic alternatives in patients who cannot be satisfactorily controlled with medical therapies

PT/OT, physiotherapy/occupational therapy

with reduced incidence of dyskinesia[17]. This fact and their possible neuroprotective effects have made them alternative first agents in treating PD. Symptoms have been well controlled in the first 5 years of treatment, with reduced incidence of dyskinesia in direct comparison to L-dopa. The duration of efficacy with dopamine agonist therapy ranges from 6 month to 3 years[18]. A recent study has shown effectiveness of dopamine agonists for up to 5 years, with reduced risk of dyskinesia by a factor of three comparing ropinirole to L-dopa[17]. The early use of these D2 agonists did not reduce the occurrence of 'wearing off' and freezing during walking to the same extent as the occurrence of dyskinesia (Table 5). When motor complications

develop, they are refractory to medical treatment, are disabling and only effectively managed with surgical interventions (pallidotomy, subthalamic or thalamic stimulation). Hypotension, nausea, vomiting, neuropsychiatric side-effects and sleep attacks may be limiting side-effects of dopaminergic agents.

Amantadine is a weak dopaminergic agent and acts by releasing existing dopamine from striatal neurons. Obviously, as the pool of dopamine-containing cells decreases, this drug loses potency. It possesses anticholinergic properties beneficial for tremor, and is used in doses of 50–100 mg three times per day. Often there is a modest response initially; efficacy is frequently lost after 3 months. In instances where dyskinesias are present, combining amantadine with L-dopa may diminish motor side-effects[19]. Dosages are reduced in the ederly.

Anticholinergics are not used much in treatment of PD. Agents such as tri-hexyphenidyl and benztropine have a preferential effect on tremor. The multitude of side-effects including cognitive dysfunction, psychosis, blurred vision, constipation, dizziness and urinary retention make these agents poor choices for older patients. They may be used more safely in young patients for the L-dopa-sparing effect when tremor is the predominant symptom.

There are several options for initial treatment of early PD. Age of disease onset, life expectancy, presence of dementia, prominent autonomic dysfunction, advanced disease with poor functional status and cost are important considerations. Due to the life expectancy of patients under the age of 60–65, a dopamine agonist is considered first-line therapy. Motor complications may be delayed by using a dopamine agonist before L-dopa. L-Dopa may be added in lower doses to a dopamine agonist with similar clinical effect to that of higher doses of L-dopa alone. This is not an issue in patients near or over 70 years; L-dopa has fewer neuropsychiatric side-effects in comparison to dopamine agonists, anticholinergics, amantadine and selegiline. Patients with prominent autonomic dysfunction tolerate L-dopa better than dopamine agonists.

Anticholinergic agents, amantadine and selegiline have little role in patients over 60 years of age, due to little therapeutic effect, cost and considerable side-effects. L-Dopa is commonly started in the 70 and over age group for quality-of-life issues and because they are less likely to develop L-dopa-induced motor complications. Functional status, however, is the most important factor when deciding to begin L-dopa, regardless of age. In patients cognitively impaired, L-dopa is the drug of choice.

Rehabilitation

Exercise is probably the most important adjunctive therapy for PD. It can prevent impairment in mobility and functional activity and has a positive effect on mood. Added flexibility and strength can be realized through regular exercise. Emphasis on stretching the extensor muscles will help prevent flexor postures. Aerobic and stretching exercises for 20–30 min/week is a reasonable goal. Yoga and Tai chi are reasonable alternatives and provide aerobic and stretching techniques. Physical therapists or PD exercise groups can be helpful in getting patients started. Fitness should be assessed to avoid cardiovascular complications, falls and injuries in those prone. Water aerobics may be helpful in some patients.

Safe homes are important in managing gait and balance problems. Carefully placed rails in bathrooms, showers and stairwells provide protection against falls. Physical therapy and gait training can be aided by certain motor or sensory tricks. Stepping over imaginary lines or rocking and marching in place can be helpful in preventing 'start hesitation or freezing'. Quadrapods and walkers are necessary when there is significant postural instability. Occupational therapy can help teach the use of special eating utensils, non-tie shoes, extended shoe horns and easily worn apparel such as clip-on ties and velcro fasteners.

Good nutrition is essential for the well-being of PD patients. There is an increased incidence of poor nutrition, weight loss and loss of muscle mass. On the other hand, a sedentary lifestyle and poor eating habits may lead to obesity. No specific diets are recommended; however, balanced meals are encouraged. Incidence of chewing and swallowing problems and inability to obtain and prepare food contribute to malnutrition. Autonomic dysfunction may be associated with constipation. Fiber and increased fluid intake help prevent this. Competition between L-dopa and dietary protein for intestinal absorption can be minimized by taking L-dopa 1 h before or after meals.

Surgical treatments

Surgery has been an increasingly popular treatment modality in patients who cannot be controlled with medical therapy. The dramatic clinical response with L-dopa led to a decline in interest in stereotactic functional neurosurgical procedures. The disabling complications of L-dopa treatment, poor response to medical treatment in advanced PD and improvements in neuroimaging and stereotactic and neurophysiologic targeting techniques have led to a renewed interest in surgical treatments. Posteroventral pallidotomy using microelectrode and neuroimaging localization and radiofrequency ablative methods has been associated with a marked reduction in drug-induced dyskinesia in contralateral limbs, and moderate improvements in rigidity and tremor[20]. There is enhanced responsiveness to L-dopa postoperatively. Unfortunately, this procedure has no enduring effect on postural instability. Bilateral pallidotomy is risky and associated with dysarthria, dysphagia and dementia. A disadvantage of ablative therapies is that they may preclude the patient from participating in future functional or restorative therapies.

High-frequency stimulation of the subthalamic nucleus has resulted in improvement of all aspects of PD, and clearly is superior to ablative lesions in the globus pallidus or subthalamic nucleus[21]. This method is now available at specialized centers through stereotactic placement of electrodes in the subthalamic nucleus.

In summary, the management of PD patients entails the use of pharmacologic agents and non-pharmacologic therapies. Surgical therapies may help those who are no longer responsive to, or suffering complications from, drug therapy. Dementia is

common and needs to be recognized early in treatment. Safety assessments should be ongoing and updated. Family education and logistic supports need to be placed, including home care and more structured living arrangements, when appropriate. Depression is common and treated with psychotherapy and medications when indicated.

SPECIAL ASSOCIATED PROBLEMS

Mental symptoms are common in up to one-third of patients. Hallucinations, dementia and delirium may be complications of PD or the pharmacologic treatments. The mental symptoms may be difficult to treat and are common reasons for placement in nursing facilities[22]. Cognitive impairments may be global hemispheric dysfunction or specific deficits in language, visuospatial relations or executive functions. Pseudodementia is part of the differential diagnosis. Anticholinergic agents, amantadine and selegiline all may contribute to delirium or psychosis and are best avoided in older patients. Dopaminergic agents and even L-dopa may need to be decreased or eliminated.

Hallucinations can occur in up to 20% of PD patients treated with anti-Parkinson drugs. L-Dopa-induced hallucinations are typically non-threatening and usually take the form of human faces/images. Patients are prone to infections, metabolic disorders such as dehydration and falls. If patients require antipsychotic therapy, clozapine is the preferred atypical neuroleptic due to lack of dopamine receptor blocking. Agranulocytosis is an associated side-effect in 1–2% of patients and not dose related, therefore weekly blood counts must be monitored. Psychiatric consultation is recommended for help with management.

Depression is common and occurs in up to 40% of PD patients. The decrease in monoamines predisposes to the development of endogenous depression. Anti-Parkinson treatment, therefore, should be the first line of treatment, reserving antidepressants for non-responders to anti-Parkinson medication. Selective serotonin reuptake inhibitors (SSRIs) are effective in PD. Co-therapy with selegiline and SSRIs is avoided due to the theoretical possibility of hypertensive crisis. Tricyclic antidepressants (TCA) may facilitate sleep, being helpful in insomnia which is common in PD. Orthostatic hypotension is a limiting side-effect. Nortriptyline has the least anticholinergic side-effects and is the least sedating, so it is preferred in PD. Doses of 20–50 mg can be helpful in treating depression and insomnia.

Sleep disorders are common in PD and present in up to three-quarters of patients[23]. Insomnia, sundowning, drug-induced nightmares, myoclonus or vocalization, rapid eye movement (REM) behavior disorder and restless legs are common features. The basis for sleep disruption is probably related to dorsal raphe serotonergic cell loss and locus ceruleus noradrenergic cell loss. REM behavior disorder is due to loss of motor inhibition that usually occurs with REM sleep. Unusual behaviors such as semipurposeful movements, aggression and wandering are observed by bed partners. These behaviors may lead to injury of the patient or spouse. REM behavior disorder in some cases may precede the diagnosis of PD. It is treated with low-dose clonazepam. TCAs and MAO inhibitors may precipitate this disorder. Nightmares may be associated with dopaminergic agents; a decrease of night-time dopaminergic agents is often helpful.

Restless leg syndrome is frequent in PD, and is associated with peculiar ill-defined symptoms in the legs. Descriptions include paresthesias, dysesthesia, aches, cramping and need to move or walk, phenomena which fragment sleep. Four criteria have been proposed by the International Restless Legs Syndrome Study Group to diagnose restless legs syndrome. These include desire to move the extremity with associated paresthesia/dysesthesia, motor restlessness, sensory symptoms mostly at rest and relieved by motion and symptoms that are worse at night[24]. Restless legs syndrome may be seen as a part of PD syndrome and may be idiopathic or drug related; it responds well to dopaminergic agents or night-time dose of L-dopa. Clonazepam and codeine are alternative treatments.

References

1. Jellinger K. Overview of morphological changes in PD. In Yahr M, Bergman K, eds. *Advances in Neurology*. New York: Raven Press, 1987;45:1–18
2. Oppenheimer D. Diseases of the basal ganglia, cerebellum and motor neurons. In Blackwood W, Corsellis J, eds. *Greenfield's Neuropathology*. London: Edward Arnold Publishers, 1976:608–51
3. McGeer P, McGeer E, Suzuki J, et al. Aging, Alzheimer disease and the cholinergic system of the basal forebrain. *Neurology* 1984;34:741–55
4. Picini P, Burn D, Ceravolo R, et al. The role of inheritance in sporadic Parkinson's disease: evidence for a longitudinal study of dopaminergic function in twins. *Ann Neurol* 1999;45:577–82
5. Schapira A. Neuroprotection and dopamine agonists. In Koller W, ed. The new role of dopamine agonists in the management of Parkinson's disease and restless legs syndrome. *Neurology* 2002;58(Suppl 1): S9–18
6. Reichart W, Doolitle J, McDowell F. Vestibular dysfunction in Parkinson's disease. *Neurology* 1982;32:1133–8
7. Weiner W, Nora L, Glanz R. Elderly patients: postural reflex impairment. *Neurology* 1984;34:945–7

8. Mayeux R, Chen J, Mirabello E, *et al*. An estimate of the incidence of dementia in idiopathic Parkinson's disease. *Neurology* 1990;40:1513–17

9. Mayeux R, Stern Y. Intellectual dysfunction and dementia in Parkinson's disease. In Mayeux R, Rosen W, eds. *The Dementias*. New York: Raven Press, 1983:211–27

10. Rajput A, Rozdilsky B. Dysautonomia in Parkinsonism: a clinicopathologic study. *J Neurol Neurosurg Psychiatry* 1976;39: 1092–100

11. Olanow C, Fahn S, Langston J, *et al*. Selegiline and mortality in Parkinson's disease. *Ann Neurol* 1996;49:841–5

12. Koller W. Treatment of early Parkinson's disease. In Koller W, ed. The new role of dopamine agonists in the management of Parkinson's disease and restless legs syndrome. *Neurology* 2002;58(Suppl 1): S79–92

13. Jankovic J. Levodopa strengths and weaknesses. In Koller W, ed. The new role of dopamine agonists in the management of Parkinson's disease and restless legs syndrome. *Neurology* 2002;58(Suppl 1): S19–32

14. Ahlskog J, Meunter M. Frequency of levodopa related dyskinesias and motor fluctuations as estimated from the cummulative literature. *Mov Disord* 2001;16:448–58

15. Olanow C, Obeso J. Preventing levodopa induced dyskinesia. *Ann Neurol* 2000;47: 167–78

16. Kaakkolas S, Gordin A, Mannisto P. General properties and clinical possibilities of new selective inhibitors of catecol-O-methyltransferase. *Gen Pharmacol* 1994; 25:813–24

17. Rascol O, Brooks D, Korczyn A, *et al*. A full year study of the evidence of dyskinesia in patients with early Parkinson's disease who were treated with ropinirole or levodopa. 056 study group. *N Engl J Med* 2000;342: 1484–91

18. Marsden C. Parkinson's disease. *J Neurol Neurosurg Psychiatry* 1994;57:672–81

19. Veragen Metman L, Del Dotto Van Den, Munckhof P, *et al*. Amantadine as treatment for dyskinesias and motor fluctuations in Parkinson's disease. *Neurology* 1998;50:1323–6

20. Laitinen L. Leksell's posterventral pallidotomy in the treatment of Parkinson's disease. *J Neurosurg* 1992;76:53–61

21. Limousin P, Krack P, Pollack P, *et al*. Electrical stimulation of the subthalamic nucleus in advanced Parkinson's disease. *N Engl J Med* 1998;339:1105–1111

22. Goetz C, Stebbins G. Risk factors for nursing home placement in advanced Parkinson's disease. *Neurology* 1993;43: 2227–9

23. Factor S, McAlarney T, Sanchez-Ramos J, *et al*. Sleep disorders and sleep effect in Parkinson's disease. *Mov Disord* 1990;5: 280–5

24. Walters A, and the International Restless Legs Syndrome Study Group. Toward a better definition of the restless leg syndrome. *Mov Disord* 1995;10:634–42

34 Alcoholism and smoking

Bhavesh S. Patel, MD, and T.S. Dharmarajan, MD, FACP, AGSF

INTRODUCTION

Alcoholism is a common yet under-recognized problem in older adults[1,2]. There appears to be little clinical or research interest in studying substance abuse in the geriatric age group. Until recently, alcoholism was considered a disorder predominantly of the young; however, alcohol abuse is far more prevalent in the geriatric population than was previously believed[2]. Alcoholism in the elderly is associated with accidents, significant co-morbidity and a shorter life span[1-3]. There appear to be two types of alcohol-related problems seen in the elderly. One is an earlier onset of alcoholism, with continued drinking throughout life, whereas the second group has a late onset of alcoholism in response to stress[1,4].

Nicotine addiction is another affliction in all ages, including older adults. A smoker has about a one in three chance of dying prematurely due to complications from smoking[5]. A discussion follows on the epidemiology, adverse effects, identification and treatment of alcohol and nicotine dependence in the geriatric population.

ALCOHOLISM

Epidemiology

Prevalence data on alcoholism in the elderly vary with criteria used and reporting bias[2,6]. Estimates suggest that 2–10% of community-living elderly in the USA, up to 4% of community-living older men and women in the UK and 10% of hospitalized geriatric patients in the UK consume excessive alcohol[7,8]. In hospitalized elderly, including those in psychiatry units, the prevalence of alcoholism ranges from 20 to 50%[9]. Two thirds of older alcoholics give a history of ethanol abuse since young age, whereas the remaining third have a late onset[1,4]. A significant genetic predisposition is said to be present for alcoholism. A positive family history increases the risk of alcoholism among relatives. Other risk factors include loss of spouse or loved one, recent retirement, social isolation, new-onset medical condition, prior history of alcoholism or substance abuse and psychiatric disorders including depression and anxiety[4,10].

Diagnostic criteria

The Diagnostic and Statistical Manual of Mental Disorder (DSM-IV) criteria are available to diagnose substance abuse and dependence. The National Guideline Clearinghouse states that DSM-IV criteria may not be adequate for diagnosis of alcoholism in the elderly. The panel recommends using terms 'at-risk drinkers' (alcohol use without demonstrable problems, but causing adverse consequences) and 'problem drinkers' (more hazardous level of consumption, meeting DSM-IV criteria for abuse and dependence)[11]. The International Classification of Diseases (ICD-10) of 'harmful use of alcohol' and alcohol dependence syndrome (ADS) is similar to the DSM-IV classification

Table 1 Alcohol and drug interactions. From references 1, 10, 11 and 13

Histamine-2 blockers (cimetidine, ranitidine, nizatidine)
Increase in blood alcohol concentration due to inhibition of gastric alcohol dehydrogenase

Benzodiazepines, barbiturates, phenothiazines and antidepressants
Additive suppression of central nervous system

Non-steroidal anti-inflammatory drugs and aspirin
Increase in bleeding time and gastritis

Warfarin
Fluctuation in International Standardized Ratio (INR), usually decreased

Anticonvulsants
Unpredictable clearance of drugs (fluctuation in serum drug levels)

Acetaminophen and isoniazid
Hepatotoxicity even with therapeutic doses in chronic alcoholics

β-Adrenergic blockers
Mask signs of delirium tremens

Cephalosporins
Disulfiram-like reaction with some cephalosporins

---

of 'alcohol abuse' and 'alcohol dependence' respectively[12].

Pharmacology, relevant to aging

Alcohol acts on specific neurotransmitter receptors and transporters to produce intoxicating effects. In the brain, it enhances γ-aminobutyric acid A (GABAA) receptors and inhibits N-methyl-D-asparate (NMDA) receptors[3]. Absorption of alcohol from the gastrointestinal tract is unchanged with aging; it occurs through the mucous membrane of the gastrointestinal tract[7]. Due to changes in body composition (age-related decrease in total body water), equivalent amounts may produce higher blood alcohol concentrations in older subjects, with increased risk for intoxication and adverse effects, in spite of efficient metabolism and elimination[2]. Levels are higher in women than men for the same amount consumed. Alcohol absorption also increases because of diminished gastric alcohol dehydrogenase (ADH), more pronounced in women. Legal limits for driving under the influence of alcohol are 80–100 mg/ml of blood alcohol concentration[3]. Alcohol interacts with several commonly prescribed medications through altered drug pharmacokinetics (e.g. delayed gastric emptying, altered protein binding and impaired hepatic enzymes)[1,2]. Alcohol may impair liver function initially but chronic consumption induces liver enzymes and increases drug clearance[1]. Excretion occurs through breath, sweat and urine. See Table 1 for alcohol–drug interactions.

Effects of alcoholism

Alcohol has adverse effects on most organ systems (Table 2). Low or moderate consumption of alcohol seems to be a beneficial measure for preventing coronary artery disease. If so, how much drinking is bad for health in adults? Experts and the National Institutional of Alcohol Abuse and Alcoholism (NIAAA) recommend that the older male and female should not consume more than one drink of alcohol per day. One standard drink is considered to be the equal of 360 ml (12 oz) of beer, 180 ml (5 oz) of wine or 45 ml (1.5 oz) of distilled spirits, all of which contain the equivalent of 12 g (0.5 oz) of alcohol[1,10,11].

Table 2 The consequences of alcoholism. From references 1, 7 and 11

Alcoholic hepatitis and cirrhosis
Blood abnormalities: thrombocytopenia, macrocytosis and elevated gamma-glutamyl transpeptidase (GGTP)
Cardiomyopathy
Cancers of head, neck, liver, breast and esophagus
Cognitive impairment and increased risk of delirium
Falls due to impaired balance and/or judgement, myopathy and neuropathy
Gastrointestinal bleeding
Injuries, including motor vehicle accidents
Insomnia
Nutritional deficiencies (e.g. thiamine, folate, nicotinic acid, vitamin B_6, magnesium, calcium,
    phosphorus, potassium), hypoglycemia and hypoalbuminemia
Osteoporosis
Pancreatitis
Peripheral neuropathy
Suicide and violent death
Urinary incontinence
Uncontrolled hypertension and stroke

The presentation of alcoholism in the elderly may be atypical. Unlike the young, geriatric individuals may present with delirium, uncontrolled hypertension, cognitive impairment, personality disorder, self-neglect or medication-related issues. Withdrawal symptoms are often mistaken for other medical conditions. Postoperative delirium, elevated gamma-glutamyl transpeptidase (GGT) and/or elevated red cell corpuscular volume may be clues to unsuspected alcoholism. Table 3 outlines signs and symptoms that may be clues to possible alcohol abuse.

Screening and diagnosis

A high index of suspicion is the best means to screen for alcoholism.

A commonly used screening test is the following CAGE questionnaire[7,13]:

(1) Need to Cut down drinking?

(2) Annoyed by criticizing of drinking?

(3) Feel Guilty about drinking?

(4) Need an 'Eye opener' (a drink first thing in the morning) to steady one's nerves?

Two or more positive responses constitute a positive screening test. Lowering of the score to one may be more sensitive and specific in the elderly[2].

The NIAAA recommends that the following three questions be asked[7]:

(1) Average number of days per week that alcohol was consumed?

(2) Number of drinks taken on a typical day?

(3) Maximum number of drinks consumed on any given occasion in the past month?

The Michigan Alcohol Screening Test – Geriatric Version (MAST-G) is a 24-item test tailored to the elderly. A score of 5 or more is suggestive of alcoholism[14]. The ten-item Alcohol Use Disorder Identification Test (AUDIT), not well studied in the geriatric population, is used to screen for less severe alcohol problems such as 'at risk', 'hazardous' or 'harmful' drinking[8]. Once this is established, further questioning should look for physical and psychological manifestations of alcoholism. Detailed information is obtained from the patient, caregiver or family members. Physical examination may reveal target organ damage (Table 2). The health provider should also search for other medical illnesses that exacerbate alcohol abuse or are exacerbated by chronic alcoholism. Laboratory

Table 3 Signs and symptoms suggestive of possible alcohol abuse. From references 7 and 13

Anxiety, irritability, restlessness and mood swings
Frequent unexplained visits to emergency departments
Non-compliance with medication and appointments
Poor hygiene, self-neglect, lack of motivation and interest
Recurrent accidents, or falls
Social isolation
Uncontrolled hypertension
Unexplained decline in functional and cognitive status
Unexpected delirium in hospitalized patients

evaluation includes liver function tests, complete blood count, serum electrolytes and serum amylase in select cases[10,15].

Management

Management is dictated by the clinical presentation.

Acute intoxication

Mild to moderate intoxication requires no specific therapy. Severe acute intoxication as defined by a depressed mental status or respiration, cardiac arrhythmia, aggressive behavior or significant blood pressure elevation needs appropriate emergency care. After stabilizing vital signs, the patient is placed in a quiet environment under close observation. Uncontrolled agitation may require cautious use of low-dose antipsychotics or short-acting benzodiazepines. Hospitalization is often necessary to detoxify the elderly with severe alcoholism[3,5].

Alcohol withdrawal: including delirium tremens, Wernicke's encephalopathy, Korsakoff's psychosis

Prompt recognition and appropriate treatment of these conditions, especially in the frail elderly, is vital to prevent mortality. Delirium tremens usually presents in 24–72 h of the last drink, but may occur a week after abstinence. Individuals with withdrawal may have tremors, fever, tachycardia, hypertension, diaphoresis, agitation, hallucination or changes in mental status. Wernicke's encephalopathy presents with ophthalmoplegia, ataxia and changes in mental status, whereas Korsakoff's psychosis has an insidious onset with profound memory loss. Correction of fluid and electrolyte depletion is essential. Intravenous thiamine (50–100 mg) should be given before any dextrose-containing solution is administered. Magnesium supplementation is an important adjunct to the treatment, the majority of alcoholics being magnesium depleted. Tapering doses of short- or intermediate-acting benzodiazepines are agents of choice for managing withdrawal. Education is imparted on further treatment options and the prognosis for continued drinking[3,5,9,16].

Chronic alcoholism

Treatment options depend on the severity of the problem. For a mild-to-moderate drinker, counseling by the primary caregiver may result in significant reduction of alcohol consumption[2,7]. Essential components of counseling include discussion on the adverse effects of alcohol, setting the limit or abstinence, coping strategies, psychosocial problems and pain management. The NIAAA has published educational materials to assist in management. Family members play an important role and should be provided access to support groups (such as Al-anon/alateen) and education[1,4]. For severe abuse, a formal alcohol treatment program may be necessary to produce a favorable outcome. There is a dearth of structured programs designated for elderly alcoholics, most are combined with programs for younger individuals[7]. The abstinence rate is about 50% after a year of treatment[2]. Once formal treatment is completed, Alcoholic Anonymous (AA), Self Management And Recovery Training (SMART) and other non-professional programs may be of help[3-5,9,16].

Pharmacotherapy could be an adjunct treatment to prevent relapse and craving for alcohol. Naltrexone (Trexan, ReVia), an opiate antagonist, helps treat alcohol dependence; its role in the elderly is not yet established. The recommended dose is 50 mg/day, common adverse effects being nausea and headache. Acamprosate, another anti-craving drug, is under study in the USA. Disulfiram (Antabuse®) is not recommended in older subjects, due to the risk of adverse effects[1]. Refractory cases may be referred for continued counseling, high-quality medical care, maintenance of functional status and palliative care[2].

The National Institutes of Health (NIH) and NIAAA have initiated the COMBINE (Combining Medication and Behavioral Interventions) clinical trial to evaluate the effectiveness of behavioral treatment with or without medications for the treatment of alcoholism. Organizations in the USA have initiated 'National alcohol screening day' and 'Alcohol awareness month' as a means of public education and increased detection by health providers.

SMOKING

Epidemiology

Nicotine dependence from cigarette use is more common than alcoholism and complicates many illnesses in the elderly[7,17]. It is a major risk factor for six of the 14 leading causes of mortality in the elderly and accounts for one in five deaths, yet one in eight elderly persons continue to smoke[6,18]. Estimates suggest that 13 million Americans over the age of 50 years and 12% of the geriatric population smoke[6,17]. Approximately two-thirds of smokers visit a physician, providing the opportunity for counseling and quitting[18]. Older smokers are less motivated to quit smoking, fear failure and see less benefit to health; this is because they are older, have smoked longer and already have co-morbidities. Older smokers also tend to be less educated, are less confident in their ability to quit, have lower income and are more likely to be female; furthermore, the negative outcomes with smoking have a lesser impact on the elderly[6].

Pharmacology

Content and absorption of nicotine varies with the type of tobacco; nicotine is absorbed from the mucous membrane and skin, and is quite lipophilic. A small amount is protein bound, with most of the excretion via the kidneys. It has complex actions on the neurologic, cardiovascular, endocrine and neuromuscular systems. Smokeless tobacco is less harmful than cigarette smoking[19-21].

Nicotine as a risk factor and the benefits of quitting

Cigarette and cigar smoking accelerates atherosclerosis, coronary and cerebrovascular events, including sudden death; there results an acceleration in coagulation and platelet aggregation with a shorter bleeding time. The body antioxidant defenses are negatively affected. Smoking has been associated with several additional disease processes, many common in older adults (Table 4). The Surgeon General's report suggests that smoking cessation is beneficial at any age and that health providers should discourage all individuals from smoking[6]. Benefits of cessation include prevention or reduction in the incidence of coronary heart disease, chronic lung diseases and cancer. An improvement in lung function and appetite as well as an overall sense of well-being are noted after abstinence[6,17].

Smoking cessation in the elderly

The Agency for Health Care Policy and Research (AHCPR) has developed clinical practice guidelines for health-care providers on smoking cessation and advice applicable to smokers, including those who do not meet

Table 4 Nicotine and related co-morbidity. From references 18–21 and 27

Cancers: oral cavity, esophagus, larynx, stomach, pancreas, lung, bladder, kidney, cervix
Cerebrovascular disease
Chronic obstructive lung disease and respiratory infections
Coronary artery disease
Drug interactions (induces cytochrome P450 system)
Hypertension
Osteoporosis
Peptic ulcer disease
Peripheral vascular disease
Risk to non-smokers
Visual problems (cataracts, macular degeneration)

DSM-IV criteria for nicotine dependence[22]. Formal smoking cessation programs tailored to the elderly are available but not well studied. Most older adults prefer quitting on their own[6,22].

Counseling

Counseling in conjunction with pharmacotherapy appears more effective for quitting smoking. It can be provided individually or in groups, and counseling strategies are available in booklets, audio/video tapes or computer programs. Behavioral smoking cessation techniques include setting a quit date, methods to diminish craving and ways to deal with stress. Smokers learn coping strategies, smoking cues, methods to break the link between cues and smoking, managing withdrawal symptoms and preventing relapse[18].

Nicotine replacement therapy

Cautious nicotine replacement therapy is effective in the elderly when combined with counseling, regular follow-up and support groups for smoking cessation, and helps alleviate withdrawal symptoms such as irritability, anxiety, restlessness, craving and difficulty with concentrating[23,24]. Nicotine replacement is based on the principles that nicotine minimizes or eliminates withdrawal symptoms and eventually breaks the conditioned association with smoking (Table 5). Nicotine replacement is available as gum, patch, spray and inhaler, with gum and patch available without a prescription in the USA. Nicotine polacrilex gum (Nicorette®), released in 1984, has to be chewed slowly, with the gum 'parked' in the mouth when not being chewed; nicotine is absorbed from the mucous membrane. Nicotine transdermal patches (Habitrol®, Nicoderm®, Nicotrol®, and Prostep®) work better than the gum in older adults; introduced in the early 1990s, they are used once daily with the strength adjusted to the number of cigarettes smoked and to co-morbidity. Manufacturers vary on suggestions to wear the patch for 16 or 24 h; both types are available in different tapering strengths. The nasal spray (Nicotrol NS) allows nicotine to be absorbed via the nasal mucosa, with nicotine levels peaking within 10 min. Nicotine inhalers (Nicotrol inhaler) appear like the cigarette; nicotine vapors are absorbed via the oral mucosa and thus absorption is similar to that of the gum[20,24].

Non-nicotine therapy

Non-nicotine preparations for smoking cessation include bupropion, clonidine, nortriptyline and lobeline (Table 6). The sustained release antidepressant bupropion (Zyban®, Wellbutrin SR®), either alone or in combination with a nicotine patch, has shown a higher abstinence rate at 1 year. The mechanism of action of bupropion is not clear; dosage varies from 150 to 300 mg orally daily. Side-effects include insomnia, headache, seizures, constipation and dreams. The drug is contraindicated in patients with seizures or anorexia nervosa and those on monoamine oxidase inhibitors[20]. Clonidine is an α_2-agonist found to decrease craving and nicotine withdrawal symptoms. The usual dose is 0.1–0.4 mg daily for 3–4 weeks, with gradual tapering of the clonidine recommended to avoid side-effects. Nortriptyline is a tricyclic antidepressant, requiring more data prior to receiving approval by the Food and Drug

Table 5 Nicotine replacement therapy. From references 18, 20 and 21

Preparation	Route/strength	Side-effects
Gum	2, 4 mg, chewed 1 piece/hour	hiccough, nausea, vomiting, jaw-ache, mouth irritation
Patch	24-h transdermal patch 7,14, 21 mg 16-h transdermal patch 5,10,15 mg 11, 22 mg	skin irritation, insomnia, unpleasant dreams
Nasal spray	1–2 doses/h 0.5 mg each nostril	Nasal/throat irritation, rhinitis, sneezing, cough
Inhaler	vapor inhalation 6–16 cartridges/day	cough, throat irritation, dry mouth

Table 6 Smoking cessation. From references 18–21 and 27

Non-pharmacologic
Obtain regular history on a routine basis
Urge smokers to quit
Provide assistance
Provide follow-up, including telephone calls
Include non-clinicians (e.g. psychosocial worker) for support
Continue vigil for recurrence

Pharmacologic
Nicotine patch, gum, oral inhaler, nasal spray
Bupropion
Clonidine*
Nortriptyline*
Lobeline*

* Not yet FDA approved

Table 7 Helpful links. From references 1, 4, 18 and 26

National Institute of Alcohol Abuse and Alcoholism (NIAAA)
http://www.niaaa.nih.gov/
Alcoholics Anonymous (AA)
http://www.alcoholics-anonymous.org
Phone: (212) 870-3400
Hope & Help for Families and Friends of Alcoholics
http://www.al-anon.alateen.org
Phone: (888) 4AL-ANON
The Public Health Service's Treating Tobacco Use and Dependence Guideline
http://www.surgeongeneral.gov/tobacco
British Health Education Authority
http://www.cochrane.org/cochrane/revabstr
Centers for Disease Control and Prevention
http://www.thecommunityguide.org

Administration (FDA). Lobeline is an alkaloid with weak nicotine-like pharmacologic properties and its efficacy is yet to be established, pending more trials. Hypnosis and acupuncture are other methods for smoking cessation, but their efficacy remains to be studied.

Nicotine replacement preparations can be safely combined with one another or with bupropion[18]. It is common to start with one drug and add a second agent if there is craving or withdrawal symptoms. Usual duration of treatment ranges from 8 weeks to 6 months. At present, it is unclear as to which form of pharmacotherapy (nicotine replacement versus bupropion) is superior. Choice may be individualized, based on preference and past experience[18]. There is also a concern regarding smoking cessation recommendations and consequent reduction in quality of life in the mind of some older individuals[25]. One-year smoking cessation rate is about 20% with nicotine replacement therapy in the elderly[25]. Smoking cessation is a cost-effective intervention and the goal is to increase help to quit smoking in the majority of smokers[6,18,26,27].

SUMMARY

Chemical dependence is under-recognized in the geriatric population and a preventable risk factor for morbidity and mortality.

Recommended screening for alcohol and nicotine dependence is desirable as a part of comprehensive geriatric assessment. Counseling and education by health-care providers are paramount in management. Research and effective strategies for prevention and treatment of the problem in the elderly are much needed. Helpful links are provided in Table 7.

References

1. Rigler SK. Alcoholism in elderly. *Am Fam Physician* 2000;61:1760–6
2. Reid MC, Anderson PA. Geriatric substance use disorders. *Med Clin North Am* 1997;81:999–1016
3. Schuckit MA. Alcohol and alcoholism. In Braunwald E, Fauci AS, Kasper DL, *et al.*, eds. *Harrison's Principles of Internal Medicine*, 15th edn. New York: McGraw-Hill, 2001:2559–62
4. Lantz MS. Alcohol abuse in the older adults. *Clin Geriatr* 2002;10:40–42
5. Benowitz NL. Tobacco. In Goldman L, Bennett JC, eds. *Cecil Textbook of Medicine*. Philadelphia: WB Saunders, 2000:33–7
6. Wilcox S, King AC. Health behavior and aging. In Hazzard WR, Blass JP, Ettinger WH, *et al.*, eds. *Principles of Geriatric Medicine and Gerontology*. New York: McGraw Hill, 1999:287–2
7. Beers MH, Berkow R, Bogin RM, *et al.* Substance abuse and dependence. In Beers MH, Berkow R, Bogin RM, *et al.*, eds. *The Merck Manual of Geriatrics*. Whitehouse Station, NJ: Merck Research Laboratories, 2000:333–1
8. Crome IB. Alcohol problems in the older persons. *J R Soc Med* 1997;90:16–22
9. Barry PP, Ackerman K. Chemical dependency in the elderly. In Hazzard WR, Blass JP, Ettinger WH, *et al.*, eds. *Principles of Geriatric Medicine and Gerontology*. New York: McGraw Hill, 1999:1357–63
10. O'Conneor PG, Schottenfeld RS. Patients with alcohol problem: review article. *N Engl J Med* 1998;338:592–602
11. National Clearinghouse for Alcohol and Drug Information. *Substance Abuse Among Older Adults*. Rockville, MD: NCADI, 1999 (800-729-6686)
12. DeHart S, Hoffmann NG. Screening and diagnosis of alcohol abuse and dependence in older adults. *Int J Addict* 1995;30:1717–47
13. Adams WL. The aging male patient, alcohol and the health of aging men. *Med Clin North Am* 1999;83:1195–1211
14. The University of Michigan Alcohol Research Center. Michigan Alcoholism Screening Test–Geriatric Version. In Cobbs EL, Duthie EH Jr, Murphy JB, eds. *Geriatrics Review Syllabus*, 5th edn. Malden, MA: Blackwell Publishing, 2002;405
15. Blazer DG. Alcohol and drug problems. In Busse EW, Blazer DG eds. *Textbook of Geriatric Psychiatry*. Washington DC: The American Psychiatry Press, 1996:341–6
16. Wiseman EJ. Drug and alcohol abuse. In Sadock BJ, Sadock VA, eds. *Kaplan and Sadock's Comprehensive Textbook of Psychiatry*. Philadelphia: Lippincott Williams & Wilkins, 2000:3081–5
17. Boyd NR. Smoking cessation: a four-step plan to help older patients quit. *Geriatrics* 1996;51:52–7
18. Rigotti NA. Treatment of tobacco use and dependence. *N Engl J Med* 2002;346:506–2
19. Burns DM. Nicotine addiction. In Braunwald E, Fauci AS, Kasper DL, *et al.* eds. *Harrison's Principles of Internal Medicine*, 15th edn. New York: McGraw-Hill, 2001:2574–7
20. Helge TD, Denelsky GY. Pharmacologic aids to smoking cessation. *Clev Clin J Med* 2000;67:818–14
21. Frishman WH, Ky T, Ismail A. Tobacco smoking, nicotine, and nicotine and nonnicotine replacement therapies. *Heart Dis* 2001;3:365–7
22. The Agency for Health Care Policy and Research. Smoking cessation clinical

practice guideline. *J Am Med Assoc* 1996; 275:1270–80

23. Patterson C. Health promotion, screening and surveillance. In Evans JG, Willliams TF, Beattie BL, *et al.*, eds. *Oxford Textbook of Geriatric Medicine*. New York: Oxford University Press, 2000:1126–35

24. Mcphee SJ, Schroeder SA. General approach to the patient: health maintenance and disease prevention & common symptoms. In Tierney LC, McPhee SJ, Papadakis MA, eds. *Current Medical Diagnosis and Treatment*. New York: McGraw-Hill, 2001:1–31

25. Connolly MJ. Smoking cessation in old age: closing the stable door? *Age Ageing* 2000; 29:193–5

26. West R, McNeill A, Raw M. Smoking cessation guidelines for health care professionals: an update. *Thorax* 2000;55:987–99

27. Gosney M. Smoking cessation. *Gerontology* 2001;47:236–40

35 Geriatric dermatology

Robert A. Norman, DO, MPH

'This traditional neglect of the skin is well-nigh unforgivable and has cruel consequences for the well being of the elderly. The great majority of persons over 70 have at least one, often two or three, skin conditions which would benefit from the attention of a knowledgeable doctor. These diseases do not kill but they are persistent pestilences which spoil the quality of life ... It is the skin more than any other organ which most clearly reveals the cumulative losses which time prints on the visage of the high and low alike.'[1]

INTRODUCTION

According to current US census statistics, the population is getting older. This means that a greater percentage of the population is in the over-65 age group. This trend is expected to continue well into the 21st century[2]. Additionally, the population of those aged over 80 is rapidly increasing. As 'baby-boomers' begin to enter into senior citizenship and the elderly get older, an increased emphasis on geriatric medicine is inevitable. Geriatric dermatology is a specialty that will receive particular attention[3].

As people age, their chances of developing skin-related disorders increase. Two types of skin aging exist: intrinsic aging, which includes those changes that are due to normal maturity and occurs in all individuals; and extrinsic aging, produced by extrinsic factors such as ultraviolet light exposure, smoking and environmental pollutants. Decreased mobility, drug-induced disorders and increased incidences of many chronic diseases are among the reasons the elderly are at heightened risk for skin diseases. Atherosclerosis, diabetes mellitus, human immunodeficiency virus (HIV) and congestive heart failure are examples of disease processes that can be detrimental to the skin. These diseases are known to impede vascular efficiency and decrease immune responses, thereby reducing the body's ability to heal.

Many histologic changes occur with aging and photoaging (Tables 1 and 2). Variation is seen in cell size, shape and staining results in epidermal dyscrasia of photoaged skin. Melanocytes decline and Langerhans' cells (intradermal macrophages) decrease in density. The dermis becomes relatively acellular, avascular and less dense and the loss of functional elastic tissue results in wrinkles. The nerves, microcirculation and sweat glands undergo a gradual decline, predisposing to decreased thermoregulation and sensitivity to burning. Nails undergo a slow decline in growth, with thinning of the nail plate, longitudinal ridging and splitting. The subcutaneous fat layer atrophies on the cheeks and distal extremities, but hypertrophies on the waist of men and thighs of women.

Many of the elderly will spend their time in nursing homes and assisted living facilities[4]. Caregivers and medical personnel can help decrease or prevent the development of many skin disorders in the elderly by addressing several factors. These include the

Table 1   Aging skin

Epidermal changes
Melanocytes
   approximately 15% decline per decade
   density doubles on sun-exposed skin
   increased lentigines
Langerhans cells
   decreased density
   decreased responsiveness

Dermal changes
   decreased collagen – 1% annual decline,
     altered fibers
   decreased density
   progressive loss of elastic tissue in the papillary dermis

Table 2   Skin changes in aging

Loss of elasticity and thinning of the skin
Clinical results – xerosis, laxity, wrinkling, uneven
   pigmentation, easy tearing, traumatic purpura,
   neoplasia

Photoaging
Clinical results – actinic keratoses, fine and coarse
   wrinkling, telangiectasia, blotchiness and pigmentary
   changes, elastotic skin with giant comedones

patient's nutritional state, medical history, current medications, allergies, physical limitations, mental state and personal hygiene.

Long-term care dermatology is truly its own art form. It is a growing specialty, drawing from the realm of both dermatology and geriatrics. In the US, those who work in long-term care serve a population of over 2.7 million patients. That is the total estimated population in nursing homes and assisted living facilities.

Preparation prior to dermatological nursing home visits is crucial. The following need to be considered: calling ahead and making sure the patient is available to be examined; filling out a skin condition checklist at the nursing station; explaining to the nursing home staff that consultations will be performed in a timely fashion but not regularly on an emergency basis; making sure that the consent form is signed by the patient, the patient's family or power of attorney, if a surgical procedure is necessary.

Nursing homes, unlike hospitals, are mostly 'low tech with high touch'. What the resident did for himself/herself in the past is now done with the assistance of others. As health-care providers, we enter the resident's home, a place that is often new and sometimes permanent. The entire group of employees and caretakers act as a surrogate family for the residents. A caring attitude and behavior make all the difference between one home and another, between a pleasant and rewarding experience and a degrading experience.

COMMON SKIN DISORDERS

Decubitus ulcers (pressure ulcers)

Decubitus ulcers are seen frequently in the elderly. The patients with high risk include the following: critical care patients, quadriplegics, terminal cancer patients, diabetics, end-stage renal, heart or liver disease patients, those with femoral fractures, the immunosuppressed, patients with incontinence, those with decreased mental status, patients who are immobile and the malnourished[4].

Decubitus ulcers usually occur over bony prominences. Pressure on tissue over extended periods of time causes ischemia and results in tissue damage. Decubitus ulcers are staged as follows: stage I – nonblanchable erythema of intact skin; stage II – necrosis with superficial to partial thickness involvement of the epidermis and/or dermis; stage III – deep necrosis with full-thickness skin loss that may extend down to, but not through, underlying fascia; stage IV – extensive necrosis into underlying fascia, possibly into muscle, bone and supporting structures[4].

Prevention should be the focus with pressure ulcers. Efforts should be made to ensure proper nourishment, increase mobility, devise repositioning schedules, reduce shearing forces, provide careful skin care, utilize pressure-reducing devices, reduce skin-to-skin contact and conduct daily skin examinations on the high-risk patient.

Table 3 Most common nursing home dermatology diagnoses (includes gender and age distribution). Total sample size 1556. Standard deviations in parentheses

Diagnosis	ICD 9 CM code	n	Male	Mean age (year)
Pruritus and other related diseases	698.0–698.9	1002	31.34	78.9 (14.1)
Diseases of the sebaceous glands (xerosis = 772)	706.0–706.8	813	29.53	80.6 (13.5)
Other dermatoses*	702.0–702.8	546	25.74	84.1 (9.8)
Basal or squamous cell carcinoma of the skin	173.0–173.9	353	29.28	84.5 (10.3)
Scabies	133.0	220	35.35	78.0 (14.7)
Contact dermatitis and other eczema	692.0–692.9	218	37.56	77.1 (14.3)
Erythematosquamous dermatitis	690	216	48.36	75.6 (16.5)
Disorders of the sweat glands	705.0–705.9	166	35.98	78.3 (14.0)
Non-thrombocytopenic purpura	287.2	145	24.65	84.8 (8.0)
Stasis dermatitis with varicosities	454.1	135	21.05	81.3 (11.3)
Candidiasis	112.0–112.9	80	21.79	80.5 (13.3)
Cellulitis, unspecified site	682.9	77	27.27	79.3 (14.1)
Dermatophytosis	110.0–110.9	71	27.12	78.4 (14.4)
Other hypertrophic and atrophic conditions of the skin[†]	701	47	24.12	83.9 (18.1)

*†Specified and unspecified hypertropic and atrophic conditions, keratoderma

Taler mentions the growing complexity of nursing home wound care[5]. The prevalence of pressure ulcers in long-term care facilities is estimated to be between 2.4 and 23%[6] and the incidence of new ulcers over a 6-month period is approximately 12%[7]. In the 1980s, Smith and colleagues showed an increasing prevalence of patients being discharged from the hospital with pressure ulcers, attributable to an aging population and the greater complexity and frailty of the patients currently treated in the acute care setting. Due to constraints on hospital utilization, up to 63% of patients transferred to nursing homes have shown pressure ulcers on admission to the facility[8].

Treatment is stage dependent. Treatments range from simple cleansing and application of protective ointments and devices to surgical debridement and packing. Newer products have shown excellent results, especially in diabetic foot ulcers. Vitamins A and K, and zinc are important in the comprehensive wound treatment protocol. Vitamin C, an antioxidant, speeds wound healing. Nutritional consultation should be considered with wound care patients to help monitor the protein and vitamin levels and maintain adequate nutrition.

Cultures with Gram stains should be taken prior to the institution of any antibiotic therapy for infected wounds. Wounds should be debrided only if the removal of the necrotic tissue speeds up the healing process. Curretting of the borders of the lesions often stimulates increased granulation and wound healing.

Xerosis

A recently completed study of nursing home patients I treat, demonstrated the two most common problems were overwhelmingly xerosis and pruritus (Table 3)[9]. Given these results, I will focus on the recognition and treatment of these entities. Of ultimate importance is the comprehensive treatment of these problems to prevent stasis dermatitis and ulcer formation.

Description

Xerosis is characterized by pruritic, dry, cracked and fissured skin with scaling. Xerosis occurs most often on the legs of elderly patients, but may be present on the hands and trunk. The appearance of xerotic skin appears like a pattern of cracked porcelain. These cracks or fissures occur from epidermal water loss. The skin splits and cracks deeply enough to disrupt dermal capillaries, and bleeding fissures may occur. Pruritis occurs, leading to secondary lesions. Scratching and rubbing activities produce excoriations, an inflammatory response, lichen simplex chronicus and even edematous patches. Subsequently, environmental allergens and pathogens can easily penetrate the skin, increasing the risk of allergic and irritant contact dermatitis as well as infection. Allergic and irritant contact dermatitis may be a cause for a persistent and possibly more extensive dermatitis despite therapy. Eczematous changes can occur with a delayed hypersensitivity response even in advanced age[10]. Secondary infection is an inherent risk with any break in the skin barrier. This cycle needs to be broken to disable the process and prevent complications.

Prevalence and predisposing factors

Xerosis preys upon the elderly. This is primarily due to the fact that aged individuals have decreased sebaceous and sweat gland activity. This reduced activity predisposes the aged skin to moisture depletion. There are a number of situations that deplete the skin's moisture. For example, xerosis tends to relapse in the winter when an environment of lower humidity predominates. Another contributor is the daily use of cleansers and/or bathing without replacing natural skin emollients[11].

Additionally, pre-existing disease states, therapies and medications make the aged individual more susceptible to xerosis. Some of these pre-existing situations include radiation, end-stage renal disease, nutritional deficiency (especially zinc and essential fatty acids), thyroid disease and neurologic disorders with decreased sweating, anti-androgen medications, diuretic therapy, HIV and malignancies[12–14].

Deficits in both skin hydration and lipid content play a key role in xerosis. Consequently, the skin's inability to retain moisture and provide an effective barrier directly impacts the development of xerosis in aged skin[15].

Once the stage is set for xerosis development, the scenarios of flaking, fissuring, inflammation, dermatitis and infection develop. The xerotic vicious cycle needs to be broken to disable the process and prevent complications. This is precisely the goal of xerosis treatment[16,17]. To achieve this goal, keratolytics, moisturizers and steroids are the primary components of xerosis treatment. The keratolytic effect of ammonium lactate 12% lotion is effective in reducing the severity of xerosis[18,19]. Individuals with sensitive skin may not tolerate some products formulated with α-hydroxy acids, due to unacceptable levels of stinging and irritation. In this case, a variant formulation for sensitive skin should be substituted[20]. Liberal use of moisturizers reduces scaling and enhances the corneodesmosome degradation process[21]. Additional treatment via application of topical steroids (class III–VI) is recommended in moderate to severe cases. Antipruritics should be added if disturbing pruritus is present.

Other additional management suggestions include the following:

(1) Reduced frequency of bathing with luke-warm (not hot) water;

(2) Minimal use of a non-irritant soap;

(3) Avoidance of harsh skin cleansers;

(4) Application of moisturizer of choice directly on skin that is still damp;

(5) Avoidance of friction from washcloths, rough clothing and abrasives;

(6) Use of air humidification in dry environments[22,23].

Aged skin is highly susceptible to the development of xerosis. The vicious cycle of the xerotic process preys on the elderly, making them an easy target for xerosis-related complications. The treatment goal focuses on breaking the xerotic cycle to prevent secondary complications.

Pruritus

Characteristic features of pruritus include scratching and inflammation. The condition is often associated with other underlying diseases. Itching is thought to be induced by the effect of histamine on the touch proprioceptors and is mediated exclusively by the peripheral nervous system. Itching evokes the desire to scratch. Scratching produces an immunology-based inflammatory response. Pruritus can be psychogenic in origin. However, there are a number of dermatologic and metabolic conditions that involve pruritus. Xerosis is the most common underlying dermatologic condition. Other dermatologic conditions include infestations, infection (fungal, bacterial or viral), lichen planus, nodular prurigo, dermatitis, eczema and miliaria. Underlying metabolic conditions that can produce pruritus include renal failure, HIV, diabetes mellitus, thyroid disease, parathyroid disease, hypervitaminosis A, iron-deficiency anemia, neuropathy, hepatic disease, malignancy and drugs.

Initial treatment focuses on relief of pruritus. The specific etiology is then determined. To maximize effectiveness, pruritis treatment strategy is then tailored to the specific underlying condition.

Description

Pruritus is a perceived itching sensation. The proprioceptors of touch are thought to be responsible for the itch sensation. Cutaneous histamine effects induce itch and are mediated exclusively by the peripheral nervous system[24]. Itching evokes the desire to scratch[25,26]. Scratching is an itch-associated response and produces an inflammatory response. This inflammation is an immunologic response[24,25].

Pruritic skin diseases are the most common dermatologic problem in the elderly[26,27].

Pathology

There is little understanding of the pathophysiology of pruritus. Pruritus is known to be a feature of inflammation. Inflammation is the result of activation of the body's immune system, normally in response to an antigen. Involved skin cells have IgE molecules on their surface. The main physiological role of IgE is to trigger acute inflammation[28]. Release of compounds such as histamine and heparin (vasoactive amines) occurs[29]. Histamine causes small blood vessels to dilate and heparin acts as an anticoagulant. Skin blood vessel walls have lymphocyte receptors on their surface, aiding the migration of lymphocytes from the blood into the tissues[30] and setting the inflammatory stage. With repetitive rubbing, scratching and touching (induced by a foreign body or self-induced), inflammatory and pigmentary cutaneous manifestations occur[31]. Some of these manifestations include excoriations, prurigo nodularis and lichen simplex chronicus[31-33].

Clinical workup and initial treatment

Immediate relief of pruritus is the focus of initial treatment efforts. The goal of these efforts is to dull the inflammatory response[34]. Treatment regimens for pruritus and products recommended are highly variable[27]. Furthermore, pruritus relief evaluation is subjective, since valid itch measurement techniques are needed for the evaluation of antipruritic therapies[25]. Mild pruritus may respond to non-pharmacologic measures such as avoiding hot water and irritants, maintaining proper humidity, using cool water compresses, trimming the nails and behavior therapy. Topical symptomatic treatments include moisturizers, emollients, tar compounds, topical corticosteroids, topical anesthetics such as benzocaine or dibucaine and pramoxine HCl (alone or combined with menthol, petrolatum or benzyl alcohol)[35].

Once temporary pruritic relief is obtained, efforts should focus on finding the underlying cause. This process begins with a thorough history, physical examination and laboratory result evaluation. The goal of pruritus therapy is to optimize treatment efficacy by tailoring the treatment to the underlying etiology. For example, doxepin cream (Prudoxin®) has been shown to be very effective in pruritus associated with eczematous dermatitis[34]. It can be used alone for acute pruritus or with corticosteroids in chronic conditions[35]. Avoidance of fragrance soap, irritating chemicals and hot water help reduce pruritus, especially in elderly patients who have the xerotic changes of aging.

Eczematous dermatitis

Asteatotic eczema, nummular eczema, seborrheic dermatitis, gravitational eczema, auto-eczematization eczema and psychogenic dermatitides fall under the category of eczematous dermatitis. Several of these disorders are commonly seen in the elderly.

Nummular eczema is characterized by pruritic, coin-shaped lesions, which may develop into scales. These lesions are most commonly found on the lower legs, upper extremities, dorsum of the hands and the trunk. A treatment regimen may include the use of medium- or high-potency topical steroids and emollients such as petroleum jelly[36]. Secondary infections should be treated with antibiotics that cover staphylococci; these include dicloxacillin and cephalexin.

Stasis dermatitis occurs with venous insufficiency, pedal edema and varicose veins. The brownish color results from hemosiderin deposition. The disease can lead to increased susceptibility to ulceration or cellulitis. An acute exacerbation of stasis dermatitis can result in an 'id' reaction or autosensitization dermatitis, producing secondary, acute,

papulovesicular, often symmetrical distribution on the extremities.

Seborrheic dermatitis presents as xerotic, erythematous, scaly or flaky skin in the scalp and on the face, trunk and/or anogenital region. The central nervous system may play a role in the severity of this disorder, due to apparent increased incidence of this form of dermatitis with Parkinson's disease, quadriplegia and emotional distress[37]. *Pityrosporum ovale* has also been implicated in this disorder. Treatment should include ketoconazole or ciclopirox applied daily. Severe cases may require oral ketoconazole or fluconazole and antistaphylococcal antibiotics if secondary infection is suspected[36].

Psychogenic dermatitides include disorders such as lichen simplex chronicus, prurigo nodularis, neurotic excoriations, and delusions of parasitosis. The lesions of lichen simplex chronicus are characterized as lichenified, red scaling plaques that are sharply demarcated[37]. This disorder usually occurs in atopic patients who obsess over pruritic lesions. These patients will habitually rub, scratch, and otherwise irritate a pruritic area until lichenification occurs. Treatment may include behavior modification along with water soaks and topical steroids for body lesions. Scalp treatment may require kenalog injections for scalp nodules and fluocinonide or clobetasol solution for resistant lesions[36].

Prurigo nodularis, like lichen simplex chronicus, may be stress related, and the lesions are secondary to habitual scratching and picking. The nodules are characteristically erythematous or hyperpigmented. They are usually scattered and discrete keratotic nodules on the extremities[37]. Triamcinolone acetonide or other topical corticosteroids may be applied to the affected areas. Stronger steroids such as betamethasone may be applied. Corticosteroid tape may be considered, also. Similar treatments may be considered for neurotic excoriations, which are excoriated papules at different stages of healing in a forest of post-inflammatory scars. Neurotic excoriations should be considered when a disease does not fit into any regular pattern; in addition, the patient may often admit to using his or her skin as an outlet for stress. The skin is often a reservoir of habitual frustrations and allows the observant and caring practitioner a chance to explore options for improvement of quality of life. Truensgaard has recommended psychotherapeutic strategies[38]. For neurotic excoriations, strategies include establishing constructive patient–doctor relationships, training patients in diversion strategies to avoid scratching, discovering daily stress that can be reduced and heightening the patient's awareness of trigger factors[38].

Patients complaining of the sensation of parasites crawling on them without evidence of the presence of parasites may have delusions of parasitosis. This condition is more attributable to a psychosis than to a dermatological problem. Drug addictions, toxins, nutritional deficiencies and arteriosclerosis may contribute to this disorder[37]. For those patients where depression is prominent, doxepin or fluoxetine may be considered; with anxiety prominence, hydroxyzine or alprazalom may be used; and pimozide or haloperidol may be considered when delusion is prominent[39]. Zyprexa and other alternative therapeutic treatments with antipsychotics can be quite helpful.

INFECTIONS OF THE SKIN

Bacterial

Staphylococcus and Streptococcus species are common causes of infections in the skin of the elderly. Often part of the normal flora, these species become problematic when skin architecture is altered through trauma, disease, malnourishment, or other processes. Insect bites and various types of dermatitis break down the skin's natural barriers and open an avenue for infection.

Impetigo caused by Streptococcus and/or Staphylococcus species presents as bullous or non-bullous forms. The majority are caused by Staphylococcus aureus, group A β-hemolytic streptococci, or a combination of both. Although impetigo can be self-limiting, it should be treated, due to possible systemic complications such as post-streptococcal glomerulonephritis. Both begin as vesicles with a very thin, fragile roof consisting only of stratum corneum.

In bullous impetigo (Staphylococcus aureus phage group II), epidermolytic toxin is produced at the site of infection, eliciting intra-epidermal cleavage below or within the stratum granulosum. Bullous impetigo is characterized by thin-walled bullae filled with clear to cloudy fluid. These bullae tend to burst, leaving an erythematous rim around lesions with honey-colored, crusty exudates.

Non-bullous impetigo develops as vesicles or pustules that rupture. An inflamed base is left which begins to form a yellowish crust[37]. The disease accounts for 10% of all impetigo and may resemble poison ivy dermatitis. The patient may develop thin, varnish-like 'honey crust' in the center of the bulla. Staphylococcus aureus nasal colonization precedes impetigo.

Non-bullous impetigo (group A β-hemolytic streptococci) starts as small vesicles or pustules that rupture to expose a red, moist base with honey crust and satellite lesions. The disease most commonly affects skin around the nose, mouth and limbs, avoiding palms and soles. Group A β-hemolytic streptococcus is carried on intact skin; trauma (abrasion, etc.) leads to infection. Anti-DNAase B rises to high levels, which is a better indicator of infection than ASO titer. Treatment consists of a 5–10-day course of oral antibiotics such as cloxacillin, dicloxacillin or cephalexin. A 5-day course of azithromycin, given as 500 mg on day 1, then 250 mg on days 2–5 is also well tolerated. Mupirocin topical ointment should be applied three times a day until lesions have cleared (ensure that the nares are included).

Viral

Varicella zoster often re-manifests itself in the elderly as herpes zoster, commonly known as shingles. This herpes virus can remain dormant for years in cutaneous neurons, and often appears in the elderly in times of stress or immunosuppression. It usually involves a single dermatome, but may include other dermatomes. Often, it presents initially as hyperesthesia with pre-eruptive pain, itching or burning. Lymphadenopathy may be present. There may be constitutional symptoms such as headache, malaise or fever. Vesicles begin to appear in the characteristic dermatomal distribution pattern, rarely crossing the midline. The vesicles arise in clusters on an inflamed base. Initially, the vesicles consist of a clear fluid which becomes purulent over a short period of time. After the appearance of the vesicles for approximately 3–5 days, the vesicles begin to crust over and dry out over the course of 2–3 weeks. Pain varies from mild irritation to severe post-herpetic neuralgia. This pain can exist long after the physical signs of the vesicular rash have disappeared. It can become almost debilitating in some cases, and has been known to persist even for years[36].

Management of herpes zoster begins with prevention of an initial varicella zoster infection by immunizing against varicella zoster with the VZV vaccine. Once herpes zoster develops, antiviral therapy should begin as quickly as possible. The effectiveness of acyclovir, valcyclovir and other similar antivirals is best when therapy is begun within the first 72 h of vesicular formation. Early therapy has been shown to reduce the duration of acute pain, accelerate healing and even reduce the frequency of post-herpetic neuralgia[40].

Associated symptoms can be relieved with the use of non-steroidal anti-inflammatory drugs (NSAIDs), bed rest, opioid analgesics, tricyclic antidepressants, capsaicin cream and even nerve blocks for severe pain. Trigeminal nerve involvement, especially the ophthalmic branch, may require referral to an ophthalmologist to reduce the chances of visual complications.

Molluscum contagiosum, generally considered a childhood disease, may also be seen in the elderly. This poxvirus causes the formation of dome-shaped, umbilicated papules. It is transmitted by skin-to-skin contact. Molluscum has been mistaken for warts or even skin cancer[37].

Patients can be treated with 5% imiquimod cream for up to 3 months. Alternative and/or additional therapies may include cryotherapy, electrodesiccation, curettage and laser surgery[40].

Fungal

Common fungal infections in the elderly are candidiasis, tinea pedis, tinea cruris and onychomycosis. Candida can be found in intertriginous areas where there is warm moisture and skin-on-skin contact. Areas often affected include inguinal, anogenital, flexural, submammary and perioral. It presents as a diffuse 'beefy-red' eruption with weeping pustules. Microscopic evaluation will show the presence of pseudohyphae and spores. Diabetes and antibiotic therapy are often implicated in the development of candidiasis[37].

Treatment includes the use of cool compresses using Burow's solution or cool water applied to affected areas several times a day to promote dryness. Miconazole, econazole or other antifungal creams should be applied twice daily until the rash resolves. After the rash has disappeared, an absorbent powder may be used as a dry lubricant[36].

Tinea pedis (athlete's foot) is a fungal infection of the foot often presenting as an erythematous dermatitis. Scaling and maceration are common, and the infection may appear in a 'moccasin' distribution pattern. Ulcerations and fissuring can occur, especially in the interdigital areas. Secondary bacterial infections may complicate the fungal infection.

Preventive measures may include the use of shower shoes and the application of benzoyl peroxide after bathing. Topical treatment may involve the use of an imidazole (i.e. clotrimazole, ketoconazole, econazole, etc.), an allylamine such as terbinafine, a napthiomate (tolnaftate), or substituted pyridone such as ciclopirox olamine. Systemic treatment for extensive and persistent infections may require the use of oral terbinafine, itraconazole or fluconazole[40].

Tinea cruris (jock itch) is an erythematous eruption in the groin area with associated pruritis and scaling dermatitis. Males are much more apt to acquire this fungal infection.

As with other fungal infections, reducing moisture in the affected area is key to helping eliminate the disease. Econazole or another antifungal cream applied for up to 2 weeks is usually effective. More severe, resistant infections may require the use of oral antifungals such as griseofulvin, itraconazole, terbinafine or fluconazole. A mixture of betamethasone dipropionate and clotrimazole may be applied to reduce inflammation[36].

Onychomycosis is often caused by a dermatophyte (tinea unguium), and less commonly caused by *Candida* species and molds. Nearly half of patients older than 70 years are affected by this disease. Onychomycosis can cause pain, predispose patients to secondary bacterial infections, and cause ulcerations in the nail bed. In distal and lateral subungual onychomycosis, the most common form of onychomycosis, this disease can present initially as a white patch on a nail. Over time the patch darkens, and the nail becomes opaque, thickens, and then begins to crack.

Management may include debridement, topical treatment with amorolfine or penlac, systemic treatment with agents such as terbinafine or itraconazole, and secondary prophylaxis using antifungal creams, benzoyl peroxide washings and good hygiene practices[40].

NUTRIENT DEFICIENCY DISORDERS

Chronic diseases and poor diet may contribute to vitamin deficiencies in the elderly. These deficiencies may have dermatologic manifestations. Deficiency in vitamin C (ascorbic acid) results in scurvy. Small hemorrhages may occur in the gingiva and skin as well as in other organ systems. Hyperkeratotic papules may be found around hair follicles causing erythema, purpura and centrally curved hairs. Niacin deficiency, and/or deficiency in other B vitamins, may result in pellagra. The skin can become extremely photosensitive. Formation of vesicles, bullae, edema and erythema may occur. This can roughen the skin's texture[37].

Optimizing dietary intake and providing palliative treatment for dermal manifestations are appropriate considerations in the management of nutritional deficiencies. Also, consideration should be given to possible underlying diseases which may contribute to or even cause the malnourished state.

VASCULAR DISORDERS

Chronic venous insufficiency is due to venous hypertension secondary to valvular incompetence. Etiologic factors include hereditary conditions, prolonged standing and venous thrombosis. The disease may manifest as edema, varicosities, brown discoloration, superficial neovascularization, dermatitis and venous ulcers (most common on the medial lower leg). Therapy includes elevating the legs, exercise, supportive stockings, surgery, mild to moderate corticosteroids, and oral antibiotics if secondary infection is present.

PARASITIC DISEASES

Pediculosis and scabies are commonly present in elderly populations. Lice can be found on the head (pediculosis capitis), the body (pediculosis corporis) and the pubic region (pediculosis or phthirus pubis). Pruritic papular eruptions occur in the infested areas. Careful examination of the hair in the affected regions will reveal nits (eggs) cemented to the hair shafts and lice. The nape of the neck is a common location for head lice to be found. Transmission is usually by direct contact with infested persons or fomites. Permethrin, an agent that affects adult lice, but not nits, is usually the first line of treatment. Nits should be combed out using a special comb. Treatment should be repeated 1 week later. Resistant strains are emerging, so treatment with lindane or malathion lotion may be considered. Shaving the affected area is effective, also.

With scabies, papules and vesicles are the most common lesions, but the burrow is the diagnostic feature. Each burrow is either a straight line or S-shaped and has a tiny vesicle overlying the site of the female mite. The diagnosis is established by mite, ova or feces identification in skin scrapings removed from vesicles, papules or burrows. Identification of burrows is often difficult, due to excoriations or secondary infections. Common sites of infestation are the areola in females and genital area in males.

Norwegian or keratotic scabies occurs when thousands of mites infest the patient's skin, rather than the usual 3–50 female mites in garden-variety scabies. Clinical manifestations differ greatly from the common scabies. When invading the scalp, it is often mistaken for seborrheic dermatitis.

Scabies can be treated with oral ivermectin, generally prescribed in two 12 mg doses taken a week apart. Fomites should be thoroughly cleaned to prevent reinfestation[36].

BENIGN AND PREMALIGNANT TUMORS

As with other organ systems, there exist many types of tumor, benign and malignant, in the skin of the elderly. Notable benign tumors are cherry angiomas, leukoplakia, seborrheic keratosis, actinic keratosis and keratoacanthoma. Common malignant neoplasms are basal cell carcinoma, squamous cell carcinoma and melanoma.

Cherry angiomas, also known as Campbell de Morgan spots or senile angiomas, are quite common. Often appearing after the age of 30 and increasing in number over time, these bright red or purple lesions can be found mainly on the trunk of many elderly individuals. Characteristically, the papular lesions are approximately 1–3 mm in diameter and consist of endothelium-lined dilated capillaries. Treatment with electrocoagulation or laser coagulation is usually for cosmetic reasons, only[40].

Leukoplakia, a premalignant neoplasm associated with alcohol and/or tobacco use, appears on mucosal surfaces as white patches that cannot be rubbed off. This lesion can progress to invasive carcinoma, particularly in the pharynx[41]. Localized areas may be treated by electro- or cryosurgery, or with topical 5-fluorouracil. Excision is best for more extensive involvement. Lymph nodes should be assessed for their involvement, also[36].

Seborrheic keratoses are extremely common lesions which are seen mainly on the trunk, face, and proximal extremities. These lesions are dark brown or black papules, which appear to be 'stuck' onto the skin. Cryosurgery or electrocautery are treatment options. A shave biopsy should be performed on any suspicious lesion to rule out melanoma[40].

Actinic keratosis is a keratotic 3–6-mm red or brown papule. It is most often found on sun-exposed areas of fair-skinned individuals. These lesions usually persist if untreated, and may present with symptoms of burning or stinging. One in five patients with multiple actinic keratoses develops squamous cell carcinoma. Reduction of sun exposure and use of sun protection (sunscreen, clothing) may reduce further development of new lesions of this type. Treatment for superficial lesions may include cryosurgery, electrodesiccation with curettage, and/or topical 5-fluorouracil.

Actinic chelitis may require carbon dioxide laser vermilionectomy[36].

Keratoacanthoma presents as an erythematous dome-shaped 1–10-cm nodule with a keratin plug in the center. This lesion, commonly found on the face and dorsum of the hands, usually spontaneously regresses within a year. An excisional biopsy should be performed to rule out squamous cell carcinoma[40].

MALIGNANT TUMORS

Basal cell carcinoma, perhaps the most common malignancy in humans, may present as one of the following: nodular-ulcerative, sclerosing (morpheaform), or superficial. Nodular-ulcerative basal cell carcinoma, the type seen most frequently, often appears as a red, translucent nodule with telangiectasia on the face. The yellow-to-white lesion of sclerosing basal cell cancer forms a plaque, while superficial basal cell cancer forms an erythematous, inflamed, psoriatic appearing lesion[5]. Risk factors for developing basal cell carcinoma include ionizing radiation therapy and a history of sun exposure. Treatment is based on location and aggressiveness of the tumor. Electrosurgery or excision is used for well-defined lesions. Problematic tumors may require radiation therapy and/or Mohs' micrographic surgery, a specialized procedure involving excision guided by sequential frozen-section mapping[36].

Squamous cell carcinoma may be caused by ultraviolet (UV) radiation or human papillomavirus (HPV). UV radiation exposure has cumulative effects that are commonly manifested in the elderly. Squamous cell carcinoma from HPV, a sexually transmitted virus, is not necessarily more common in the elderly. Additionally, these tumors have been known to arise in burn scars and other previously traumatized tissues. Squamous cell carcinoma can appear as an erythematous, sharply demarcated, scaling, erosive plaque. Keratinized lesions are usually well-differentiated and firm. The non-keratinized lesions are softer and granulomatous with poorer differentiation. Cryotherapy and/or 5-fluorouracil may be used for treatment of carcinoma *in situ*. Excision of the lesion is recommended for invasive carcinoma[40].

Malignant melanoma is becoming more common in all populations, but it has increased in incidence with increasing age. The four main types of melanoma are superficial spreading melanoma, nodular melanoma, lentigo maligna (*in situ* and invasive) and acral lentiginous melanoma.

Superficial spreading melanoma, the most common type (70–80%), tends to be > 6 mm in diameter and spreads laterally. Over time, nodules begin to appear within the lesion. Nodular melanoma is a brown or black papule that grows rapidly. This lesion usually extends vertically into the skin rather than laterally (horizontally).

Lentigo maligna, an *in situ* carcinoma and lentigo maligna melanoma, the invasive form, are often seen in elderly individuals. Caucasians with years of heavy sun exposure are particularly susceptible to this form of skin cancer. It appears as a brownish macule with some irregularities of border and symmetry. Nodule formation may indicate increased invasion.

Acral lentiginous melanoma is found primarily on the hands and feet. It can be found in the nails, and is common in darker pigmented people. This lesion is a brown macule that expands slowly over years.

In general, the depth of the melanoma is the crucial prognostic factor. Patients treated for lesions less than 0.76 cm in depth have 5-year survival rates of > 95%, however, patients treated for lesions of > 4 cm in depth have 5-year survival rates of < 50%. Any lesion suspected to be a melanoma should be biopsied. Shave biopsies are not recommended, because they may not show the full depth of the lesion. Consider a punch biopsy in a cosmetically important area if the lesion is large. The recommended biopsy is complete excision of the lesion into the subcutaneous fat.

Lymph node involvement should be assessed. Patients with histories of melanoma should be followed closely, and first-degree relatives should be screened[36].

PURPURA

Purpura can be defined as any of a group of conditions characterized by ecchymoses or other small hemorrhages in the skin, mucous membranes or serosal surfaces. Purpura may be caused by decreased platelet counts (thrombocytopenia), platelet abnormalities, vascular defects, trauma or drug reactions[42].

The elderly are especially susceptible to hemorrhage into the skin. As people age, there is a gradual reduction in the number of blood vessels and elastic fibers. There are also losses in dermal collagen and fat, causing a thinning of the skin and reduced protection from external trauma[42].

Many of the elderly are on medications which can cause thrombocytopenia (platelet counts below $100\,000/mm^3$) leading to purpura. Post-traumatic bleeding is common when platelet counts are less than $50\,000/mm^3$. Spontaneous bleeding can occur when platelet counts fall below $20\,000/mm^3$. Drugs commonly associated with thrombocytopenia include penicillins, quinine, quinidine, thiazide diuretics, methyldopa and heparin[43].

Thrombocytopenic purpura presents as petechiae and/or ecchymoses in association with decreased platelet counts. The petechiae are small, non-palpable, non-blanchable, reddish macules. The ecchymoses are larger (> 0.5 cm) bluish to black lesions. These lesions tend to lighten in color over time, due to enzymatic degradation of the pooled blood.

Treatment should focus on the underlying cause. Administration of oral glucocorticoids and immunoglobulins may be necessary. If platelet counts are extremely low (< $10\,000/mm^3$), platelet transfusion may be needed[40].

Skin tears most often result from a purpura torn open by inadvertent trauma. This is one of the most difficult problems to treat, especially with patients on steroids. Important measures include skin protectors and designing the living environment to prevent injuries.

BULLOUS PEMPHIGOID

The disease usually appears as tense bullae on erythematous or normal skin of the extremities and the lower abdomen. It occurs primarily in women over 50 years of age. The patient may have pruritus for weeks or months before the onset of blistering. Bullous pemphigoid may be associated with furosemide, penicillins and antipsychotic drugs.

Treatment includes potent topical steroids and oral tetracycline. Alternatively, dapsone, nicotinamide, azathioprine, cyclosporine or chlorambucil may be used. For severe cases, systemic corticosteroids are often required. With severe progressive disease, intravenous pulse corticosteroids, plasmapharesis, intravenous immunoglobulins or intravenous pulse cyclophosphamide should be considered[44].

CONCLUSION

As evident by the many disease processes mentioned above, geriatric dermatology encompasses a vast array. Major players are xerosis and pruritus. The perceived itch of pruritis induces scratching and is often associated with several underlying dermatologic and systemic diseases. However, pruritus can be psychogenic in origin. Xerosis is the most common underlying dermatologic condition. Several infectious – metabolic, hepatic, hematologic – and other systemic conditions are associated with pruritus. Immediate relief of pruritus is the initial treatment goal. After initial pruritic relief, a thorough history, physical examination and laboratory testing work-up is necessary to find the underlying treatable cause. An effective pruritic treatment strategy is tailored to the underlying etiology. For specific underlying etiology categories, several pharmacologic treatment choices are suggested.

Many other geriatric dermatologic problems are not mentioned in this paper. Alopecia, photosensitivity disorders, paraneoplastic syndromes and erythroderma are among the other diseases that deserve attention. Many of the diseases are localized to the skin, but illnesses originating in other organ systems are often made manifest on the skin. As stated before, chronic diseases such as diabetes mellitus and HIV compound the diagnoses and treatment of dermatologic problems. Since the human population is living longer, chronic diseases will become more prevalent, as will the diseases of the skin.

References

1. Kligman AM. Foreword. In Gilchrest B. *Skin and Aging Processes*. Boca Raton, FL: CRC Press,1984

2. US Bureau of the Census. Population projections of the United States by age, sex, race, and Hispanic origin: 1995–2050. *Current Population Reports*. Washington, DC: US Government Printing Office, 1996:25–1130

3. Norman R. The aging of the world's population. In Norman R, ed. *Geriatric Dermatology*. New York: Parthenon Publishing, 2001:1–4

4. Norman R. Dermatological problems and treatment in long-term/nursing-home care. In Norman R, ed. *Geriatric Dermatology*. New York: Parthenon Publishing, 2001: 5–16

5. Taler G. Management of pressure ulcers in long-term care. Advances in wound care. *Prev Heal* 1997;10:30

6. Taler G. Pressure ulcers. In *Clinical Practice Guidelines*. Columbia, MD: American Medical Directors Association, 1996

7. Taler G, Richardson JP, Fredman L, Lazur A. The wound unit: a specialized unit for pressure sore management in a long term care facility. *Md Med J* 1994;43:165–9

8. Smith DM, Winsemius DK, Besdine RW. Pressure sores in the elderly: can this outcome be improved? *J Gen Intern Med* 1991;6: 81–93

9. Norman R. Xerosis and pruritus. *Ann Longterm Care* 2001;9:35–40

10. Aoyama H, Tanaka M, Hara M, *et al*. Nummular eczema: an addition of senile xerosis and unique cutaneous reactivities to environmental aeroallergens. *Dermatology* 1999;2:135–9

11. Harding R, Mayo C, Rawlings A. Stratum corneum lipids: the effect of ageing and the seasons. *Arch Dermatol Res* 1996;288: 765–70

12. Weismann K, Wadskov S, Mikkelsen HI, *et al*. Acquired zinc deficiency dermatosis in man. *Arch Dermatol* 1978;114:1509–11

13. Rowe A, Mallon E, Rosenberger P, *et al*. Depletion of cutaneous peptidergic innervation in HIV-associated xerosis. *J Invest Dermatol* 1999;112:284–9

14. Simon M, Bernard D, Minondo AM, *et al*. Persistence of both peripheral and non-peripheral corneodesmosomes in the upper stratum corneum of winter xerosis skin versus only peripheral in normal skin. *J Invest Dermatol* 2001;116:23–30

15. Engelke M, Jensen J, Ekanayake-Mudiyanselage S, Proksch E. Effects of xerosis and ageing on epidermal proliferation and differentiation. *Br J Dermatol* 1997; 137:219–25

16. Paepe K, Derde M, Roseeuw D, Rogiers V. Incorporation of ceramide 3B in dermato-cosmetic emulsions: effect on the transepidermal water loss of sodium lauryl sulphate-damaged skin. *J Eur Acad Dermatol Venereol* 2000;14:272–9

17. Thaipisuttikul Y. Pruritic skin diseases in the elderly. *J Dermatol* 1998;25:153–7

18. Jennings M, Alfieri D, Ward K, Lesczczynski C. Comparison of salicylic acid and urea versus ammonium lactate for

the treatment of foot xerosis. A randomized, double blind, clinical study. *J Am Podiatry Med Assoc* 1998;88:332–6

19. Kempers S, Katz H, Wildnauer R, Green B. An evaluation of the effect of an alpha hydroxy acid-blend skin cream in the cosmetic improvement of symptoms of moderate to severe xerosis, epidermolytic hyperkeratosis, and ichthyosis. *Cutis* 1998; 61:347–50

20. Wolf B, Paster A, Levy S. An alpha hydroxy acid derivative suitable for sensitive skin. *Dermatol Surg* 1996;22:469–73

21. Gammal C, Pagnoni A, Kligman A, Gammal S. A model to assess the efficacy of moisturizers – the quantification of soap-induced xerosis by image analysis of adhesive-coated discs (D-Squames). *Clin Exp Dermatol* 1996;21:338–43

22. Rawlings A, Harding C, Watkinson A, *et al.* The effect of glycerol and humidity on desmosome degradation in stratum corneum. *Arch Dermatol Res* 1995;287:457–64

23. Lazar A, Lazar P. Dry skin, water, and lubrication. *Dermatol Clin* 1999;9:45–51

24. Johansson O, Virtanen M, Hilliges M. Histaminergic nerves demonstrated in the skin. A new direct mode of neurogenic inflammation. *Exp Dermatol* 1995;4:93–6

25. Wahlgren C. Measurement of itch. *Semin Dermatol* 1995;14:277–84

26. Woodward D, Nieves A, Spada C, *et al.* Characterization of a behavioral model for peripherally evoked itch suggests platelet-activating factor as a potent pruritogen. *J Pharmacol Exp Ther* 1995;272:758–65

27. Fleischer A Jr. Pruritus in the elderly: management by senior dermatologists. *J Am Acad Dermatol* 1993;28:603–9

28. Seidenari S, Giusti G. Objective assessment of the skin of children affected by atopic dermatitis. *Acta Dermato-venereol* 1995;75:429–33

29. Rukwied R, Lischetzki G, McGlone F, *et al.* Mast cell mediators other than histamine induce pruritus in atopic dermatitis patients: a dermal microdialysis study. *Br J Dermatol* 2000;142:1114–20

30. Graham J. (1997) A guide to atopic eczema. Honours Project. Edinburgh: Napier University Department of Biological Sciences, 1997. Available: http://www.biol.napier.ac.uk/BWS/COURSES/projects/eczema/itching.htm

31. Leung C. Pruritis. In *Handbook of Dermatology & Venereology*, 2nd edn. 1997. Available: http://www.hkmj.org.hk/skin/

32. Kosko D. Dermatologic manifestations of human immunodeficiency virus disease. *Lippincotts Prim Care Pract* 1997;1:50–61

33. Robertson K, Mueller B. Uremic pruritus. *J Health Syst Pharm* 1996;53:2159–70

34. Drake L, Millikan L. The antipruritic effect of 5% Doxepin cream in patients with eczematous dermatitis: Doxepin study group. *Arch Dermatol* 1995;131:1403–8

35. Herting R. Dermatology: pruritis. In *University of Iowa Family Practice Handbook*, 3rd edn. 1997:1–13. Available: http://www.vh.org/Providers/ClinRef/FPHandbook/Chapter13/01–13.html

36. Habif T, Campbell J Jr, Quitadamo M, Zug K. *Skin Disease: Diagnosis and Treatment.* St Louis: Mosby, 2001:18–415

37. Moschella S. Skin diseases of the elderly. In Norman R, ed. *Geriatric Dermatology.* New York: Parthenon Publishing, 2001: 17–34

38. Truensgaard K. Psychotherapeutic strategy and neurotic excoriations. *Int J Dermatol* 1991;30:198–203

39. Fried RG. Evaluation and treatment of 'psychogenic' pruritus and self excoriation. *J Am Acad Dermatol* 1994;30:993–9

40. Fitzpatrick T, Johnson R, Wolff K, Suurmond D. *Color Atlas and Synopsis of Clinical Dermatology*, 4th edn. USA: McGraw-Hill, 2001:196–966

41. Braunwald E, Fauci A, Kasper D, *et al. Harrison's Principles of Internal Medicine*, 15th edn. USA: McGraw-Hill, 2001:560

42. Habif T. *Clinical Dermatology – a Color Guide to Diagnosis and Therapy*, 3rd edn. St Louis: Mosby, 1996:598.

43. Cotran R, Kumar V, Collins T. *Robbins – Pathological Basis of Disease*, 6th edn. Philadelphia: WB Saunders, 1999:634–6

44. Korman NJ. Bullous pemphigoid. The latest in diagnosis, prognosis and therapy. *Arch Dermatol* 1998;134:1137–41

36 Disorders of the ear

M. Kanagala, MD, and Alan S. Berkower, MD, PhD

INTRODUCTION

Disorders of the ear are common with aging. Hearing loss is the third most common chronic disability in older adults[1-3]. The disorder typically begins in the fourth decade and clinically manifests in older age[4]. Because of aging trends, the disorder assumes increasing significance as a public health problem. Physicians tend to view the problem as benign and patients tend to believe that hearing loss is an inevitable consequence of aging[4]. Hearing loss is not a universal phenomenon; nevertheless, most older persons do have some degree of hearing loss. The attitude of the health-care provider towards hearing disability is quite different from that towards visual impairment, in that the former is given less importance[5]. Health-care providers and society need to recognize the impact of the problem and make appropriate referrals for evaluation.

IMPACT OF THE PROBLEM

Overall, nearly 10% of the adult population have some degree of hearing loss[5]. In the 65–75-year age group the prevalence is about 25%, increasing as age advances to involve over half the adults; the prevalence may be as high as 70–80% in the nursing home population[1,2,4-6]. The primary consequence of hearing impairment is on communication. Additionally, social isolation, diminished educational attainment and accidents are a consequence[7]. Psychosocial dysfunction is poorly appreciated, even though the independence, social relationships and quality of life of those affected are threatened, with disability leading to irritability, frustration and depression. Further, affected patients fail to complain about the problem for fear of the social stigma[1,3]. Despite the high prevalence, and its impact, only 5–18% of the hearing impaired are adequately evaluated[4].

Definitions relevant to the understanding of disorders of the ear are listed in Table 1[5,6,8-12].

ANATOMY

The human ear consists of three components – the external, middle and inner ear – in addition to the auditory pathways.

External ear

This comprises the auricle, external auditory meatus and the outer aspect of the tympanic membrane. The outer part of the auditory canal is cartilaginous; the lining skin is thick and contains hair follicles, sebaceous and ceruminous glands. Dermal and subcutaneous layers are well developed[12]. The inner part of the external auditory canal is bony in structure, and lined by thin skin which firmly attaches to underlying bone, containing scanty hair follicles and ceruminous glands. Thin hair, known as vellous hair, covers the entire canal, except at the cartilaginous lateral part, where the hair is coarse and long (referred to as tragi).

Table 1 Definitions of terms relevant to hearing disorders. From references 5, 6 and 8–12

Frequency
The rate at which the compression and rarefaction of air particles occur is the frequency of sound. A single compression and rarefaction is a cycle. Frequency is the number of such cycles per second. The unit of measurement is the hertz (Hz)

Intensity
The pressure exerted by the sound and expressed as *watts* or *dynes/cm²*. The smallest increase in intensity a normal human ear appreciates is termed a *decibel* (dB)

Audiogram
Graphic representation of hearing loss in threshold sensitivity at each test frequency

Speech reception threshold
Intensity at which the person identifies 50% of equally balanced two-syllable words presented to each ear

Speech discrimination score
Percentage of correct responses to 25 phonetically balanced words presented to each ear at the level of 30–40 decibels

Auditory brainstem response
Audiometric measure of electric response by the auditory nerve to the sound stimulus

Electrocochleography
Measure of cochlear microphonic potentials, summating potentials and whole nerve action potentials from the auditory nerves

Tympanometry
Graphic measure of middle ear compliance

Tinnitus
Abnormal noise perception in the absence of an external acoustic stimulus

Vertigo
Dizziness associated with an illusion of motion

Middle ear

This consists of the tympanic membrane and the middle ear cavity containing three bony ossicles (malleus, incus and stapes) and two muscles (stapedius and tensor tympani). The middle ear pressure is maintained equal to that of the external ear by the Eustachian tube connecting to the nasopharynx; this mechanism preserves the maximum compliance of the tympanic membrane. Integrity of the ossicular chain and dexterity of the joints is essential for normal transmission of sound waves[1].

Inner ear

This is contained in a dense bony capsule consisting of cochlea, vestibule and three semicircular canals and is responsible for hearing and maintaining balance. The end organ for hearing is the hair cell, located in the cochlea. High frequencies are perceived in the basal turn of the cochlea, while low frequencies are perceived at the cochlear tip. Cells of the auditory pathways are highly specialized in function and cannot replicate. Sound waves are transmitted from the ossicular chain through the oval window and processed through the endolymph of the inner ear before eliciting an action potential at the level of the hair cell.

AGE-RELATED CHANGES

Atrophy of the sebaceous glands causes a decrease in epithelial oiliness and skin hydration. Additionally, atrophy of the lining skin predisposes to easy trauma. A decrease in the number of ceruminous glands along with altered nature of secretions, and desquamated epithelial cells, predispose to cerumen accumulation (wax) in older subjects[1,12]. Dryness of the epithelium results in increased pruritus[13]. Degenerative changes occur in the synovial joints of the ossicular chain in the middle ear, resulting in calcification and obliteration of the joint space with impaired mobility. Age-related changes by themselves have minimal effect on sound transmission; co-morbidity or medications are often contributory and magnify the problem. The major changes in the inner ear are mostly degenerative, with hair cell and neuronal loss secondary to atherosclerosis. These may be the basis for hearing impairment and balance-related disorders. Aside from atherosclerosis, numerous factors contribute to the degenerative process; these include diet, dyslipidemias, exposure to noise, drugs and genetic factors[6,13].

The human ear can appreciate a wide range of frequencies, from 20 to 20 000 Hz. The ear is most sensitive to speech frequencies, which are typically between 500 and 2000 Hz. Although hearing loss begins in a subtle manner in middle age, it is hardly noticeable or detectable until the loss of frequencies falls below 8000 Hz. The disability becomes apparent as the loss involves the speech frequencies between 500 and 2000 Hz[8,10].

EXTERNAL, MIDDLE AND INNER EAR DISORDERS

External ear

Impacted cerumen

This is very common in the elderly and a result of aging changes, as described earlier. This may contribute to pain, fullness in the ear and conductive deafness. Significant cerumen accumulation, causing even up to 90% occlusion, may occur without interfering with hearing, yet further occlusion may result

in a substantial deficit[6]. Cerumen becomes drier because of decreased glandular activity in the elderly: the coarser hair in the external canal traps the cerumen leading to impaction. Decrease in hearing acuity of as much as 40–45 dB can result from cerumen obstructing transmission of sound[14]. If the cerumen is soft, gentle irrigation of the external auditory canal with normal saline at body temperature suffices. Use of keratolytic agents for hard cerumen will be necessary prior to irrigation. An additional option is microscopic aural toilet. Cautious use of irrigation measures is recommended in the presence of ongoing or past middle ear infections.

Dermatitis

As a result of aging changes, the external ear is predisposed to dryness, itching and dermatitis. Corrective measures include moisturizing or lubricating agents such as glycerin or mineral oil applications. Alcohol-based mixtures should be avoided, as they increase dryness. Middle ear infection should be excluded prior to instituting the measures.

Infections (otitis externa)

Fungal Predisposition to fungal infections includes cerumen impaction and hearing aid use with entrapment of moisture[15,16]. Itching is the predominant symptom. Serous or serosanguinous discharge may be evident. Corrective measures include debridement of the retained material or fungal ball, use of antifungal topical applications and keeping the external auditory canal dry. In most cases, systemic antifungal therapy is not required.

Bacterial Acute pain, often with foul-smelling discharge, may be evident. Tragal tenderness, erythema and edema of the external auditory canal may also be encountered. Treatment includes aural toilet coupled with topical antibiotic solutions, with or without steroids. Malignant otitis externa is a serious bacterial infection (usually *Pseudomonas aeruginosa*) in diabetics and immunocompromised patients. It is rapidly progressive and locally destructive. Systemic antibiotics are indicated, tailored to results of cultures. Surgical intervention may be necessary.

Neoplasms

Osteomas and chondromas that cause conductive deafness are rare; disorders that involve the external ear include actinic keratosis, basal cell carcinoma, and squamous cell carcinoma.

Perforation of the tympanic membrane

This may result from either trauma or infection involving the tympanic membrane. Hearing loss and recurrent infections may follow. Surgical correction is an option[6].

Middle ear

Infections (otitis media)

These are less common in the elderly; they may be serous or suppurative[15,17].

Serous The acute type is secondary to middle ear pressure changes or upper respiratory infections, usually viral. The course is self-limited, requiring treatment of the underlying etiology. The chronic type has a potential for long-term consequences impacting the hearing mechanism. The usual etiological factors are recurrent viral infections and/or chronic unrelieved obstruction requiring drainage and ventilation of the middle ear.

Suppurative Predisposing factors are upper respiratory bacterial infections, penetrating injuries or postoperative infections. The usual complaints include excruciating pain, discharge and conductive deafness, with occasional bleeding. Treatment includes systemic and topical antibiotics and aural toilet. When infection is cleared, surgical correction may be required to restore the hearing mechanism.

Miscellaneous

These include ossicular chain dysmotility or dislocation, rarely neoplasms (e.g. squamous cell carcinoma, glomus jugulare) and otosclerosis; the last entity typically involves middle-aged women, and causes conductive deafness.

Inner ear

Infections

In the inner ear, infections are less common than non-infectious problems[15].

Labyrinthitis This is of viral or bacterial etiology, and is usually preceded by upper respiratory viral syndromes, causing acute vertigo, nausea, vomiting and dysequilibrium syndrome, lasting several days. Treatment includes labyrinthine sedatives (e.g. meclizine) and symptomatic measures, including fall precautions. Bacterial infections are usually seen in the postoperative setting following middle or inner ear surgery[12,17].

Vestibular neuronitis Symptoms resemble labyrinthitis with spells of vertigo lasting 24 h or more. Central nervous system compensation occurs within days, provided adequate visual and proprioceptive input is available. Treatment is similar to that for labyrinthitis. Vestibular rehabilitation provides significant help in these cases.

Non-infectious causes

Systemic diseases Hypertension, diabetes mellitus, hyperlipidemia and atherosclerosis are some of the causes that affect the circulation, metabolism or oxygen delivery, resulting in labyrinthine dysfunction.

Acoustic neuroma This is a rare cerebellopontine angle tumor seen mostly in late middle age, causing unilateral vestibular and/or auditory dysfunction. Cranial nerve involvement, particularly trigeminal and

Table 2   Common causes of conductive deafness

Impacted cerumen
External ear infections
Serous otitis media
Otosclerosis
Tumors

Table 3   Common causes of sensorineural hearing loss

Presbycusis
Drug induced
Noise induced
Acoustic neuroma
Meniere's disease
Inner ear infections

Table 4   Drug-induced hearing loss*

Loop diuretics: furosemide, ethacrynic acid, bumetanide
Antimicrobials: aminoglycosides, vancomycin, erythromycin
Cytotoxic drugs: cisplatin
Anticonvulsants: phenytoin, ethosuximide
Salicylates: aspirin
Quinine sulfate

*The list is not complete and is used for illustration only

facial, can be associated findings. Early detection is important, since symptoms are reversible with surgical intervention[8,17].

Meniere's disease   This is characterized by sudden episodes of intense vertigo, lasting minutes to hours, associated with nausea and vomiting, often resulting in falls. Additional features of unilateral or bilateral fluctuating hearing loss ultimately result in gradual deterioration of hearing. Peripheral nystagmus is usually demonstrable. Treatment includes labyrinthine sedatives (e.g. meclizine 25–50 mg every 6–8 h), scopolamine patch (every 3 days), antiemetics, salt and fluid restriction and systemic steroids for acute episodes. Refractory cases can be dealt with by surgery[5,17].

A discussion on deafness follows, although it is worth mentioning that several of the aforementioned ear disorders are common causes of deafness.

DEAFNESS

Deafness can be broadly classified as conductive, sensorineural, mixed and/or central auditory processing disorders[1,5,15,16].

Conductive deafness

Conductive hearing loss is seen in all age groups, with bone conduction better than air conduction. The presence of an air–bone gap in the audiogram is pathognomonic; the disorder usually results from either external or middle ear pathology and is often correctable. People with conductive deafness can hear better in noisy surroundings. Common causes are listed in Table 2.

Sensorineural deafness

This is the common type seen in the elderly, characterized by better air conduction than bone conduction; nevertheless, compared to normal, there is a reduction in bone conduction mostly involving high frequencies (Tables 3 and 4). People with sensorineural deafness are handicapped by poor speech discrimination and worsening hearing in noisy surroundings (in contrast to conductive deafness). Presbycusis, a common prototype, is discussed below.

Mixed

This includes a combination of characteristics of both conductive and sensorineural deafness.

Central auditory processing disorder

This is a relatively common, often unrecognized cause of deafness in the geriatric age group. The usual pathology is either in the auditory cortex or in central neuronal connections, with an intact peripheral hearing apparatus. The entity is seen in neurodegenerative conditions such as dementia.

Presbycusis

Presbycusis is the common type of hearing loss seen in the elderly, characterized by slowly progressive, bilateral, painless, symmetrical, high-frequency hearing loss, usually a result of multifactorial etiology[6]. The usual presentation is deteriorating functional status, social withdrawal, depression or cognitive impairment. Self-reporting of this disability is uncommon. Four subtypes are recognized.

Sensory presbycusis is characterized by gradual high-frequency hearing loss with the pathology in the organ of Corti in the basal turn of the cochlea. *Neural* presbycusis is characterized by disproportionate loss of speech discrimination to the amount of pure tone loss and is secondary to a reduced number of cochlear neurons in the presence of a functioning organ of Corti. *Strial* presbycusis is characterized by hearing loss in all frequencies secondary to atrophic changes in the stria vascularis, with preservation of good speech discrimination capability. *Cochlear* conductive presbycusis is characterized by loss of speech discrimination in proportion to the degree of hearing loss, with a clear histopathological correlate to be identified[1,4,5].

Evaluation for presbycusis is aimed at identification and assessment of the degree of hearing loss and disability, including a detailed history and physical examination to rule out systemic disease. A focused examination of the ear and auditory function should follow. Cognitive dysfunction should raise a high index of suspicion for hearing disorders. Screening tests are listed in Table 5. Frequencies vital to understanding speech range between 500 and 2000 Hz[6]. Pure tone audiometry is the gold standard for assessment of hearing loss and indicates the nature and degree of hearing loss. Specific tests for identifying the site of a lesion should be considered where applicable, e.g. speech reception threshold (SRT), speech discrimination scores, acoustic reflex, electrocochleography

Table 5 Screening tests for hearing impairment

Screening with audioscope
Tuning fork test
Spoken voice test
Whisper voice test
Finger friction test
Hearing Handicap Inventory for the Elderly (HHIE)

Table 6 Assessment of hearing loss handicap

	Level (dB)	Description
Normal	up to 25	no difficulty in communication
Mild	25–40	problem in understanding soft speech
Moderate	40–55	problem in understanding normal speech
Severe	55 and above	problems with loud and/or amplified speech

and brainstem evoked potentials. For assessment of the degree of handicap, see Table 6[1,4,5].

Management of presbycusis primarily involves the use of hearing aids. Cochlear implants in association with speech reading and aural rehabilitation can be considered, since sensorineural hearing loss is usually permanent. The use of assistive listening devices for hearing impaired people in specific situations is helpful.

HEARING AIDS

Hearing aids are the principle source of improving communicating ability and reducing social handicap. They are effective and well tolerated in both conductive and sensory hearing loss, but are nevertheless underutilized. With improving technology, most types of hearing loss can be helped with these aids. Barriers to utilization of hearing aids are listed in Table 7. Hearing aids are not inexpensive, often entailing a cost of over $1000 for each device[3,6].

Binaural usage of hearing aids is preferable, because of improvements in speech reception

Table 7 Barriers to the use of hearing aids in older adults

Failure to accept the disability (denial)
Lack of motivation
Fear of social stigma
Poor counseling
Low expectation of benefits
Financial reasons

Table 8 Types of hearing aid

Body worn hearing aids
  large in size, non-cosmetic, helpful in severe hearing impairment
Behind the ear type[*]
  sits behind the ear; flexible mold; easier to use if dexterity impaired
In the ear type[*]
  sits in the lateral ear canal; moderate dexterity required; high cost
In the canal type[*]
  fits snugly in the ear canal; hardly noticeable; needs greater dexterity; entails higher cost

[*]For moderate to severe hearing impairment, better speech discrimination

and ability to function in groups and noisy surroundings, balanced hearing, sound localization and loudness summation. The patient has to be counseled that the hearing aid does not restore normal hearing but enables better communication capability. The components of a hearing aid[3,4,5,10] include the following:

(1) *Microphone* Converts acoustic signals to electrical signals;

(2) *Amplifier* Selectively processes and amplifies output signals;

(3) *Receiver* Converts electrical signals back to acoustic signals;

(4) *Ear mold and tubing* Deliver acoustic signals to patient's ear.

The various types of hearing aid are listed in Table 8. With improving technology, aids are available in a variety of cosmetically acceptable forms. The 'in the canal type' aid is small and hardly visible, but difficult to maneuver for those with limited dexterity. Batteries have to be changed periodically and may have economic impact. Larger hearing aids may be more suitable for those with severe hearing loss.

Cochlear implants can be considered in situations where hearing aids provide inadequate rehabilitation. These are neural prostheses that convert sound energy to electrical energy and stimulate the cochlear or auditory nerve directly[5].

Speech reading is the use of visual clues for better understanding not only by recognizing lip movements but also interpreting facial expressions, body language and gestures. All people, whether hearing impaired or not, use speech reading to some extent subconsciously to enhance understanding. Speech reading is taught along with auditory training and hearing aid orientation[1,4,5].

Assistive listening devices are situation-specific amplifiers; since all hearing aids amplify both noise and speech, difficulty is experienced by the hearing impaired in noisy surroundings such as public halls, concerts, meetings, etc. The only solution to this problem is moving the microphone close to the sound source (speaker) and using electromagnetic loops or infrared transmission to the earpiece worn by the hearing impaired person. Assistive listening devices can provide visual and vibrotactile alerts[1,3-5].

IMPROVE COMMUNICATION SKILLS

One can learn to better communicate with hearing-impaired older adults in several ways. Avoid a fast tempo, rather attempt to speak clearly and towards the better ear, after seeking the subject's attention. Avoid yelling and instead take steps to minimize the background noise. The speaker should not cover the lips with hands or by other means. Gestures are helpful wherever applicable. And if one must repeat, do so using a different sentence[4].

Table 9   Common causes of tinnitus

Medications, e.g. diuretics, aminoglycosides, aspirin, quinine
Infections of external, middle and inner ear
Metabolic: hyperlipidemias, thyroid disease
Meniere's disease
Nutritional deficiencies, e.g. zinc
Impacted cerumen
Central nervous system neoplasms, e.g. cerebellopontine tumors
Abnormal movements of the palate (palatoclonus)
Vascular disease: arterial and venous, arteriovenous malformations

TINNITUS

Over 10% of the population in the USA suffer from tinnitus; although it may occur at any age, most commonly affected are the 40–80-year age group. Of those affected, 20% have tinnitus severe enough to affect the quality of life. Tinnitus can be differentiated from auditory hallucination by not being complex sounds such as voices or music. It is unilateral in half the cases, and the origin can be at any locus along the neural axis from the cochlear nucleus to the auditory cortex. Characteristics can vary and may be low or high in pitch, loud or soft, paroxysmal or constant[5,10,11,18].

Tinnitus may be subjective or objective. The subjective type is more common and characterized by noise perception when there is no stimulation of the cochlear nerve, and is not audible to the health provider. The objective type is internal, and may be audible to the health provider; an identifiable cause is usually found – often pulsatile in nature. The causes of tinnitus are listed in Table 9.

Evaluation

Evaluation includes a history focusing on the nature of onset (acute versus chronic), whether unilateral or bilateral and presence or absence of associated symptoms (e.g. hearing loss, vertigo, ear fullness). Review of medications, prescribed and over the counter, is essential. A focused examination of the head and neck in addition to an otological examination should follow Evaluation should also include assessment of auditory function by pure tone and speech audiograms, and speech discrimination score. Ancillary testing includes head and neck imaging studies, electrocochleography and occasionally invasive angiography[11].

Management

Management varies with etiology, with no single specific treatment. The majority of patients usually find a way to compensate for their tinnitus in a healthy, socially acceptable way. One may begin with offering counseling regarding the benign nature of the disorder and explaining the pathophysiologic basis. Any reversible otological or medical condition should be addressed. Eliminating incriminating medications should be considered[18]. Three basic modalities of treatment are options. Medical therapy includes several drugs with limited success, including anxiolytics, antidepressants and sedative–hypnotics, with need for awareness of adverse effects in the elderly. Surgery has a limited role. Non-medical management includes cognitive therapy and counseling, noise masking at the ear or environment level and tinnitus retraining therapy[11].

VERTIGO

Complaints of dizziness or vertigo are close to 90% in the over-65 age group, with many geriatric subjects affected by some type of balance disturbance. Balance is maintained by accurate interpretation of vestibular, visual and somatosensory stimuli. Sense of imbalance usually results from an absence of two or more sensory inputs, poor central nervous system integration or faulty motor response[12]. Recovery entails the need for intact processes, and is often delayed in the elderly because of co-existing deficits. Vertigo is a diagnostic challenge in view of remarkable attempts at central nervous system compensation and lack of physical findings.

Evaluation elicits an etiologic factor in over two-thirds of subjects by a thorough history, accurate description of episodes, presence or absence of sense of motion and accompanying symptoms related to vestibular disease[1,12]. Review of co-morbidities, in particular vascular disease and medications, should be explored. Physical examination includes blood pressure monitoring (including check for orthostasis), cardiopulmonary, neurologic and neuro-otologic examinations. Tests for visual acuity coupled with vestibular function should be considered.

Vertigo can result from acute labyrinthine dysfunction. These conditions include benign positional vertigo, Meniere's disease, labyrinthitis and acoustic neuroma. Acute central vestibular dysfunction resulting from vascular disease such as transient ischemic attacks, cerebellar or brainstem infarcts, and cerebellopontine angle tumors can be the etiology. Systemic disease and medications that affect vestibular function can also cause vertigo.

Benign positional vertigo is a common and easily diagnosed disorder in the elderly and is most disabling in terms of symptomatology and functional status. The pathology is development of otoconia (calcium deposits in the inner ear), which creates a turbulence of the endolymph and stimulation of the sensory organ within the semicircular canals. When the affected canal is placed in a dependent position, gravity displaces endolymph and sensory epithelium to a new position, resulting

Table 10 Indications for referral to the otolaryngologist

Unilateral hearing loss
Hearing loss associated with tinnitus or vertigo
Sudden-onset hearing loss
Conductive type of hearing loss
Fluctuating hearing loss
Intractable ear pain
Ear infections in diabetes and immunocompromised patients
Recurrent ear infections

in neuronal activity that is interpreted by the brainstem as a rotation. Clinical manifestations include brief episodes of intense vertigo, lasting usually less than a minute, associated with nausea, noticeable with change of posture, either while lying down or getting up from a recumbent posture. Elicitable nystagmus with reproducible symptomatology helps make the diagnosis. Confirmation is by using the bedside head-tilting test (Hallpike maneuver). Management involves vestibular sedatives, early ambulation and regular exercises. Vestibular rehabilitation can help alleviate symptoms. Many cases resolve spontaneously in weeks to months. Refractory cases may be referred to a neuro-otologist for otolith repositioning[1,12].

In summary, disorders of hearing, tinnitus and vertigo are frustrating to the patient and diagnosis may be difficult for the primary care provider. Appropriate and timely referrals may help in diagnosis and in improving both function and quality of life (Table 10).

References

1. Rees TS, Duckert LG, Carey JP. Auditory and vestibular dysfunction. In Hazzard WR, Blass JP, Ettinger WH, Halter JB, Ouslander JG, eds. *Principles of Geriatric Medicine and Gerontology*, 4th edn. New York: McGraw Hill, 1999:617–31
2. Keller BK, Morton JL, Thomas VS, Potter JF. The effect of visual and hearing impairments on functional status. *J Am Geriatr Soc* 1999; 47:1319–25
3. Fook L, Morgan R. Hearing impairment in older people: a review. *Postgrad Med J* 2000;76:537–41
4. Bade PF. Hearing impairment. In Cobbs EL, Duthie EH, Murphy JB, eds. *Geriatric Review Syllabus: A Core Curriculum in*

Geriatric Medicine, 5th edn. Malden, MA: Blackwell Publishing for the American Geriatrics Society 2002;170–5

5. Lalwani AK, Snow JB. Disorders of smell, taste and hearing. In Braunwald E, Fauci AS, Kasper DL, Hauser SL, Longo DL, Jameson JL, eds. *Harrison's Principles of Internal Medicine*. New York: McGraw-Hill, 2001: 178–87

6. Marcincuk MC, Roland PS. Geriatric hearing loss: understanding the causes and providing appropriate treatment. *Geriatrics* 2002;57:44–59

7. Steel KP. New interventions in hearing impairment. *Br Med J* 2000;320:622–5

8. Feldman AS, Grimes CT. Audiology. In Ballenger JJ, ed. *Diseases of the Nose, Throat, Ear, Head and Neck*, 14th edn. Philadelphia: Lea and Febiger, 1991; 1029–52

9. Bordley JE, Brookhouser PE, Tucker GF Jr, eds. The ear: measurement of hearing. In *Ear, Nose and Throat Disorders in Children*. New York: Raven Press, 1986: 149–73

10. Cohn ES. Hearing loss with aging. *Clin Geriatr Med* 1999;15:145–61

11. Fortune DS, Haynes DS, Hall JW. Tinnitus: current evaluation and management. *Med Clin North Am* 1999;83:153–62

12. Patt BS. Otologic disorders. In Duthie EH Jr, Katz PR, eds. *Practice of Geriatrics*, 3rd edn. Philadelphia: Saunders, 1998: 449–56

13. Meyerhoff W. Age related disorders of the ear, nose, and throat. *Geriatrics* 2002;57:43

14. Moore AM, Voytas J, Kowalski D, Maddens M. Cerumen, hearing and cognition in the elderly. *J Am Med Dir Assn* 2002;3:136–9

15. Weber PC, Klein AJ. Hearing loss. *Med Clin North Am* 1999;83:125–37

16. Silverman CA. Audiologic assessment and amplification. *Primary Care* 1998;25: 545–82

17. Hearing loss. In Beers MH, Berkow R, eds. *The Merck Manual of Geriatrics*, 3rd edn. Whitehouse Station, NJ: Merck Research Laboratories, 2000:1317–28

18. Caicedo E, Preciado D, Harris G, Ondrey F. Aging and inner ear dysfunction. In Lunenfeld B, Gooren L. eds. *Textbook of Men's Health*. London: Parthenon Publishing, 2002:499–512

37 Disorders of the eye

Kenneth B. Juechter, MD

It is estimated that there are 13.5 million Americans over the age of 45 with visual impairment, and more than two-thirds are over the age of 65[1]. Current aging trends suggest that a larger number of elderly will have visual impairment. A significant number of individuals in this population are legally blind. Among the disabilities that affect the geriatric population, visual loss ranks with the most feared. Cataracts, glaucoma, macular degeneration and diabetic retinopathy are the most common of these disorders. Nevertheless, each of these may be favorably influenced in outcome by timely discovery and appropriate treatment.

AGING AND THE EYE

As with other body tissues, the eye structures undergo involutional changes with aging. Eyelids become more lax, leading to ectropion or entropion. Tear production decreases causing dry eye syndrome. The lens, isolated from nerves and blood vessels and dependent on nutrition from aqueous fluid produced by the ciliary body, continues to grow and add lens fibers throughout life. Aging results in darkening and hardening of the lens nucleus (sclerosis), decrease in accommodative function for near vision (referred to as presbyopia), and often clouding of vision associated with cataract formation. The vitreous gel becomes less viscous, resulting in separation of its collagen fibers and often partial or complete

separation from the loose attachments to the retina. This may result in symptoms of flashes and formation of 'floaters'. Less commonly, retinal tears also result, creating the potential for detachment. The retina also loses cells, decreasing visual function.

VISUAL IMPAIRMENT AND LEGAL BLINDNESS

The age-related changes and many diseases of the eye can lead to visual impairment and blindness. The term 'low vision' describes residual vision that is useful, but less than normal. It may result from any one of many ocular or neurologic disorders. The International Classification of Diseases 9 (ICD-9-CM) divides visual impairment into five categories[2]. These include:

(1) *Moderate visual impairment* best-corrected visual acuity 20/70 to 20/160

(2) *Severe visual impairment* best corrected visual acuity 20/200 to 20/400, or the visual field is 20° or less

(3) *Profound visual impairment* best-corrected visual acuity 20/500 to 20/1000, or the visual field is 10° or less

(4) *Near total visual loss* best corrected visual acuity is 20/1000 or less

(5) *Total blindness* no light perception

Severe visual impairment in both eyes is the minimum requirement to be considered legally blind in the USA. The categories above should be used instead of the terms 'blindness' or 'legal blindness' to describe visual impairment accurately.

Other factors in addition to visual acuity may affect function and impact on the normal activities of daily living. Glare and decreased contrast sensitivity (often associated with cataracts, retinal and optic nerve dysfunction and glaucoma) can influence performance. Scotomas or visual field defects that can be related to such disorders as cerebrovascular accidents, optic nerve loss and focal retinal loss may impact visual ability.

CATARACT

Prevalence and risk factors

A cataract is a degradation of the optical quality of the crystalline lens through loss of clarity or change in color. Cataract is the leading cause of blindness in the world and one of the major causes of visual impairment in the USA. The Baltimore Eye Survey found cataract to be the leading cause of blindness in the group over age 40. Also, unoperated cataract was four times more common among African-Americans than Caucasian Americans. A Baltimore area study of nursing home residents found cataract to be the leading cause of blindness[3].

Many factors appear to increase the risk of cataract formation. Among these are ultraviolet B light exposure, prolonged inhaled or systemic corticosteroid use, diabetes, blunt trauma, chronic uveitis, prior intraocular surgery, hypertension, smoking, alcohol use, ionizing radiation and chemical or electrical ocular surface injuries. A population-based study found the 5-year risk for any cataract was 60% lower among participants who reported 10 years' use of multivitamins or supplements containing vitamins C or E[3]. However, the Age Related Eye Disease Study of high-dose supplementation with vitamins

C and E, β-carotene and/or zinc found no effect of treatment on the development or progression of lens opacities over 6 years[4].

Pathophysiology

The lens of the eye consists of an outer capsule, a cortical layer and an inner nucleus. Cataracts may be typed subcapsular, cortical or nuclear, depending on the location of change. A combination of some or all layers with change is not unusual. Subcapsular cataracts are usually posterior and disable early. Cortical cataracts involve liquefaction of lens cells, often causing glare symptoms; when advanced, this cataract appears white. Nuclear cataracts are located centrally, vary in color from yellow to dark brown and result in differing degrees of haze; these cataracts progress slowly.

Management

Visually significant cataracts, once formed, can be treated only by surgery. The decision to operate usually depends on the visual needs and wishes of the patient. Surgery is recommended when the symptoms of visual loss caused by the cataract impair the ability of the patient to perform activities of daily living, thus reducing quality of life. The appropriate time for surgical intervention varies considerably, depending on the needs of the patient. Since visual impairment often progresses slowly over a long period, many patients may be unaware of the loss. Contrast sensitivity, glare testing and visual acuity can be helpful in assessment, as can a careful history of functional status. Surgery is indicated when visual function no longer meets the needs of the patient and cataract removal offers a reasonable possibility of improvement. It may also be indicated when the cataract interferes with the evaluation and treatment of retinal disease, such as diabetic retinopathy, or if the lens causes intraocular

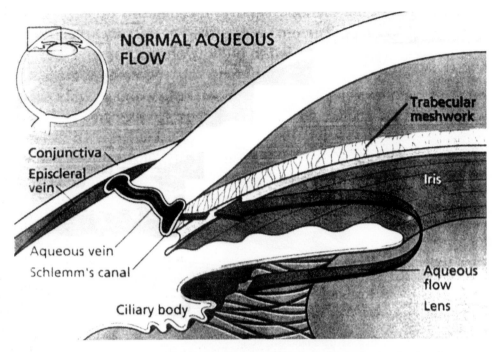

NORMAL AQUEOUS FLOW

Trabecular meshwork

Conjunctiva

Episcleral vein

Iris

Aqueous vein

Schlemm's canal

Ciliary body

Aqueous flow

Lens

Figure 1 Diagrammatic cross section of the anterior segment of the normal eye, showing the site of aqueous production (ciliary body) and sites of resistance to aqueous outflow (trabecular meshwork – Schlemm's canal system and episcleral venous plexus). Adapted with permission of American Academy of Ophthalmology from American Academy of Ophthalmology. *Basic and Clinical Science Course Section 10: Glaucoma*. San Francisco: American Academy of Ophthalmology, 2001–2002

inflammation, or contributes to narrow-angle or open-angle glaucoma[3].

Anesthesia for cataract surgery is local with monitored care. General anesthesia is used infrequently. Local anesthesia may be retrobulbar, peribulbar, periocular or topical. Perioperative sedation is often provided in conjunction with local techniques.

The most common method of surgery is phacoemulsification with a small incision and a foldable intraocular lens implant. This technique usually does not require sutures, as the wound is self sealing. Extracapsular cataract extraction (ECCE) with a larger sutured incision is less often used. Although the laser is not used for cataract removal, it may be used to open the posterior capsule if this becomes clouded postoperatively. Cataract surgery is a highly successful procedure, with complications resulting in serious loss of vision rare.

GLAUCOMA

Pathophysiology and risk factors

The term 'glaucoma' represents a group of eye diseases that may be associated with a progressive loss of vision. In the eye, aqueous humor is produced by the ciliary body from the arterial side of the circulation. The fluid passes through the posterior chamber, the pupil and the anterior chamber to exit mostly by the trabecular meshwork in the angle of the chamber, returning to the venous side of the circulation (Figure 1). This is analogous to the production and reabsorption of cerebrospinal fluid. This flow may be impaired gradually over time while the angle remains open (Figure 2) or suddenly with a narrow or closing angle (Figure 3). In glaucoma these changes may be associated with optic neuropathy, causing visual loss.

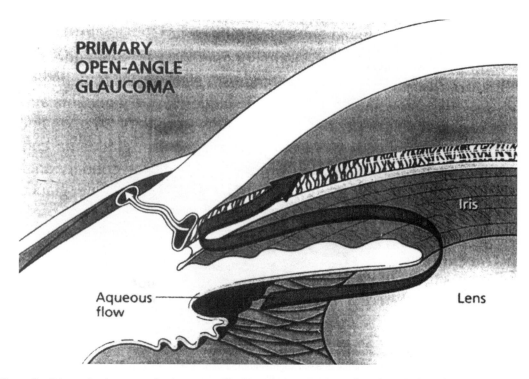

Figure 2   Schematic of open-angle glaucoma with resistance to aqueous outflow through the trabecular meshwork – Schlemm's canal system in the absence of gross anatomic obstruction. Small white arrow shows normal path of outflow and indicates that resistance in this illustration is relative, not total. Adapted with permission of American Academy of Ophthalmology from American Academy of Ophthalmology. *Basic and Clinical Science Course Section 10: Glaucoma.* San Francisco: American Academy of Ophthalmology, 2001–2002

Glaucoma is one of the leading causes of blindness, particularly among African-Americans. Many people are not aware that they have or are at risk for glaucoma. Risk factors include family history, race, age, increased intraocular pressure, hypertension, diabetes and myopia. The primary care physician may contribute significantly to the discovery of undiagnosed individuals or those at risk by including an assessment of risk factors in the history, and an evaluation of the condition of the optic nerve along with measurement of ocular pressure in the physical examination. Although 95% of adult patients will fall in a pressure range of 10–22 mmHg, a significant number will have glaucoma at this level of pressure. Indeed, some with pressures above this range will not develop optic neuropathy associated with glaucoma. Therefore, evaluation of the condition of

the optic nerve by ophthalmoscopy is necessary as well. The nerve head has a depression called the cup, with a peripheral rim. If the cups are asymmetric, with one larger than the other, or if the size is over 50% of the whole disc, or if the cup changes configuration or size over time, glaucoma should be suspected.

Open angle glaucoma

The most common type of glaucoma (over 90%) is open angle. This is a multifactorial optic neuropathy in which there is a characteristic acquired loss of retinal ganglion cells and atrophy of the optic nerve[5]. In early stages there are often no symptoms. Advanced loss of peripheral vision may be a presenting finding. Treatment is aimed at lowering intraocular pressure since this has been shown to be effective in slowing progression

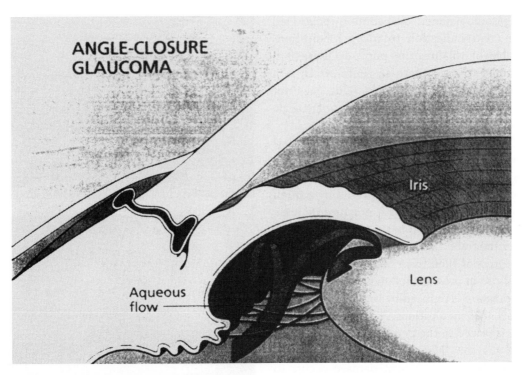

Figure 3 Schematic of angle-closure glaucoma with pupillary block leading to peripheral iris obstruction of the trabecular meshwork. Adapted with permission of American Academy of Ophthalmology from American Academy of Ophthalmology. *Basic and Clinical Science Course Section 10: Glaucoma.* San Francisco: American Academy of Ophthalmology, 2001–2002

of the disease. This can be done by medical treatment, laser surgery or incisional surgery or a combination of these. Since open angle glaucoma is a chronic disease, long-term therapy is needed. Medications commonly used include β-adrenergic antagonists, α_2-adrenergic agonists, carbonic anhydrase inhibitors and prostaglandin analogs. Topical miotics or adrenergic derivatives are used less frequently. Systemic carbonic anhydrase inhibitors may be used for short-term treatment. Laser treatment of the trabecular meshwork can help lower pressure. If these methods do not provide an adequate drop towards target pressure, a level expected to slow or stop nerve damage, then incisional filtering surgery is indicated. This creates an alternative route for the aqueous to leave the eye.

Corticosteroid use in topical, periocular, inhaled or systemic forms may be associated with increased intraocular pressure resulting in open angle glaucoma. Therefore, any patient on such therapy should be regularly monitored for the onset of corticosteroid-induced glaucoma.

Angle closure glaucoma

Angle closure glaucoma constitutes about 10% of all glaucomas. Risk factors include hyperopia (farsightedness), family history of angle closure, advancing age, female gender and Eskimo or Far East Asian extraction[6]. If the onset is acute, the patient may present with pain, ocular redness, blurred vision and even nausea and vomiting mimicking a gastrointestinal disorder. The red eye has a non-reactive mid-dilated pupil, thus differentiating it from conjunctivitis or iritis. An intermittent acute attack may be associated with halos around lights and blurred vision in an episodic manner. Glaucoma is mentioned as a contraindication to many medications capable of dilating the pupil as there is a potential to precipitate an acute attack in a patient with a narrow angle. This does not refer to the far more common open angle type of glaucoma.

Acute angle closure is a medical emergency. Initial treatment is aimed at reducing the severe elevation of intraocular pressure. The attack is usually precipitated by a pupil block of aqueous causing a pressure increase in the posterior chamber, forcing the iris to cover the trabecular meshwork, thus blocking the egress of fluid from the eye (Figure 3). A rapid rise in pressure follows. After diagnosis, the pressure is reduced by topical, oral and/or intravenous medications. A laser iridotomy or hole is placed in the peripheral iris, creating a path for the fluid to bypass the pupil. If treated before permanent damage occurs to the chamber angle, the iridotomy may provide long-term control. Subsequently, the fellow eye is also treated by laser, since the disease is bilateral with a high risk of attack.

MACULAR DEGENERATION

Risk factors and types

Age-related macular degeneration (ARMD) is a leading cause of loss of central vision and legal blindness in the elderly, particularly Caucasians. Incidence and progression increase with age. Other risk factors include family history, smoking and probably hypertension, cardiovascular disease, dietary factors[7] and sun exposure.

ARMD may be of the dry or wet type, classified by the absence or presence of neovascularization. The early stages of ARMD are characterized by the formation of drusen (Figure 4) which may vary in size and consistency. These abnormal deposits accumulate under the retinal pigment epithelium (RPE) and appear clinically as yellow lesions in the outer retina. Attenuation and atrophy of the

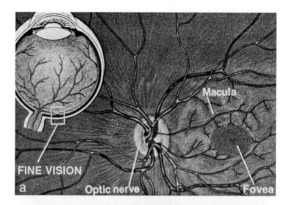

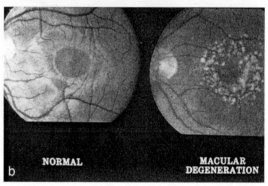

Figure 4 (a) Normal posterior retina; (b) normal versus macular degeneration. Adapted with permission of American Academy of Ophthalmology from American Academy of Ophthalmology. *Basic and Clinical Science Course Section 10: Glaucoma.* San Francisco: American Academy of Ophthalmology, 2001–2002.

RPE may also be noted. While small hard drusen with minimal RPE change has a relatively low risk of progression, larger, irregular drusen with RPE abnormalities carries a higher risk for evolving into advanced disease of either the geographic, atrophic non-neovascular form (dry) or the neovascular type (wet). The wet type of ARMD may seem abrupt in onset when a subretinal hemorrhage occurs from vessels that have extended into the subretinal space from the underlying choroid. Visual loss is often more severe than in the more common dry type.

Management

Management of ARMD includes patient instruction, photocoagulation therapy and micronutrient considerations. Patients, especially those with identified risk factors, should be instructed to test each eye individually, looking for distortions (metamorphopsia), central or paracentral blind spots (scotomas) or any decrease in vision. In advanced disease, patients need low vision evaluation for optical aids and visual rehabilitation. Also, the patient with severe, and especially sudden, visual loss may have significant clinical depression when faced with the additional difficulties in activities of daily living. It should be emphasized that visual loss is limited to the central field. Good peripheral vision allowing ambulatory function is usually maintained. The disease does not progress to total blindness.

Thermal laser photocoagulation and the more recent photodynamic therapy may have a favorable effect on the final visual outcome of selected patients with the wet type of ARMD. These patients need rapid access to a retinologist to evaluate the need for laser treatment.

The role of micronutrients, long considered controversial, has been enhanced by release of the 6-year data of the ARMD Study recently[8]. The report showed a statistically significant protective effect of antioxidant and/or zinc formulation for stabilization of vision in eyes with extensive intermediate-sized drusen, one large drusen or non-central geographic atrophy in one or both eyes or advanced ARMD in one eye. The antioxidants used in the study were vitamins C and E and β-carotene, alone or combined with minerals zinc and copper. Current, but unproven recommendations include encouraging a diet high in fruits and green leafy vegetables, added supplementation with selenium, lutein and manganese, and controlling risk factors such as hypertension and smoking.

DIABETIC RETINOPATHY

Diabetic retinopathy is one of the leading causes of blindness in the elderly, with most patients having type 2 diabetes. Nearly all patients with diabetes of 20 or more years' duration will have some degree of retinopathy[9]. However, it has been shown that significant retinopathy may be present at the time of first diagnosis of type 2 diabetes. Therefore, ophthalmology evaluation for retinopathy is indicated at discovery of diabetes with subsequent periodic examinations depending on findings. Visual loss is related to hemorrhages from retinal neovascularization and/or macular edema from vascular leakage. Poorly controlled blood glucose and hypertension are risk factors for progression of retinopathy. It is well established that timely laser treatment of retinopathy favorably affects visual outcome.

SPECIAL CONSIDERATIONS IN OLDER ADULTS

Giant cell arteritis

Severe, unilateral visual loss may occur in one-third to one-half of patients with giant cell arteritis. This is an emergency as the second eye may be involved within hours or days of the first. The most frequent cause of blindness is anterior ischemic optic neuropathy (AION), but non-embolic central artery occlusion is the presentation in about 10% of patients. Cranial motor nerve paralysis, most commonly the third cranial nerve with outward deviation of the eye, ptosis and pupil sparing, should raise suspicion in the elderly, especially if associated with pain. Appropriate diagnostic studies and high-dose corticosteroid treatment are indicated if giant cell arteritis is suspected.

Amaurosis fugax

Amaurosis fugax, a sudden, severe, painless transient loss of vision, may occur from emboli that temporarily obstruct the ophthalmic or central retinal artery. The monocular dimming of vision is often described as a curtain coming down or over the eye. The attack usually lasts only a few minutes, with vision then returning to the pre-attack level. Ophthalmoscopic evaluation may show an embolus in the retinal artery. Assessment of both cardiovascular and cerebrovascular systems is indicated.

Blepharitis

Blepharitis is a chronic ocular inflammation that involves the eyelid margin primarily and is a common cause of chronic ocular irritation[10]. It is thought to be associated with aging. The anterior ciliary and/or posterior Meibomian margin may be involved. Other ocular surface problems such as conjunctivitis, tear deficiency and keratitis are not uncommon. Staphylococcal blepharitis has scaling and crusting along the cilia (lashes). Seborrheic blepharitis may be present with a similar dermatitis on the face or scalp. Meibomian gland dysfunction of the inner margin may show pouting or plugging of the gland openings with increased local vascularity. These patients may also have rosacea and seborrheic dermatitis. Non-Sjögren's keratoconjunctivitis sicca may be associated. Patient complaints include irritation, burning and tearing. Eyelid hygiene is the basic initial treatment with warm compresses and lid cleaning. Topical antibiotics and a short course of topical steroids may be needed. Associated dermal conditions should be addressed. Atypical or non-responsive eyelid infection suggests the possible presence of carcinoma and should be evaluated for biopsy.

Dry eye syndrome

The term 'dry eye' refers to a group of disorders characterized by reduced tear production or excessive tear evaporation associated with ocular discomfort, which may result in ocular surface damage[11]. This is a common condition that occurs more frequently in the elderly. Failure to diagnose and treat the condition can result in ocular epithelial metaplasia and erosions. Rarely, corneal ulcerations, scarring, thinning and neovascularization can cause severe visual disability.

The symptoms of dry eye such as a sandy grittiness, foreign body sensation, irritation, burning, tearing and blurred vision may be increased by diuretics, antihistamines, anticholinergics and psychotropics. Environmental conditions including wind, heating, air-conditioning and air travel may increase evaporation and aggravate the condition. Air-borne irritants and allergens may also worsen symptoms. Systemic disease such as Sjögren's syndrome, with inflammation of the lacrimal gland, and blepharitis associated with rosacea may result in insufficient tears. Additionally, lid malpositions including ectropion, entropion and lagophthalmos may result in enhanced tear loss and dryness.

Treatment options need to be addressed with the patient emphasizing the chronic nature of the disorder and setting realistic expectations for therapy. Understanding is important to management. Aqueous tear deficiency is treated with eliminating adverse exogenous factors and aqueous enhancement mainly by artificial tears and ointment. Artificial tears vary in consistency and should be tailored to patient needs. Associated systemic disease may require anti-inflammatory and/or immunosuppressive therapy. Surgical therapies used, when a medical approach is insufficient, include correction of lid abnormalities and punctual occlusion. Severe cases may require tarsorrhaphy (partial closure of the lids).

Ectropion, entropion, ptosis

The eyelid is supported in position by the attachment of the tarsal plate to the medial and lateral bony orbit via palpebral tendons.

This lid sling loses elasticity with age, due to many factors including gravity, rubbing and pulling. The resulting laxity may lead to either ectropion or entropion. The looseness may result in an outward evertion of the lid – involutional ectropion, with exposure of the ocular surface tissues, drying and even keratinization. On the other hand, the stretching along with contraction of the orbicularis muscle may cause the tarsus and lid margin to rotate inward – involutional entropion, resulting in rubbing of the lower eyelashes against the conjunctiva and cornea. Cicatrization of the eyelid skin can add to ectropion just as scarring of the conjunctiva may result in cicatricial entropion. Treatment of ectropion and entropion is surgical and aimed at correcting the causes of the lid malposition. Temporary relief may be obtained in some patients by the use of artificial tears and lubricating ointments, taping the lid into position and possible use of antibiotic drops and ointments for secondary infections.

Involutional ptosis is due to a laxity of the aponeurosis of the levator palpebrae muscle resulting from a thinning or dehiscence of that tissue. The lid may approach or cover the visual axis, necessitating a head-back or lid-lifting maneuver by the patient to see. In these patients, surgical correction is indicated to restore visual function.

Ophthalomological disorders are widely prevalent in the elderly and perhaps under-recognized and undertreated; they contribute significantly to a decrease in function, resulting in diminished quality of life. A Task Force on Aging formed by the American Academy of Ophthalmology recently made recommendations to increase geriatric expertise among ophthalmologists in order to improve the delivery of care to the elderly[12].

References

1. American Academy of Ophthalmology. *Vision Rehabilitation for Adults, Preferred Practice Pattern.* San Francisco: American Academy of Ophthalmology, 2001
2. *The International Classification of Diseases, 9th Revision, Clinical Modification*, 2nd edn. ICD.9.CM. vol 1. Washington, DC: US Department of Health and Human Services, Public Health Service – Health Care Finance Administration, 1980:315
3. American Academy of Ophthalmology. *Cataract in the Adult Eye, Preferred Practice Pattern.* San Francisco; American Academy of Ophthalmology, 2001
4. Age-Related Eye Disease Study Research Group. A randomized, placebo-controlled clinical trial of high dose supplementation with vitamins C and E and beta-carotene for age-related cataract and vision loss. AREDS Report No. 9. *Arch Ophthalmol* 2001;119: 1439–52
5. American Academy of Ophthalmology. *Primary Open-angle Glaucoma, Preferred Practice Pattern.* San Francisco: American Academy of Ophthalmology, 2000
6. American Academy of Ophthalmology. *Primary Angle-Closure, Preferred Practice Pattern.* San Francisco: American Academy of Ophthalmology, 2000
7. American Academy of Ophthalmology. *Age-Related Macular Degeneration, Preferred Practice Pattern.* San Francisco: American Academy of Ophthalmology, 2001
8. Age-Related Eye Disease Study Research Group. A randomized, placebo-controlled clinical trial of high dose supplementation with vitamins C and E and beta-carotene and zinc for age-related macular degeneration and vision loss. *Arch Ophthalmol* 2001;119:1417–36
9. American Academy of Ophthalmology. *Diabetic Retinopathy, Preferred Practice*

Pattern. San Francisco: American Academy of Ophthalmology, 1998

10. American Academy of Ophthalmology. *Blepharitis, Preferred Practice Pattern*. San Francisco: American Academy of Ophthalmology, 1998

11. American Academy of Ophthalmology. *Dry Eye Syndrome, Preferred Practice Pattern*. San Francisco: American Academy of Ophthalmology, 1998

12. Lee AG, Liesegang T. Increasing geriatrics expertise in ophthalmology. *Ophthalmology* 2002;109:635–6

38 The cardiovascular system and aging

Lekshmi Dharmarajan, MD, FACP, FACC, and May Luz F. Bullecer, MD

INTRODUCTION

Demographic trends in the USA and across the world show a consistent increase in the older population. Cardiovascular disease is the most frequent cause of death in the geriatric age group[1]. Awareness of age and disease-related alterations in the cardiovascular system helps provide appropriate care to minimize morbidity and mortality. Congestive heart failure, coronary artery disease, cardiac dysrhythmias, valvular abnormalities and hypertension increase with age; however, presentations of these diseases may differ in the older individual compared to the young.

AGE-RELATED CARDIOVASCULAR ALTERATIONS

Structure

Cardiac mass increases as a result of hypertrophy of myocytes as well as an increase in non-cellular components[2]. Thickening in the interventricular septum is more pronounced than in the left ventricular free wall. Left atrial enlargement is observed. Reduction in the number of pacemaker cells by as much as 90% by the age 75, along with amyloid deposition and fibrosis in the conduction system, contribute to the occurrence of arrhythmias[2,3]. Valvular fibrosis and calcification usually involve the aortic and mitral valves[2]. Increased collagen deposition, calcification, smooth muscle cell proliferation and elastin breakdown lead to vascular thickness and stiffening. The presence of stiff vasculature and diminished β-adrenergic receptor reactivity in the elderly result in reduced vasodilatation. There is an increase in epicardial and pericardial fat, more pronounced in women. Most of the above changes can be demonstrated by echocardiography.

Physiology

The direct effects of age *per se* on the cardiovascular system are physiologically trivial. Systolic function is relatively preserved, while diastolic changes are more pronounced, with prolonged diastolic relaxation time, affecting ventricular filling. The resting cardiac output and stroke volume change little with age, but response to exercise progressively declines. A noticeable increase in pulse wave velocity (from vascular stiffening) occurs, resulting in elevated systolic blood pressure[2]. Maximal oxygen consumption decreases by 50% between ages 20 and 80 years in healthy sedentary individuals, explained by a reduction in cardiac reserve function[2]. Diminution of β-receptor responsiveness manifests as a suboptimal heart rate response, more pronounced during exercise. The exact reason for the decreased β-adrenergic response is unclear, and is possibly related to a decrease in adenylate cyclase or increased G protein activity[4]. An attempt to maintain cardiac output with exercise is made by an increase in stroke volume, as the heart rate increment is inadequate. The formulae to calculate maximum heart rate for age[4] are:

Men: maximum heart rate = 220 – age
Women: maximum heart rate
= 190 – (0.8 × age)

CARDIOVASCULAR DISORDERS IN OLDER ADULTS

Heart failure

Heart failure (HF) remains the leading cause of hospitalization, involving nearly five million people in the USA, with 5–10% of geriatric subjects affected[5]. Advanced HF is associated with significant mortality[5].

The syndrome of HF is characterized either by a failure in filling and relaxation of the left ventricle with normal ejection fraction (diastolic dysfunction) or by an increase in end-diastolic pressure with impaired emptying of the left ventricle, with the ejection fraction less than 45% (systolic dysfunction). HF manifests in the elderly as shortness of breath and fatigue or atypically as mental status changes, abdominal pain, anorexia, cough and nocturia, or any combination of the above[5–7].

Underlying postulated mechanisms for HF include alterations in myocardial thickness and relaxation, diminished β-receptor density, vascular stiffness, valvular abnormalities, altered mitochondrial energy metabolism[8] and activation of the neurohormonal systems[5,9]. Neurohormones implicated include the renin–angiotensin–aldosterone system, norepinephrine, epinephrine, atrial natriuretic

Table 1 Mechanisms and causes of heart failure

Types
Systolic dysfunction: ejection fraction less than 45%
Diastolic dysfunction: ejection fraction more than 45%

Postulated mechanisms
Impaired cardiac relaxation
Diminished β-adrenergic response
    attenuated heart rate and contractility
    compromised β$_2$-mediated peripheral vasodilatation
Vascular stiffening
Valvular abnormalities
Altered myocardial mitochondrial energy metabolism
Neurohormonal

Causes of heart failure
Coronary heart disease
Hypertension
Valvular diseases
Cardiac dysrhythmias
Cardiomyopathy
Thyroid disease
Infections
Severe anemia

peptide, tissue necrosis factor α, antidiuretic hormone, growth hormone, cortisol, adrenomedullin and endothelin[5,6].

The causes of HF in the elderly are many. Coronary heart disease remains the predominant cause, accounting for two-thirds of cases[5,6]. Hypertension, valvular diseases, cardiac dysrhythmias, cardiomyopathy (alcohol, drugs, idiopathic), thyroid disease, anemia and infection are other etiologies[8] (Table 1).

Based on the degree of symptoms, the New York Heart Association (NYHA) classification is used to describe the functional status of the patient[5]:

(1) Class I: no limitation; ordinary physical activity does not result in fatigue, dyspnea, angina or palpitations;

(2) Class II: slight limitation of physical activity, asymptomatic at rest, but ordinary physical activity precipitates symptoms;

(3) Class III: significant limitation of physical activity; while comfortable at rest,

less than ordinary activity results in symptoms;

(4) Class IV: symptoms at rest.

A recent approach to the classification of HF emphasizes both evolution and progression in four stages[6]:

(1) Stage A: identifies patients at high risk for HF but who have no cardiac structural disorders (e.g. hypertension, diabetes mellitus, alcohol abuse);

(2) Stage B: includes patients who never developed HF but have cardiac structural changes (e.g. left ventricular hypertrophy or dilatation, valvular disease, prior myocardial infarction);

(3) Stage C: refers to those with symptomatic HF and structural heart disease (e.g. dyspnea or fatigue from systolic dysfunction requiring treatment);

(4) Stage D: identifies those with end-stage heart disease, markedly symptomatic at rest in spite of interventions for HF (e.g. patients frequently hospitalized and candidates for hospice care or transplant).

Diagnosis and management

The diagnosis of HF warrants a thorough history including review of drugs (prescribed and over-the-counter) and physical examination, keeping in mind that the older adults may present atypically. Electrocardiogram, chest X-ray, thyroid function tests and radionuclide scan help in the diagnosis. The gold standard and most informative test is the two-dimensional echocardiogram with Doppler flow studies[5,6,9]. The echocardiogram helps decipher pericardial, myocardial and valvular abnormalities in addition to quantifying ejection fraction and determining systolic and diastolic function[9].

Lifestyle modification for HF involves initiation of dietary sodium restriction to 2 g/day and in the presence of hypervolemia and/or hyponatremia, fluid restriction to approximately 1000 ml/day. Fluid restriction can be monitored based on weights. Cessation of smoking, alcohol consumption, and avoidance of processed foods (which have high salt content) should be emphasized.

Drug therapies for HF with left ventricular systolic dysfunction include angiotensin converting enzyme (ACE) inhibitors, which have been proven to improve morbidity and mortality in patients with ischemic and non-ischemic left ventricular systolic dysfunction, including asymptomatic patients. In the USA the ACE inhibitors approved for management of congestive heart failure (CHF) include captopril, lisinopril, enalapril, fosinopril, quinapril, ramipril and trandolapril. Treatment is initiated with a low dose and titrated gradually to the maximum tolerated dose. Close monitoring of blood pressure, renal function and potassium levels is recommended in the initial weeks of treatment and subsequently less often. Concomitant use of diuretics may add to azotemia and electrolyte abnormalities.

β-Blockers, although initially considered inappropriate for use in HF, have been clearly shown to be beneficial on the basis of chronic blockade of the adrenergic system. They improve ejection fraction, increase survival and are best initiated after stabilization of the patient with HF. They are recommended in all stable patients with heart failure due to left ventricular dysfunction unless contraindicated; in the presence of acute decompensation, the dose may be decreased or withheld on a temporary basis[5,6]. Carvedilol, an α- and β-blocker, is known to offset the harmful effects of catecholamines in the cardiovascular system; additional benefits are from antiproliferative and antioxidant effects[10]. Metoprolol and bisoprolol have also been found to be beneficial in HF.

Diuretics are the most effective treatment for symptoms of acute fluid overload and the only means of rapid salt and water excretion.

Loop diuretics (e.g. furosemide) are used as primary agents, while supplementary thiazides (e.g. metolazone) are added for synergy for fluid overload not responsive to loop diuretics alone. In acute situations loop diuretics are used intravenously and in larger doses particularly in the presence of renal insufficiency[6,8,9]. Infusion therapy of loop diuretics may overcome diuretic resistance[9]. Aldosterone antagonists have recently been recognized as beneficial in stable NYHA class III–IV HF with ejection fraction less than 35%, serum creatinine below 2.5 mg/dl and potassium less than 5.0 mmol/l. Spironolactone may be added to the regimen of ACE inhibitors, loop diuretics, digoxin and vasodilators[11]. When spironolactone is concomitantly administered with ACE inhibitors, potassium levels need to be monitored[11].

Digoxin offers symptomatic improvement in NYHA class II–IV, enhancing quality of life and function; it reduces hospitalization but does not decrease mortality. Benefit is observed in HF with or without sinus rhythm. Digoxin has a narrow therapeutic index; the dose has to be adjusted for renal function, and levels must be checked when toxicity is suspected[5,9].

Angiotensin II receptor blockers (ARB) have been studied in the elderly with results not different with respect to morbidity and mortality compared to captopril. At present their use is suggested only in patients who are unable to tolerate ACE inhibitors due to cough; angioedema is a rarer phenomenon. The combination of ACE inhibitors and ARB has been shown to improve hemodynamics[10,12]. However, the combination of ACE inhibitors, ARBs and beta-blockers had safety concerns in the Valsartan Heart Failure Trial[13]. Hydralazine–isosorbide, a vasodilator combination, is a substitute for those who cannot tolerate ACE inhibitors, especially with renal insufficiency and hyperkalemia. Calcium channel blockers do not offer added benefits for heart failure[5]. Antiarrhythmic agents are recommended when worsening of clinical condition is brought about by atrial or ventricular arrhythmias. Amiodarone is safe in the management of atrial arrhythmias with concomitant heart failure. Inotropic drugs (dobutamine) dosed as intermittent outpatient infusions have no proven benefit on mortality, and in fact may be harmful. Anticoagulation in the absence of atrial fibrillation or intracardiac thrombus is still controversial. The role of anticoagulation in HF is being studied[5].

Recently, nesiritide, a recombinant B-type natriuretic peptide, with venous and arterial dilator properties, has been approved for the management of acute heart failure. While B-type natriuretic peptide is produced from the ventricles, A-type arises from the atria and C-type from the vascular endothelium. The B-type peptide increases glomerular filtration and causes natriuresis. Benefit in heart failure is attained through diuresis, natriuresis and vasodilation. An association has been observed between the blood concentration of B-type peptide measured by rapid assay and severity of CHF. The main adverse effect of therapy is hypotension[14,15].

Diastolic heart failure

Diastolic dysfunction accounts for half of the HF cases in older subjects but nevertheless is not well studied; data from randomized trials are inadequate[16,17]. Causes of diastolic HF include left ventricular hypertrophy (from hypertension or aortic stenosis), chronic coronary heart disease and cardiomyopathy (hypertrophic, infiltrative, or restrictive cardiomyopathy and constrictive pericarditis).

The objective of treatment is to address the risk factors responsible. Long-term management with definite diastolic HF includes prevention and treatment of congestive symptoms, control of hypertension, maintaining sinus rhythm and prevention of cardiac ischemia[7]. While diuretics and nitrates have a

Table 2 Management of heart failure

	Target doses
Non-pharmacologic	
Cessation of cigarette smoking and alcohol consumption	
Dietary salt restriction	
Avoidance of processed foods	
Pharmacologic	
ACE inhibitors	
captopril	50 mg tid
enalapril	20 mg/day
fosinopril	40 mg/day
lisinopril	40 mg/day
ramipril	10 mg/day
quinapril	40 mg/day
trandolapril	4 mg/day
β-Blockers	
carvedilol	25 mg bid
metoprolol	100–200 mg/day
bisoprolol	10 mg/day
Diuretics	
furosemide	40–80 mg/day
hydrochlorothiazide	25 mg/day
metolazone	2.5–10 mg/day
spironolactone	25 mg/day

role, concern for decrease in preload and consequent reduced cardiac output is emphasized. ACE inhibitors, through their neuro-hormonal effects, attenuate ventricular hypertrophy; β-blockers reduce heart rate and thereby improve diastolic filling; calcium channel blockers may be used for their antihypertensive, anti-ischemic and anti-chronotropic action[17] (Table 2).

Cardiac resynchronization, a new option, produces substantial improvement in individuals with moderate to severe heart failure and intraventricular conduction delay; this biventricular pacing helps improve symptoms and decreases frequency of hospitalization[18,19].

End-of-life care

This includes appropriate education of the patient and caregiver regarding the illness, discussion of treatment options available and preparation for the anticipated outcome. In particular, the responses to cardiac arrest or other non-cardiac catastrophes (e.g. cerebrovascular accident) should be discussed. Hospice services are available for those dying of HF with the focus on relief of symptoms and suffering. Care may include the use of intravenous diuretics and inotropic agents and consideration for anxiolytics. Continuity of care between in-patient and out-patient settings should be preserved[7].

Coronary heart disease

Prevalence of coronary heart disease (CHD) increases in older subjects, attributed to advances in diagnosis. Measures to modify risk factors are instituted earlier today, as are treatment interventions[20]. Approximately 80% of fatal myocardial infarctions occur in those more than 65 years, with women having less favorable outcome[20,21]. Angina pectoris is common but the presentation is often atypical[21].

The underlying pathophysiology of acute coronary syndromes is the disruption and/or rupture of atherosclerotic plaques resulting in coronary thrombosis and obstruction[15]. Coronary occlusion and resultant myocardial ischemia without infarction is termed unstable angina[20].

The risk factors for CHD that are modifiable include hypertension, smoking, dyslipidemia, diabetes mellitus, elevated homocysteine levels and possibly inflammatory processes; non-modifiable factors are age, male gender, and premature CHD in family.

Hypertension, particularly systolic, is the most significant risk factor. Control of hypertension has been shown to decrease cardiovascular morbidity and mortality[20,22]. Isolated systolic hypertension is common in the elderly. Efforts to normalize blood pressure are important (see Chapter 48). Smoking is a risk factor in approximately 25% of individuals aged 65 and over; it has a propensity to increase tissue factor expression (proinflammatory effect) and cause direct endothelial injury, mechanisms that promote thrombogenicity and atherosclerosis[20,23]. Dyslipidemia is a well-recognized risk factor (discussion follows). Diabetes mellitus, mostly type 2, occurs in a fifth of older individuals[22]. The process of atherosclerosis may be accelerated through non-enzymatic glycation of lipoproteins[24]. Hyperhomocysteinemia is common in the elderly and is linked to the development of vascular disease in the heart, brain and elsewhere[25]. Homocysteine levels increase with age, male gender, renal insufficiency, deficiency of B vitamins (folic acid, B_{12}, B_6), use of certain drugs (e.g. nitrous oxide, phenytoin, methotrexate), diseases (e.g. hypothyroidism) and inherited enzyme deficiencies[25,26]. Chronic infections and C reactive protein (CRP) increasingly appear to be associated with CHD. *Chlamydia pneumoniae*, *Streptococcus viridans* and *Helicobacter pylori* are some of the infectious agents that have been linked[27] (Table 3).

The elderly with myocardial ischemia most often present with dyspnea rather than chest pain; approximately 40% have silent ischemia. Atypical symptoms such as confusion, lethargy, abdominal pain or nausea (interpreted as of gastrointestinal origin) and shoulder pain (falsely attributed to musculoskeletal origin) are not uncommon[28,29].

Diagnostic evaluation for CHD includes a thorough history whenever possible. The findings on physical examination may be non- specific; signs of atherosclerosis may be evident in other organ systems. The electrocardiogram (ECG) may show non-specific ST–T changes or ST segment depression rather than elevation[29]. Serial ECGs and cardiac enzymes (troponin I, creatine phosphokinase) help exclude or rule in a diagnosis of an acute myocardial infarction. Non-invasive investigations (exercise testing, with optional nuclear imaging and echocardiography with or without pharmacologic agents) are used for diagnosis and prognosis[29]. Coronary arteriography is the gold standard for evaluation of

Table 3 Impact of risk factors on coronary heart disease

Smoking
Increased thrombogenicity
Increased atherosclerosis
Decreased oxygen delivery

Hypertension
Increased afterload
Increased myocardial demand

Dyslipidemia
Increased atherogenesis and plaque formation

Diabetes mellitus
Accelerated atherosclerosis
Augmented platelet adhesiveness
Increased levels of tissue factor

Hyperhomocysteinemia
Endothelial injury
Collagen deposition in atherosclerotic plaque
Prothrombotic effect

Obesity
Increased adaptive hemodynamic demands

Chronic infections and CRP
Inflammatory cytokines increase degradative enzymes
Increased thrombogenesis

CRP, C reactive protein

CHD; however, in the elderly its role has limitations in that there is an increased occurrence of significant coronary atherosclerosis with the clinical anatomic correlation not as accurate as in the young[29].

Education of the patient as well as the caregiver is important. Again, lifestyle modification is important. Measures include smoking cessation, moderation of alcohol intake, exercise and appropriate diet. Treatment of concomitant risk factors, e.g. dyslipidemia, diabetes mellitus, hypertension and hyperhomocysteinemia, should be addressed.

In unstable angina where intravascular thrombosis is a major concern, antithrombotic treatment plays an important role in addition to the use of aspirin, clopidogrel, β-blockers and nitrates. Heparin dose is weight adjusted with initial bolus of 60–70 units/kg (maximum 5000 units) followed by an infusion of

12–15 units/kg, to attain activated partial thromboplastin time of one and a half to twice the control for at least 48 h[30]. Glycoprotein IIB/IIIA inhibitors and low molecular weight heparin may reduce acute events, but their exact role and efficacy in the elderly is ill defined[29]. Use of these agents is individualized to high risk patients without contraindications[30]. Calcium channel blockers, e.g. diltiazem and verapamil, are used only when β-blockers are contraindicated[29].

Management of acute myocardial infarction (AMI) in the elderly requires an astute individualized approach. Age by itself is not a contraindication for reperfusion therapy either by thrombolysis or coronary angioplasty. Administration of thrombolytic therapy within 6–12 h of ischemic chest pain and ST elevation or left bundle branch block improves mortality[31,32]. However, most geriatric patients are asymptomatic and do not present with a typical ECG finding, causing delay in diagnosis; besides, there is a greater risk of bleeding, especially with recombinant tissue plasminogen activator (rtPA) rather than streptokinase[33]. Percutaneous transluminal coronary angioplasty in AMI is as effective as thrombolytic therapy with less risk of intracranial bleeding, but it is not readily available in most centers.

Ideally, non-enteric coated aspirin (160–325 mg) chewed and swallowed is administered promptly in AMI and subsequently the enteric or non-enteric form is continued on a daily basis. Ticlodipine or clopidogrel may be used in those unable to tolerate aspirin or unresponsive to aspirin (class IIb indication)[32]. Clopidogrel should be added at the earliest in non-ST-segment elevation myocardial infarction[30]. Intravenous β-blockers (atenolol and metoprolol) within the first 12 h have been shown to improve mortality, and reduce reinfarction and arrhythmias[33]. ACE inhibitors are recommended in the presence of anterior wall myocardial infarction, AMI with left ventricular systolic dysfunction and ejection fraction

Table 4 Aortic stenosis in the elderly

Etiology
Most common: degenerative
Less common: rheumatic or congenital

Features
Anacrotic pulse may be absent
Hypertension may co-exist
Aortic murmur may radiate to the apex
Murmur may not be typical

Presentation
Asymptomatic, syncope, angina, HF

Diagnosis
ECG shows LVH in 50% of cases
Chest radiography: valve calcification in lateral view
2D echocardiography
   cusp thickening and calcification
   jet velocity
   transvalvular gradient
   valve area

Management
Surgical valve replacement
   mechanical
   bioprosthetic
Valvuloplasty – poorer option

HF, heart failure; ECG, electrocardiogram; LVH, left ventricular hypertrophy; 2D, two-dimensional

less than 40%. ACE inhibitors should be prescribed even with normal left ventricular function, in the presence of high risk CHD[30]. Nitrates are given for relief of ischemic symptoms, HF, large anterior infarction or hypertension[31,32], although long-term use does not influence prognosis. Antiarrhythmics are not routinely given.

The US Preventive Services Task Force (USPSTF) in its guidelines states there is good evidence for the use of aspirin for primary prevention in patients at increased risk of CHD. The use of aspirin is associated with increased risk of gastrointestinal bleeding and hemorrhagic strokes. Risks, benefits and patient preferences influence final decision; it is favorable in those with a 5 year CHD risk of over 3%[34]. The dose of aspirin for primary prevention is not clear from trials; doses have ranged from 75 mg to 500 mg once a day. It is believed that for prevention of myocardial infarction low doses of aspirin (less than 100 mg per day) suffice; it is unclear if the dose of aspirin relates to the risk of bleeding[35].

Valvular heart disease

Cardiac murmurs, particularly systolic, are frequently audible on routine evaluation in the presence or absence of significant heart disease[36]. A murmur is generated whenever the blood flow is high and also when the flow is normal but the valve is stenosed or incompetent, criteria commonly present in older adults. Murmurs are graded based on intensity from grade I through VI, I being the mildest and VI the most profound[36]. Although any valve may be affected, aortic stenosis and mitral regurgitation are particularly common.

Aortic stenosis is common in the older age group, but relatively less recognized because of vague and gradual progression of symptoms[37]. The characteristic harsh systolic murmur may not be appreciated. Aortic stenosis is usually due to degenerative calcification of the trileaflet valve or secondary calcification of a pre-existing bicuspid aortic valve, the latter more common in the below 60 age group[37]. The cardinal manifestations are syncope, angina and HF. While limitation of exercise tolerance is the usual initial presentation, the presence of HF heralds a poor prognosis[22,37]. More important, the manifestation of aortic stenosis differs from that in the young, in that the elderly may not manifest the anacrotic pulse, hypertension may be co-existent, the aortic murmur may radiate to the apex instead of the neck or may even be absent, and when present it may not have the classic midsystolic ejection qualities[24]. Aortic sclerosis, the term used for thickening and calcification of the aortic valve, without significant obstruction, may represent the same process in its mildest form without functional consequences[37]. Two-dimensional echocardiogram with pulse Doppler helps to assess the severity of stenosis and flow gradient. Asymptomatic individuals may be monitored and surgery deferred until symptoms develop or the flow gradient exceeds 50 mmHg, when surgery needs consideration[22,38]. Prophylaxis for infective endocarditis is indicated as per standard guidelines (e.g. American Heart Association recommendations). Symptomatic patients should be referred for surgical valve replacement regardless of age, except when risk for surgery is high from co-morbidity[33]. Valves may be mechanical or bioprosthetic; where a mechanical valve is inserted anticoagulation therapy is indicated for life. Valvuloplasty is a poorer second option (Table 4).

Mitral regurgitation is observed in approximately half of the older subjects from annular calcification, and is mostly found incidentally[37]. The prevalence increases with age. Other causes of mitral regurgitation are mitral valve prolapse and ischemia induced, e.g. papillary muscle dysfunction or rupture. Mitral valve prolapse is associated with increased occurrence of atrial fibrillation and HF[22]. The most frequent etiology of significant mitral regurgitation necessitating surgery in the geriatric age group is mitral valve prolapse[22,37]. Diagnosis is entertained in the presence of a holosystolic murmur, prominent at the apex that radiates to the axilla or at times anteriorly to the precordium, and confirmation is by two-dimensional echocardiogram with Doppler. Medical management includes endocarditis prophylaxis, periodic echocardiograms and symptomatic relief of pulmonary congestion. Mitral valve repair has a lower operative risk compared to valve replacement, with good outcome, and is the procedure of choice in the older age group[37].

Aortic regurgitation occurs from aortic valvular sclerosis or aortic root dilatation as a result of atherosclerosis and/or hypertension. Medical or surgical intervention is seldom required; however, in the presence of progressive left ventricular dysfunction, ACE inhibitors may be used to reduce afterload. Endocarditis prophylaxis is again indicated. In the presence of acute chest pain with a new finding of aortic regurgitation, aortic dissection should be excluded[37].

Mitral stenosis is often unsuspected in the elderly until symptoms of pulmonary congestion and/or atrial fibrillation develop[17]. Medical treatment with diuretics, anticoagulation and control of ventricular rate in the presence of atrial fibrillation and endocarditis prophylaxis are appropriate[37].

Cardiac dysrhythmias

Changes in the conduction system predispose to dysrhythmias, frequently in the presence of cardiac disease. Asymptomatic unifocal or multifocal premature ventricular contractions (PVCs) are most common on 24-h Holter monitoring, and may not warrant treatment[39]. The important dysrhythmias include ventricular tachycardia, associated with increased risk of myocardial infarction and death, while atrial fibrillation, atrioventricular block and sinus bradycardia are linked to future cerebrovascular accidents[39].

Ventricular tachycardia

Three or more consecutive premature ventricular contractions comprise ventricular tachycardia[40]. It is considered sustained if duration exceeds 30 seconds. Non-sustained ventricular tachycardia occurs in 4% of older subjects without cardiac disease; when asymptomatic, treatment is deferred in such cases, due to risk of drug-induced proarrhythmia. On the other hand, in symptomatic ventricular arrhythmias with accompanying cardiac disease, therapy is suggested utilizing β-blockers or amiodarone, and an implantable defibrillator for those unresponsive to drug therapy[41]. Prophylactic implantation of a defibrillator improves survival in those with prior myocardial infarction associated with severe left ventricular dysfunction[42].

Atrial fibrillation

Atrial fibrillation affects 2.2 million Americans, which is likely to be an underestimate of the actual prevalence, because of the absence of symptoms and undersampling during trials[43]. Structural age- and/or disease-related cardiac changes (e.g. left atrial enlargement, left ventricular hypertrophy), hypertension, CHD, hypoxemia, hyperthyroidism, fever, alcohol consumption and electrolyte abnormalities are predisposing factors. Atrial fibrillation is the most common persistent arrhythmia in the geriatric population[41].

Atrial fibrillation increases the risk of stroke by four to five times over that of the general population due to increased stasis, thrombus formation in the left atrium and possibly induction of a hypercoagulable state[43]. In a recent study lone atrial fibrillation (in the absence of morphologic heart disease) in subjects over 60 years old was associated with a higher risk for stroke and development of chronic atrial fibrillation[43]. Management of atrial fibrillation includes identification and correction of reversible causes, conversion to and maintenance of sinus rhythm, rate control and most importantly stroke prevention.

Antiarrhythmics (class Ia: quinidine, procainamide; class Ic: flecainide, propafenone; class III: sotalol, amiodarone, dofetilide) are used with caution for conversion to and maintenance of sinus rhythm[44]. Rate control can be achieved with the use of β-blockers, calcium channel blockers and/or digoxin especially in the presence of left ventricular dysfunction. Stroke prevention is accomplished with aspirin for those less than 60 years and without risk factors. Warfarin is used in the presence of risk factors and in those more than 75 years, to maintain an

Table 5 Management of atrial fibrillation

Search for risk factors
Reversible
  alcohol
  drugs
  electrolyte abnormalities
  hypoxemia
  thyroid disorders
Irreversible
  age
Modifiable
  coronary heart disease
  hypertension
  left atrial enlargement
  left ventricular systolic dysfunction

Conversion to sinus rhythm
Chemical cardioversion (class Ia, Ic, class III
  antiarrhythmics)
Electrical cardioversion

Stroke prevention
Aspirin
  age < 60 without risk factors
  age 60–75 without risk factors*
Warfarin
  any age with risk factors
  age > 75 with or without risk factors
Rate control
β-blockers
Digoxin
Calcium channel blockers

* Warfarin may also be given

international normalized ratio between 2 and 3 (Table 5)[44]. Implantable pacemakers and defibrillators are new therapeutic options in the prevention and treatment of atrial fibrillation and enhance quality of life[45].

Bradyarrhythmias

The reduction in the number of pacemaker cells, diminished sensitivity to β-adrenergic stimulation as well as the use of multiple drugs, e.g. digoxin, β-blockers (oral or ocular preparations), calcium channel blockers, clonidine, etc. predispose the elderly to heart blocks and sinus pauses. When sick sinus syndrome (tachycardia–bradycardia) presents as sinus arrest and syncope, pacemaker insertion is indicated. A permanent pacemaker

improves cardiovascular function and quality of life[41]; dual chamber pacing is the favored mode, and maintains physiologic synchrony, reducing the incidence of strokes and HF[41]. Pacemaker syndrome is usually associated with VVI (ventricularly paced, sensed, inhibited) pacing due to loss of atrioventricular synchrony and manifests as dyspnea, palpitations, flushing and syncope[46]; it is uncommon with dual chamber pacing.

MISCELLANEOUS CONDITIONS RELEVANT TO AGING

Dyslipidemia

Increased low-density lipoprotein (LDL) cholesterol promulgates atherogenesis not only in early stages of atherosclerosis, but also in the presence of heart disease[20]. Other abnormal lipid states such as elevated triglycerides and low levels of high-density lipoprotein (HDL) are also atherogenic. The most common cause of mortality in the geriatric population is cardiovascular disease; it is conceivable that correction of lipid abnormalities is beneficial in this regard from extrapolated data[20].

The role of serum cholesterol concentration in aging has been studied; an increased ratio of total cholesterol to HDL is associated with a greater risk for all-cause mortality in ages 65 and over[47], while low HDL is a predictor of new coronary events[48]. Is it then advantageous to decrease cholesterol in this age group? While all sources do not concur (e.g. American College of Physicians), data support the application of The National Cholesterol Education Program Guidelines for the young old (65–75 years), where screening is recommended for serum cholesterol and lipid fractions even in the absence of established CHD. More recently, the Adult Treatment Panel (ATP) III has made definite recommendations for the elderly; no age limit has been set for treatment[49,50]. The current belief is that older adults get the same or more benefit following treatment as younger individuals. The ATP III report suggests better identification of those at risk; type 2 diabetes without CHD confers similar risk to that of CHD. A fasting lipoprotein profile is now recommended for screening, with an HDL level less than 40 mg/dl (instead of 35) recognized as a risk factor and above 60 mg/dl as protective. The LDL goal is 100 mg/dl or lower in patients with CHD and diabetes without CHD. The panel also believes that statins will be required by many older patients, especially those with CHD[49,50]. In the absence of CHD but with risk factors, assessment of co-morbid status and life expectancy should be weighed against the benefits and risks of therapy. When HMGCoA reductase inhibitors (statins) are used, drug–drug interactions become a consideration in older subjects who are on several medications for co-morbid conditions[48].

Hormone replacement therapy

In the early 1980s, hormone replacement therapy (HRT) was used not just for menopausal symptoms and osteoporosis but also for possible protection from CHD. Estrogen is known to enhance endothelium-dependent coronary vasodilatation, raise HDL and triglyceride levels, reduce LDL and decrease plasminogen activator inhibitor type 1 (which improves fibrinolysis)[51]. In the late 1980s and early 1990s trials such as the Heart and Estrogen/Progestin Replacement Study (HERS) and Estrogen Replacement in Atherosclerosis (ERA), both for secondary prevention, published data on the lack of benefit for CHD and in fact an augmented risk for cardiac events, particularly in the first year of estrogen treatment[52]. The Nurses' Health Study, an observational study, also supports the initial increased risk of coronary events; however, on long-term follow-up,

coronary benefits have been demonstrated. A study in Japan claims that the estrogen-related increase in plasma triglycerides may result in increased levels of small LDL particles that are more susceptible to oxidation and are likely atherogenic[53]. Recent data from the WHI study[54] has indicated that the use of estrogen and progestin was associated with an absolute increase in risk of cardiovascular events and strokes at 5.2 years; these risks have to be weighed against the benefits of estrogen for postmenopausal symptoms and osteoporosis. At this time, HRT is not a recommendation for the primary or secondary prevention of CHD[54]. Based on available data and until further clarification, HRT may be a consideration for menopausal symptoms and osteoporosis but not for CHD.

Vascular disease

The belief that a vascular disease in one location should prompt investigation for vascular involvement at other sites has resulted in enhanced awareness of extracardiac vascular disease[55] involving the carotids, renal arteries, or peripheral vasculature. There is a linear relationship between the prevalence of peripheral vascular disease and aging, with 10% in ages 65 and older, and 20% in those 80 and above[56].

Peripheral arterial disease

Peripheral arterial disease is an atherosclerotic occlusive disorder distal to the aortic bifurcation[55]. The risk factors associated with CHD are again implicated (see Table 3); however, cigarette smoking is considered the most important[57]. Manifestations of arterial insufficiency include intermittent claudication, paresthesias, exertional muscle or limb weakness, compromised wound healing and, in advanced disease, rest pain[55]. On examination there may be evidence of diminished or absent pulses, vascular bruit, compromised capillary refill, loss of hair, muscle atrophy, skin changes, non- healing ulcers and gangrene. Absence of the dorsalis pedis or posterior tibial pulse is not always significant in older adults. A unilateral finding may be more suggestive. Clinical correlation is recommended. An ankle–brachial index (ABI) of 0.9 or lower suggests an occlusive lesion; 0.5 or lower connotes multilevel arterial disease; less than 0.26 indicates severely compromised status. In diabetics a higher resting ABI of 1.2–1.3 may be observed, due to medial vessel calcification[55]. Other non-invasive tests include duplex ultrasound and Doppler color flow imaging, magnetic resonance imaging/angiography, and digital imaging. Non-surgical management focuses on risk factor modification, e.g. smoking cessation, progressive treadmill exercise programs, drugs (aspirin, pentoxifylline, cilostazol) and gene therapy (still under investigation)[55,58]. Definitive treatment is surgical or catheter-based revascularization.

Aneurysms

A localized increase of the arterial diameter by 1.5 times its normal is referred to as an aneurysm[59]. While an abnormal arterial wall matrix may be the basis, the etiology is not definite[59]. Aneurysms are usually incidental findings, mostly involving the abdominal and thoracic aorta, and popliteal and iliac vessels. Most patients are asymptomatic and can be followed by serial sonography or computed tomography scans for rate of growth every 6 months or yearly[60]. Increased risk of rupture is noted in thoracic aortic aneurysms of 6 cm or greater and abdominal aortic aneurysms of 5 cm or more[59,61]. A recent British study revealed that ultrasonic surveillance is a management option for abdominal aortic aneurysms of 4 to 5.4 cms and repair for larger ones. Elective operative mortality is as low as 2% (in the real world closer to 5 to 8%), in carefully selected patients[62]. Life expectancy must be a consideration.

Venous thromboembolism

Venous thrombosis is common in advanced age, especially aggravated by concomitant risk factors such as HF, stroke, major surgery, prolonged immobilization, malignancy, obesity, venous insufficiency and prior venous thrombosis[22]. Acquired and hereditary coagulation inhibitor deficiencies and mutation in factor V Leiden which is responsible for activated protein C resistance (most common hereditary risk factor) are described in the elderly[63]. The dreaded complication of deep venous thrombosis is pulmonary embolism. Prophylaxis with the use of unfractionated heparin, low molecular weight heparin and/or warfarin are available options. In a tenth of cases of idiopathic deep venous thrombosis, an occult malignancy, usually adenocarcinoma, is present. Routine screening and evaluation for malignancy, e.g. mammography, Pap smear, gastrointestinal and prostate evaluation, are suggested when applicable.

Cardiac amyloidosis

The senile heart is commonly infiltrated with amyloid[64]. Deposits may take the form of isolated atrial amyloidosis, or diffuse deposition in the heart, and involve the conduction system. Patients may remain asymptomatic, with amyloidosis found only in autopsies, or manifest with HF, atrial fibrillation or heart blocks, sometimes lethal. Primary amyloidosis results from clonal plasma cell proliferation and is associated with multiple myeloma[64]. In a third of cases the heart is involved. When HF develops in patients with senile amyloidosis the prognosis is generally better compared to that caused by primary amyloidosis. The median survival for senile amyloidosis and heart failure is 5 years, whereas it is a few months for primary amyloidosis with heart failure[64]. The echocardiogram is a useful tool in diagnosis, but endomyocardial biopsy is definitive.

References

1. *Health and Aging Chartbook*. DHHS Publication (PHS). United States: US Department of Health and Human Resources, CDC, 1999:99–1232

2. Lakatta EG. Circulatory function in younger and older humans in health. In Hazzard WR, Blass JP, Ettinger WH, *et al.*, eds. *Principles of Geriatric Medicine and Gerontology*, 4th edn. New York: McGraw Hill, 1999:645–60

3. Dharmarajan TS, Ugalino JT. The aging process. In Dreger D, Krumm B, eds. *The Hospital Physician Geriatric Medicine Board Review Manual*. Wayne, PA: Turner White Communications 2000;1:1–12

4. Taffet GE. Age related physiological changes. In Cobbs EL, Duthie EH, Murphy JB, eds. *Geriatric Review Syllabus*, 4th edn. Dubuque, Iowa: Kendall/Hunt Publishing, 1999:10–23

5. Gomberg-Maitland M, Baran DA, Fuster V. Treatment of congestive heart failure. *Arch Intern Med* 2001;161:342–52

6. Hunt SA, Baker DW, Chin MH, *et al.* ACC/AHA guidelines for the evaluation and management of chronic heart failure in the adult: executive summary. *J Am Coll Cardiol* 2001;38:2101–13

7. Meier-Ernest HK, Gaasch WH. What is diastolic heart failure and how do we treat it? *Am College Cardiology Curr J Rev* 2001;10:52–4

8. Rich MW. Heart failure. In Hazzard WR, Blass JP, Ettinger WH, *et al.*, eds. *Principles of Geriatric Medicine and Gerontology*, 4th edn. New York: McGraw Hill, 1999: 679–700

9. Packer M, Cohn JN, Abraham WT, *et al.* Consensus recommendations for the management of CHF. *Am J Cardiol* 1999; 83:1A–38A

10. Metra M, Giubbini R, Nodari S, *et al.* Differential effects of beta-blockers in patients with heart failure. *Circulation* 2000;102:546–51

11. Pitt B, Zannad F, Remme WJ, *et al.* The effect of spironolactone on morbidity and mortality in patients with severe heart failure. *N Engl J Med* 1999;341:709–17

12. Califf RM, Cohn JN. Cardiac protection evolving role of angiotensin receptor blockers. *Am Heart J* 2000;139:S15–S22

13. Cohn JN, Tognoni G. A randomized trial of the angiotensin-receptor blocker Valsartan in chronic heart failure. *N Engl J Med* 2001;345:1667–75

14. Poole-Wilson PA. Treatment of acute heart failure: out with the old, in with the new. *J Am Med Assoc* 2002;287:1578–80

15. Baughman KL. B-Type natriuretic peptide – a window to the heart. *N Engl J Med* 2002;347:158–9

16. Kitzman DW. Diastolic dysfunction in the elderly genesis and diagnostic and therapeutic implications. *Cardiol Clin* 2000;18: 597–617

17. Elesber AA, Redfield MM. Approach to patients with heart failure and normal ejection fraction. *Mayo Clin Proc* 2001;76: 1047–52

18. Abraham WT, Fisher WG, Smith AL, *et al.* Cardiac resynchronization in chronic heart failure. *N Engl J Med* 2002;346:1845–53

19. Hare JM. Cardiac resynchronization therapy for heart failure. *N Engl J Med* 2002; 346:1902–5

20. Grundy SM. The role of cholesterol management in coronary artery disease risk reduction in elderly patients. *Endocrinol Metab Clin* 1998;27:655–75

21. Wei JY. Coronary heart disease. In Hazzard WR, Blass JP, Ettinger WH, *et al.*, eds. *Principles of Geriatric Medicine and Gerontology*, 4th edn. New York: McGraw Hill, 1999:661–8

22. Blazing MA, Galanos AN, O'Connor CM. Cardiovascular diseases and disorders. In Cobbs EL, Duthie EH Jr, Murphy JB, eds. *Geriatric Review Syllabus: a Core Curriculum in Geriatric Medicine*, 4th edn. Dubuque, Iowa: 1999:199–207

23. Goldstein MG, Niaura R. Methods to enhance smoking cessation after myocardial

infarction. *Med Clin North Am* 2000;84:
63–80

24. Goldberg RB. Cardiovascular disease in diabetic patients. *Med Clin North Am* 2000;84:81–93

25. Booth GL, Wang EEL. Preventive health cares 2000 update: screening and management of hyperhomocysteinemia for the prevention of coronary artery events. *Can Med Assoc J* 2000;163:21–9

26. Seshadri N, Robinson K. Homocysteine vitamins and coronary artery disease. *Med Clin North Am* 2000;84:215–37

27. Morrow DA, Ridker PM. C-reactive protein, inflammation, and coronary risk. *Med Clin North Am* 2000;84:149–61

28. Aronow WS, Tresch DD. Management of the older patient with acute myocardial infarction: difference in clinical presentations between older and younger patients. *J Am Geriatr Soc* 1998;46:1157–62

29. Freisinger GC, Ryan TJ. Coronary heart disease stable and unstable syndromes. *Cardiol Clin* 1999;17:93–122

30. Braunwald E, Antman EM, Beasley JW, *et al.* ACC/AHA Guideline update for the management of patients with unstable angina and non-ST-segment elevation myocardial infarction: a report of the American College of Cardiology/American Heart Association Task Force on Practice guidelines (Committee on the Management of Patients with Unstable Angina). 2002 (available at: http://www.acc.org/clinical/guidelines/unstable/unstable.pdf)

31. Ryan TJ, Anderson JL, Antman EM, *et al.* ACC/AHA Guidelines for the management of patients with acute myocardial infarction. *J Am Coll Cardiol* 1996;28: 1328–402

32. Ryan TJ, Antman EM, Brooks NH, *et al.* 1999 update: ACC/AHA guidelines for the management of patients with acute myocardial infarction. A report of the American College of Cardiology/American Heart Association Task Force on Practice guidelines (Committee on Management of Acute Myocardial Infarction). *J Am Coll Cardiol* 1999;34:890–911

33. Rich MW. Therapy of acute myocardial infarction in older persons. *J Am Geriatr Soc* 1998;46:1302–7

34. Berg AO, Allan JD, Frame PS, *et al.* Aspirin for the primary prevention of cardiovascular events: recommendation and rationale. US Preventive Services Task Force. *Ann Int Med* 2002;136:157–60

35. Lauer MS. Aspirin for the primary prevention of coronary events. *N Engl J Med* 2002;346:1468–74

36. Hara JH. Valvular heart disease. *Primary Care Clin Office Pract* 2000;27:725–40

37. Hinchman DA, Otto CM. Valvular disease in the elderly. *Cardiol Clin* 1999;17: 137–58

38. Rohenhek R, Binder T, Porenta G, *et al.* Predictors of outcome in severe, asymptomatic aortic stenosis. *N Engl J Med* 2000;343:611–17

39. Frishman WH, Heiman M, Karpenos A, *et al.* Twenty-four-hour ambulatory electrocardiography in elderly subjects: prevalence of various arrhythmias and prognostic implications (report from the Bronx Longitudinal Aging Study). *Am Heart J* 1996;132:297–302

40. Aronow WS. Therapy of older persons with ventricular arrhythmias. *Ann Longterm Care* 2000;8:35–44

41. Lampert R, Ezekowittz MD. Management of arrhythmias. *Clin Geriatr Med* 2000;16: 593–616

42. Moss AJ, Zareba W, Hall WJ, *et al.* Prophylactic implantation of a defibrillator in patients with myocardial infarction and reduced ejection fraction. *N Engl J Med* 2002;346:877–83

43. Chugh SS, Blackshear JL, Shen WK, *et al.* Epidemiology and natural history of atrial fibrillation: clinical implications. *J Am Coll Cardiol* 2001;37:371–8

44. Fuster V, Ryden LF, Asinger RW, *et al.* ACC/AHA/ESC Guidelines for the management of patients with atrial fibrillation: executive summary (A report of the American College of Cardiology/American Heart Association Task Force on Practice Guidelines and the European Society of

Cardiology Committee for Practice Guidelines and Policy Conferences). *J Am Coll Cardiol* 2001;38:1231–65

45. Cooper JM, Katcher MS, Orlov MV. Implantable devices for the treatment of atrial fibrillation. *N Engl J Med* 2002;346: 2062–8

46. Ross RA, Kenny RA. Pacemaker syndrome in older people. *Age Ageing* 2000;29:13–15

47. Chyou PH, Eaker ED. Serum cholesterol concentrations and all cause mortality in older people. *Age Ageing* 2000;29:69–74

48. Aronow WS. Drug therapy for older persons with hypercholesterolemia and vascular disease: the value of secondary prevention. *Ann Long term Care* 1999;7:135–9

49. Cleeman JI. Executive Summary of the Third Report of the National Cholesterol Education Program (NCEP) Expert Panel on Detection, Evaluation, and Treatment of High Blood Cholesterol in Adults (Adult Treatment Panel III). *J Am Med Assoc* 2001;285:2486–97

50. Sherman FT. New guidelines on high cholesterol ATP III report concludes it's never too late to consider treating our older patients. *Geriatrics* 2001;56:3–4

51. Heim LJ, Brunsell SC. Heart disease in women. *Primary Care Clin Clin Office Pract* 2000;27:741–66

52. Grady D, Hulley SB. Hormones to prevent coronary disease in women: when are observational studies adequate evidence? *Ann Intern Med* 2000;133:999–1000

53. Wakatsuki A, Ikenoue N, Okatani Y, *et al.* Estrogen induced small low-density lipoprotein particles may be atherogenic in postmenopausal women. *J Am Coll Cardiol* 2001;37:425–30

54. Rossouw JE, Anderson GL, Prentice RL, *et al.* Risks and benefits of estrogen plus progestin in healthy postmenopausal women: principal results from the Women's Health Initiative Randomized Controlled Trial. *J Am Med Assoc* 2002;288:321–33

55. Powers KB, Vacek JL, Lee S. Non invasive approaches to peripheral vascular disease. What's new in evaluation and treatment? *Postgrad Med* 1999;106:52–64

56. Newman AB. Peripheral arterial disease: insights from population studies of older adults. *J Am Geriatr Soc* 2000;48:1157–62

57. Meijer WT, Grobbee DE, Hunink MGM, *et al.* Determinants of peripheral arterial disease in the elderly. The Rotterdam Study. *Arch Intern Med* 2000;160:2934–8

58. McNamara DB, Champion HC, Kadowitz PJ. Pharmacologic management of peripheral vascular disease. *Surg Clin North Am* 1998;78:447–64

59. Gorton ME. Current trends in peripheral vascular surgery. When is surgical intervention the best option? *Postgrad Med* 1999;106:87–94

60. Gorski Y, Ricotta JJ. Weighing risks in abdominal aortic aneurysm best repaired in an elective, not an emergency procedure. *Postgrad Med* 1999;106:69–80

61. Bell R, Rosenthal RA. Surgery in the elderly. In Hazzard WR. Blass JP, Ettinger WH, *et al.*, eds. *Principles of Geriatric Medicine and Gerontology*, 4th edn. New York: McGraw Hill, 1999:391–411

62. Thompson RW. Detection and management of small aortic aneurysms. *N Engl J Med* 2002;346:1484–6

63. Andre E, Siguret V, Alhenc-Gelas M, *et al.* Venous thrombosis in older people: prevalence of the factor V gene mutation Q506. *J Am Geriatr Soc* 1998;46:1545–9

64. McCarthy RE, Kasper EK. A review of amyloidosis that infiltrate the heart. *Clin Cardiol* 1998;21:547–52

39 The gastrointestinal system

C.S. *Pitchumoni*, MD, FACP, FRCP(C), MACG, MPH,
Ajit J. *Kokkat*, MD, *and* T.S. *Dharmarajan*, MD, FACP, AGSF

INTRODUCTION

Older adults frequently present with gastrointestinal symptoms; the primary care providers are often faced with the dilemma of deciding whether these manifestations are age-related or secondary to disease. Common gastrointestinal disorders present atypically. Advanced age is no longer a barrier to investigation and treatment of disease. Knowledge of alterations in morphology and function with aging is essential to differentiate physiological changes from pathological processes (Table 1).

APPETITE, TASTE AND SMELL

Food intake is a motivated behavior enjoyed primarily through the senses of olfaction, taste, vision and hearing, all of which may be impaired in older adults. Significant olfactory loss from neuronal involvement consistently occurs as one ages. By the ninth decade, the olfactory threshold increases by about 50%, contributing to poorer smell recognition[1]. The ability to detect and discriminate between salt, sweet, sour and bitter tastes diminishes; each may be variably affected[2]. The circulating concentration of cholecystokinin, a gastrointestinal satiety hormone, is increased and linked to the anorexia of aging[3]. However, there appears to be no difference in either the hunger and desire to eat or satiety prior to meals between healthy older and younger subjects[4]. Dietary supplements and physical exercise by themselves do not improve

Table 1 Aging and the gastrointestinal system

Appetite
Desire to eat and satiety are intact
Cholecystokinin levels high
Taste detection and discrimination impaired
Poor smell recognition

Oral cavity
Fragile teeth, gingival recession, tooth discoloration
Tongue strength decreases
Taste buds not diminished in number, fewer lingual papillae
Basal salivary flow decreases, stimulated flow unchanged

Esophagus
Upper esophageal sphincter pressure lower
Gastric acid reflux common

Stomach
Acid secretion generally intact, decline from disease/drugs
Decreased mucosal prostaglandin synthesis
Emptying time generally preserved
Delayed emptying due to disease/drugs
Impaired gastric blood flow

Intestine
Enterocyte height and absorptive area unchanged
Nutrient and drug absorption generally preserved
Impaired absorption of calcium
Lactose intolerance common
Neuronal density reduced
Orocecal transit time constant
Insignificant decrease in anal sphincter tone

Hepatobiliary system
Decreased liver mass and volume
Reduced hepatic blood flow
Phase 1 metabolism declines, phase 2 relatively preserved
Liver function tests unchanged
Albumin synthesis generally preserved
Supersaturation of bile with cholesterol

Pancreas
Marginal displacement downwards
Decreased pancreatic mass, patchy fibrosis
Exocrine function unaffected

appetite[5]. Anorexia may be a manifestation of dementia, dysphagia, depression, dehydration or many other disorders. Patients with dementia find it difficult to make appropriate food choices, recognize items as food (agnosia) and feed themselves independently. They may have blunted thirst or hunger drives[6]. Depression is often underdiagnosed and screening for this disorder is indicated in subjects with altered appetite with no satisfactory explanation. Flavor enhancement and modification of the environment with provision of social interaction contribute to the joy of eating.

ORAL CAVITY

Teeth discoloration is common in older adults, possibly due to years of staining from bacteria, tea or tobacco[4]. Root canals narrow and roots become fragile. Gingival recession and cracking of enamel result in unsightly teeth. Incisal edges and cusps of teeth wear away with age, at the rate of $30\,\mu$m/year[4,7]. Tongue strength decreases, more so in females. The number of taste buds remains unchanged, although the number of lingual papillae may decrease[2]. Older adults are unable to open their mouths as wide or chew as strongly as younger subjects, due to progressive sarcopenia of the muscles of mastication[4]. Saliva helps in lubrication, cleaning and neutralization of acid regurgitated into the esophagus. As fat and fibrous tissue replace up to 25% of the secretory parenchyma of the salivary glands, basal salivary flow decreases while stimulated salivation remains unchanged, even with an edentulous state[4,8]. A dry mouth is often the result of medications such as antihistamines, diuretics and tricyclic antidepressants, or disease. Sugarless gum and sour candy are useful measures to alleviate this symptom.

ESOPHAGUS

Swallowing is a complex neuromuscular interaction requiring split-second co-ordination, involving oral, pharyngeal and esophageal phases. The oral phase is voluntary and involves mastication, formation of the food bolus and propulsion of the bolus posteriorly[9]. The pharyngeal phase is a reflex that transfers the bolus from the pharynx to the esophagus, involving tongue retraction, pharyngeal contraction, laryngeal closure and cricopharyngeal muscle relaxation. The esophageal phase involves a peristaltic wave that moves the bolus from the cervical esophagus to the stomach under the influence of the brainstem and the intrinsic myenteric plexus in the esophagus. With age, there is a decline in the number of myenteric ganglion cells and thickening of the esophageal smooth muscle layer[10]. The term 'presbyesophagus' was coined to describe abnormalities in esophageal motility (decreased contractile forces, polyphasic waves, partial sphincter relaxation and esophageal dilatation) thought to be age-related but more likely attributable to disease; the term has fallen out of favor[10]. Upper esophageal sphincter (UES) and lower esophageal sphincter (LES) activity are barriers against reflux of acid from the stomach. The UES maintains a high-pressure zone between the esophagus and pharynx, protecting the airway against entry of gastroesophageal refluxate. UES pressure is significantly lower in the elderly compared to the young[11]. Pharyngeal swallow may prevent aspiration by inducing glottal closure, sealing off the airway and clearing the pharynx of refluxate from the esophagus. A larger amount of liquid is required to trigger pharyngeal swallow in older adults[11]. The frequent presence of hiatal hernia in the elderly repositions the gastroesophageal junction above the diaphragm and is associated with decreased LES function[2]. These physiological changes in the elderly account for increased incidence of acid reflux.

Dysphagia

The presence of dysphagia in the elderly warrants evaluation. The history must include the onset, duration and progression of symptoms such as cough during mealtime and results of prior diagnostic tests in addition to a review of medications. A comprehensive neurologic examination is essential. Anatomic integrity and function of dentition, tongue, palate and pharynx must be evaluated. Examination of the neck may reveal adenopathy or an enlarged thyroid gland. Modified barium swallow with videofluoroscopy is the gold standard for studying the swallowing process[9]. This technique provides a motion recording while the patient swallows liquid barium, barium paste or solid food coated with barium, useful to evaluate for aspiration, pooling, bolus transit and motor function[9,12]. Fiberoptic endoscopic evaluation of swallowing via a fiberoptic nasolaryngoscope detects aspiration; accuracy is improved by concurrent use of methylene blue[9]. Scintigraphy bolus analysis helps evaluate for silent aspiration. Manofluorography (manometry with videofluoroscopy) measures the pressure gradient of the pharyngoesophageal junction during swallowing and is useful in neurogenic dysphagia[9].

Dysphagia can be oropharyngeal (transfer) or esophageal (transport). Oropharyngeal dysphagia secondary to cerebrovascular or degenerative brain disease is more frequent than transport dysphagia. Oropharyngeal dysphagia primarily affects the oral and pharyngeal phase of swallowing. Management is usually complicated by the presence of cognitive and/or motor impairments. Causes include disorders affecting the central nervous system (e.g. stroke, Parkinson's disease, Alzheimer's disease, trauma), the neuromuscular junction (e.g. myasthenia gravis) and muscle (e.g. myopathy secondary to endocrine disorders such as hyperthyroidism, hypothyroidism and Cushing's syndrome, or muscle dystrophy). Vitamin B_{12} deficiency can lead to vascular disease and pseudobulbar palsy secondary to corticobulbar tract dysfunction. Drugs can cause dysphagia either by affecting cognition and neuromuscular transmission or by inducing myopathy; examples include antidepressants, corticosteroids, aminoglycosides and anticholinergics. Esophageal causes of dysphagia include motility disorders, esophagitis and structural disorders (Table 2). Zenker's diverticulum is thought to result from decreased compliance of the cricopharyngeal muscle; manifestations (halitosis, regurgitation of undigested food, aspiration pneumonia, cough during meals) usually occur in the elderly[10].

Rehabilitation therapy involves strategies that employ the patient's natural compensatory mechanisms to accomplish adequate intake of food in a safe manner (safe swallow). Speech and swallow evaluation can determine the best consistency of diet for the individual; choices are level I (puree), level II (soft solids), level III (chopped), level IV (all foods except sliced roast beef, sliced poultry and bread) and level V (regular)[13]. One may apply a 'no thin liquids' restriction to patients at risk for aspiration. Thickeners may be added to achieve a honey-like consistency. Patients who cannot swallow thick liquids or puree effectively may be candidates for feeding tube placement.

Gastroesophageal reflux disease

Although symptoms from gastroesophageal reflux disease (GERD) are similar across age groups, complications such as esophagitis, stricture and Barrett's esophagus (replacement of the squamous epithelium of the esophagus by columnar epithelium) occur more often in older adults[14]. This fact, along with the possibility of carcinoma, necessitates consideration for endoscopy in older patients with GERD[14]. Older adults with decreased gastric acidity and reduced esophageal sensitivity are less likely to experience heartburn[14,15]. Patients complain of water brash, belching and nausea without emesis. Alarm symptoms such as dysphagia, weight loss, gastrointestinal bleeding and anemia are common and warrant immediate

Table 2 Etiology of esophageal (transport) dysphagia in older adults. From reference[9]

Etiology	Brief description
Motility disorders	
Diffuse esophageal spasms	multiple spontaneous large-amplitude contractions
	dysphagia, chest pain and regurgitation
	corkscrew appearance on barium swallow
Achalasia	degeneration of esophageal ganglion cells
	rare in the elderly
Scleroderma	smooth muscle atrophy, incompetent lower esophageal sphincter
	decreased peristalsis in distal esophagus
	predisposition to reflux, aspiration, cancer
Esophagitis	
Gastroesophageal reflux disease	most common cause of esophagitis
Infection	odynophagia often present
	herpes virus and *Candida* the usual basis
Radiation	may result from 4500–6000 rad over 6–8 weeks
Structural disorders	
Zenker's diverticulum	pharyngoesophageal diverticulum
	halitosis, regurgitation of saliva and food
Epiphrenic diverticula	located in the lower esophagus
	usually asymptomatic
Strictures, webs, rings	dysphagia to solid foods
	webs, e.g. Plummer–Vinson syndrome (post-cricoid, acquired)
	rings, e.g. Schatzki's rings (lower esophagus, common)
Neoplastic disease	squamous cell tumors, adenocarcinomas

investigation. Extraesophageal manifestations such as asthma, cough, chest pain, aspiration pneumonia and dental erosions may be atypical presentations which should suggest GERD[14]. Upper gastrointestinal symptoms warrant evaluation for a cardiac basis, as cardiovascular disease is also common in the elderly. Management of GERD involves lifestyle modifications and pharmacological treatments (Table 3). Proton pump inhibitors are effective in the management of even severe forms of GERD. Antireflux surgery is useful in a small number of patients, when response to medical treatment is poor. Prior to surgery, endoscopy (to exclude Barrett's esophagus) and manometry (to document adequate peristalsis) should be performed. There is no difference in morbidity, mortality and length of hospital stay in older adults undergoing open or laparoscopic Nissen fundoplication compared to younger patients[14].

Pill esophagitis

Drug-induced esophagitis results more often from direct injury due to prolonged contact than via systemic effects. Predisposing factors are inadequate fluid intake while swallowing the medication, pill size and shape, and supine posture during ingestion[12]. Drugs commonly implicated include enteric coated non-steroidal anti-inflammatory drugs (NSAIDs), alendronate, tetracyclines, potassium chloride, vitamin C, quinidine and iron tablets[9]. Barium swallow may suggest clustered ulcers or a stricture at the level of the gastroesophageal junction with endoscopy revealing pill fragments or ulcers with heaped-up margins[10]. Preventive measures include adequate water ingestion (180–240 ml), avoidance of lying down for at least 30 minutes post-pill intake and discontinuance of the offending drug if odynophagia or retrosternal chest pain occurs[12].

Table 3 Treatment of gastroesophageal reflux disease in the elderly. From reference 14

Lifestyle modifications
Weight reduction, if overweight
Stop smoking, as nicotine decreases LES pressure
Promote gastric emptying via a low-fat, high-protein diet
Minimize use of citrus juices, coffee, chocolate, tomatoes and alcohol
Elevate head of bed during sleep
Refrain from eating for 2–3 h prior to sleep

Medication review
Minimize use of drugs that decrease LES pressure, e.g. theophylline, anticholinergics and calcium channel blockers
Adequate water intake with drugs known to cause pill esophagitis, e.g. alendronate and potassium

Antacids
Use for immediate short-term symptomatic relief
Side-effects: sodium and magnesium overload, diarrhea, constipation and aluminum accumulation in renal failure

H_2-receptor blockers
Famotidine, cimetidine, ranitidine, nizatidine
Use prior to activity causing symptoms
Side-effects: delirium, drug interactions through cytochrome P450 system (e.g. cimetidine)

Proton pump inhibitors
Omeprazole, lansoprazole, pantoprazole, rabeprazole, esomeprazole
Use 15–20 min prior to eating

Prokinetic agents
Cisapride, associated with fatal arrhythmias (taken off the market)
Metoclopramide or domperidone, useful when abdominal bloating, nausea and vomiting are prominent
Side-effects of metoclopramide: tremors, dyskinesia, agitation and insomnia

LES, lower esophageal sphincter

STOMACH

While the data on acid production by the stomach in older adults is controversial, in general, the healthy elderly do not demonstrate a significant decrease in gastric acid secretion with age alone[4,16–19]. Atrophic gastritis appears to be responsible for the reduction of acid secretion associated with aging[19]. Atrophic gastritis is associated with pernicious anemia, especially in Northern European countries, and *Helicobacter pylori* infection, and is characterized by low serum pepsinogen and high serum gastrin levels[18]. Pernicious anemia is associated with parietal cell antibodies (non-specific) and antibodies to intrinsic factor (specific). Diminished gastric mucosal prostaglandin synthesis along with reduced secretion of bicarbonate and a reduction in gastric blood flow predispose older adults to NSAID-induced mucosal damage[4]. Data on gastric emptying and aging are inconsistent[4,19,20]. Explanations for delayed gastric emptying in older adults include higher prevalence of autonomic dysfunction and hypersensitive small intestinal receptors with increased inhibitory feedback[4]. Stimulation of small intestinal receptors leads to suppression of antral pressure waves, reduction of fundic tone and stimulation of pyloric pressure waves, all of which slow gastric emptying[20]. Radiolabeled liquid and solid meals demonstrate slowing of liquid emptying but unchanged solid-phase emptying with advancing age. Previously reported delays in gastric emptying were perhaps due to concurrent disease or medication use[19].

Gastroparesis

Gastroparesis is common in the elderly. Early satiety in older adults may be explained by reduced distensibility of the stomach with

Table 4   Features of the geriatric peptic ulcer. From references 6, 17, 19

Abdominal pain frequently absent or obscure
Substernal or precordial chest pain may mimic angina
Anorexia, weight loss and vomiting may be the presentation
More likely to develop complications compared to the young
Dysphagia can occur if ulcer is at gastroesophageal junction
Giant gastric ulcers may be the manifestation
Ulcer bleeding may initially present as cardiac or cerebral ischemia
Malignancy must be excluded

early filling of the antrum. Delayed gastric emptying is well recognized in diabetic autonomic neuropathy but also noticed is a delay during hyperglycemia and acceleration during hypoglycemia[20]. Gastroparesis can result in nausea, abdominal fullness and vomiting, erratic oral drug absorption, postprandial hypotension and alterations in glycemic control. Reversible causes scuh as drug side-effects, electrolyte abnormalities and hypothyroidism should be excluded. Investigations to measure gastric emptying include scintigraphy, ultrasound and radioisotopic breath tests; upper endoscopy can rule out gastric outlet and proximal small bowel obstruction[20]. Prokinetic agents (e.g. metoclopromide, domperidone and erythromycin) are used to treat symptomatic individuals.

Peptic ulcer disease

Geriatric patients account for over 80% of deaths from peptic ulcer disease in the USA[19]. Definite causes of peptic ulcer disease include *H. pylori* infection, NSAID use and Zollinger– Ellison syndrome. *H. pylori* disrupts the gastric mucus layer and cellular tight junctions of the mucosa. Eradication of *H. pylori* infection in all patients with gastric or duodenal ulcer in active or remission phase improves clinical outcome and reduces ulcer recurrence, symptoms and ulcer-associated chronic gastritis[21]. Although institutionalized older adults are at high risk for *H. pylori* infection, no specific hygienic or behavioral measures are currently recommended for minimizing *H. pylori* transmission in nursing homes[21]. Treatment regimens usually combine a proton pump inhibitor with two of the following antibiotics: amoxicillin, clarithromycin and a nitroimidazole (metronidazole/ tinidazole) for 1-week therapy; this regimen is effective and well tolerated by the elderly. The [^{13}C]urea breath test is the best non-invasive diagnostic method for confirming eradication of *H. pylori* infection after completion of therapy[21].

A high consumption of NSAIDs for a variety of musculoskeletal disorders occurs in the geriatric population. Chronic NSAID use results in direct superficial mucosal damage, reduced mucosal prostaglandin production, inhibition of mucus and bicarbonate secretion and decreased mucosal blood flow[19]. Risk of complications appears greatest in the initial three months. Bleeding in NSAID-induced ulcers may be painless; giant painless gastric or duodenal ulcers are characteristically seen (Table 4)[19]. The major complications of peptic ulcer disease include hemorrhage, perforation and gastric outlet obstruction. The underlying chronic anemia makes the episode of acute gastrointestinal (GI) bleeding life-threatening in a number of patients. Empiric use of anti-ulcer medication without diagnostic investigation is inappropriate; endoscopy is recommended in older adults to exclude malignancy[19]. Management strategies are listed in Table 5.

INTESTINE

Enterocyte height and jejunal absorptive area do not change with age[22]. Nutrient and drug

Table 5   Management of peptic ulcer disease in older adults. From reference19

Strategy	Comments
Life style	minimize use of NSAIDs, alcohol and tobacco
Antacids	sodium overload in renal and cardiovascular disease
	magnesium causes diarrhea; caution in renal failure
	aluminum causes constipation and osteomalacia
	calcium carbonate binds dietary phosphorus
Sucralfate	forms ulcer-adherent complex that is protective
	has aluminum, causes constipation, osteomalacia
	alters drug kinetics by drug adsorption
H_2 receptor antagonists	inhibit histamine-induced gastric acid secretion
	cimetidine and ranitidine interact with cytochrome P450 system; famotidine and nizatidine less likely
Misoprostol	synthetic prostaglandin E_1 analog
	reduces NSAID-induced ulcer risk
	causes dose-related diarrhea
Proton pump inhibitors	examples include omeprazole, lansoprazole, pantoprazole, rabeprazole, esomeprazole
	inhibit the parietal cell H^+/K^+ ATPase enzyme system
	profound acid suppression causes hypergastrinemia
Surgery	reserved for refractory ulcers and complications
	experience with laparoscopic approach limited

absorption are generally unaffected by aging except for certain micronutrients, e.g. calcium and zinc[2]. Small bowel responsiveness to vitamin D is diminished, due to decreased concentration of vitamin D receptors; this impairs active transport of calcium, resulting in increased parathyroid hormone levels and subsequent bone loss[4]. Lactose intolerance is common and predisposes to reduced dietary calcium intake; consumption of low-lactose, high-calcium alternatives such as cheese and yogurt should be encouraged[23]. Small intestinal motility is usually intact[22]. Deposition of elastin and collagen reduces the compliance of the aging colon[24]. Neuronal density in the colon is reduced, but colonic transit time is not altered[2]. Constipation is a common occurrence in older adults; the subject is discussed in Chapter 27. An insignificant decrease in anal sphincter tone occurs; fecal incontinence is always pathological.

Bacterial overgrowth syndrome

Normally, the upper gastrointestinal tract has relatively few bacteria. Gastric acid, normal small intestinal motility and luminal immunoglobulin A (IgA) protect against the development of small intestinal bacterial overgrowth (SIBO). Anatomic changes such as strictures, postgastrectomy states, Crohn's disease and jejunal diverticulosis predispose to bacterial overgrowth[22]. Bacteria deconjugate bile acids, causing fat malabsorption, and utilize dietary carbohydrates and vitamin B_{12}. Older adults, without any clinically apparent predisposition or nutrient deficiency, presenting with non-specific symptoms such as anorexia, nausea and diarrhea, may have SIBO with colonic-type bacteria, e.g. Enterobacteriaceae[25]. Even if the hydrogen breath test is positive (suggesting occult SIBO), in the absence of malabsorption, treatment with antibiotics is not indicated[26].

Drug-induced diarrhea

A careful review of all the medications being consumed is essential in those presenting with diarrhea. Drugs lead to diarrhea by disrupting fluid and electrolyte absorption and excretion, damaging the intestinal mucosa or altering defenses. Diarrhea due to drugs that cause intestinal hypermotility (e.g. erythromycin, tacrine) is uncommon. On the other hand, secretory diarrhea results from drug activation of adenylate cyclase, which increases cyclic AMP, leading to active secretion of anions, e.g. bisacodyl and misoprostol. Alternatively, drugs inhibit $Na^+K^+ATPase$ activity with resultant fluid loss, e.g. digoxin and colchicine[27]. Osmotic diarrhea may occur with antacids containing magnesium and laxatives such as lactulose and sorbitol. NSAIDs, antineoplastic agents and methyldopa can cause mucosal damage, resulting in diarrhea. The number and quality of T helper and suppressor cells decline with advancing age; use of immunosuppressive drugs (e.g. corticosteroids) further impairs mucosal immune mechanisms[27].

Reduction of acid secretion (e.g. proton pump inhibitors, H_2 blockers) promotes gastric bacterial colonization. Anticholinergic agents (e.g. benztropine, tricyclic antidepressants) decrease intestinal motility, encouraging bacterial overgrowth. Antibiotics decimate the usual intestinal flora, leaving an ecological vacuum to be filled with organisms that may prove harmful, such as *Clostridium difficile*, *Clostridium perfringens*, *Salmonella* and *Shigella*. Of these, *C. difficile* is the most common cause of nosocomial intestinal infections, colonizing 21% of hospitalized patients and found in a fifth of antibiotic-associated diarrhea[28]. Probiotics involve the introduction of competing, non-pathogenic organisms, e.g. *Lactobacillus* strains and *Saccharomyces boulardii* into the gut to restore microbial balance, resulting in improvement of *C. difficile* colitis when used in combination with metronidazole or vancomycin. Spurious diarrhea from fecal impaction must always be ruled out; other causes of diarrhea applicable to the general population also deserve consideration.

Diverticulosis

Diverticular disease, frequent in older adults, is found in a third of persons over age 50 and in two-thirds over age 80[17]. Reduced dietary fiber and lack of exercise may contribute to high intraluminal pressures in the sigmoid colon which promote formation of diverticula, especially at sites where blood vessels penetrate the muscular layer[16]. Thus, changes in dietary habits particularly in Western societies have contributed to the increased prevalence of the disorder. Diverticulosis is mostly asymptomatic but may cause recurrent lower abdominal pain. Diverticulitis presents usually with left lower quadrant abdominal pain, fever and leukocytosis; barium enema and colonoscopy are to be avoided in the acute setting. Mild cases respond to oral trimethoprim–sulfamethoxazole or ciprofloxacin and metronidazole or clindamycin. Moderate to severe cases require intravenous ampicillin, metronidazole and an aminoglycoside; surgery is needed for obstruction, worsening sepsis or fistulae[16]. In contrast, diverticular bleeding is bright red in color, sudden and painless, and typically stops spontaneously[17,29]. Diagnostic techniques involve the use of scintigraphy, angiography and colonoscopy. Therapy includes radiographic selective embolization, and colonoscopic electrocoagulation, injection therapy and hemoclipping. Surgery is an option when other methods fail[30].

Gastrointestinal bleeding

The approach to GI bleeding in the elderly stresses resuscitation as the first priority with careful attention to fluid balance, hemodynamics and clinical status. The medication list as always should be reviewed particularly for aspirin, NSAIDs and warfarin. The ligament of Treitz forms the anatomic separation of the upper and lower GI tract. Nasogastric tube aspiration of blood suggests upper GI bleed; return of bilious fluid is reassuring. Elevation of serum urea nitrogen from absorption of hemoglobin breakdown products in the proximal small bowel may occur. The presence of occult blood in stools with or without iron deficiency warrants a search for gastrointestinal neoplasms. Colonoscopy is the first procedure to evaluate an asymptomatic geriatric patient with occult blood in the stool[29].

Common causes of upper GI bleed are peptic ulcer disease, erosive gastritis, esophagitis,

Table 6   Etiology of gastrointestinal (GI) bleeding in the elderly

	Common	Less common
Upper GI bleeding	peptic ulcer erosive gastritis esophagitis varices Mallory–Weiss tear	vascular ectasia aortoenteric fistula esophageal cancer gastric cancer duodenitis
Lower GI bleeding	diverticular disease vascular ectasia intestinal ischemia hemorrhoids benign polyps colon cancer	infectious colitis inflammatory bowel disease radiation colitis rectal ulcers

varices and Mallory–Weiss tear; rare causes include vascular ectasia, aortoenteric fistula, gastric cancer and duodenitis (Table 6)[29]. Surgical history of aortic aneurysm repair could be the clue for an aortoenteric fistula. Upper endoscopy, the procedure of choice, is diagnostic and therapeutic. Heat coagulation of the bleeding site in an ulcer and injection of vasoconstrictors and sclerosing agents in bleeding varices help promptly arrest the bleeding. An ulcer with an adherent clot or visible vessel has a high risk of rebleeding and warrants close observation. Gastric lavage with iced water is of dubious benefit[29]. Therapeutic endoscopy reduces the need for emergency surgery, combined with H_2 receptor antagonists or proton pump inhibitors. Where NSAID therapy is essential in a bleeder, consider the use of cyclooxygenase 2 (COX2) selective inhibitors or the addition of a proton pump inhibitor[17]. In our experience, upper GI bleeding in patients with feeding tubes was usually due to esophagitis, possibly from increased gastroesophageal reflux, and H_2 blocker therapy did not appear to be protective[31]. The role of proton pump inhibitor therapy in preventing esophagitis-related bleeding in this subset of patients is yet to be established.

Common causes of lower GI bleeding include diverticular disease, vascular ectasia, intestinal ischemia, neoplasms and hemorrhoids; rare causes include infectious colitis, inflammatory bowel disease, radiation colitis

and rectal ulcers[29]. Vascular ectasia are degenerative lesions found mostly in the cecum and right colon, associated with aging and cardiac disease, with risk of rebleeding. Ischemic colitis is characterized by bloody diarrhea and left lower quadrant abdominal cramps; the splenic flexure, descending colon and sigmoid colon are frequently affected. A plain radiograph of the abdomen may reveal colonic submucosal edema or 'thumbprinting' in ischemic colitis. Colonoscopy is the appropriate test to evaluate lower GI bleeding that allows thermocoagulation and snare polypectomy. A radionuclide technetium-99 bleeding scan may be performed if endoscopy cannot be performed or is unremarkable, to guide further angiographic evaluation[29].

Occult GI bleeding can be investigated with repeat upper endoscopy and colonoscopy, push enteroscopy (endoscope pushed into small bowel), enteroclysis (nasoenteric tube containing barium advanced under fluoroscopic guidance) and mesenteric angiography[29]. Small bowel and gastric vascular ectasia account for the majority of cases of occult GI bleeding.

HEPATOBILIARY SYSTEM

Aging is associated with a decreased liver mass and volume along with an age-related reduction in hepatic blood flow[32]. Although the metabolic function of the liver appears to decline with age, there is no difference in liver cell enzyme activity between old and young subjects[32]. Liver function tests remain unchanged and albumin synthesis is generally preserved. The cytochrome P450 enzymatic system *per se* is generally intact, although phase 1 metabolism (oxidation, reduction, hydrolysis), which is dependent on hepatic blood flow, declines with increasing age[17]. Phase 2 metabolism (conjugative processes) is less affected. Blood levels of alcohol are higher after ingestion because of a reduction in total body water and hepatic blood flow; however, the rate of alcohol metabolism is unchanged.

Gallstones are frequent incidental radiological findings in older adults for which no treatment is necessary. If they are symptomatic, elective cholecystectomy is a safe procedure. Choledocholithiasis is common (possibly from the gradual narrowing of the distal common bile duct or periampullary diverticula), for which endoscopic retrograde cholangiopancreatography with sphincterotomy is the treatment of choice[17]. Acalculous cholecystitis can occur in critically ill elderly patients.

Drug-induced liver disease

The increased prevalence of drug-induced hepatotoxicity can be attributed to polypharmacy (prescription and over-the-counter drugs) along with the age-related hepatic changes described above[32]. Altered plasma protein binding, with increased free drug levels and smaller volumes of distribution contribute to drug toxicity. NSAIDs induce mild hepatotoxicity which resolves when the drug is stopped. α-Methyldopa, amiodarone, tacrine, isoniazid, rifampin and pyrazinamide are other examples of drugs that cause hepatotoxicity[33]. Liver function tests should be checked within the first few weeks of starting new medications. Larger doses of acetaminophen may cause liver damage when associated with excessive alcohol consumption (depletion of glutathione)[16]. Abnormal liver function tests

should prompt consideration for a drug basis as etiology. Adverse drug effects may be minimized by reducing dosage with combination therapy, monitoring drug concentrations, improving nutritional status, regular review for side-effects, and surveillance of liver chemistries[32].

Hepatitis

Hepatitis A infection is rare, but risk of death from fulminant liver failure increases with advancing age; the vaccine is recommended for travelers to endemic areas, food handlers and patients with chronic liver diseases. Outbreaks of hepatitis B have been described in nursing home residents after shared use of bath brushes, non-disposable syringes and shaving appliances[31]. Interferon α for treatment of chronic hepatitis B in older adults should be initiated on an individual basis after due consideration of risks and benefits. Hepatitis C occurs with about the same frequency in the elderly as compared to the young, but the course is more indolent with lower serum aminotransferase levels[16]. Advanced age is not a contraindication for antiviral therapy in chronic hepatitis C infection, but most clinical trials did not include a significant number of older adults. Autoimmune hepatitis is usually mild, but severe disease should be treated with corticosteroids alone or in combination with azathioprine.

PANCREAS

Although there is a modest decline in pancreatic mass and a downward displacement with age, exocrine function as judged by cerulein-stimulated trypsin, chymotrypsin and lipase secretion is not affected[17]. An age-related pancreatic fibrosis occurs which is patchy[34]. The echogenicity of the pancreas increases with advancing age, possibly due to fibrosis and fatty infiltration, and the pancreatic duct diameter increases; this is considered pathological if it is over 3 mm[35]. Pancreatic β-cell secretion is inappropriately low in the presence of insulin resistance, as assessed by C-peptide concentrations[36]. Ammann described 'senile pancreatitis', a painless disorder characterized by pancreatic calcifications observed on routine abdominal radiographs in older adults[37].

CANCERS OF THE GASTROINTESTINAL TRACT

The incidence of adenocarcinoma in the older Caucasian population is rapidly increasing and nearly equals the incidence of squamous carcinoma. Predisposing factors include alcohol, tobacco and chronic gastric reflux (with Barrett's esophagus). Significant co-morbidity necessitates palliative therapy with radiation, laser ablation, esophageal prosthesis insertion or gastrostomy tube placement[17]. Gastric cancers are mostly adenocarcinomas and are common in Asia and South America[16]. *H. pylori* is associated with gastric lymphoma, gastric atrophy and intestinal metaplasia (a premalignant condition), and gastric cancer; partial to complete remission of gastric mucosa-associated lymphoma occurs with *H. pylori* therapy irrespective of age[21]. *H. pylori* screening and eradication is currently not recommended for cancer prevention in asymptomatic people with no known risk factors[21]. Tumors of the small bowel are rare and include adenocarcinomas, carcinoid tumors and lymphomas. Patients with celiac sprue and recurrence of symptoms despite adherence to a gluten-free diet should be investigated for malignancy, usually lymphoma[22]. As the prevalence of colon cancer increases with age, the positive predictive value of screening tests for colon cancer is high[17]. Colonoscopy is performed to screen for polyps and for surveillance of patients with adenomatous polyps[38]. The need for colonoscopy should be individualized based on indications, life expectancy and quality of life[38]. Recently, the US Preventive Services Task Force (USPSTF) issued recommendations on screening for colorectal cancer[39]. The USPSTF strongly recommends that adults over the age of 50 be screened for colorectal cancer, stating that benefits from screening outweigh potential harm. It further added that there is insufficient data as to which screening procedure is best in terms of cost, benefits and potential harm[39].

Hepatocellular carcinoma is associated with exposure to carcinogens and cirrhosis from several causes, e.g. chronic hepatitis B and C infection and hemachromatosis. Screening involves the use of ultrasound and testing for serum α-fetoprotein. Hepatic lobectomy and liver transplantation are feasible in selected patients; chemoembolization and percutaneous sclerosis of the tumor with absolute alcohol are palliative methods[31]. Pancreatic cancer is the most common cause of malignant biliary obstruction in the elderly; survival is often measured in months and otherwise healthy subjects should be offered curative resection[17].

ABDOMINAL PAIN

Abdominal pain is a frequent presentation in older adults; acute pain may generally be classified into four categories: peritonitis (appendicitis, diverticulitis, perforation), bowel obstruction (strangulated bowel, volvulus), vascular (ruptured or leaking aneurysm, mesenteric infarction) and non-specific (drug-related, angina, pneumonia)[40]. Most elderly patients with abdominal pain in one study had significant disease requiring hospitalization, with infection and obstruction the most likely basis[40]. Drug-induced pain is common (e.g. NSAIDs, erythromycin), and correlates with high prevalence of polypharmacy in the elderly. The source of abdominal pain may be extra-abdominal, such as pneumonia or myocardial infarction; these causes are associated with high mortality and should always be excluded. Finally, abdominal illness could be atypical in presentation, often necessitating the use of radiographic techniques such as ultrasound and/or CT scan to obtain a diagnosis[40]. Surgical consultation should not be delayed, as eventual need for surgery is much more likely in older adults than in the young[40].

SUMMARY

Normal aging is accompanied by several changes in the gastrointestinal system. Physiological changes may be difficult to differentiate from disease[2]. Anorexia, hypoalbuminemia, abnormal liver function and fecal incontinence are pathological. Dysphagia is common in the elderly, associated with morbidity and mortality, and warrants evaluation; optimal management strategy involves a customized approach[41]. Physicians may tend to pay less attention to conditions such as GERD, considered benign, especially in the presence of comorbid conditions; on the other hand, heartburn may cause difficulties in differential diagnosis from cardiac pain, resulting in a missed diagnosis of the cardiac or gastrointestinal problem[42]. Thus, opportunities exist for the primary health care provider of older adults to interact with the gastroenterologist or other consultants to maximize patient benefit[42]. Review of medications should be an integral part of the assessment. Treatment should not be denied on the basis of age alone; quality of life often guides management decisions.

References

1. Dharmarajan TS, Ugalino JT. The aging process. In Dreger D, Krumm B, eds. *Hospital Physician Geriatric Medicine Board Review Manual*. Wayne, PA: Turner White Communications, 2000;1:1–12

2. Dharmarajan TS, Pitchumoni CS, Kokkat AJ. The aging gut. *Practical Gastroenterol* 2001;25:15–27

3. Morley JE, Thomas DR. Anorexia and aging: pathophysiology. *Nutrition* 1999;15:499–503

4. Blechman MB, Gelb AM. Aging and gastrointestinal physiology. *Clin Geriatr Med* 1999;15:429–38

5. de Jong N, Paw MJ, de Graf C, *et al*. Effect of dietary supplements and physical exercise on sensory perception, appetite, dietary intake and body weight in frail elderly subjects. *Br J Nutr* 2000;83:605–13

6. Dharmarajan TS, Ugalino JT, Kathpalia R. Anorexia in older adults: consequence of aging or disease? *Practical Gastroenterol* 2000;23:82–92

7. Christensen GJ. The inevitable maladies of the mature dentition. *J Am Dent Assoc* 2000; 131:803–4

8. Bergdahl M. Salivary flow and oral complaints in adult dental patients. *Community Dent Oral Epidemiol* 2000;28:59–66

9. Domenech E, Kelly J. Swallowing disorders. *Med Clin North Am* 1999;83:97–113

10. Sallout H, Mayoral W, Benjamin SB. The aging esophagus. *Clin Geriatr Med* 1999; 15:439–56

11. Shaker R, Hogan WJ. Reflex-mediated enhancement of airway protective mechanisms. *Am J Med* 108:8S–14S

12. Ouatu-Lascar R, Triadafilopoulos G. Oesophageal mucosal diseases in the elderly. *Drugs Aging* 1998;12:261–76

13. Ancheta JI, Reding MJ. Stroke diagnosis and treatment: a multidisciplinary effort. In Hazzard WR, Blass JP, Ettinger WH Jr, *et al.*, eds. *Principles of Geriatric Medicine and Gerontology*, 4th edn. New York: McGraw-Hill, 1999:1239–56

14. Mullick T, Richter JE. Chronic GERD. Strategies to relieve symptoms and manage complications. *Geriatrics* 2000;55:28–43

15. Fass R, Pulliam G, Johnson C, *et al*. Symptom severity and oesophageal chemosensitivity to acid in older and young patients with gastro-oesophageal reflux. *Age Ageing* 2000;29:125–30

16. Schaefer DC, Cheskin LJ. Gastrointestinal diseases and disorders. In Cobbs EL, Duthie EH Jr, Murphy JB, eds. *Geriatric*

Review Syllabus, 4th edn. Dubuque, Iowa: Kendall/Hunt Publishing, 1999:249–55

17. Quirk DM, Friedman LS. Approach to gastrointestinal problems in the elderly. In Yamada T, Alpers DH, Laine L, *et al.*, eds. *Textbook of Gastroenterology*, 3rd edn. Philadelphia: Lippincott Williams and Wilkins, 1999:1015–33

18. Oksanen A, Sipponen P, Karttunen R, *et al.* Atrophic gastritis and *Helicobacter pylori* infection in outpatients referred for gastroscopy. *Gut* 2000;46:460–3

19. Borum ML. Peptic-ulcer disease in the elderly. *Clin Geriatr Med* 1999;15:457–71

20. Kong MF, Horowitz M. Gastric emptying in diabetes mellitus: relationship to blood-glucose control. *Clin Geriatr Med* 1999;15:321–38

21. Pilotto A, Mario FD, Franceschi M. Treatment of *Helicobacter pylori* infection in elderly subjects. *Age Ageing* 2000;29:103–9

22. Nagar A, Roberts IM. Small bowel diseases in the elderly. *Clin Geriatr Med* 1999;15:473–86

23. Goulding A, Taylor RW, Keil D, *et al.* Lactose malabsorption and rate of bone loss in older women. *Age Ageing* 1999;28:175–80

24. Camilleri M, Lee JS, Viramontes B, *et al.* Insights into the pathophysiology and mechanisms of constipation, irritable bowel syndrome and diverticulosis in older people. *J Am Geriatr Soc* 2000;48:1142–50

25. Riordan SM, McIver CJ, Wakefield D, *et al.* Small intestinal bacterial overgrowth in the symptomatic elderly. *Am J Gastroenterol* 1997;92:47–51

26. Lewis SJ, Potts LF, Malhotra R, *et al.* Small bowel bacterial overgrowth in subjects living in residential care homes. *Age Ageing* 1999;28:181–5

27. Ratnaike RN, Jones TE. Mechanisms of drug-induced diarrhea in the elderly. *Drugs Aging* 1998;13:245–53

28. Pochapin M. The effect of probiotics on *Clostridium difficile* diarrhea. *Am J Gastroenterol* 2000;95:S11–S13

29. Rosen AM. Gastrointestinal bleeding in the elderly. *Clin Geriatr Med* 1999;15:511–25

30. Poulos JE, Zachary PE, Ramrakhiani S. Diverticular hemorrhage: pathogenesis, diagnosis and treatment. *Pract Gastroenterol* 2002;26:13–22

31. Yadav D, Kokkat A, Dharmarajan TS, Pitchumoni CS. Upper GI bleeding in PEG patients: is esophagitis the commonest cause? *J Am Med Dir Assoc* 2001;2:A7 (abstr)

32. Varanasi RV, Varanasi SC, Howell CD. Liver diseases. *Clin Geriatr Med* 1999;15:559–70

33. Kumar SK, Dharmarajan TS, Pitchumoni CS. Drug-induced liver disease in older adults. *Practical Gastroenterol* 2001;25:43–60

34. Pitchumoni CS, Glasser M, Saran RM, *et al.* Pancreatic fibrosis in chronic alcoholics and nonalcoholics without clinical pancreatitis. *Am J Gastroenterol* 1984;79:382–8

35. Glaser J, Stienecker K. Pancreas and aging: a study using ultrasonography. *Gerontology* 2000;46:93–6

36. Gama R, Medina-Layachi N, Ranganath L, *et al.* Hyperproinsulinemia in elderly subjects: evidence for age-related pancreatic beta-cell dysfunction. *Ann Clin Biochem* 2000;37:367–71

37. Ammann RW. Chronic pancreatitis in the elderly. *Gastroenterol Clin North Am* 1990;19:905–14

38. Miller KM, Waye JD. Approach to colon polyps in the elderly. *Am J Gastroenterol* 2000;95:1147–51

39. Berg AO, Allan JD, Frame PS, *et al.* Screening for colorectal cancer: recommendation and rationale. US Preventive Services Task Force. *Ann Intern Med* 2002;137:129–31

40. Dang C, Aguilera P, Dang A, Salem L. Acute abdominal pain: four classifications can guide assessment and management. *Geriatrics* 2002;57:30–42

41. Akhtar AJ, Shaikh A, Funnye AS. Dysphagia in the elderly patient. *J Am Med Dir Assoc* 2002;3:16–20

42. Pitchumoni CS, Lin M, Dharmarajan TS. Gastroesophageal reflux disease in the elderly. *Pract Gastroenterol* 2002;26:13–29

40 Renal and electrolyte disorders in older adults

T.S. Dharmarajan, MD, FACP, AGSF, Durairaj Venkatasamy, MD, and Robin O. Russell, MD

INTRODUCTION

Demographic trends the world over in developing as well as other countries show an increasing number of people attaining old age as a result of improved health care, nutrition, sanitation and preventive health management. Six per cent of the world population is over age 65; in the USA, a fifth of the population will be in the same category by the year 2030[1].

With economic and social development, disease patterns in the geriatric population have shifted from infection to chronic disease These include cardiac, cerebral and renal diseases, as well as others. Aging is also associated with a decline in homeostatic reserves in most systems, the kidney being a prime example[2]. Age-related physiological changes are further compounded by diseases such as hypertension and diabetes mellitus. The evaluation and management of renal and electrolyte disorders in the elderly has become a challenge to the primary care physician. The following review will describe the morphologic and physiologic alterations associated with aging and discuss pertinent disease processes.

STRUCTURAL CHANGES IN THE AGING KIDNEY

With advancing age there is a 10–43% decline in renal size and weight. Total kidney mass drops from 250–270 g in young adults to 180–200 g by the eighth decade[3]. The predominant decrease is in the renal cortex: the total number of functioning glomeruli declines; hyalinized glomeruli increase from 1–2% in young adults to over 10% after age 70, with sclerosis increasing up to 30% in some healthy persons beyond 80 years[3]. Glomerular basement membrane (GBM) thickening, followed by hyaline deposition, eventually leads to glomerulosclerosis, predominantly cortical. Glomerular mesangial cells increase with matrix expansion, from 8% of total glomerular volume in middle age to 12% by the eighth decade. Minute diverticuli are seen in the collecting duct system, the importance of which is unclear; they may play a role in the development of pyelonephritis by harboring organisms[4]. The arcuate arteries (branches of interlobar arteries) become angulated and irregular while the smaller vessels are spared. A high percentage of direct communication exists between afferent and efferent arterioles in the areas of glomerulosclerosis[5]. Autopsy angiograms and histopathology demonstrate spiraling in afferent arterioles, and aglomerular cortical and juxtamedullary arterioles with aging[5]. Despite changes in morphology, glomerular permeability does not change appreciably[6].

Tubular changes include a decrease in number, tubular epithelium atrophy and

Table 1 Renal changes with aging

Morphologic changes
Decrease in total kidney mass, cortex more than medulla
Decrease in total number of glomeruli and tubules
Sclerosis of glomeruli with hyperfiltration of remaining glomeruli
Thickening of glomerular basement membrane and tubular basement membrane
Increase in mesangial matrix
Tubular dilatation and diverticula formation
Interstitial fibrosis
Hyalinosis of arterial walls
Shunting of blood from afferent to efferent arterioles

Functional changes
Decreased glomerular filtration rate
Increased filtration fraction
Decreased renal blood flow, cortex more affected
Impaired sodium conservation and excretion
Impaired urinary concentration and dilution
Impaired ability to excrete an acid load
Impaired potassium excretion
Decreased tubular reabsorption of glucose (TmG decreased)
Decreased tubular reabsorption of phosphate

TmG, tubular maximum for glucose

dilatation of tubules. The tubular basement membrane thickens and the interstitium reveals evidence of fibrosis[6]. Increased connective tissue is noted in the medullary interstitium compared to the cortex[7]. Although uncertain, diet, toxins, immune-mediated injury, mesangial fatigue, change in the composition of the GBM and hydraulic or hemodynamic factors are thought to play roles in the genesis of glomerular aging[8] (Table 1).

FUNCTIONAL CHANGES IN THE AGING KIDNEY

Glomerular function

Between the ages of 30 and 60, renal blood flow falls progressively at a rate of 10% per decade. Effective renal plasma flow falls from approximately 600 ml/min in the third decade to 300 ml/min by the ninth decade[5]. However, the filtration fraction (glomerular filtration rate (GFR)/renal blood flow) increases with age, mainly due to redistribution of blood flow from the cortex to the medulla. Renal functional reserve, defined as the difference between the GFR at rest and the maximum GFR under stimulation (protein meal)[8], goes down with age, as shown in experimental animals. While the aging renal vasculature does respond to stimuli that cause vasoconstriction and vasodilatation, the latter response is blunted. The Baltimore Longitudinal Study of Aging reported a mean estimated fall in GFR of 8 ml/min per decade[6] or nearly 1 ml/year, the rate of decline unique to each person. This decline is not inevitable. Variability in renal function with age includes a milder decline in GFR in a third of subjects, no alteration in some, and even a mild increase in a small proportion, indicating that age alone does not influence these developments. The reason for this variation is unclear, but it is possible that diseases, diet, race and other factors may play a role[3].

Due to a gradual decrease in muscle mass with age (sarcopenia), less creatinine is generated, resulting in a serum creatinine level lower than would be expected for the decrease in GFR. In other words, serum creatinine levels in elderly subjects signify a lower creatinine clearance than would similar levels in young subjects. This fact is even more relevant in older women with a lower muscle mass. Creatinine clearance may be calculated by the Cockcroft–Gault formula:

$$\text{Creatinine clearance} = \frac{140 - \text{age (years)} \times \text{body weight (kg)}}{72 \times \text{serum creatinine (mg/dl)}}$$

For females, multiply the value by 0.85.

Although the above formula is practical, studies have shown an error of from 33 ml/min underestimation to 18 ml/min overestimation[9]; hence, the time-honored clinical application of 24-h urine estimates for creatinine clearance remains useful[5].

Tubular function

Impaired tubular reabsorption of sodium occurs with aging. When deprived of sodium, the adaptive decrease in urinary excretion of sodium takes longer to achieve in older subjects compared to the young[6]. In other words, if dietary sodium is restricted, urinary sodium losses may continue temporarily. The exact mechanism is unclear: low baseline and stimulated renin and aldosterone levels with aging may cause decreased tubular sodium reabsorption. High levels of circulating atrial natriuretic peptide (ANP) lead to salt wasting by the aging kidney through a direct natriuretic effect; further, impaired synthesis and release of renin and aldosterone is also contributory. The age-related decrease in GFR favors solute diuresis in the remaining functioning nephrons. Hence, a drastic decrease in salt intake in geriatric patients should be avoided to prevent symptomatic volume depletion[7]. In the same manner, older adults have difficulties in handling sodium excess. With impaired ability to excrete an acute sodium load, salt retention, volume overload and hypertension may result. The excess sodium may gradually be excreted over several days. In summary, the elderly take longer to achieve sodium balance, either to conserve or to excrete sodium.

The ability to concentrate and dilute urine declines with aging. In one study the maximum urinary osmolality achieved after water deprivation for 12 h was higher in younger than in older adults[3]. The concentration defect may result from decreased medullary tonicity resulting from a less efficient countercurrent system, due to medullary washout[8]. The implication of this defect would be the need to focus on volume repletion as a life-saving measure, if necessary with intravenous infusion, especially if the blood pressure is low. Older individuals who are volume depleted may continue to manifest an altered mental status with gradual recovery only over a few days.

Table 2 Hormones and the aging kidney

Renin: basal and stimulated levels low (decreased synthesis and release)
Aldosterone: basal and stimulated levels low
Atrial natriuretic peptide: basal levels elevated
Vasopressin: adequate response to osmotic challenge
Calcitriol (1,25 (OH)2 D3): low levels (decreased 1 α-hydroxylase activity)
Parathyroid hormone: levels elevated
Erythropoietin: no change
Insulin: decreased degradation by the kidney

Following fluid administration, urinary osmolality in older adults is not lowered to the same extent as it is in the younger age group. Impaired GFR (decreased free water clearance), failure of arginine vasopressin (AVP) suppression, and defective solute transport in the loop of Henle may be the reasons for the diluting defect. The renal diluting defect renders the elderly susceptible to the development of dilutional hyponatremia with water administration.

Tubular capacity for glucose is reduced, but this is not clinically significant. As there is a relative decrease in GFR, the reabsorptive load for glucose is lessened at the proximal tubule[8] (Table 1).

Endocrine function

Renin–angiotensin–aldosterone system

Well-documented studies show an invariable age-related decline in plasma renin levels beyond the sixth decade (Table 2). Both renin synthesis and renin release are decreased. Plasma angiotensin II levels do not differ despite low levels of renin and aldosterone activity[5]. The decrease in renin may be due to diminished synthesis, impaired release or reduced conversion of inactive to active renin. Diminished renin activity in turn results in lower intrarenal levels of angiotensin II, which controls renal hemodynamics[3]. An age-associated decline occurs in both basal and stimulated renin and aldosterone levels. Decreased activity of the renin–angiotensin–aldosterone system contributes to the syndrome of hyporeninemic hypoaldosteronism in older subjects, a common cause of hyperkalemia (see section on potassium).

Atrial natriuretic peptide

Older individuals when compared to young healthy adults have 3–5 times higher basal levels of ANP. The stimulated levels of ANP are also higher as a result of altered metabolism and diminished clearance. Nevertheless, the response to elevated levels of ANP is blunted, due to diminished end-organ response and post-receptor defects[3].

Vasopressin

Both the basal and stimulated circulating vasopressin levels in response to osmolar stimuli are increased in the elderly, although clinical effects are not evident. The basis for an inadequate response could be either a receptor or a post-receptor end-organ defect[3]. There is no change in the kinetics of vasopressin with aging.

Calcitriol

Levels of calcitriol are low, due to age-related decreased activation of 1 α-hydroxylase, which converts 25-hydroxyvitamin D_3 (25 (OH) D3) to 1,25-dihydroxyvitamin D_3 (calcitriol; 1,25 (OH)2 D3), the active form of vitamin D.

Parathyroid hormone

Both basal levels and maximum secretory capacity of parathyroid hormone (PTH) increase progressively with age, due to constant stimulation by low serum calcium levels.

Erythropoietin

Age and gender appear to have no influence on plasma levels of erythropoietin[10]. Diminished levels are usually the result of renal failure, with a resulting anemia that is responsive to treatment with erythropoietin.

RENAL AGING: MECHANISMS AND MODIFICATIONS

Mechanisms for renal aging may be mediated by several factors. Autocoids play a major role in the regulation of cell proliferation and synthesis of cellular matrix. Angiotensin II and endothelin regulate cell proliferation while nitric oxide and ANP may inhibit cell growth and matrix synthesis[6]. Tumor growth factor-β (TGF β) m-RNA overexpression is associated with age-related interstitial fibrosis and has a role in the development of glomerulosclerosis, as demonstrated in experimental models and diabetic nephropathy. Altered equilibrium in the prostacyclin and thromboxane systems, defective intracellular second messenger and diminished cyclic AMP response or reactive oxygen intermediates may contribute to the pathophysiological changes in the aging kidney[6]. Nitric oxide, which mediates vasodilatation, is inactivated by superoxide anions. Hypertension may play a role by causing endothelial dysfunction.

Western diets are characterized by high protein intake and the resultant increase in renal blood flow (RBF) may lead to a decrease in renal function; however, chronic dietary protein and sodium restriction may result in significant improvement in histopathology, declining function and proteinuria. Studies in mice have revealed the beneficial effects of angiotensin converting enzyme inhibitor therapy with an aging kidney on glomerular size and number, and the amount of glomerular mesangial matrix, thereby leading to reduction in glomerulosclerosis[3]. Treatment with lipid-lowering agents (lovostatin and clofibrate) has shown considerable decrease in proteinuria and glomerular injury in the obese Zucker rat, a model with similarities to human type 2 obese diabetics, suggesting a role for abnormal lipid metabolism in the pathogenesis of renal disease[3].

FLUID AND ELECTROLYTE ALTERATIONS

Sodium and water metabolism

Body water proportion declines from 60–65% in early middle age to 50% by age 75; the decline is more pronounced in women[11]. Philips and colleagues, in a classic study, demonstrated that 24-h fluid deprivation was followed by impaired response to thirst in the elderly despite high serum osmolality, hypernatremia and high antidiuretic hormone (ADH) levels[12]. Younger subjects in the same study responded appropriately to thirst. Patients with Alzheimer's disease demonstrated defective vasopressin release in addition to the concentrating defect and decreased thirst[13]. The decreased ability of the kidney to concentrate urine is not from a secretory defect of ADH but is probably due to receptor or post-receptor dysfunction. Besides having defective concentrating ability, the older kidney is also unable to dilute urine to the same extent as the younger. The implication of impaired concentrating and diluting ability is that older adults are prone to both hyper- and hyponatremia. Hypernatremia is more prevalent in the elderly compared to the young and results from gastrointestinal losses (use of cathartics, diarrhea and vomiting), urinary losses (diuretics, postobstructive and osmotic) and febrile losses from the skin. Impaired thirst, presence of dementia and restricted mobility make them even more vulnerable.

Impaired diluting function in older subjects increases the risk of hyponatremia. Causes of hyponatremia include situations where ADH is stimulated (drug induced, pneumonia, neoplasms, intracranial disease, etc.), renal sodium losses (diuretics), gastrointestinal losses (diarrhea), and retention of salt and water (congestive heart failure, nephrotic syndrome and cirrhosis). In particular, geriatric subjects on thiazides and nonsteroidal anti-inflammatory drugs (NSAIDs) are predisposed to the development of

Table 3 Hyponatremia in older subjects

Exclude
Pseudohyponatremia (hyperglycemia)
Factitious hyponatremia (hypertriglyceridemia or high serum protein levels)

Hypervolemia
Congestive heart failure
Cirrhosis of the liver with ascites
Nephrotic syndrome

Euvolemia
Syndrome of inappropriate ADH secretion
Medications: psychotropic agents, carbamazepine, vincristine, cyclophosphomide narcotics*
Diseases: pneumonia, cancer of the lung, intracranial processes, severe pain*
Postoperative state: stress-related ADH secretion
Diuretics, particularly thiazides

Hypovolemia
Renal losses, including diuretics
Gastrointestinal losses (diarrhea, vomiting)

ADH, antidiuretic hormone. *The list is selective and only for illustration

hyponatremia; thiazides interfere with free water excretion, acting at the cortical diluting site[14] (Tables 3 and 4).

The decreased ability to conserve or excrete sodium is discussed under tubular function.

Potassium homeostasis

The interplay of physiological and pathological changes compounded with iatrogenic causes frequently result in altered potassium levels in older adults. The incidence of hyperkalemia rises progressively with age, reaching 5% by the eighth decade. Studies support a relationship between age and a predisposition to drug-induced hyperkalemia[15]. The rate of rise as well as the maximum level of aldosterone attained in response to a potassium infusion are lower in older adults compared to the young[16].

The elderly are predisposed to dangerous hyperkalemia from drug–drug and drug–disease interactions. In the presence of congestive heart failure (CHF) or hypovolemia, which result in diminished delivery of

Table 4 Hypernatremia in older subjects

Predisposing factors (diminished fluid intake)
Dementia, depression, psychosis
Restricted mobility
Impaired thirst
Fluid restriction
Altered sensorium (delirium)
Dysphagia
Medications that alter sensorium

Gastrointestinal losses
Vomiting, nasogastric suction, bowel preparations

Urinary fluid losses
Excess free water excretion (diuretics)
Osmotic fluid loss (hyperglycemia)
Post-obstructive diuresis

Dermal fluid losses
Fever, excessive sweating

Table 5 Causes of hyper- and hypokalemia in older adults

Hyperkalemia
Predisposition
  suppressed renin–angiotensin–aldosterone system
Medications
  potassium preparations, potassium-sparing diuretics,
    ACE inhibitors, heparin, NSAIDs, trimethoprim*
Diseases
  obstructive uropathy, type IV renal tubular acidosis,
    diabetes mellitus, renal failure (acute and chronic),
    rhabdomyolysis
Extracellular shift
  β-blockers, hyperglycemia, metabolic acidosis*

Hypokalemia
Medications
  diuretics and laxatives*
Others
  urinary losses (diuretics, relief of obstruction, osmotic),
    gastrointestinal losses (diarrhea, vomiting),
    hypomagnesemia (diuretics, alcoholism,
    malnutrition)
Intracellular shift
  insulin therapy, B$_{12}$ vitamin replacement, β-agonists,
    metabolic alkalosis

ACE, angiotensin converting enzyme; NSAIDs,
non-steroidal anti-inflammatory drugs
*The list is selective and used for illustration only

sodium and water to the distal renal tubule, potassium secretion is impaired at the distal site. The major protective mechanism, aldosterone activity, is diminished with a decline in renal as well as colon Na-K-ATPase activity[4], compounding the problem. Hyperkalemia commonly results from the use of intravenous or oral potassium preparations, angiotensin converting enzyme (ACE) inhibitors, NSAIDs, heparin and non-selective β-blockers. Other events may be superimposed, e.g. gastrointestinal bleeding (a major source of gut potassium), or obstructive uropathy (a cause of type IV renal tubular acidosis). In summary, administration of potassium supplements with or without drugs that predispose to hyperkalemia should be judicious in the elderly.

Hypokalemia is also noted in older adults; likely causes include the use of thiazides, laxatives or cathartics, gastrointestinal losses (diarrhea) and hypomagnesemia. Hypokalemia may manifest as constipation, ileus and apathy or may predispose to cardiac arrythmias, especially in the elderly on digoxin (Table 5).

Acid–base balance

While acid secretion in the elderly does not differ from that in the young, challenge with an acid load fails to increase acid excretion to a similar degree. With aging an intrinsic tubular defect in ammonium excretion largely accounts for the decrease in total acid excretion while titratable acid excretion is intact[3]. Many medications prescribed in the geriatric population may precipitate the development of acid–base disorders. Acetazolamide, aspirin, laxatives and NSAIDs may lead to metabolic acidosis, while vomiting induced by digoxin, theophylline and chemotherapeutic agents may cause metabolic alkalosis[8].

Calcium and phosphate metabolism

In general the serum calcium level does not change with age, but PTH levels increase after age 60, reaching as high as two times that in the young[7]. The plasma level of 25(OH) D3, an index of vitamin D activity, is frequently low, especially in home-bound and institutionalized elderly, and is pronounced in the winter months. As a result of diminished exposure to sunlight, the aging skin has a reduced capacity to produce provitamin D_3 (the precursor to 25 (OH) D3). Lower levels of 1,25 (OH)2 D3 are due to decreased 1 α-hydroxylase activity, with declining age or renal disease as the basis. In addition to diminished 25(OH) D3 and 1,25 (OH)2 D3 production in the liver and kidney, respectively, there is a reduction in vitamin D receptor activity in the gastrointestinal tract with aging, resulting in diminished calcium absorption[8]. Most older adults fail to ingest adequate amounts of calcium; lactose intolerance, not uncommon in this age group, may account for inadequate ingestion of dairy products. The above factors predispose the geriatric population to the development of osteoporosis and osteomalacia. Thiazide diuretics used as therapy for hypertension improve serum calcium levels by decreasing calciuria, thereby maintaining a positive calcium balance[8].

Studies have shown a decrease in renal tubular reabsorption of phosphate with increasing age in addition to impaired renal tubular adaptation to a low phosphate diet. This change is due to a defect in Na–PO_4 co-transport in the proximal convoluted tubule. Decreased levels of circulating growth hormone and insulin-like growth factor-I with aging may potentially contribute to increased phosphaturia[17]. Increased urinary excretion of phosphate combined with decreased intestinal phosphate absorption (from diminished vitamin D activity) leads to negative phosphate balance and osteomalacia[3].

RENOVASCULAR DISEASE

Renovascular disease and diabetic nephropathy together account for half the cases of end stage renal disease (ESRD) worldwide (European Dialysis and Transplant Association and United States Renal Data System)[18]. Renovascular causes of ESRD are predominantly hypertensive nephrosclerosis and atheromatous renovascular disease. The latter, which may be unilateral or bilateral, includes ischemic atheroscelerosis, atheroembolism and acute occlusion of the renal arteries. Frequently, atheromatous renovascular disease (RVD) is overlooked; it affects a third of elderly ESRD patients in the USA[18].

The most common cause of renal artery stenosis is atheromatous disease. In random necropsies renal artery occlusion of > 50% increased from 5% under 64 years to 42% over 75 years. Bilateral stenosis was noted in half the cases[18]. Occlusion in atheromatous disease typically occurs at the ostia of the renal arteries half the time[18]. RVD should be considered a possibility in geriatric patients who present with hypertension and progressive renal failure, an unremarkable urinary sediment, minimal to no proteinuria, and signs and symptoms suggestive of atherosclerosis in extrarenal sites[18]. Vascular disease elsewhere is typically noted in the heart, brain, carotids or extremities. New-onset hypertension in older adults and well-controlled hypertensives presenting with uncontrolled hypertension requiring higher doses of medication warrant evaluation for RVD[19] (Table 6).

Renal artery occlusion from cholesterol emboli is being more frequently recognized today in the geriatric population. Renal atheroembolism may be spontaneous, may follow vascular surgery involving major arteries or may complicate fibrinolytic therapy for acute myocardial infarction[18]. Cholesterol embolism may present as acute renal failure with fever, increased erythrocyte sedimentation rate, decreased complement, eosinophilia, eosinophiluria and hematuria (without casts) or as a progressive decline in GFR over weeks associated with episodic labile hypertension. In the latter entity, eosinophiluria is not a feature. Cholesterol crystals may be seen on fundoscopic examination; biopsies of kidney, muscle or skin may also reveal cholesterol emboli[18].

Table 6 Renovascular diseases

Types
Nephrosclerosis
Ischemic nephropathy
Atheroembolism
Atherosclerotic renovascular disease (unilateral or
    bilateral)

Diagnostic clues for hypertensive nephrosclerosis
Longstanding hypertension with target organ damage:
    retinopathy, left ventricular hypertrophy, renal insuffi-
    ciency or failure
History of hypertension prior to the onset of proteinuria
Absence of any other basis for primary renal disease
Family history of hypertension, Black race
Negative renal biopsy for parenchymal disease

Supporting evidence for renovascular disease
New-onset hypertension at age > 50 years
Hypertension and progressive renal failure
Inactive urine sediment and mild proteinuria
Evidence of atherosclerosis at other sites
Radiologic features
Prior surgical procedure involving major artery/
    anticoagulation
Biopsy in case of atheroembolism

As intraglomerular angiotensin II plays a role in renal hemodynamics, treatment with ACE inhibitors may result in renal functional deterioration in bilateral renovascular disease. ACE inhibitors may unmask renal artery stenosis (RAS) if the occlusion is > 70% bilaterally or unilaterally in a single functioning kidney[19].

Diagnosis of RAS by renal isotope scintigraphy following a captopril challenge has a sensitivity and specificity of 90%[20,21]. Furosemide is also used in discriminating the presence of significant renal artery obstruction from patent arteries[22]. Magnetic resonance angiography has a similar range of accuracy[23]. Carbon dioxide digital angiography and duplex scanning using color Doppler ultrasound are other newer diagnostic methods for diagnosing RAS[19].

Patients with RAS and severe or difficult to treat hypertension, presenting with recurrent sudden pulmonary edema and progressive renal failure, may benefit from percutaneous transluminal angioplasty (PTLA) with stenting[24]. The value of invasive angiography and PTLA with stenting in the management of ostial RAS is recognized[24].

RENAL PARENCHYMAL DISEASES

Glomerular diseases

Glomerular diseases present in several ways. These include the acute nephritic syndrome, rapidly progressive glomerulonephritis (RPGN), nephrotic syndrome, asymptomatic hematuria, and/or proteinuria and chronic progressive glomerulonephritis. In contrast to young adults the geriatric population has a high prevalence of type 2 diabetic nephropathy, amyloidosis, renal paraneoplastic syndromes and complications due to adverse effects of therapeutic agents[25].

Acute nephritic syndrome

The acute nephritic syndrome in the elderly is commonly caused by cutaneous streptococcal infection while in the young, pharyngeal infection is the usual source. Urinary abnormalities are minor, whereas hypertension and fluid retention or exacerbation of CHF are common. ACE inhibitors are ineffective in treating this form of hypertension, as the pathogenesis is a hypervolemic hyporeninemic state[25].

Rapidly progressive glomerulonephritis

RPGN, common in older adults, presents as glomerulonephritis with rapid and progressive deterioration in renal function. Microscopic polyangiitis along with glomerular crescents are the pathological findings in RPGN. Causes include Henoch–Schönlein purpura, Wegener's granulomatosis, Goodpasture's syndrome and organ-limited Pauci immune crescentic glomerulonephritis. The majority of elderly patients with RPGN are anti-neutrophilic cytoplasmic antibody (ANCA)-positive, while 10–15% have autoantibodies to GBM antigens. The diagnosis of crescentic glomerulonephritis leading to rapid progression of renal failure is often confused with acute tubular necrosis. When diagnosis is in doubt, renal biopsy should be performed[8]. The prognosis of RPGN is poor unless treated early with high-dose parenteral methylprednisone and cyclophosphamide. The elderly are at high risk for lethal infections when immunosuppressive therapy is used[25]. Plasmapheresis appears to be of questionable benefit.

Nephrotic syndrome

This syndrome is defined as 'proteinuria over 3.5 g/1.73 m^2 per day with hypoalbuminemia, and variably with edema and hyperlipidemia'. A fifth of adult nephrotic syndrome cases[25] occur in the elderly. Renal biopsy helps to differentiate membranous glomerulopathy from proliferative glomerulonephritis and aids in management, as the response to treatment with steroids is much better in the former. Of nephrotic syndrome cases, 60% are from membranous glomerulopathy, minimal change disease or amyloidosis. Of these, the most common is membranous glomerulonephritis (MGN), idiopathic in the majority. The Medical Research Council Glomerulonephritis Registry of 317 patients over 60 years old reported that the nephrotic syndrome resulted from MGN in a third of cases; minimal change disease and amyloidosis accounted for a tenth of cases each[3]. Malignancies of the lung, stomach, breast, colon, prostate and less frequently lymphoma and melanoma can cause MGN. Remission of the underlying cancer may be followed by disappearance of the nephrotic syndrome, while relapse may be associated with tumor recurrence. In a third of patients the nephrotic syndrome can precede the presentation of cancer itself. Physical examination and diagnostic evaluation should focus on the etiology. Idiopathic minimal change disease is the second most frequent cause of nephrotic syndrome in the geriatric age group and responds well to steroid therapy. Another common etiology is medication, particularly NSAIDs, which cause minimal change disease. ACE inhibitors, penicillamine, gold, mercurial compounds and anticonvulsants have been reported to cause membranous glomerulopathy[25].

Miscellaneous

Amyloidosis of the AL (primary) type causes nephrotic syndrome; extrarenal manifestations of amyloidosis are not common in this population[25]. Proteinuria may be mild. Paraproteinemia or paraproteinuria is found in up to two-thirds of patients with primary amyloidosis presenting as the nephrotic syndrome[25]. By virtue of bladder involvement, amyloidosis may produce isomorphic (non-distorted red blood cell) hematuria[25]. The prognosis is poor and many will develop progressive renal insufficiency. In the elderly with unexplained proteinuria, urine and plasma protein electrophoresis in addition to bone marrow aspiration or biopsy will help exclude underlying multiple myeloma. Congo red staining and electron microscopy of renal biopsy material may help identify amyloidosis.

Fibrillary glomerulonephritis may present with hematuria, hypertension, nephrotic syndrome and progressive renal failure leading to ESRD in less than 5 years. These Congo red-negative, intraglomerular immunoglobulin fibrils are not amyloid but are locally produced abnormal paraproteins which stain like polyclonal immunoglobulins[8].

Chronic viral infections deserve consideration, particularly hepatitis B, as a cause of membranous glomerulopathy, and hepatitis C as a cause of membrano-proliferative glomerulonephritis[25]. IgA nephropathy and systemic lupus erythematosus are rare causes of glomerulonephritis in the older adult.

Tubulointerstitial diseases

Tubulointerstitial disease, i.e. involvement of both tubules and interstitium of the kidney, occurs from several causes. Co-morbidity, polypharmacy and alteration in immunological status predispose the elderly to this entity. Tubulointerstitial nephritis (TIN) may be acute or chronic. Bacterial pyelonephritis and drug-induced interstitial nephritis are common causes of acute TIN. Benign prostatic hyperplasia (BPH) in males, and altered vaginal anatomy and flora in females, increase patient susceptibility. Atypical presentation of acute bacterial pyelonephritis is not uncommon: delirium, septicemia with hypotension and acute renal failure (ARF) may be the clinical presentation. Response to antibiotic treatment is typical; in its absence, obstruction or perinephric abscess should be excluded[26].

Drug-induced hypersensitivity as a cause of TIN presents with arthralgia, rash, fever, eosinophiluria and ARF. Formerly methicillin was a common cause. Today other penicillins, sulfonamides, NSAIDs, fluoroquinolones, diuretics and several other drugs are well known to be associated with this disorder[8]. NSAIDs are safe if used within the therapeutic dosage for a short period with adequate monitoring. Chronic TIN, on the other hand, is not a hypersensivity phenomenon and results from long-term use of analgesics. The presentation ranges from renal insufficiency to renal failure; appropriate use and/or withdrawal of offending agents is important to arrest progression of the entity[26].

Rare causes of TIN include neoplastic diseases such as lymphomas, leukemias and multiple myeloma; unexplained anemia, hypercalcemia and renal impairment should raise suspicion of a neoplastic basis.

RENAL FAILURE IN OLDER ADULTS

Acute renal failure

Age-related changes with diminished reserves, compounded by systemic diseases such as cardiac failure, diabetes mellitus, hypertension and obstructive uropathy, in addition to risk factors such as dehydration and the use of nephrotoxic medications or radiocontrast agents, render geriatric patients

susceptible to ARF. Gram-negative sepsis accounts for a third of ARF. The incidence of ARF appears to rise with age[27]. Impaired nitric acid synthesis increases tubular cell susceptibility to ischemic damage with advancing age[28].

Broadly, ARF in the geriatric population may result from diminished perfusion (consequent to ischemia, medications or toxins and septic states). Hypovolemia from poor intake or excessive losses, especially in nursing home residents with acute febrile illness and concomitant use of diuretics and laxatives, may be causative factors in ARF. Hypernatremia is seen in a quarter of febrile patients who are dehydrated[29,30]. Diagnosis of hypovolemic ARF in older adults may be difficult at times, due to the unreliable clinical signs and symptoms of dehydration in this age group. Identification of ARF by fractional excretion of sodium (FENa) estimation is not definitive in the geriatric population with decompensated CHF, cirrhosis or sepsis, or following diuretic or contrast administration[31]. Miscellaneous ischemic causes include cholesterol emboli, acute bilateral renal artery occlusion and aortic cross clamping.

While cholesterol embolization causes ARF over a few weeks, contrast-induced ARF occurs over days. Acute bilateral renal artery thrombosis is rare and is characterized by very high serum levels of lactic dehydrogenase and high urinary FENa. Aortic cross clamping for abdominal aortic aneurysm repair in the elderly causes renal microembolization without clinical hypotension.

Several mechanisms play a role in the development of drug-induced ARF. Reduction in urinary prostaglandin E_2 in older hypertensives increases risk of NSAID-induced ARF[32]. Aminoglycoside administration without dosing adjustment for decreased renal function, particularly in dehydrated individuals, results in high blood levels and dose-related toxic renal injury. Radiocontrast agents used for angiograms or computed tomography scans are well recognized to be nephrotoxic in diabetics with pre-existing renal insufficiency. The injudicious use of loop diuretics may worsen azotemia.

Rhabdomyolysis resulting in ARF may occur from prolonged immobilization. Additional co-morbid processes include viral syndromes, neurological disease, tourniquet use in orthopedic hip surgery, disordered thermoregulation (hypo- and hyperthermia) and the use of certain neuroleptic agents[33].

Crescentric glomerulonephritis is a common cause of glomerular disease presenting as ARF. Idiopathic and anti-GBM-associated rapidly progressive glomerulonephritis[33], post-streptococcal glomerulonephritis and Wegener's granulomatosis are recognized causes of ARF. Clinical suspicion of glomerular disease warrants a renal biopsy to determine an etiology, as some of these entities are treatable.

ARF can also result from obstruction. Sudden onset of obstruction may result from medications, particularly those with anticholinergic actions (diphenhydramine, tricyclic antidepressants) or opiates, and from processes such as constipation resulting in fecal impaction. This may be superimposed on pre-existing obstructive uropathy from prostatic disease or a diabetic neurogenic bladder. Lower urinary tract obstruction should always be excluded in older men with unexplained ARF.

Dialysis and hemofiltration are well tolerated by the elderly, resulting in good renal functional recovery and survival. Hemodialysis is preferred to peritoneal dialysis in the management of ARF. Timely initiation of dialysis prevents complications such as gastrointestinal bleeding, CHF and infection, which adversely affect recovery from ARF. While intermittent hemodialysis is widely used, continuous hemofiltration is another available modality of treatment in critical care units for geriatric patients with ARF[34].

Obstructive uropathy

In the USA, obstructive nephropathy leading to ESRD accounts for 2% of cases[35], while post-mortem studies reveal hydronephrosis in approximately 4% of older patients[35]. BPH is less prevalent in Japan than in Europe and the USA[35]. By age 85, 90% of men have identifiable BPH. Half the men beyond age 60 are symptomatic, and by 75, one-fourth of them require some form of intervention for symptoms related to BPH[36]. African-American men manifest symptoms many years earlier than Caucasians. The presentation of BPH may be hesitancy, frequency, nocturia or overflow incontinence. Hydronephrosis is present in less than 10% and up to a third present with renal insufficiency, with uremia in many. As the periurethral area of prostatic tissue enlarges first, urinary symptoms can manifest even before the enlarged prostate is detected clinically[35]. Severe bladder mucosal and muscular hypertrophy from prostatic hyperplasia may even cause bilateral ureterovesical obstruction with or without bladder neck obstruction. Other causes of obstruction in older adults include neurogenic bladder, interstitial cystitis and bladder fibrosis from radiation or any other cause. Chronic inflammation and fibrosis of the trigone can lead to vesicoureteric reflux[35]. Relief of obstruction and reversibility depend on the duration of obstruction and severity of damage to the kidneys. During the period of obstruction, older patients are at increased risk of volume overload leading to CHF, hyperkalemia, metabolic acidosis and urinary tract infection secondary to frequent instrumentation. At the same time these patients are at risk of dehydration from diuresis when the obstruction is relieved.

Functional obstruction in women rarely occurs from compression or stretching of the ureterovesical junction during bladder distension. Lower urinary tract or ureterovesical junction dysfunction unusually follows obstruction after surgery for urinary incontinence, severe atrophic vaginitis with urethral stenosis, large cystoceles with or without uterine prolapse and huge uterine fibroids[37].

When there is doubt, a post-void residual urine volume must be measured to rule out urinary retention; this can be achieved by post-void bladder catheterization or by ultrasonogram. The normal residual is only a few milliliters. The post-void residual goes up with age; in any case volumes over 50 ml are abnormal and if much higher, need evaluation. Additional diagnostic studies in obstructive uropathy (to be individualized) include ultrasound examination of kidneys and pelvis, ystoscopy, cystometric studies and, in women, a pelvic examination.

Urolithiasis is seen in the geriatric population. Nephrolithiasis may be from calcium oxalate, uric acid and struvite (triple phosphate) stones. Uric acid stones are seen secondary to hematologic malignancies while struvite stones occur as a consequence of urinary tract infections by urea-splitting organisms. Hyperparathyroidism, use of drugs such as acetazolamide (for glaucoma), calcium antacids, loop diuretics and low urine volume may potentiate stone formation in the elderly[38].

Chronic renal failure

Chronic renal failure in the elderly commonly results from atherosclerotic renovascular disease, diabetes mellitus, hypertension, chronic glomerulonephritis, multiple myeloma, and obstructive uropathy due to benign prostatic hyperplasia. The presentation in older subjects may differ from that in the young, and includes decompensated CHF, worsening control of hypertension or gastrointestinal bleeding or delirium, rather than with classic uremic symptoms[3].

As per the United States Renal Data System, diabetic nephropathy accounted for about 35% of ESRD in the USA[39]. A similar trend has been noted by the European Dialysis and Transplant Association[39]. In type 2 diabetic nephropathy, deterioration of renal function is inevitable after the development of clinical proteinuria. Uncontrolled hypertension, poor glycemic status, dyslipidemia and cigarette smoking are factors that appear to contribute to the rapid decline in renal function. Studies in type 2 diabetics suggest a genetic link between hypertension and diabetic kidney disease[40]. In a multi-center study over 5 years, the beneficial effect of ACE inhibitors was clearly apparent in ameliorating progression from microalbuminuria to clinical proteinuria and in preserving renal function as shown by measured serum creatinine levels[41].

Anemia of renal disease

Anemia develops with both acute and chronic renal failure; it is typically a normochromic, normocytic anemia of chronic disease. Renal anemia occurs in approximately a fifth of patients with a serum creatinine of 2.0 mg/dl or less and in the vast majority of individuals with a serum creatinine greater than 4.0 mg/dl. Anemia substantially impairs the quality of life, is a contributor to the higher incidence of cardiovascular disease in association with chronic kidney disease and results in an increase in hospitalizations and death[42].

The basis for anemia of renal disease is the diminished production of erythropoietin (EPO), a 165 amino-acid glycoprotein hormone. EPO is mainly produced in the interstitial cells near the proximal tubules of the kidneys, and is responsible for the development of red cell precursors and maturation of erythroid cells. Hypoxia and anemia are recognized stimuli for production of EPO[42]. The gene for EPO was cloned in 1985; recombinant human erythropoietin (rHuEPO) resembles endogenous EPO immunogenetically and biologically. EPO is marketed in the US as Epogen® for use in ESRD patients requiring dialysis and as Procrit® for all other indications, including renal disease related anemia prior to institution of dialysis; outside the US it is available as Eprex®. A longer acting novel erythropoiesis-stimulating protein, darbepoietin-α (Aranesp®) is also now available for weekly or every other week administration, in a dose of 0.45 µg/kg/week[43]. EPO is initially administered in a dose of 50 to 100 units/kg and titrated to keep the hematocrit between 33 and 36. Failure of adequate response and the return of anemia in some patients on EPO has been ascribed to a pure red cell aplasia from neutralizing antierythropoietin antibodies[44]. While on EPO, iron replacement must be ensured, either through the oral or parenteral route; injections of iron are most often resorted to, as a lack of response to EPO from newly acquired iron deficiency usually develops while on EPO. Hence, close follow-up of hematocrit utilizing ferrokinetics is essential to ensure the optimum correction of anemia and efficient use of the hormone[42].

It should be recognized that while renal anemia typically occurs from diminished production of EPO, other causes may well be contributory. The presence of microcytic or macrocytic red cell indices may be a clue to additional non-renal etiologies. These include blood loss (from dialysis and other sites), iron deficiency, nutritional causes (e.g. folate deficiency) and any additional basis such as the anemia of chronic disease. A full evaluation for anemia is thus warranted in all patients with renal disease, rather than assuming that it is solely of renal etiology.

Dialysis

The number of older adults on dialysis is increasing substantially the world over. Early institution of dialysis is advisable to help avoid symptoms of uremia and organ dysfunction. The United States National Kidney Foundation advises the initiation of dialysis when creatinine clearance declines to 15 ml/min in all patients, as opposed to waiting longer, as in the past[45]. Based on this criterion the incidence of patients needing dialysis could increase from 300 per million to 1000 per million in the geriatric group; over half the ESRD population in the USA is over age 60[46].

In the year 2000, two-thirds of new patients on dialysis were over age 65. Diabetes and hypertension appeared to be the etiology of half the cases of ESRD in the geriatric population. Poor nutritional status (hypoalbuminemia) suggests a bad prognosis.

The growth in number of older patients on dialysis has been rapid. This is mainly attributed to an increase in referral and acceptance rates of geriatric patients, in spite of the high prevalence of associated comorbid conditions[46]. The fact that geriatric individuals are better treated today for conditions such as hypertension, diabetes, and coronary artery disease increases their chances of survival into an older age and the probability of developing chronic renal failure[46].

Continuous ambulatory peritoneal dialysis (CAPD) is preferred in those who have diffuse vascular disease causing difficulty in creation and maintenance of vascular access; further, hemodialysis may not be well tolerated in those with cardiac disease and associated hypotension and arrhythmias. About 12% of patients over age 60 are on CAPD compared to 46% in the younger age group[47]. The incidence of peritonitis and the organisms responsible for it are similar in both age groups; but poor nutrition, increased hospitalizations from treatment failure and frequent transfer to hemodialysis are noted more in older patients. The cardiovascular death rate is higher with peritoneal dialysis compared to hemodialysis and is thought to be secondary to hypoalbuminemia and hyperlipidemia, common in peritoneal dialysis subjects[48].

In the geriatric population it is advisable to create the vascular access early. Hemodialysis is usually associated with better survival compared to CAPD, and is technically easier. In-center hemodialysis provides an opportunity for the isolated, older, depressed subject to socialize. Age is not a contraindication for initiating dialysis, as many geriatric patients improve their health and quality of life. Absolute contraindications for dialysis include advanced dementia and metastatic cancer (exception: multiple myeloma)[5]. Although they do well, withdrawal from dialysis in geriatric patients is usually a result of dissatisfaction with life. The most common cause of death in the older dialysis patient is cardiovascular, followed by withdrawal from dialysis. Factors predisposing to withdrawal include age over 65, White race, female gender, diabetes mellitus and nursing home residence[49]. Obtaining advance directives at the time of initiating dialysis is valuable and the self decision of withdrawal from dialysis by the cognitively preserved patients should be honored, respecting their autonomy[47].

Renal transplantation

Of patients awaiting renal transplantation in the USA in 1997, 7% were over age 65. Many transplant centers consider the biologic age of the recipient to be more important than the chronologic age[50]. Pretransplant evaluation for vascular disease (especially cardiac) and malignancy is essential. Voiding cystourethrogram, not a routine for younger patients, may be necessary. As immune function declines with age, a lower dosage of immunosuppressive agents is required to avoid graft rejection. Death in renal transplant recipients is usually from cardiovascular disease and infection, rather than graft loss due to rejection[50]. Kidneys from older donors may survive for a shorter time, as the glomeruli are more sclerosed and prone to ischemia during organ harvesting. Of relevance is the fact that older recipients may be offered a kidney from older donors. Cadaveric donors are rejected if kidney biopsy reveals sclerosis in more than 20% of glomeruli. A few centers may choose to place two kidneys from older donors[49]. A quarter of US transplant centers do not consider age as a criterion for exclusion of donors, while 70% of the centers exclude donors over age 70[51].

DRUGS AND THE KIDNEY

Adverse drug reactions are 3–10-fold more frequent in older adults due to changes in volume of drug distribution, drug half-life and altered elimination of the parent drug and its metabolites. Physiologic age-related changes alter pharmacokinetics and pharmacodynamics[52]. The older kidney is susceptible to damage from both appropriate and inappropriate use of drugs. There is a need to adjust the dosage for renal function, if the medication or active metabolite is excreted by the kidney, through glomerular filtration or tubular secretion.

Drugs principally excreted by the kidney, such as digoxin, aminoglycosides, vancomycin, lithium, procainamide, nitrofurantoin, amantadine and meperidine, among others, require appropriate dosing for renal function in the elderly. Ideally, the dose is calculated based on an estimation of creatinine clearance (Cockroft–Gault formula) and by monitoring plasma drug levels where available (e.g. aminoglycosides and vancomycin). Dose reduction is achieved by altering either the maintenance dose or the interval between doses.

While hypersensitivity reactions are not age related, older adults are susceptible to other forms of drug-induced nephrotoxicity such as alteration in renal hemodynamics and development of azotemia from decreased renal blood flow (ACE inhibitors, cyclosporine), salt and fluid retention or poor control of blood pressure (NSAIDs), type IV renal tubular acidosis with hyperkalemia (NSAIDs) and acute renal failure (ARF) from aminoglycosides even when used appropriately. Hypovolemia, underlying renal insufficiency, concomitant use of other nephrotoxic drugs (e.g. diuretics) and inappropriate dose or interval between doses predispose the aged to aminoglycoside toxicity[53].

In particular, the use of NSAIDs by geriatric patients for a variety of chronic painful muscle, joint and bone disorders predisposes them to several disturbances in renal function[54]. These include a reduction in the glomerular filtration rate and worsening of function, acute and chronic interstitial nephritis, nephrotic syndrome, chronic renal insufficiency and even ESRD. Immune complex glomerulonephritis occurs less commonly with use of NSAIDs. Salt and water retention and hyperkalemia are well known phenomena. The predisposition of older subjects to adverse effects from NSAIDs appears related to a variety of drug–disease interactions (as comorbid conditions frequently include hypertension, heart failure, renal insufficiency and liver disease) and drug–drug interactions (as geriatric patients are typically on several additional medications). Renal dysfunction can also occur from the use of the more recently introduced selective COX-2 inhibitors[54].

In summary, the health-care provider should pay attention to the pharmacokinetics and pharmacodynamics of drugs based on renal function, particularly in the elderly; appropriate prescribing will minimize adverse reactions.

CONCLUSION

Aging is associated with a variety of morphologic and physiologic changes involving the kidney. Several co-morbid processes in the presence of diminished renal reserves along with adverse drug events often combine to produce a variety of renal parenchymal, fluid and electrolyte disturbances. Enhanced awareness of renal age-related alterations and disease will help manage many of these disturbances.

References

1. Lubitz JD, Eggers PW, Gornick ME, Villafranca NP. Demography of aging. In Cobbs EL, Duthie EH Jr, Murphy JB, eds. *Geriatric Review Syllabus*, 4th edn. Dubuque, Iowa: Kendall/Hunt Publishing, 1999:1–5
2. Dharmarajan TS, Ugalino JT. The aging process. In Dreger D, Krum B, eds. *Hospital Physician Geriatric Medicine Board Review Manual*. Wayne, PA: Turner White Communications, 2000;1:1–12
3. Palmer BF, Levi M. Renal function and disease in the aging kidney. In Shrier RW, Gottschalk CW, eds. *Diseases of the Kidney*, 6th edn. Boston: Little, Brown, 1997:2293–317
4. McLachlan MSF. The ageing kidney. *Lancet* 1978;2:143–5
5. Epstein M. Aging and the kidney. *J Am Soc Nephrol* 1996;7:1106–22
6. Puyol DR. The aging kidney. *Kidney Int* 1998;54:2247–65
7. Chou SY, Lindeman RD. Structural and functional changes of the aging kidney. In Jacobson HR, Striker GE, Klahr S, eds. *The Principles and Practice of Nephrology*, 2nd edn. St Louis: Mosby, 1995:510–14
8. Zawada ET Jr, Boice JL, Santella RN. Kidney and aging. In Massry SG, Glassock RJ, eds. *Massry & Glassock Text Book of Nephrology*, 3rd edn. Baltimore: Williams & Wilkins, 1995:1138–47
9. Malmrose LC, Gray SL, Pieper CF, *et al.* Measured versus estimated creatinine clearance in a high-functioning elderly sample: MacArthur foundation study of successful aging. *J Am Geriatr Soc* 1993;41: 715–21
10. Spivak JL. Polycythemia vera and other myeloproliferative diseases. In Fauci AS, Braunwald E, Isselbacher KJ, *et al.*, eds. *Harrison's Principles of Internal Medicine*, 14th edn. New York: McGraw-Hill, 1998: 679–84
11. Beck LH. Changes in renal function with aging: *Clin Geriatr Med* 1998;14:199–209
12. Philips PA, Rolls BJ, Ledingham JGG, *et al.*, Reduced thirst after water deprivation in

healthy elderly men. *N Engl J Med* 1984; 311:753–9

13. Albert SG, Nakra BRS, Grosberg GT, Caminal ER. Vasopressin response to dehydration in Alzheimer's disease. *J Am Geriatr Soc* 1989;37:843–7

14. Clark BA, Shannon RP, Rosa RM, Epstein FH. Increased susceptibility to thiazide-induced hyponatremia in the elderly. *J Am Soc Nephrol* 1994;5:1106–11

15. Lawson DH. Adverse reactions to potassium chloride. *Q J Med* 1974;43:433–40

16. Mulkerrin E, Epstein FH, Clark BA. Aldosterone responses to hyperkalemia in healthy elderly humans. *J Am Soc Nephrol* 1995;6:1459–62

17. Mulroney SE, Woda C, Haramati A. Changes in renal phosphate reabsorption in the aged rat. *Proc Soc Exp Biol Med* 1998;218:62–7

18. Campdera FJG, Luno J, Garcia de Vinuesa S, Valderrabano F. Renal vascular disease in the elderly. *Kidney Int* 1998;54:s-73–7

19. Henrich WL. Renal artery disease in the elderly. In Oreopoulos DG, Hazzard WR, Luke R, eds. *Nephrology and Geriatrics Integrated*. Boston: Kluwer Academic Publishers, 2000:67–75

20. Van De Ven PJG, Beutler JJ, Kaatee R, *et al*. Angiotensin converting enzyme inhibitor-induced renal dysfunction in atherosclerotic renovascular disease. *Kidney Int* 1998;53:986–93

21. Wilcox CS. Use of angiotensin-converting-enzyme inhibitors for diagnosing renovascular hypertension. *Kidney Int* 1993;44: 1379–90

22. Moller BE, Dumas A, Roth D, *et al*. Furosemide–[131]I-Hippuran renography after angiotensin-converting enzyme inhibition for the diagnosis of renovascular hypertension. *Am J Med* 1991;90:23–9

23. Farrugia E, King BF, Larson TS. Magnetic resonance angiography and detection of renal artery stenosis in a patient with impaired renal function. *Mayo Clin Proc* 1993;68:157–60

24. Blum U, Krumme B, Flugel P, *et al*., Treatment of ostial renal artery stenosis with vascular endoprothesis after unsuccessful baloon angioplasty. *N Engl J Med* 1997; 336:459–65

25. Glassock RJ. Glomerular disease in the elderly population. In Oreopoulos DG, Hazzard WR, Luke R, eds. *Nephrology and Geriatrics Integrated*. Boston: Kluwer Academic Publishers, 2000:57–66

26. Sands JM, Vega SR. Renal disease. In Hazzard WR, Blass JP, Ettinger WH Jr, *et al.*, eds. *Principles of Geriatric Medicine and Gerontology*, 4th edn. New York: McGraw-Hill, 1999:777–96

27. Groeneveld AB, Tran DD, Van der Meulen J, *et al*. Acute renal failure in the medical intensive care unit: predisposing, complicating factors and outcome. *Nephron* 1991;59:602–10

28. Reckelhoff JF, Manning RD Jr. Role of endothelium-derived nitric oxide in control of renal microvasculature in aging male rats. *Am J Physiol* 1993;265(suppl): 1126–31

29. Weinberg AD, Pals JK, Levesque PG, *et al*. Dehydration and death during febrile episodes in the nursing home. *J Am Geriatr Soc* 1994;42:968–71

30. Mourey RL, Johnson J, Stolley P. Risk factors for dehydration among elderly nursing home residents. *J Am Geriatr Soc* 1988;36: 213–18

31. Zarich S, Fang LST, Diamond JR. Fractional excretion of sodium: exceptions to its diagnostic value. *Arch Intern Med* 1985;145:108–12

32. Lamy PP. Renal effects of non steroidal antiinflammatory drugs. Heightened risk to the elderly? *J Am Geriatr Soc* 1986;34: 361–7

33. Lameire N, Nelde A, Hoeben H, Vanholder R. Acute renal failure in the elderly. In Oreopoulos DG, Hazzard WR, Luke R, eds. *Nephrology and Geriatrics Integrated*. Boston: Kluwer Academic Publishers, 2000:91–111

34. Lameire N, Van Biesen W, Vanholder R, Colardijn F. The place of intermittent hemodialysis in the treatment of acute renal failure in the ICU patient. *Kidney Int* 1998; 53(suppl66):s110–19

35. Klahr S. The geriatric patient with obstructive uropathy. In Oreopoulos DG, Hazzard WR, Luke R, eds. *Nephrology and Geriatrics Integrated*. Boston: Kluwer Academic Publishers, 2000:167–77

36. O'Brien WM. Benign prostatic hypertrophy. *Am Fam Phys* 1991;44:162–71

37. Sustaria PM, Staskin DR. Hydronephrosis and renal deterioration in the elderly due to abnormalities of the lower urinary tract and ureterovesical junction. In Oreopoulos DG, Hazzard WR, Luke R, eds. *Nephrology and Geriatrics Integrated*. Boston: Kluwer Academic Publishers, 2000:155–65

38. Goldfarb DS, Parks JH, Coe FL. Renal stone disease in older adults. *Clin Geriatr Med* 1998;14:367–81

39. Humphrey LL, Ballard DJ, Frohnert PP, *et al*. Chronic renal failure in non-insulin dependent diabetes mellitus. A population based study in Rochester, Minnesota. *Ann Intern Med* 1989;111:788–96

40. Gall MA, Rossing P, Jensen JS, *et al*. Red cell Na^+/Li^+ countertransport in non-insulin-dependent diabetics with diabetic nephropathy. *Kidney Int* 1991;39:135–40

41. Ravid M, Savin H, Jutrin I, *et al*. Long term stabilizing effect of angiotensin-converting enzyme inhibition on plasma creatinine and on proteinuria in normotensive type II diabetic patients. *Ann Intern Med* 1993;118:577–81

42. Anand S, Nissenson AR. Renal anemia management in the chronic kidney disease population. *Ann Long-Term Care: Clin Care Aging* 2002;10:43–52

43. Locatelli F, Olivares J, Walker R, *et al*. Novel erythropoiesis stimulating protein for treatment of anemia of chronic renal insufficiency. *Kidney Int* 2001;60:741–7

44. Casadevall N, Nataf J, Viron B, *et al*. Pure red cell aplasia and antierythropoietin antibodies in patients treated with recombinant erythropoietin. *New Engl J Med* 2002;346:469–75

45. Winchester JF, Rakowski TA. End-stage renal disease and its management in older adults. *Clin Geriatr Med* 1998;14:255–63

46. Lindeman RD. Renal diseases and disorders. *Clin Geriatr* 2002;10:41–52

47. Winchester JF. Peritoneal dialysis in older individuals. In Oreopoulos DG, Hazzard WR, Luke R, eds. *Nephrology and Geriatrics Integrated*. Boston: Kluwer Academic Publishers, 2000:127–35

48. Foley RN, Parfrey PS. Cardiac disease in chronic uremia: clinical outcome and risk factors. *Adv Ren Replace Ther* 1997;4:234–48

49. Husebye DG, Kjellsrand CM. Old patients and uremia: rates of acceptance to and withdrawal from dialysis. *Int J Artif Organs* 1987;10:166–72

50. Bia MJ. Older transplant recipients; older transplant donors – what are the issues? In Oreopoulos DG, Hazzard WR, Luke R, eds. *Nephrology and Geriatrics Integrated*. Boston: Kluwer Academic Publishers, 2000:149–54

51. Bia MJ, Ramos EL, Donovitch GM, *et al*., Evaluation of living donors: the current practice of U.S. transplant centers. *Transplant* 1995;60:322–7

52. Platt WMD. Age dependent changes of the kidneys: pharmacologic implications. *Gerontology* 1999;45:243–53

53. Moore RD, Smith CR, Lipsky JJ, *et al*. Risk factors for nephrotoxicity in patients treated with aminoglycosides. *Ann Intern Med* 1984;100:352–7

54. Lindeman RD, Kelleher CL. Renal diseases and disorders. In Cobbs EL, Duthie EH, Murphy JB, eds. *Geriatrics Review Syllabus: A Core Curriculum in Geriatric Medicine*, 5th edn. Malden, MA: Blackwell Publishing for the American Geriatrics Society, 2002;374–84

41 Endocrine disorders in the elderly

Monisha Medhi, MD, *and Merville C. Marshall Jr*, MD, FACP, FACE

INTRODUCTION

The elderly population is increasing globally. The prevalence of certain endocrine diseases, such as hypothyroidism and diabetes mellitus, is increased in the elderly. Endocrine disease in elderly subjects may present without classic signs and symptoms, and may present as non-specific symptoms including fatigue, anorexia, weight loss, failure to thrive, loss of motivation and difficulty in concentration. The physician has to distinguish among age-related changes, altered endocrine function that is secondary to coincident non-endocrine disease, and true endocrinopathy.

AGE-RELATED CHANGES

Carbohydrate metabolism

Glucose intolerance and insulin resistance increases with age[1,2]. Fasting plasma glucose increases by 1–2 mg/dl per decade and 2-h postprandial plasma glucose increases by 8–20 mg/dl per decade after the age of 30–40 years. Although insulin secretion may decline with age, the defect underlying age-related glucose intolerance appears to be a decrease in insulin-mediated peripheral glucose metabolism. There is disagreement as to whether the insulin response to a glucose load is unchanged[3,4] or increased[1,5] with aging. However, a recent review[6] concluded that the purported increase in insulin resistance in peripheral tissue was not significant

when confounders were controlled, the largest one being obesity. Also, hepatic glucose sensitivity to insulin and beta-cell sensitivity are unaltered with aging[6].

The physiologic response to hypoglycemia is unaltered with age. However, there may be physical or mental disability as well as environmental impediments that can affect an appropriate response to hypoglycemia in the elderly. Also, the glucose level at which the maximum physiologic response occurs is lower in the elderly[7].

Anterior pituitary and hypothalamic axis

The hypothalamic–pituitary axis remains intact with age, with no alterations in circadian rhythms. However, dynamic studies of the pituitary in hospitalized patients over 75 years reveal normal basal hormone levels but diminished peak responses of growth hormone (GH), luteinizing hormone (LH), follicle stimulating hormone (FSH) and thyroid stimulating hormone (TSH) to stimulation, when compared to younger patients[8]. GH and insulin-like growth factor decline with increasing age, with an estimated decrease of 14% per decade after the age of 20 years[9]. The exact cause of the age-related decline is not clear; however, obesity and hyperglycemia also inhibit GH secretion and can contribute to the observed decline[10]. GH therapy can improve body composition, but not cognitive function, strength and systemic endurance[11].

Thyroid

The age-related changes in thyroid volume are controversial. Some studies have found decreasing glandular volume with age[12], whereas others have reported increase in weight by the age of 70 years to approximately 35–40 g[13,14]. The discrepancy may be related to regional differences in the amount of dietary iodine intake. There is a marked increase in the nodularity of the gland with age. It is estimated that up to 90% of women over the age of 72 years and 60% of men over the age of 80 years have thyroid nodules[15]. Another study, though, reports the prevalence of thyroid nodules as only 25%[16].

TSH levels remain in the normal range throughout life[17]. Twenty-four-hour basal TSH secretions of healthy octogenarians show normal diurnal variation, with normal or slightly decreased production[18]. The thyroidal uptake of iodine as measured by radioactive iodine uptake, corrected for age-related decrease in renal and thyroid iodide clearance, is decreased[19]. Thyroxine (T_4) production decreases by 25% with age[20]. However, a decrease in metabolic clearance of T_4 results in normal serum T_4 levels. Plasma thyroxine binding globulin (TBG) levels are unchanged in healthy individuals.

Early studies of non-selected heterogeneous populations indicated a decline in serum tri-iodothyronine (T_3) with age[21]. Recent investigations in selected populations of healthy elderly persons showed serum T_3 levels remaining in the normal range[17].

Adrenal

Serum cortisol levels change little with age, due to an equivalent decrease in both secretion and clearance of cortisol. Dynamic testing of the hypothalamic–pituitary–adrenal (HPA) axis is normal[22]. The morning peak of cortisol secretion occurs several hours earlier in the elderly[23]. However, the rise in cortisol levels in response to acute stress, such as surgery, is often protracted in the elderly. Chronic illness affects the HPA axis as well. Patients with diabetes mellitus and hypertension have also been found to have an exaggerated and prolonged response to corticotropin releasing hormone stimulation[24]. It is not known whether these elevated levels contribute to the increased prevalence of hypertension, glucose intolerance, muscle atrophy, osteoporosis and impaired immune function observed in the elderly.

Serum levels of dehydroepiandrosterone (DHEA) and its sulfate (DHEAS) decline linearly with age. DHEAS has been inversely associated with cardiovascular mortality in some studies. However, this has not been a consistent finding, and one large study found no relationship between DHEAS and cardiovascular mortality[25]. Also, there is little evidence that DHEAS supplements have significant clinical benefits.

DIABETES MELLITUS

Diabetes mellitus is a disorder of carbohydrate metabolism due to a relative or absolute deficiency of insulin. In the USA, nearly half of all the persons known to have type 2 diabetes mellitus are over 65 years of age[26]. The prevalence increases with age; 17% of persons over age 65 have diabetes mellitus[27]. The vast majority of all diabetic patients have type 2 (non-insulin-dependent) diabetes mellitus. However, with the improved care and survival of younger patients with type 1 (insulin-dependent) diabetes mellitus, the number of type 1 diabetes mellitus patients among the elderly will rise. Moreover, approximately 10% of patients in whom diabetes mellitus develops and who are over the age of 70 years have type 1[28]. The presentation of symptomatic elderly patients with diabetes may be significantly different from the classic triad of polyuria, polydipsia and weight loss. Diminished thirst perception may be a reason for lack of polydipsia, and is also one of the reasons for the increased frequency of hyperosmolar states in the elderly. Polyuria may be manifest by urinary incontinence rather than a complaint of frequent urination. Altered cognition may also be a presenting symptom.

Diagnosis

Diabetes mellitus is diagnosed in one of three ways[29], and any given method must be confirmed by repeat testing:

(1) Symptoms of diabetes plus a casual plasma glucose concentration of ≥ 200 mg/dl (11.1 mmol/l). 'Casual' is defined as any time of day without regard to time since last meal. The classic symptoms of diabetes include polyuria, polydipsia and unexplained weight loss.

(2) Fasting plasma glucose concentration of ≥ 126 mg/dl (7.0 mmol/l). 'Fasting' is defined as no caloric intake for at least 8 h.

(3) Two-hour plasma glucose concentration of ≥ 200 mg/dl (11.1 mmol/l) during an oral glucose tolerance test (OGTT). The test should be performed as described by the World Health Organization (WHO)[30], using a glucose load containing the equivalent of 75 g anhydrous glucose dissolved in water. The OGTT is not recommended for routine use.

Goals of therapy

The therapeutic goal in a diabetic patient is to achieve an acceptable serum glucose level, prevent acute symptoms or complications of uncontrolled hyperglycemia, avoid hypoglycemia and prevent or delay the progression of the chronic complications of diabetes. Diabetic complications in the elderly are compounded by the fact that many of the organ systems affected by diabetes (kidneys, eyes, blood vessels, nerves) are also affected by aging itself.

A fasting glucose level of < 120 mg/dl, a postprandial serum glucose level of < 140 mg/dl, and a hemoglobin A_{1c} level of < 7% are generally accepted criteria of good control. The Diabetes Control and Complications Trial (DCCT) in 1993[31], the Kumamoto Trial in 1995[32] and the United Kingdom Prospective Diabetes Study (UKPDS) in 1998[33] demonstrated the efficacy of glycemic control in preventing microvascular complications in type 1 diabetes mellitus[31] and type 2 diabetes mellitus[32,33]. Hypoglycemia is considered to be more hazardous in the elderly than in the younger patient, because of the risk of myocardial infarctions and cerebral vascular accidents. Nonetheless, the American Diabetes Association[34] reminds us, correctly, that 'age per se should not be an excuse for suboptimal control of blood glucose...' It is our practice to try to maintain serum glucose levels between 100 and 180 mg/dl in the elderly diabetic patient.

Medical nutrition therapy

Dietary therapy remains the foundation of diabetes management. The nutritional guidelines recommended for the adult diabetic patient are equally appropriate for the older and younger person with diabetes. Nutritional intervention in elderly patients can be particularly challenging. Factors that can adversely affect nutrition in the elderly include impaired food shopping capabilities or food preparation skills (due to cognitive dysfunction or physical disabilities), limited finances, poor motivation, co-existing illness, age-related decline in taste perception, poor eating habits and lack of sufficient education. Appropriate meal planning can significantly improve glycemic control in the elderly diabetic patient[35]. Excessive caloric restriction should be avoided in the lean patient.

Table 1 Oral agents for the therapy of diabetes mellitus

Agent	Mechanism of action	Comments
Insulin secretagogs		
Second generation sulfonylureas glipizide, glyburide, glicazide, glimepiride	stimulate insulin secretion	generally preferred for lean patients; can cause hypoglycemia; first generation agents (e.g. chlorpropramide, tolbutamide, tolazamide) not recommended, because of drug interactions, prolonged half-lives, and risk for SIADH
Meglitinides repaglinide, nateglinide	stimulate insulin secretion for a short interval of time	rapid onset and offset of action; used only as preprandial agents; no effect upon fasting glucose; lower incidence of hypoglycemia than sulfonylureas
Insulin sensitizers		
Thiazolidinediones pioglitazone; rosiglitazone	improve insulin sensitivity primarily at muscle and adipose tissue	Liver function tests must be monitored every 2 months during the first year of therapy; can cause weight gain and edema; contraindicated in congestive heart failure
Biguanide metformin	improves insulin sensitivity primarily at the liver	generally preferred for obese patients; often aids weight loss; major side-effects are diarrhea, nausea, dyspepsia; lactic acidosis is rare; contraindicated in renal disease
Others		
α-glucosidase inhibitors acarbose, miglitol	inhibit absorption of carbohydrates in the small intestine	used only as a preprandial agent; will cause bothersome flatulence; if insulin-induced hypoglycemia occurs, oral feeding will not be effective within 2 h of medication

SIADH, syndrome of inappropriate antidiuretic hormone

Exercise therapy

Exercise is clearly salutary for all patients; it has beneficial effects on glucose intolerance, blood pressure control, weight control, lipid profile and cardiovascular status[36,37]. Several factors need to be considered when prescribing exercise for the elderly. First, older adults are sedentary and cannot be expected to undergo a drastic change in lifestyle. Therefore, a simple walking program, or even just getting out of the house to go shopping, is beneficial, both psychologically and physically. Before an exercise prescription is given, variables such as functional status, health needs, and medical problems of the individual patient need to be addressed. All diabetic patients should be aware of their glucose levels before exercise[38]. Patients treated with oral agents or insulin are at particular risk for exercise-induced hypoglycemia and must monitor themselves carefully in the initial phase of an exercise program.

Pharmacological therapy

The elderly diabetic patient whose glucose levels remain consistently above 200 mg/dl, despite dietary compliance and physical activity, is a candidate for pharmacologic

Table 2 Insulins

Type of insulin	Peak action	Comments
Rapid acting Lispro, aspart	1–2 h	for mealtime dosing to target postprandial glucose peaks
Short acting Regular (R)	4–6 h	for pre-meal dosing to target postprandial glucose peaks
Intermediate acting Neutral protamine Hagedorn (NPH), Lente	8–12 h	if used as a single dose, generally the preferred timing is a bedtime dose to target fasting hyperglycemia. For multiple doses: a morning dose and a bedtime dose are given. Bedtime dosing is preferred to evening dosing, to avoid nocturnal hypoglycemia
Long acting Ultralente	8–20 h	can be used in place of intermediate acting insulins in selected patients; can be used on an every 12-h regimen to treat patients on continuous feedings
Very long acting Insulin glargine	'peakless'	used as a once a day insulin, in place of twice a day intermediate acting insulins, to provide a basal level of insulin for 24 h; lower incidence of hypoglycemia than intermediate acting insulins
Premixed insulins 70/30 (70% NPH, 30% R) 50/50 (50% NPH, 50% R) 75/25 (75% NPH, 25% lispro)		Options for patients who cannot or will not mix insulin; offers the convenience of a single injection but less flexibility for optimal control; different ratios and combinations are available in different countries

therapy. As is true for the administration of all drugs in the elderly, medications should be initiated at low doses in the older patient. Table 1 provides a brief overview of the drugs available. Patients who fail to respond to a combination of oral agents are candidates for insulin therapy.

Physicians should not be dissuaded from initiating insulin therapy in older diabetic patients simply because of age. Although insulin therapy in the elderly often entails special considerations, the principles of insulin therapy are essentially the same in older and younger adults with diabetes[39]. Synthetic human insulin is widely used and preferred to animal insulin. There are many algorithms for starting insulin therapy (e.g. 0.2–0.5 U/kg body weight)[40], but the optimal total dose of insulin needed for good glycemic control will vary from patient to patient. The initial dose is always somewhat arbitrary. The older diabetic patient is more likely to have diminished eyesight or disabling arthritis, which can impair self-administration of insulin. A variety of devices are available to aid such patients. These include magnifiers designed to wrap around insulin syringes to enlarge the numbers on the syringe, syringe-filling devices that click so that the patient can hear and count the numbers of units being drawn into syringes, and 'talking glucometers' that permit self-monitoring by the visually impaired. It is perhaps more true for the elderly diabetic that compromise must be made between optimal control and the feasibility of, or compliance with, a given regimen for a given patient. Some of the available insulin formulations are detailed in Table 2.

All insulin users should carry medical identification that alerts others to the fact that the wearer uses insulin. Patients also should be instructed to carry at least 15 g of carbohydrate to be eaten in the event of a hypoglycemic reaction. Family members, roommates and all patient care providers should be instructed in the use of glucagon injections for situations when a patient cannot be given carbohydrate orally.

Acute complications

Hypoglycemia

Hypoglycemia is a complication of insulin or any of the insulin secretagogues (sulfonylureas and meglitinides). Hypoglycemic symptoms in the elderly tend to present predominantly as neuroglycopenic symptoms: impaired concentration, personality changes, focal neurologic deficits, seizures or syncope. Adrenergic symptoms (tremulousness, anxiety, diaphoresis, palpitations and hunger) are diminished in part due to a loss of autonomic nerve function. Elderly patients who become hypoglycemic may be at greater risk for myocardial infarction or cerebrovascular accident. Thus, the potential threat and risks of hypoglycemia are greater in older diabetics then in younger patients. Avoiding hypoglycemia in the elderly diabetic patient demands careful vigilance on the part of the health-care team.

Diabetic ketoacidosis and hyperglycemic hyperosmolar state

Diabetic ketoacidosis (DKA) and hyperglycemic hyperosmolar state (HHS) are the most serious acute complications of diabetes mellitus. The terms 'hyperglycemic hyperosmolar non-ketotic coma' and 'hyperglycemic hyperosmolar non-ketotic state' have been replaced by the term 'hyperglycemic hyperosmolar state'[41] to reflect the facts that: alterations in sensorium may be present even in the absence of coma; and HHS may consist of moderate to variable degrees of clinical ketosis. These conditions are characterized by a relative or absolute hypoinsulinemia. Although DKA is classically identified with type 1 diabetes mellitus, and HHS with type 2 diabetes mellitus, reviews have stressed the concept of these conditions representing two ends of a continuum[42,43]. A considerable proportion of patients with HHS reside in nursing homes. The predilection of the elderly to HHS may be secondary to age-related impaired maintenance of serum osmolality, decreased thirst sensation, or decreased cognitive function interfering with fluid intake. The institutionalized bedridden elderly patient may lack free access to fluids and may be at greater risk for HHS, especially if glucose levels are infrequently monitored. Table 3 briefly outlines the characteristics of DKA and HHS[44].

The principle objective in treating HHS is to correct the hyperosmolar state. Hyperosmolarity and dehydration are the primary causes for coma and death. Insulin therapy and fluid replacement are of paramount importance. Because most patients are hypovolemic upon presentation, fluid replacement is initiated with isotonic saline. If hypovolemia is not present, hypotonic (0.45%) saline is preferable, because it delivers more free water. As much as 4–6 liters of fluid may be needed within the first 12 h of therapy. Caution is indicated in the elderly patient with heart failure or renal insufficiency to avoid fluid overload. Along with frequent clinical and laboratory assessment, bladder catherization and monitoring of central venous pressure or pulmonary capillary wedge pressure may be warranted to assess fluid status more accurately.

Insulin therapy is usually started with a bolus of 10–20 U of regular (R) insulin, followed by a maintenance dose of 5–10 U/h given intravenously. A decline in serum glucose of approximately 10%/h is a reasonable goal. When serum glucose returns to normal, hourly intravenous insulin therapy can give way to less intensive subcutaneous insulin therapy. Ultimately, the majority of patients

Table 3   Features of diabetic ketoacidosis (DKA) and hyperglycemic hyperosmolar state (HHS)

	DKA	HHS
Incidence	4–9% of hospital discharges; less common in the elderly, but can occur with significant stress	< 1% of all diabetic admissions; most common in the elderly, often in the absence of a known history of diabetes; can also occur in hospitalized patients
Precipitating event	infection, omission of insulin, myocardial infarction	infection, concomitant illness, drugs (e.g. steroids, thiazides)
Mental status	alert to stupor/coma	stupor/coma
Usual glucose level	300–600 mg/dl	600–1000 mg/dl
Arterial pH	< 7.30	> 7.30
Serum bicarbonate	< 15 mEq/l	> 18 mEq/l
Serum ketones (acetoacetate)	positive	negative or small
Anion gap	> 12	< 10
Effective plasma osmolality	variable	> 320 mOsm/kg
Mortality	< 5%	~15%

admitted with a diagnosis of HHS can be managed without insulin and are discharged with adequate glycemic control as the result of dietary and/or oral glucose-lowering agents.

Chronic complications

The diabetic patient is uniquely predisposed to accelerated atherosclerosis, which leads to macrovascular complications of diabetes (coronary artery disease, cerebrovascular accidents and peripheral vascular disease). This may be due to any combination of hyperlipidemia, hyperglycemia, insulin resistance or the increased prevalence of hypertension in the diabetic patient. Dyslipidemia (increased low-density lipoprotein cholesterol, increased triglyceride, and decreased high-density lipoprotein cholesterol) is a common clinical problem in diabetic patients that greatly increases the risk for macrovascular complications. Many authorities recommend aggressive treatment of hyperlipidemia in elderly patients, although this is still a controversial issue[45].

Diabetic nephropathy is the most common cause of end-stage renal disease[46]. Microalbuminuria, which is the first sign of diabetic nephropathy, is a problematic screening tool in the elderly, as proteinuria increases with age even in the absence of diabetes. Age-specific norms for microalbuminuria should be helpful in the future. The presence of microalbuminuria warrants attention to optimizing glycemic control and control of hypertension, if present. Angiotensin converting enzyme inhibitors are proven therapy for type 1 diabetics with microalbuminuria and may be useful for type 2 diabetics with microalbuminuria. Angiotensin-receptor blockers are also beneficial in diabetic nephropathy.

Persons with diabetes have a 25-fold greater risk of blindness than non-diabetic individuals[47]. In addition to routine examinations to assess the presence of glaucoma and cataracts, all patients with newly diagnosed or newly recognized type 2 diabetes mellitus should undergo dilated ophthalmoscopic examination to evaluate for retinopathy. There are many different manifestations of diabetic neuropathy, but the most common is peripheral neuropathy, which typically presents with paresthesia, dysesthesia, hypesthesia or anesthesia. Screening and education for diabetic foot problems should be undertaken more vigorously in the elderly than in younger persons with diabetes, because the elderly are at higher risk due to the combination of vascular and neuropathic disease. The first therapeutic modality for peripheral neuropathy is improved glycemic control. Gabapentin and amitriptyline are adjunct therapy for persistent neuropathic pain.

Impotence secondary to autonomic neuropathy or vascular insufficiency has several therapeutic modalities including vacuum erection devices, intracavernous injections of vasoactive drugs, sildenafil and penile prosthesis; however, patient acceptance of these modalities varies amongst individuals. Sildenafil is effective in about one-third of diabetics with erectile dysfunction. It is important to warn patients taking nitrates of the increased risk of hypotension when using sildenafil.

Diabetic chiropathy or rheumatologic complications of diabetes can be a cause of functional impairment in the older diabetic patient and include: carpal tunnel syndrome, Dupuytren's contracture, trigger finger and limited joint mobility[48].

THYROID DISEASES

Screening recommendations

There is no consensus among thyroidologists regarding the utility of screening for thyroid dysfunction in the absence of symptoms. It is reasonable to measure TSH in older individuals who present with atypical symptoms of thyroid disease such as exacerbation of cardiac symptoms, change in mental status, falling or onset of depression. Given the 2–10% incidence of unrecognized hyperthyroidism and hypothyroidism in the elderly, many advocate routine screening of this population with a TSH assay.

Hypothyroidism

The prevalence of thyroid disease in the elderly is approximately twice that in younger individuals, with hypothyroidism ranging from 2 to 7%[27]. Hypothyroidism in the elderly is most often due to Hashimoto's thyroiditis or prior radioactive iodine ablative therapy for Graves' disease. Iodine-induced hypothyroidism (Wolff– Chaikoff effect) after the excessive intake of iodine or iodine-containing substances (e.g. medications such as amiodarone, which have a high iodine load) can be seen in the presence of underlying autoimmune thyroid disease, especially in iodine replete areas.

Clinical features

The resemblance between overt hypothyroidism and some of the changes occurring with older age frequently make this a difficult diagnosis. The elderly are more likely to present with cardiovascular symptoms (e.g. congestive heart failure or angina) or neurologic findings (e.g. cognitive impairment, confusion, depression, paresthesias, deafness and psychosis). Fatigue (67.7%) and weakness (52.5%) were the two most common complaints in elderly patients aged more than 70 years with documented hypothyroidism[49]. Physical findings are frequently non-specific, although puffy face, delayed tendon reflexes and myoedema support the diagnosis.

Myxedema coma is the end stage of untreated hypothyroidism. Disorders that may precipitate myxedema coma include heart failure, pneumonia, pulmonary edema, excessive fluid administration, or administration of sedative or narcotic drugs to a patient with severe hypothyroidism. It is characterized by progressive weakness, stupor, hypothermia, hypoventilation, hypoglycemia, hyponatremia, water intoxication, shock and death. Hypothermia (body temperature as low as 75°F 24°C) is frequently not recognized by the ordinary clinical thermometer that only registers as low as 93°F (34°C). A laboratory-type thermometer that registers a broader scale must be used. Although rare now, in the future myxedema coma may occur more frequently with the increasing use of radioiodine for the treatment of Graves' disease, and resulting permanent hypothyroidism. Since it occurs most frequently in older patients with underlying pulmonary and vascular disease, the mortality rate is extremely high.

Diagnosis

Primary hypothyroidism is confirmed by an elevated serum TSH and a low free T_4 or total T_4. Measurement of T_3 is unnecessary and potentially misleading, because T_3 decreases with non-thyroidal illness. Serum TSH alone should not be used to make a diagnosis, because it will not always differentiate symptomatic from subclinical hypothyroidism. The pulsatile nature of TSH release along with a nocturnal rise in serum TSH can falsely lead to a diagnosis of subclinical hypothyroidism. Corticosteroids and dopaminergic drugs reduce TSH. Patients on these medications may require additional tests with free T_4 and reverse T_3 levels to differentiate between hypothyroidism and non-thyroidal illness.

Low voltage and bradycardia on electrocardiography, normocytic or macrocytic anemia, hypercholesterolemia and elevated serum creatinine phosphokinase are additional features of hypothyroidism. Hyponatremia secondary to the syndrome of inappropriate antidiuretic hormone secretion (SIADH) is usually seen in patients with myxedema coma.

A radioactive iodine uptake has no role in the diagnostic workup for hypothyroidism. Antithyroglobulin antibody or antimicrosomal antibody titers can aid in diagnosing an autoimmune etiology of hypothyroidism. A very high titer of antimicrosomal antibody, e.g. > 1 : 1600, along with an elevated TSH and a normal T_4, have been shown to be a marker of progression to overt hypothyroidism in 80% of patients within 4 years[50].

Treatment

The treatment for hypothyroidism is L-thyroxine. The doses of thyroid hormone required for adequate replacement decrease in older adults[51,52]. Elderly patients should be started on 25–50 µg of levothyroxine, and the dose should be increased by 25 µg every 3–4 weeks until serum TSH returns to the normal range. In patients with cardiovascular disease, lower doses can be used to initiate therapy. Desiccated thyroid extract and other preparations containing T_3 should be avoided, because T_3 levels rise rapidly and patients often complain of palpitations. Overtreatment, as documented by a suppressed TSH, should be avoided because of the increased risk of osteoporosis and potential adverse effects on the cardiovascular system. Once thyroid functions are normal at a given dose, annual follow-up is adequate. All other medications that the patient may be taking should be re-evaluated, as the metabolic clearance of other drugs will change once hypothyroidism is corrected.

Myxedema coma is an acute medical emergency and should be treated in the intensive care unit. Patients usually require intubation and mechanical ventilation. Associated illnesses such as infections or heart failure must be sought and treated appropriately. Because patients with myxedema coma absorb all drugs poorly, it is imperative to give levothyroxine intravenously. An initial dose of 300–400 µg of levothyroxine is administered intravenously, followed by 50 µg of levothyroxine intravenously daily. There is an inherent risk of precipitating angina, heart failure or arrhythmias in older patients with underlying coronary artery disease. Active rewarming of the body is contraindicated, because it may induce vasodilatation and vascular collapse. The clinical guides to improvement are a rise in body temperature and the return of normal cerebral and respiratory function. If, the patient is known to have normal adrenal function before the coma, adrenal support is probably not necessary. If, however, no data are available, the possibility of concomitant adrenal insufficiency (due to autoimmune adrenal disease or pituitary insufficiency) does exist. Full adrenal support should be administered, e.g. hydrocortisone, an initial dose of 100 mg intravenously, followed by 50 mg intravenously every 6 h. The dose is tapered over a week while monitoring the clinical status. Adrenal support can be withdrawn sooner if pretreatment plasma cortisol is 20 µg/dl or greater, or if results of a cosyntropin test are within normal limits.

Hyperthyroidism

Hyperthyroidism affects 2% of the older population[27]. Toxic multinodular goiter is the most common cause of hyperthyroidism in the elderly. The incidence of Graves' disease declines after the age of 60 years[53]. Iodine-induced hyperthyroidism (Jodbasedow phenomenon) can be seen in iodine-deficient areas, among patients with non-toxic multinodular goiter following administration of iodine (e.g. amiodarone, contrast agents containing iodine used for angiograms, etc.). Because of the age-related decrease in the clearance of thyroid hormone, a patient who has been taking the same dose of thyroid hormone for many years may become hyperthyroid.

Elderly hyperthyroid patients tend to present with symptoms or complications related to the most vulnerable organ system – usually the cardiovascular system (atrial fibrillation, congestive heart failure, angina and acute myocardial infarction) or the central nervous system (apathy, depression, confusion or lassitude). Patients over the age of 75 years have the greatest risk of mortality from cardiovascular or cerebrovascular causes[54]. The hypercatabolic state also causes muscle wasting, particularly of the quadriceps, thereby increasing the risk of falls. Findings suggestive of hyperthyroidism include increased frequency of bowel movements, weight loss despite increased appetite, fine finger tremor, eyelid retraction and increased perspiration. Gastrointestinal symptoms may differ from those seen in the younger patients, with constipation seen more often than hyperdefecation. Anorexia and failure to thrive may be the only symptoms in the

elderly. 'Apathetic hyperthyroidism' is a unique presentation in the elderly[55], characterized by fatigue and apathy, and a lack of ocular findings, goiter and tachycardia.

The most common physical signs of hyperthyroidism in the elderly are atrial fibrillation, fine skin, tremor and hyperactive reflexes. Sinus tachycardia is less frequent. The thyroid feels normal in size or is not palpable in two-thirds of the patients. Lid lag and ophthalmopathy are less common, not only because Graves' disease is less common in the elderly, but also because even with Graves' disease ophthalmopathy occurs less frequently in the elderly.

Diagnosis

A suppressed TSH (measured by a sensitive immunoradiometric or chemiluminescent assay) along with a high total T_4, free T_4, or free T_4 index estimate confirms the diagnosis. If T_4 levels are normal with a suppressed TSH one must consider T_3 toxicosis and obtain a serum total T_3 level. This may be a more difficult diagnosis because concomitant non-thyroidal illnesses are common and can depress serum T_3. In the patient with debilitating non-thyroidal illness, a serum T_3 which is not suppressed (e.g. $T_3 > 100$ ng/dl) should prompt an investigation for hyperthyroidism[56]. The 24-h radioactive iodine uptake is usually elevated in hyperthyroidism.

Treatment

Thyroid ablation with I-131 is the treatment of choice in the elderly, because it is efficient, uncomplicated and inexpensive. In patients with ischemic heart disease, pretreatment with propylthiouracil or methimazole and β-blockers before thyroid ablation is recommended to prevent a transient release of thyroid hormone, consequent to radioactive iodine therapy (radiation thyroiditis) and the exacerbation of cardiac symptoms. Surgery has a limited role, because of its increased morbidity in the elderly. Following radioactive iodine treatment, patients become euthyroid over a period of 6–12 weeks. They should receive careful follow-up, because hypothyroidism develops in 80% or more of patients who have been adequately treated with radioactive iodine.

Subclinical hypothyroidism

A moderate elevation of TSH to 10–20 mU/l with a normal serum T_4 in subjects without overt symptoms of hypothyroidism is considered subclinical hypothyroidism. The estimated prevalence in the elderly is 4–14%[27]. It is still not known whether treating this entity is beneficial in older patients. Two-thirds of these patients will remain chemically euthyroid for at least 4 years. Low titers of antimicrosomal antibodies may identify patients at lowest risk for progression to overt hyperthyroidism. A therapeutic trial with levothyroxine may be offered to patients. No association has been reported between subclinical hypothyroidism and lipid abnormalities and cardiovascular disease[57]; however, improvements in left ventricular function during exercise[58], and systolic time intervals as well as non-specific symptoms have occurred[59] on therapy in patients with subclinical hypothyroidism.

Subclinical hyperthyroidism

A suppressed TSH with a normal T_4 and T_3 in the absence of debilitating non-thyroidal illness or medications interfering with TSH secretion is considered subclinical hyperthyroidism. The estimated prevalence in the elderly is 4%[27]. This may be due to autonomous function of a multinodular goiter or nodule. A low serum TSH concentration is associated with a three-fold higher risk of atrial fibrillation in the subsequent decade[60] and also increased bone loss[61]. However, an isolated low TSH level in an elderly person does not have a high predictive value for hyperthyroidism. In a geriatric practice in the UK, only 2% of patients with a low TSH level

progressed to thyrotoxicosis in 12 months[62]. In the Framingham study, only 12% of patients with low TSH had hyperthyroidism[63]. These patients require monitoring, especially if presented with an iodine load. A therapeutic trial may be attempted with antithyroid drugs in patients with new-onset atrial fibrillation or unexplained weight loss, in the presence of subclinical hyperthyroidism.

Multinodular goiter

The prevalence of multinodular goiter increases with age. If swallowing and breathing are not compromised and thyroid function tests are normal, the goiter can be observed without treatment. Levothyroxine suppressive therapy rarely shrinks the gland, although it may prevent further enlargement. Suppressive therapy is not recommended, because of the risk of osteoporosis. Also, overt hyperthyroidism may occur if the gland develops autonomous function.

Thyroid function in non-thyroidal illness

Acute or chronic illness may have striking effects on circulating thyroid hormone levels. The high frequency of these changes makes it inadvisable to screen patients for thyroid dysfunction in the setting of acute illness unless there is a strong suspicion of intrinsic thyroid disease. These changes occur via modifying the peripheral metabolism of T_4 or by interference with T_4 binding to TBG. Decreased deiodination of T_4 to T_3, resulting in a low serum T_3 level and decreased clearance of reverse T_3, resulting in an elevated reverse T_3 level, are virtually universal accompaniments of significant illness or starvation. The serum total T_4 and free T_4 (as measured by radioimmune assay or free T_4 index estimate) are also often decreased. However, when the free T_4 has been measured by equilibrium dialysis, it has been reported to be normal or even elevated in the most sick patients. Low total and free T_4

concentrations have been associated with more severe illness and higher mortality rates in several studies. Treatment with thyroid hormones in this circumstance is not recommended and may in fact worsen the situation.

Pituitary TSH secretion is also diminished in severe systemic illness and may, in fact, be a primary event in the development of hypothyroxinemia in these patients. Furthermore, certain drugs commonly used in critically ill patients (e.g. dopamine, glucocorticoids) also inhibit TSH release. During recovery from non-thyroidal illness, patients may have a transiently and modestly elevated serum TSH level. Thus, these changes may represent a protective adaptation to severe illness.

Thyroid cancer

Thyroid nodules are common in the elderly. Ninety per cent of these nodules are benign, but the prognosis for elderly patients with malignant nodules may be worse than that for younger patients with malignant nodules. The following increase the risk for malignancy and should prompt early referral to an endocrinologist:

(1) Age more than 60 years

(2) Male sex

(3) History of thyroid cancer

(4) History of radiation

(5) Presence of a single nodule

(6) Rapid growth of a thyroid nodule

(7) Fixation of a nodule to surrounding tissue

(8) Firm, hard, and irregular surface of thyroid swelling

(9) Hoarseness

(10) Dysphagia

The approach is similar to the workup in a younger patient. Fine-needle aspiration is the most useful diagnostic tool in the assessment of a thyroid nodule. The prognosis correlates with the size of the tumor. The outcome in elderly patients may therefore be substantially improved by early evaluation of nodules in patients who are good surgical candidates. Papillary carcinoma is more common in young and middle-aged patients, and has an excellent prognosis in these patients. It has a poorer prognosis in the elderly, possibly because it is detected at a more advanced stage. Follicular carcinoma accounts for 15% of thyroid cancers and usually occurs in middle-aged and older patients. Follicular cancer is more aggressive than papillary carcinoma. Many tumors have elements of both, are classified as papillary–follicular carcinoma and have the same prognosis as papillary carcinoma.

Thyroid lymphoma in a patient with long duration of Hashimoto's disease occurs infrequently. Metastatic malignancy can be found in the thyroid gland. Lung, breast and renal carcinomas are the tumors most often associated with metastases to the thyroid gland.

The therapy for thyroid malignancy is surgical excision. Postoperative follow-up with whole body scans, serum thyroglobulin levels and radioactive iodine therapy should be supervised by an endocrinologist.

ADRENAL DISORDERS

Adrenal hypersecretion

While adrenal hypersecretion (Cushing's syndrome) is uncommon in the elderly, it can be easily overlooked, because it mimics the normal aging process. Signs such as hypertension, glucose intolerance, weight gain and osteoporosis are less specific in the elderly than in younger patients, but the diagnostic workup is the same as in younger patients.

Adrenal insufficiency

Symptoms of adrenal insufficiency in younger patients (failure to thrive, weakness, weight loss, confusion and arthralgias) are common complaints in adrenally intact elderly patients. The most specific sign of adrenal insufficiency in the elderly is hyperpigmentation. The diagnostic workup for adrenal insufficiency is similar to that of a younger patient. The laboratory findings in the elderly in adrenal insufficiency are similar to those found in the young: azotemia, hypoglycemia, hyponatremia, hyperkalemia and eosinophilia. Elderly patients, however, generally require lower replacement doses of cortisol, due to the decrease in the metabolic clearance rate.

Adrenal incidentaloma

Management of incidentally discovered adrenal masses is controversial, and a wide range of recommendations exists about which tests are necessary and which patients should have surgery. The critical questions are: is the mass benign or malignant? and is the mass functional or non-functional? A recent US National Institutes of Health conference[64] suggested the following algorithm. If an adrenal mass larger than 1 cm in diameter is found on imaging in an asymptomatic patient, biochemical screening should be done for latent hormone hypersecretion syndromes, including hyperaldosteronism, hypercortisolism, pheochromocytoma, hyperandrogenism and hyperestrogenism (the latter two instances are quite rare). Any hormone-secreting adrenocortical tumor should be excised. A non-secreting mass of ≥ 5 cm should be excised, because the likelihood of malignancy increases with size. For patients with non-secretory tumors smaller than 5 cm and no signs suggestive of malignancy, an observation approach should include follow-up with a computed tomography scan 3 months after diagnosis[65].

References

1. Fink RI, Revers RR, Kolterman OG, *et al.* The metabolic clearance of insulin and the feedback inhibition of insulin secretion are altered with aging. *Diabetes* 1985;34:275
2. Broughton DL, James OWF, Albert KG, *et al.* Peripheral and hepatic sensitivity in healthy elderly subjects. *Eur J Clin Invest* 1991;21:13
3. Chen M, Bergan RN, Pacini G, *et al.* Pathogenesis of age related glucose intolerance in man: insulin resistance and reduced beta cell function. *J Clin Endocrinol Metab* 1985;60:13
4. Defronzo RA. Glucose intolerance and aging: evidence of tissue insensitivity to insulin. *Diabetes* 1979;28:1095
5. Fink RI, Kolterman OG, Griffin J, *et al.* Mechanism of insulin resistance in aging. *J Clin Invest* 1983;71:1523
6. Elahi D, Muller DC. Carbohydrate metabolism in the elderly. *Eur J Clin Nutr* 2000;54 Suppl 3:S112–20
7. Meneilly GS, Cheung E, Tuokko H. Altered responses to hypoglycemia of healthy older people. *J Clin Endocrinol Metab* 1994; 78:1341
8. Impallomeni M, Yeo T, Rudd A, *et al.* Anterior pituitary function in elderly inpatients over the age of 75 years. *Q J Med* 1987;242:505
9. Iranmanesh A, Lizarralde G, Veldhuis JD. Age and relative adiposity are specific negative determinants of the frequency and amplitude of growth hormone (GH) secretory outburst and the half-life of endogenous GH in healthy men. *J Clin Endocrinol Metab* 1991;73:1081
10. Daughaday W, Rotwein P. Insulin-like growth factors I and II: peptide, messenger ribonucleic acid and gene structures, serum and tissue concentrations. *Endocr Rev* 1989;10:68
11. Papadakis MA, Grady D, Black D, *et al.* Growth hormone replacement in healthy older men improves body composition but not functional ability. *Ann Intern Med* 1996;124:708
12. Gregerman RI, Davis PJ. Effects of intrinsic and extrinsic variables on thyroid economy. In Werner SC, Ingbar SH, eds. *The Thyroid*, 4th edn. Hagerstown, MD: Harper & Row, 1978:223
13. Hegedus L, Perrid H, Poulsen LR, *et al.* The determination of thyroid volume by ultrasound and its relationship to body weight

age and sex in normal subjects. *J Clin Endocrinol Metab* 1983;56:260

14. Morley JE. The aging endocrine system. Postgrad Med 1983;73:107

15. Irvine RE, Hodkinson HM. Thyroid disease in old age. In Broclehurst JC, ed. *Textbook of Geriatric Medicine and Gerontology*. London: Churchill Livingstone, 1978:461

16. Denham MJ, Wills EJ. A clinico-pathological survey of the thyroid gland in old age. *Gerontology* 1980;26:160

17. Tietz NW, Shuey DF, Wekstein DR. Laboratory values in fit aging individuals: sexagenarians through centenarians. *Clin Chem* 1992;38:1167

18. Lewis GF, Alessi CF, Imperial JG, *et al.* Low serum free thyroxine index in ambulating elderly is due to a resetting of the threshold of thyrotropin feedback suppression. *Clin Endocrinol Metab* 1991;73:843

19. Hansen JM, Skovsted L, Siersboek-Nielssen JK. Age-dependent changes in iodine metabolism and thyroid function. *Acta Endocrinol (Copenh)* 1975;79:60

20. Herman J, Heinen E, Kroll HJ, *et al.* Thyroid function and thyroid hormone metabolism in elderly people: low T3 syndrome in old age. *Klin Wochenschr* 1981;59:315

21. Herman J, Rusche HJ, Kroll HJ, *et al.* Free triiodothyronine and thyroxine serum levels in old age. *Horm Metab Res* 1974;6:239

22. Pavlov EP, Harman SM, Chrousos GP, *et al.* Response of plasma adrenocorticotrophin, cortisol and dehydro-epiandrosterone to ovine corticotrophin-releasing hormone in healthy aging men. *J Clin Endocrinol Metab* 1986;62:767

23. Sherman B, Wysham C, Pfohl B. Age-related changes in the circadian rhythm of plasma cortisol in man. *J Clin Endocrinol Metab* 1985;61:439

24. Greenspan S, Rowe J, Maitland L, *et al.* The pituitary–adrenal glucocorticoid response is altered by gender and disease. *J Gerontol* 1993;48:M72

25. Trivedi DP, Khaw KT. Dehydroepiandrosterone sulfate and mortality in elderly men and women. *J Clin Endocrinol Metab* 2001;86:4171

26. Harris MI. Epidemiology of diabetes mellitus among the elderly. *Clin Geriatr Med* 1990;6:703–19

27. Greenspan SL, Resnick NM. Basic and clinical endocrinology. In Greenspan FS, Strewler GJ, eds. *Geriatric Endocrinology*, 5th edn. Norwalk CT: Appleton & Lange, 1997:770–87

28. Morley JE, Kaiser FE. Unique aspects of diabetes mellitus in elderly. *Clin Geriatr Med* 1990;6:693–711

29. The Expert Committee on the diagnosis and classification of diabetes mellitus. *Diabetes Care* 1998;21(suppl 1):S5–S19

30. World Health Organization. *Diabetes Mellitus: Report of a WHO Study Group*. Geneva: World Health Organization, 1985

31. The Diabetes Control and Complications Trial Research Group. The effect of intensive treatment of diabetes on the development and progression of long-term complications in insulin-dependent diabetes mellitus. *N Engl J Med* 1993;329:977–86

32. Yasuo O, Hideki K, Eiichi A, *et al.* Intensive insulin therapy prevents the progression of diabetic microvascular complications in Japanese patients with non-insulin-dependent diabetes mellitus: a randomized prospective 6 year study. *Diabetes Res Clin Pract* 1995;28:103–17

33. UK Prospective Diabetes Study (UKPDS) Group. Intensive blood glucose control with sulphonylureas or insulin compared with the conventional treatment and risk of complications in patients with type 2 diabetes (UKPDS 33). *Lancet* 1998;352:837–53

34. American Diabetes Association. Nutritional principles for the management of diabetes and related complications (technical review). *Diabetes Care* 1994;17:490–518

35. Coulston AM, Mandelbaum D, Reaven GM. Dietary management of nursing home residents with non-insulin-dependent diabetes mellitus. *Am J Clin Nutr* 1990;51:67–71

36. Koivisto VA, Yki-Jarvinen H, Defronzo RA. Physical training and insulin sensitivity. *Diabetes Metab Rev* 1986;1:445–81

37. Schneider SH, Vitug A, Ruderman NB. Atherosclerosis and physical activity. *Diabetes Metab Rev* 1986;1:513–53

38. Kligman EW, Pepin E. Prescribing physical activity for older patients. *Geriatrics* 1992;47:33–47

39. Rosenstock J. Management of type 2 diabetes mellitus in the elderly: special considerations. *Drugs Aging* 2001;18:31

40. Genuth S. Insulin in non-insulin dependent patients. In Mazzaferri EL, Bar RS, Kreisberg RA, eds. *Advances in Endocrinology and Metabolism*, vol 3. St Louis: Mosby-Year Book, 1992:84

41. Ennis ED, Stahl EJVB, Kreisberg RA. The hyperosmolar hyperglycemic syndrome. *Diabetes Rev* 1994;2:115–26

42. Siperstein MD. Diabetic ketoacidosis and hyperosmolar coma. *Endocrinol Metab Clin North Am* 1992;21:415–33

43. Wachtel TJ, tetu-Mouradian LM, Goldman DL, *et al.* Hyperosmolarity and acidosis in diabetes mellitus. *J Gen Intern Med* 1991; 6:497–502

44. Kitabchi AE, Kreisberg RA, Umpierrez GE, *et al.* Management of hyperglycemic rises in patients with diabetes. *Diabetes Care* 2001;24:131–61

45. Expert Panel on Detection, Evaluation, and Treatment of High Blood Cholesterol in Adults (Adult Treatment Panel II). Summary of the second report of the National Cholesterol Education Program (NCEP). *J Am Med Assoc* 1993;269:3015–23

46. Eggers PW. Effect of transplantation on the Medicare end-stage renal disease program. *N Engl J Med* 1988;318:223–7

47. Friedman SM, Rubin ML. Diabetic retinopathy: newer therapies to prevent blindness. *Geriatrics* 1992;47:71–85

48. Spanheimer RG. Skeletal and rheumatological complications of diabetes. In Mazzaferri EL, Bar RS, Kreisberg RA, eds. *Advances in Endocrinology and Metabolism*, vol 4. St Louis: Mosby-Year Book, 1993:55

49. Doucet J, Trivalle C, Chassagne P, *et al.* Does age play a role in clinical presentation of hypothyroidism? *J Am Geriatr Soc* 1994; 42:984

50. Rosenthal ML, Hunt WC, Garry PJ, *et al.* Thyroid failure in the elderly: microsomal antibodies discriminant for therapy. *J Am Med Assoc* 1987;258:209

51. Rosenbaum MJ, Barzel US. Levothyroxine replacement dose for primary hypothyroidism decreases with age. *Ann Intern Med* 1982;96:53

52. Swain CT, Herman T, Molitch ME, *et al.* Aging and the thyroid: decreased requirement for thyroid hormone in older hypothyroid patients. *Am J Med* 1983;75:206

53. Iverson K. Thyrotoxicosis in aged individuals. *J Gerontol* 1953;8:65

54. Osman F, Gammage MD, Franklyn JA. Hyperthyroidism and cardiovascular morbidity and mortality. *Thyroid* 2002;12:483

55. Lahey FA. Non-activated (apathetic) type of hyperthyroidism. *N Engl J Med* 1931; 204:747

56. Engler D, Donaldson E, Stockigt J, *et al.* Hyperthyroidism without triiodothyronine excess: an effect of severe nonthyroidal illness. *J Clin Endocrinol Metab* 1978;46:77

57. Tunbridge WM, Evered D, Hall R, *et al.* The spectrum of thyroid disease in the Whickham area with particular reference to thyroid failure. *Clin Endocrinol* 1977;7:495

58. Forfar JC, Wathen CG, Todd WT, *et al.* Left ventricular performance in subclinical hypothyroidism. *Q J Med* 1985;57:857

59. Cooper DS, Halpern R, Wood LC, *et al.* L-Thyroxine therapy in subclinical hypothyroidism: a double blind placebo-controlled trial. *Ann Intern Med* 1984;101:18

60. Sawin CT, Geller A, Wolf PA, *et al.* Low serum thyrotropin concentrations as a risk factor for atrial fibrillation in older persons. *N Engl J Med* 1994;331:1249

61. Greenspan SL, Greenspan FS. The effect of thyroid hormone on skeletal integrity. *Ann Intern Med* 1999;130:750–8

62. Parle JV, Franklyn JA, Cross KW, *et al.* Prevalence and follow-up of abnormal thyrotropin (TSH) concentrations in elderly in the United Kingdom. *Clin Endocrinol (Oxf)* 1991;34:77

63. Swain CT, Geller A, Kaplan MM, *et al.* Low serum thyrotropin (thyroid stimulating hormone) in older persons without hyperthyroidism. *Arch Intern Med* 1991;151:165

64. Bornstein SR, Stratakis CA, Chrousos GP. Adrenocortical tumors: recent advances in basic concepts and clinical management. *Ann Intern Med* 1999;130:759–71

65. Herrera MF, Grant CS, van Heerden JA, *et al.* Incidentally discovered adrenal tumors: an institutional perspective. *Surgery* 1991;110:1014–21

42 Pulmonary disorders

Mehmet K. Albulak, MD, FCCP, and Etta M. Eskridge, MD, PhD

INTRODUCTION

People 65 years and older represent 12.67% of the US population. Pulmonary diseases are among the most common causes of morbidity and mortality in the elderly[1] (Table 1). As the population continues to age we will encounter pulmonary disorders more often in geriatrics practice.

PULMONARY PHYSIOLOGY

Lung physiology in the elderly

Pulmonary functions improve progressively until the age of 20–25, after which it enters a plateau phase, followed by a progressive decline[2]. Lung physiology is affected, in addition to aging, by tobacco smoke, air pollution, occupational exposures and prior illnesses. The major changes with aging include the following.

Decreased elastic recoil

The inflated lung tends to collapse inward and the chest wall tends to expand outward. Elastic recoil is generated by multiple components such as elastic fibers, collagen fibers, smooth muscle, pulmonary blood volume, bronchial structures and surface-active material. Elastic recoil of the lung progressively declines with aging[3]. As a result, the compliance of the lung (distensibility of the lung for a given inflating pressure) increases. The etiology of the decreased elastic recoil is not

Table 1 Five leading causes of death, all races, both sexes, 65 years and over, 1998. From reference 1

	Number
Heart disease	605 673
Malignant neoplasm	384 186
Cerebrovascular disease	139 144
Chronic obstructive pulmonary disease	97 896
Pneumonia and influenza	83 989

clear. Earlier it was attributed to declining elastin content of the lung; however, further studies have supported the notion that neither the elastin nor the collagen content of the lung changes with aging.

Stiffening of the chest wall

As the rigidity of the rib cage increases, chest wall compliance falls with aging and the contribution of the diaphragm to expansion of the thoracic cavity increases. Compliance of the total respiratory system is decreased in the elderly, because stiffening of the chest wall counterbalances the increased compliance of the lung[2]. The end result of decreased compliance of the respiratory system is increased work in breathing.

Respiratory muscle strength

The endurance of the respiratory muscle declines with aging; however, respiratory muscle endurance can be enhanced by exercise[4].

461

Other changes

Lung height increases until the age of 60. The kyphotic curve and anteroposterior (AP) diameter also increase with aging. Although some emphysematous changes also take place, the increased AP diameter is not from those changes. The elderly may develop panacinar-type emphysema; this process is usually limited and has no clinical significance. The diameter of cartilaginous bronchioles declines after the age of 40. In contrast, alveolar ducts and respiratory bronchioles increase in size at the expense of alveolar volume (senile emphysema or aging lung)[2].

Pulmonary function tests

Total lung capacity decreases with age; individual height also declines, therefore, when corrected for height, total lung capacity does not change significantly (Table 2). Residual volume increases, due to small airway closure during exhalation, resulting in air trapping. Functional residual capacity also increases with age, but this increase is usually small.

Spirometry is the most commonly used test to evaluate pulmonary function. In flow-volume recording, the terminal portion of the curve shows progressively lower flows and increased concavity with aging. Additionally, peak expiratory flow rates decline with age because of increased peripheral airway resistance. After the age of 50, the annual decline of the flow is about 4 l/min in men and 2.5 l/min in women. Pa_{O_2} and alveolar–arterial P_{O_2} (A–a) gradient also change with the aging process (Table 3).

The most commonly measured parameters during spirometry are forced expiratory volume in 1 s (FEV_1) and forced vital capacity (FVC). Both increase up to the age of 20 in women and 25 in men, plateau until the age of 30 and then decline progressively. As aging progresses the decline of FEV_1 and FVC accelerates and is usually greater in men. The FEV_1/FVC ratio also decreases with aging. Spirometry is the primary test for the diagnosis

of chronic obstructive pulmonary disease. Frequently, an FEV_1/FVC ratio less than 70% indicates obstructive airway disease. However, it may be normal in some older individuals[2]. Therefore, the diagnosis of chronic obstructive pulmonary disease in the elderly requires a history and physical examination consistent with obstructive airway disease in addition to spirometric measurements. Overall airway resistance does not change, since the increase in peripheral airway resistance is counterbalanced by the decline in central airway resistance.

Control of breathing

Normal subjects respond to hypoxemia and hypercapnia with increased minute ventilation (tidal volume multiplied by number of breaths per minute). The response to hypoxemia and hypercapnia decreases with age. This blunted response is mostly due to the inability to mount an increase in tidal volume and originates from the central nervous system[2].

Table 2 Changes in pulmonary functions with aging

	Change
Total lung capacity	decreased
Vital capacity	decreased
Residual volume	increased
Functional residual capacity	increased
Peak expiratory flow rate	decreased
Forced vital capacity (FVC)	decreased
Forced expiratory volume in 1 s (FEV_1)	decreased
Ratio of FEV_1/FVC	decreased
Pa_{O_2}	decreased
A–a gradient	increased

Table 3 Room air blood gases at sea level

Age (years)	Pa_{O_2} (mmHg)	$(A–a)P_{O_2}$ (mmHg)
20	84–95	4–17
40	78–90	10–24
60	72–84	17–31
70	70–81	21–34
80	67–79	25–38

Exercise capacity

Maximum oxygen uptake declines with aging. The decline in sedentary individuals is double the rate of the decline in those who are physically active. Reduced cardiac output plays a major role in the reduction of maximum oxygen uptake[2].

CHRONIC OBSTRUCTIVE PULMONARY DISEASE

Chronic obstructive pulmonary disease (COPD) is defined as a disease state characterized by the presence of airflow obstruction due to chronic bronchitis or emphysema[5]. The airflow obstruction is generally progressive, may be accompanied by airway hyperreactivity and is partially reversible. Chronic bronchitis is defined as the presence of chronic productive cough for 3 months in each of 2 successive years in a patient in whom other causes of chronic cough are excluded[5]. Emphysema is defined as abnormal enlargement of the air spaces distal to terminal bronchioles, accompanied by destruction of their walls and without obvious fibrosis[5]. Centriacinar emphysema develops in smokers, affecting most commonly and severely the upper lung zones. While COPD occurs in cigarette smokers, only 15% of smokers develop symptomatic airflow obstruction.

Epidemiology

COPD is the fourth leading cause of death in the USA and a growing health problem[2]. A large portion of the patients suffer from chronic bronchitis[5]. It is more common among men, and mortality is higher in Whites. After the age of 65, males have a substantially higher number of office visits because of COPD. Delayed occurrence of respiratory symptoms because of a large pulmonary reserve, and attribution of dyspnea to old age or being unfit, result in late presentation and thus delayed recognition of the problem.

Pathophysiology

Airflow obstruction in COPD patients is generated by one or more of the following mechanisms: secretion due to mucous gland hyperplasia, bronchial wall thickening, smooth muscle hypertrophy and loss of airway supportive structures (tethering effect of the lung parenchyma). Age-related changes are additive to the reductions caused by COPD. The airflow limitation produces hyperinflation and increased work of breathing. The etiology of hypoxemia in COPD patients is ventilation–perfusion mismatch and an overall decline in gas exchange surface[6].

Diagnosis

Most patients have at least a 20-pack-year smoking history. Dyspnea usually starts in the fifth decade and progresses gradually. In late stages the patients may become orthopneic. Additionally, individuals may complain about wheezing, cough, clear sputum production or occasional blood-streaked sputum. Increased sputum volume or color changes may indicate superimposed infections. With the development of right heart failure the patients may also develop peripheral edema. In addition to tachypnea and orthopnea the patients may demonstrate pursed-lip breathing, use of accessory muscles, increased AP diameter, decreased breath sounds and a prolonged expiratory phase. Most of the symptoms occur when the FEV_1 is less than 50% of the predicted value.

Pulmonary function tests

Diagnosis of airflow obstruction in the elderly requires a reduced FEV_1 and FEV_1/FVC ratio and the proper clinical setting[6]. FEV_1/FVC ratio reduction alone is not sufficient for the diagnosis of COPD. Total lung capacity (TLC) and residual volume (RV) are usually elevated in COPD, particularly in those with emphysema. In general, diffusion capacity is normal in individuals with chronic bronchitis but reduced in patients with emphysema.

Roentgenographic manifestations

In most cases the chest X-ray is normal. The two roentgenographic abnormalities that are most suggestive of chronic bronchitis are thickened bronchial walls and prominent lung markings. The roentgenographic signs of emphysema include the classic triad of over-inflation, oligemia and bullae formation.

Other laboratory findings include hypoxemia, hypercapnia, secondary polycythemia and increased bicarbonate levels.

Treatment

Dyspnea is the most common complaint for which the patients seek medical attention. The goal of therapy is improvement of well-being; symptom relief may improve quality of life in the elderly. Leaning forward in a seated position with elbows or forearms supported by the thighs, or adopting a supine position provides partial relief to those with dyspnea. Pursed-lip breathing improves oxygen saturation, increases tidal volume, reduces respiratory frequency and provides some relief. Extremes of the environment (hot and humid or cold and dry air) may cause increased dyspnea. Many patients prefer moderate temperatures and humidity as well as a natural breeze or fan. Bronchodilator medications can be delivered by metered-dose inhalers, inhalers with spacer devices, dry-powder inhalers and jet or ultrasonic nebulizers. The open-mouth technique is proper for metered-dose inhalers. Forty per cent of elderly patients do not use metered-dose inhalers properly despite repeated instruction[6]. With spacer devices aerosol delivery improves, although in some cases the nebulizer systems are a better choice for the elderly.

The following interventions are used in COPD.

Smoking cessation

This is the single most important intervention.

β-Adrenergic agents

Short-acting inhaled β-adrenergic agonists are the most effective bronchodilators. These agents relax the airway smooth muscle, improve airflow and reduce symptoms rapidly. For persistent symptoms they can be used every 4–6 h or can be replaced with long-acting agents such as salmeterol. Their onset of action is quicker than that of anticholinergic drugs. However, they can produce cardiovascular and peripheral nervous system side-effects. Oral preparations are not more effective and can cause significant side-effects. A slight increase in resting heart rate, and increased frequency of ventricular premature complexes can be seen with β-adrenergic use. The arrhythmogenic effect of β-adrenergic stimulation may be further increased with hypokalemia, particularly in patients taking digitalis and diuretics[7]. In stable patients, β-adernergic agonists have additive effects when used with anticholinergics.

Anticholinergic agents

Ipratropium bromide is clinically effective and poorly absorbed, therefore it does not cause major side-effects. Some side-effects are dry mouth, worsening of angle-closure glaucoma, urinary retention/difficulty, nausea and palpitation[7]. Its onset of action is later than that of β-adrenergic agonists, with greater and more sustained peak effect. As a result, combining β-adernergic agonists and anticholinergic agents minimizes side-effects and provides a rapid and more sustained effect.

Methylxanthines

Methylxanthines are a third-line therapy in chronic obstructive pulmonary disease for symptomatic patients. Sustained-release theophylline provides modest bronchodilatation, improves respiratory muscle function and stimulates the respiratory center. It is particularly helpful in patients with poor compliance and nocturnal symptoms, or those unable to use aerosol therapy. In the elderly the initial dose should be 200 mg once a day, increased gradually to maintain a target blood level of 8–12 µg/ml[6]. With high serum concentration, life-threatening events may occur. Theophylline interacts with other medications, therefore the dose needs to be adjusted accordingly in the event of starting a new medication. Methylxanthines cause frequent cardiovascular side-effects and should be used in selected patients.

Corticosteroids

A trial of oral corticosteroid therapy is reasonable in functionally limited, dyspneic patients. During this trial, prednisone 30–40 mg is given once daily for a 2-week period. FEV_1 values are measured in the beginning and at the end of the trial. Twenty-five per cent improvement in FEV_1 is considered a good response. Therefore, steroids should be reduced to the lowest maintenance dose. The benefit of inhaled steroids is controversial at this time[8,9]. The side-effects of chronic steroid therapy are particularly troublesome in the elderly. Examples include osteoporosis, diabetes mellitus, hypertension, mood swings, loss of attention span and cataracts.

Oxygen

In patients with Po_2 less than 55 mmHg or 55–59 mmHg with dependent edema, P pulmonale (p wave ≥ 2.5 mm in lead II) or a hematocrit more than 56%, continuous oxygen therapy is recommended. Continuous oxygen therapy reduces mortality and provides symptomatic relief in dyspneic patients.

Pulmonary rehabilitation

The short-term benefits of rehabilitation include the improved strength of the specific muscle groups trained, improved exercise capacity and improved functional status. However, the pulmonary function tests do not change significantly as a result of training[5].

Vaccination

Patients with COPD should be immunized for influenza and *Streptococcus pneumoniae*.

Antibiotic therapy

In the event of acute exacerbation, depending on the clinical setting, the patients may benefit from antibiotic therapy.

Surgical options

Lung volume reduction surgery is a new approach to improve pulmonary function and control respiratory symptoms. At this time it is considered experimental. Finally, patients 65 years and older are generally not considered candidates for lung transplantation[10].

PULMONARY INFECTIONS

Pneumonia is the fifth leading cause of mortality and was responsible for 82 989 deaths in the USA in 1998[1]. It is a common cause of hospitalization and prolonged hospital stay, and a significant number of intensive care unit admissions in the elderly. The majority of pneumonia-related mortality occurs in patients older than 70 years of age. Bacterial pneumonia increases in incidence from 1 : 100 000 in the age group of 35–44 years to 25 : 100 000 in the age group of 65–74 years. Several factors affect the prognosis (Table 4).

Risk factors and comorbid conditions

The virulence of the organism, the dose of the inoculum and the host's immune system determine the outcome for all infectious diseases. Humoral immunity declines with aging. Despite significant reduction in IgG4

Table 4 Prognostic factors in pneumonia

Delayed or missed diagnosis due to atypical clinical
  presentation
Long-term care facility residence
Cytotoxic therapy
Radiation therapy
Steroid use
Heart disease
Impaired consciousness
Neurologic dysfunction

and IgM levels, older individuals do not experience increased infection rates with encapsulated organisms such as pneumococcus[11]. The number of T-helper cells, the T-cell response to interleukin (IL)2 and the CD4/CD8 ratio all decline, and the number of T-suppressor cells increases with aging. However, the incidence of *Pneumocystis carinii* pneumonia (PCP) or cytomegalovirus infections does not change. On the other hand, the increased incidence of tuberculosis observed in the elderly may be related to T-cell dysfunction. Mechanical defense mechanisms are also impaired in the elderly. Impaired cough reflex, decreased mucociliary clearance, diminished gag reflex and impaired glottic closure may all play a role in inoculation of organisms into the lower respiratory tract.

Oropharyngeal colonization with respiratory pathogens is a well-known risk factor for the development of pneumonia. A decrease in salivary clearance of potential pathogens may be a major risk factor for the development of colonization[12]. Alcohol consumption may impair ciliary function, surfactant production and both neutrophil and macrophage functions. Smoking, on the other hand, impairs mucociliary clearance. Although it is not a common problem among the elderly, alcoholism is the strongest relative risk factor for developing pneumonia. Other co-morbid conditions include heart disease, bronchial asthma and other lung diseases, immunosuppressive therapy (steroid, cytotoxic agents, radiation therapy), institutionalization in nursing homes and advanced age. Diabetic

patients with bacteremic pneumococcal pneumonia have a higher mortality rate then non-diabetic patients. One-third of the patients with stroke develop pneumonia, most likely due to dysphagia and aspiration. The presence of a feeding tube increases this risk. Poor nutritional status may also affect the immune response to infections. Patients with low body mass index or low serum albumin demonstrate increased mortality[11,13,14].

Diagnosis

Patients at extreme older age, with underlying systemic or central nervous system disease, may have atypical clinical presentations. Many elderly patients with pneumonia have respiratory manifestations. However, underlying systemic or central nervous system diseases may obscure these signs and symptoms, making diagnosis more difficult. Change in functional status, new episodes of falls, acute change in mental status, worsening of an underlying problem (diabetes mellitus, congestive heart failure, COPD) or failure to thrive should alert the physician for further investigation[15]. Often pneumonia cases are misdiagnosed initially or the diagnosis is established later in the course of the disease. Tachypnea and tachycardia are fairly sensitive but not specific findings in older patients with pneumonia. Other manifestations of pneumonia include cough, dyspnea, sputum production, fever, chills and pleuritic chest pain. Absence of fever has been demonstrated in up to 40% of cases, and 15% of bacteremic patients have been found to be afebrile; therefore, blood cultures should be obtained in all cases of pneumonia. Additionally, the patients may suffer from dehydration, hypotension or renal function impairment. Those with tuberculosis may present with altered mental status, gradual debilitation or decreased ability to perform daily activities in addition to the typical signs and symptoms of tuberculosis. A positive purified protein derivative (PPD) response is less common in the elderly.

Studies in nursing home residents reveal that approximately 20–35% of 60-year-old patients and less than 10% of 90-year-old patients have a positive reaction to tuberculin testing, despite repeated booster testing in a population in which previous exposure to the disease is currently postulated to be almost 90%[15].

A chest X-ray is required to confirm the diagnosis of pneumonia and useful for follow-up. However, in neutropenic patients and in the early phase of aspiration the chest X-ray may not demonstrate any infiltrate.

Treatment

Treatment of pneumonia differs for out-patients and in-patients and for those with or without modifying factors[11,15] (Table 5). Hospital-acquired pneumonia, defined as pneumonia occurring ≥ 48 h after admission, excluding any infection that is incubating at the time of admission, and management of nosocomial pneumonia are beyond the scope of this text[16].

Pneumonia in a nursing-home population

Etiologic agents for nursing home-acquired pneumonia is poorly defined because of the limited number of studies. The most common cause of pneumonia in this population has been aspiration because of dementia or stroke[15]. Aspiration pneumonia develops after the inhalation of colonized oropharyngeal material. In one study, 18% of nursing home-acquired pneumonia was found to be due to aspiration. Risk of aspiration pneumonia is lower in edentulous patients and in the elderly in an institutionalized setting receiving aggressive oral care. Some of the risk factors for aspiration pneumonia are dysphagia, disruption of the gastroesophageal junction, poor oral care, stroke and sedatives. Gastric, post-gastric and nasogastric tubes have similar risks for aspiration pneumonia[17]. Over the long term, aspiration pneumonia is the most common cause of death in patients fed by gastric tube, although these tubes are useful for delivering the prescribed nutrition. Levofloxacin or piperacillin–tazobactam or ceftazidime is recommended for empirical treatment of nursing home-acquired pneumonia. In case of severe periodontal disease, putrid sputum or alcoholism, levofloxacin plus clindamycin or piperacillin–tazobactam or imipenem is the choice of antibiotic.

Non-resolving and slowly resolving pneumonia

Non-resolving pneumonia is defined as an infiltrate on the chest X-ray that begins with signs and symptoms suggesting pulmonary infection but is slow to resolve following optimal therapy[18]. Arbitrarily, a minimum of 10 days' antibiotic therapy and a radiographic infiltrate that has not resolved in the expected period of time can be considered slowly resolving. Those over 50 years of age account for two-thirds of these cases. Whether aging itself or associated chronic illnesses are responsible for delayed resolution is a complex issue.

Impaired immune response such as ineffective cough, impaired mucociliary clearance, impaired cell mediated immunity, reduced levels of antibodies and diminished neutrophil reserve due to aging are all thought to be partly responsible for prolonged resolution. Associated comorbid illnesses such as COPD, renal failure, diabetes mellitus, cancer and stroke affect local clearance mechanisms and systemic immunity and cause prolonged resolution. Organisms infecting the elderly such as Gram-negative enteric bacteria are virulent organisms and may cause slow resolution. However, *Streptococcus pneumoniae* accounts for 40–60% of cases in the elderly and is therefore responsible for the majority of slowly-resolving pneumonia cases[18]. An atypical presentation, or a delayed diagnosis or initiation of therapy may also contribute to delayed resolution.

Table 5   Treatment of pneumonia[11]

Out-patient with no cardiopulmonary disease and/or modifying factors

Organism
   Streptococcus pneumoniae, Mycoplasma pneumoniae, Chlamydia pneumoniae, Hemophilus influenzae, Legionella
Therapy
   azithromycin or clarithromycin or doxycyclin (only if the patient is allergic or intolerant to macrolide)

Out-patient with cardiopulmonary disease and/or modifying factors
Organism
   Streptococcus pneumoniae, Mycoplasma pneumoniae, Chlamydia pneumoniae, Hemophilus influenzae, enteric
      Gram-negatives
Therapy
   β-lactam (cefuroxime, amoxicillin/clavulanate) plus macrolide or doxycyclin or antipneumococcal
      fluoroquinolone alone

*In-patient, outside the ICU with no cardiopulmonary disease and/or modifying factors (including being
   from a nursing home)*
Organism
   Streptococcus pneumoniae, Hemophilus influenzae, Mycoplasma pneumoniae, Chlamydia pneumoniae
Therapy
   intravenous azithromycin alone or β-lactam and doxycyclin or antipneumococcal fluoroquinolone alone

*In-patient, outside the ICU with cardiopulmonary disease and/or modifying factors (Including being from a
   nursing home)*
Organism
   Streptococcus pneumoniae, Hemophilus influenzae, Mycoplasma pneumoniae, Chlamydia pneumoniae, enteric
      Gram-negatives, aspiration
Therapy
   Intravenous β-lactam (ceftriaxone, cefotaxime, ampicillin/sulbactam) plus intravenous or oral macrolide or
      doxycyclin or antipneumococcal fluoroquinolone

Modifying factors
Penicillin-resistant pneumococci
   age > 65 years
   β-lactam therapy within the past 3 months
   immune-suppressive illness
   multiple medical co-morbidities
   exposure to a child in a day-care center
Enteric Gram-negatives
   residence in a nursing home
   underlying cardiopulmonary disease
   multiple medical co-morbidities
   recent antibiotic therapy
Pseudomonas aeruginosa
   structural lung disease
   corticosteroid therapy
   broad-spectrum antibiotic therapy
   malnutrition

ICU, intensive care unit

Clinical improvement precedes radiographic improvement. Age and co-morbid illnesses such as alcoholism, COPD or smoking may delay resolution of chest X-ray abnormalities beyond a 1-month period. In any case, most patients clear their chest X-ray abnormalities by 3 months. Complete failure to resolve or radiographic deterioration should suggest a non-infectious process or an unusual organism.

Table 6 Mechanism of thrombus formation (Virchow's triad). From reference 32

---

1. Venous stasis
Left-sided heart failure
Shock
Obesity, intra-abdominal tumors
Right-sided heart failure
External pressure from leg casts or bandages
Post-surgical or paraplegic state
Varicose veins
Prolonged travel

2. Endothelial injury

3. Alteration in coagulation
Factor V Leiden (the most common inherited cause)
Prothrombin gene mutation
Protein C deficiency
Protein S deficiency
Antithrombin III deficiency
Antiphospholipid antibodies
Intrinsic abnormality of the blood (multiple myeloma)
Neoplasms (7.6% idiopathic venous thromboembolism
    and 17.1% recurrent idiopathic venous
    thromboembolisms are due to underlying
    neoplastic process)[20]
Myeloproliferative disorders
Nephrotic syndrome
Inflammatory bowel disease

Prevention

Avoiding alcohol and tobacco use and vaccination for influenza and pneumococcus are important measures. For hospitalized patients, removal of a nasogastric or endotracheal tube as soon as clinically feasible, adequate hand washing between patient contacts and provision of adequate nutritional support are some helpful interventions.

VENOUS THROMBOEMBOLISM

Clinical manifestations of venous thromboembolism are deep venous thrombosis and pulmonary embolism. Deep venous thrombosis occurs in the deep veins of the lower extremities, proximal to and including the popliteal veins; pulmonary embolism occurs as a complication of deep venous thrombosis[19]. Symptomatic and asymptomatic pulmonary embolism occurs in 50–60% of cases of deep venous thromboembolism. More than half of the cases are never diagnosed[19]. Most of the attributable mortality occurs before the diagnosis is made, therefore preventive measures in the high-risk population are important.

The source of thrombus in pulmonary embolism is the lower extremities in more than 90% of the cases. Thrombi confined to the calf veins generally do not embolize (Table 6).

Diagnosis

Symptoms and signs

Pulmonary embolism cannot be diagnosed solely from the history and physical examination. Common symptoms are dyspnea with or without associated anxiety, as well as pleuritic chest pain and hemoptysis. Tachypnea and tachycardia are the most common signs. Lightheadedness, syncope and hypotension are other common symptoms[19] (Table 7).

Electrocardiography

Eighty-seven per cent of patients have electrocardiogram (ECG) abnormalities including T wave changes, ST segment abnormalities, and left or right axis deviation. Manifestations of acute cor pulmonale (S1 Q3 T3 pattern, right bundle branch block, P pulmonale or right axis deviation) were shown by 26% of patients with submassive pulmonary embolism and 32% of those with massive pulmonary embolism[19].

Arterial blood gas analysis

Hypoxemia is common in acute pulmonary embolism. In a retrospective analysis of patients with proven pulmonary embolism, Pao_2 was greater than 80 mmHg in 29% of patients. The alveolar–arterial gradient is usually elevated but it can be normal in some[19].

Table 7   Clinical risk classification for venous thromboembolism, from reference 21

High-risk
    chest pain or dyspnea of unknown origin
    unexplained hypoxemia or increased alveolar–arterial oxygen gradient
    chest X-ray finding suspicious for pulmonary embolism
Low risk
    dyspnea or pleuritic chest pain, but attributable to other causes
    abnormal X-ray or blood gas, but attributable to other causes

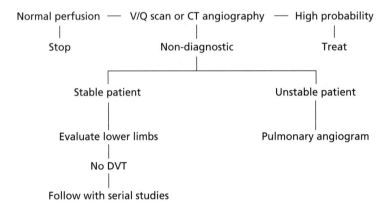

Figure 1   Diagnostic approach to pulmonary embolism, from reference 19. V/Q, ventilation–perfusion; CT, computed tomography; MRI, magnetic resonance imaging; DVT, deep venous thrombosis

Chest X-ray

The majority of patients with pulmonary embolism have an abnormal but non-specific chest radiograph. Common findings are atelectasis, pleural effusion, pulmonary infiltrates and elevation of a hemidiaphragm. A normal chest X-ray in the setting of severe dyspnea and hypoxemia without evidence of bronchospasm is strongly suggestive of pulmonary embolism[19].

D-Dimer

In patients with suspected pulmonary embolism, low plasma D-dimer concentration less than 500 ng/ml measured by enzyme-linked immunosorbent assay has a 95% negative predictive power[19].

The ventilation–perfusion scan

The ventilation–perfusion (V/Q) scan is diagnostic in a minority of cases. However, pulmonary embolism often exists in the presence of a non-diagnostic V/Q scan and high clinical suspicion. A non-diagnostic V/Q scan is common in patients with cardiopulmonary disease.

Pulmonary angiography

Pulmonary angiography is indicated if the V/Q scan is non-diagnostic, and clinical suspicion is high. It is invasive and expensive, and requires an experienced physician, but pulmonary angiography remains the most accurate test for pulmonary embolism.

Spiral computed tomography

Its positive predictive value is about 60–89% and its negative predictive value is 81%. Limitations are poor visualization of peripheral areas, horizontally oriented vessels in the right middle lobe and lingula and false positives from lymph nodes[22]. An advantage is the ability to define other pathologies.

Echocardiography

Although non-specific, dysfunction of the right ventricle frequently accompanies massive pulmonary embolism or recurrent pulmonary embolism. In one study it was demonstrated that akinesia of the mid-free wall with apical sparing had 77% sensitivity and 94% specificity for the diagnosis of acute pulmonary embolism[19] (Figure 1).

Treatment

Prevention

Prevention of deep venous thrombois can be accomplished with heparin, intermittent compression or fitted elastic stockings and ambulation. Bleeding is seldom a complication of low-dose heparin, but may cause wound hematoma in the postoperative state; therefore, intermittent compression stockings are more commonly used in this setting, immediately after surgery[23].

Treatment of venous thromboembolism

Death from recurrent PE is about 25% in untreated patients. Venous thromboembolism does recur even with adequate therapy (5–7%), but attributable mortality is less than 5%. Treatment is accomplished with heparin. Body weight-based dosing of intravenous heparin is preferred to other heparinization methods. Initial dose is 80 u/kg and maintenance infusion is 18 u/kg/hr. The dose should be adjusted according to APTT levels[21]. Warfarin is initiated on the first day of heparin therapy. The usual initial dose of warfarin is 5 mg/day and dose titrated to target international normalized ratio (INR) of 2.5 (2–3). Other precautions for patients with venous thromboembolism include bed rest until APTT/INR are therapeutic and fitted elastic stockings when the patient becomes ambulatory.

Thrombolytic therapy

There is no proven mortality effect with thrombolytic therapy and no proven reduction in long-term disability after massive pulmonary embolism with thrombolytic therapy[22]. The best candidates are those at low risk for bleeding with hemodynamically unstable pulmonary embolism or massive ileofemoral deep venous thrombosis. Absolute contraindications include previous hemorrhagic stroke, intracranial neoplasm, recent cranial surgery or trauma and active or recent internal bleeding[24].

Inferior vena cava filters

Some of the indications are failure of anticoagulation therapy, chronic recurrent embolism with pulmonary hypertension, surgical pulmonary embolectomy, contraindication for anticoagulation and massive pulmonary embolism[24].

LUNG CANCER

Lung cancer is the leading cause of cancer deaths in men worldwide. The overall 5-year survival rate is about 13.4%. Lung cancer mortality increases rapidly with aging. For the year 2000 the estimated number of deaths was about 157 000 in the USA. Smoking is the leading cause of lung cancer and is responsible for up to 90% of the cases. One out of eight cigarette smokers develop lung cancer[25]. Passive smokers are also at risk. About 25% of lung cancers in non-smokers are believed to be due to environmental tobacco exposure[25]. Following smoking cessation the risk of developing lung cancer declines to the level of a non-smoker in 10–20 years[25]. Some of the other risk factors for lung cancer include exposure to asbestos, arsenic, polycyclic aromatic hydrocarbons and radon. Asbestos is the most common occupational cause of lung cancer. Cigarette smoking and asbestos exposures have a synergistic effect on lung cancer development. The risk increases 80 to 90-fold in this population. Dietary and inherited factors may also have an effect on cancer development.

Clinical manifestations

At initial presentation, about 95% of patients have symptoms. These symptoms may be due to the tumor itself such as cough, wheezing, hemoptysis, dyspnea (more common in the elderly) or chest pain. Sometimes the symptoms are secondary to intrathoracic expansion of the tumor, for example hoarseness (left recurrent laryngeal nerve involvement), pleural effusion, superior vena cava syndrome or Horner's syndrome. The patients may be symptomatic because of metastatic disease such as bone pain or central nervous system symptoms. Lung cancer can also present with paraneoplastic syndromes. Small cell lung cancer may cause Cushing's syndrome or the syndrome of inappropriate antidiuretic hormone. Squamous cell carcinoma is known for hypercalcemia. Hypertrophic pulmonary osteoarthropathy is rare in small cell lung cancer, but is seen in other cancers.

Lung cancer screening

The likelihood of diagnosing lung cancer using sputum cytology and chest X-ray is about 77%[25]. In the 1970s the National Cancer Institute sponsored three large lung cancer-screening trials. On the basis of these trials it was concluded that there was no role for lung cancer screening[26]. Low-dose spiral computed tomography (CT) scan has been under investigation as a screening test for early lung cancer. Although spiral CT scan of the chest is more sensitive than chest X-ray in detecting lung cancer, it raised new issues. In a recent study, investigators detected at least one nodule in 51% of the patients. Although the majority of these nodules are benign, establishing the etiology may result in morbidity from invasive procedures. Additionally, radiation exposure, participants' anxiety and the cost of spiral CT are some of the other issues with such screening programs[27,28].

Diagnosis

Chest X-ray may demonstrate atelectasis, abnormal mediastinal contour or a peripheral nodule. Spiculated or poorly defined margins, eccentric calcification, doubling time from 1 to 18 months and large size are some of the features of neoplastic lesions. CT scan of the chest is the procedure of choice to obtain information about the morphology of the lesions as well as for staging. Positron emission tomography scanning is a new modality to investigate mediastinal involvement and metastatic disease[29]. Other studies include bone scan and magnetic resonance imaging.

Sputum cytology obtained on five consecutive mornings, fiberoptic bronchoscopy, percutaneous fine-needle aspiration or mediastinoscopy can be used to obtain tissue for definitive diagnosis.

Treatment

Proper staging is the initial step before the treatment. Tumor node metastasis (TNM) classification is used for non-small cell lung cancer (NSCLC) staging[30]. Small-cell lung cancer is staged as 'limited' or 'extensive' disease. Chemotherapy is the treatment of choice for small cell lung cancer. Median survival is about 10–14 months for limited disease. On the other hand, surgical resection of the tumor is preferred for NSCLC, although morbidity and mortality may be higher in the older population. There is no established role for preoperative radiation therapy, with occasional exceptions. Postoperative radiation therapy for stage II and III squamous cell lung cancer produces a significant reduction in recurrence. Palliative radiation is beneficial for pain control, hemoptysis, superior vena cava syndrome and atelectasis. Combination chemotherapy has 20–50% partial response rates for non-surgical NSCLC cases.

Solitary pulmonary nodule

This is a common problem in the elderly and is defined as a single well-circumscribed lesion 1–3 cm in size, within the lung. Criteria for a benign diagnosis include detection of fat or a benign pattern of calcification on CT scan within the nodule, stability of the nodule over a 2-year period, younger age (usually under 35) and no exposure to tobacco or other lung carcinogens. Lesions more than 2 cm are more likely to be malignant. If the probability of cancer justifies the surgical risk, the patient should be referred for surgery; otherwise, a positron emission tomography scan and/or fine-needle aspiration are the diagnostic tests for further investigation[26,31].

References

1. Murphy SL. *Deaths: Final Data for 1998. National Vital Statistics Reports.* Hyattsville, MD: CDC, 2000;48:24–7

2. Crapo RO. The aging lung. In Mahler DA, ed. *Pulmonary Disease in the Elderly.* New York: Marcel Dekker, 1993:1–21

3. Knudson RJ. Physiology of the aging lung. In Crystal RG, West JB, eds. *The Lung.* New York: Raven Press, 1991:1749–59

4. Tolep K. Effect of aging on respiratory skeletal muscles. *Clin Chest Med* 1993;14: 363–78

5. American Thoracic Society. Statement: standards for the diagnosis and care of patients with chronic obstructive pulmonary disease. *Am J Respir Crit Care Med* 1995;152: S77–120

6. Mahler DA. Chronic obstructive pulmonary disease. In Mahler DA, ed. *Pulmonary Disease in the Elderly.* New York: Marcel Dekker, 1993:159–83

7. McEvoy GK, ed. *AHFS Drug Information.* Bethesda, MD: ASHP, 1997:930–5, 940–5

8. Calverley PMA. Inhaled corticosteroids are beneficial in chronic obstructive pulmonary disease. *Am J Respir Crit Care Med* 2000; 161:341–4

9. Barnes PJ. Inhaled corticosteroids are not beneficial in chronic obstructive pulmonary disease. *Am J Respir Crit Care Med* 2000; 161:341–4

10. Fessler HE, Wise RA. Lung volume reduction surgery. *Am J Respir Crit Care Med* 1999;159:1031–5

11. American Thoracic Society. Statement: guideliness for the management of adults with community-acquired pneumonia. *Am J Respir Crit Care Med* 2001;163:1730–54

12. Palmer LB, Albulak K, Fields S, *et al.* Oral clearance and pathogenic oropharyngeal colonization in the elderly. *Am J Respir Crit Care Med* 2001;164:464–8

13. Bartlett JG, Breiman RF, Mandell LA, File TM Jr. Guidelines from the Infectious Disease Society of America. Community-acquired pneumonia in adults. *Clin Infect Dis* 1998;26:811–38

14. Fine MJ. A prediction rule to identify low-risk patients with community-acquired pneumonia. *N Engl J Med* 1997;336: 243–50

15. Rello J, Gallego M. Pneumonia in the elderly. In Niederman MS, Sarosi GA, Glassroth J, Eds. *Respiratory Infections,* 2nd edn. Philadelphia: Lippincott Williams & Wilkins, 2001:271–83

16. American Thoracic Society. Statement: hospital-acquired pneumonia in adults. *Am J Respir Crit Care Med* 1995;153:1711–25

17. Marik PE. Aspiration pneumonitis and aspiration pneumonia. *N Engl J Med* 2001;344: 665–71

18. Feinsilver SH, Hertz G. Nonresolving and slowly resolving pneumonia. *Clin Chest Med* 1993;14:555–71

19. American Thoracic Society. Clinical practice guideline: the diagnostic approach to acute thromboembolism. *Am J Respir Crit Care Med* 1999;160:1043–66

20. Prandoni P. Deep-vein thrombosis and the incidence of subsequent symptomatic cancer. *N Engl J Med* 1992;327:1128–32

21. Hyers HM. Venous thromboembolism, state of the art. *Am J Respir Crit Care Med* 1999;159:1–14

22. Tapson VF. Pulmonary embolism, new diagnostic approaches. *N Engl J Med* 1997;336:1449–51

23. Hyers TM, Agnelli G, Hull RD, *et al.* Antithrombotic therapy for venous thromboembolic disease. *Chest* 2001;119:S176–93

24. Tapson VF, Fulkerson WJ, Saltzman HA. Venous thromboembolism. *Clin Chest Med* 1995;16:229–389

25. Lee-Chiong TL. Lung cancer in the elderly. *Clin Chest Med* 1993;14:453–78

26. American Thoracic Society. Statement: pretreatment evaluation of non-small-cell lung cancer. *Am J Respir Crit Care Med* 1997;156:320–32

27. Jett JR. Spiral computed tomography screening for lung cancer is ready for prime time. *Am J Respir Crit Care* 2001:163:812–15

28. Patz EF. Low-dose spiral computed tomography screening for lung cancer: not ready for prime time. *Am J Respir Crit Care* 2001;163:812–15

29. Erasmus JJ, Patz EF Jr. Positron emission tomography imaging in the thorax. *Clin Chest Med* 1999;20:715–23

30. Mountain CF. Revisions in the international system for staging lung cancer. *Chest* 1997;111:1710–16

31. Ost D. Evaluation and management of the solitary pulmonary nodule. *Am J Respir Crit Care Med* 2000;162:782–7

32. Hirsh J, Raschke R, Warkentin TE, *et al.* Heparin. *Chest* 1995;108:S258–68

43 Infections in the elderly

Marilou O. Corpuz, MD, FACP

AGE-RELATED CHANGES RELEVANT TO INFECTIONS

It is recognized that the elderly have increased susceptibility to infection compared to younger adults. The state of dysregulated immune function, also referred to as immunosenescence[1], contributes to this higher risk. It is still unclear as to why older adults have a lowered resistance. It is difficult to separate the contribution of chronic diseases that plague many older people from the immune dysfunction inherent in aging.

Malnutrition is a common occurrence in the elderly. Deficiencies of nutrients such as pyridoxine, folate and zinc, which occur with malnutrition, have been associated with depressed humoral immunity and delayed skin test reactivity[2].

Studies have suggested that aging is associated with immune dysfunction, especially by a depression of cell-mediated immunity and anergy to common skin test antigens[3,4]. There are many reasons for the reduced function of T lymphocytes in the elderly. Although the total number of T lymphocytes may remain the same with different ages, the number of T cells responsive to antigenic stimulation, as well as clonal proliferation, is reduced in the elderly[5,6]. The response time to peak activity of the lymphocytes is delayed, and the membrane viscosity of the T lymphocytes is altered, leading to a decreased responsiveness to antigens[7]. The production of interleukin-2, which promotes T-cell clonal proliferation and increases response to antigens, is reduced as one ages.

More recent studies have shown that humoral function is also depressed in older subjects. Both *in vitro* and *in vivo* studies have shown the inability to produce immunoglobulins efficiently in the geriatric population. This is attributed to defects in thymic cell helper function, inherent defects in B-cell function or a lack of circulating B cells[8].

Reasons other than impairment of cell-mediated and humoral immunity exist and cause more frequent infections in the elderly. Physiologic functions such as altered cough reflex, poor circulation and reduced wound healing contribute to specific infections[4,9]. Chronic illnesses, use of immunosuppressive medications and socioeconomic factors may contribute to infections.

Certain infections occur more frequently in the elderly (e.g. urinary tract infections, pneumonia, skin and soft tissue infections, intra-abdominal infections, endocarditis, meningitis, tuberculosis, listeriosis and herpes zoster) and are often associated with higher mortality.

Table 1 Factors contributing to higher morbidity and mortality in the elderly. From reference 1

Reduced reserve capacity
Reduced host resistance
Presence of co-morbid chronic medical illness
Delays in diagnosis and therapy
Inability to tolerate invasive procedures
Poor or delayed response to antibiotics
Higher rates of adverse reactions to drugs
Greater risk and incidence of nosocomial infections

Table 2 Estimated prevalence of bacteriuria according to age and level of care. From references 14 and 17

Age (years)	Care	Women(%)	Men(%)
< 65	home	5	<1
65–79	home	17–20	6–10
80+	home	33–40	13–20
65+	nursing home	25–27	17–25
65+	acute hospital	30–40	30–34
65+	chronic disease hospital	40–50	35

Many factors predispose to this risk for death and complications, as outlined in Table 1.

Possible explanations for the higher morbidity and mortality in the older age group include low physiologic reserves due to the biologic changes that accompany aging[10]. The elderly are at greater risk for hospitalizations, which subsequently places them at risk for nosocomial infections. Adverse drug reactions may occur from use of multiple medications and altered pharmacokinetics. Diagnosis and treatment may be delayed because of the difficulty in recognition of infection in the aged patient. Signs and symptoms of inflammation may be blunted or altered. Fever and leukocytosis may be absent in patients with serious infections[9,10].

In frail elderly patients, mean baseline temperatures are lower than in the younger age group[11]. Based on multiple studies, fever in the elderly can be defined as a persistent oral or tympanic membrane temperature of $\geq 37.2°C$ or persistent rectal temperature of $\geq 37.5°C$, or an increase over baseline temperature of $\geq 1.3°C$[10]. In infectious processes, animal models show that fever may be an important host defense mechanism. Approximately 20–30% of older individuals with serious infections present with a blunted or absent fever response, which heralds a poorer prognosis than a strong febrile response[10,11]. The significance of fever in the elderly patient is that it is most likely to be due to a serious bacterial or viral infection, unlike in the young where it is associated with benign viral illness[10,11].

The atypical presentation of infections in the elderly is well established. A worsening in mental status may be the primary finding[12,13]; likewise, anorexia, falls, weakness and/or urinary incontinence may be the presenting findings[1,12].

URINARY TRACT INFECTIONS

Urinary tract infections (UTIs) are the most common infections in the elderly, often with serious consequences. The prevalence of bacteriuria increases with age, level of care and decreasing functional capacity (Table 2).

The clinical features of UTIs in older persons may be similar to those in the young. However, the features may be more difficult to interpret in older individuals. Signs and symptoms of lower UTIs such as urinary frequency, nocturia, urgency or dysuria may occur as a result of underlying bladder abnormalities, such as neurogenic bladder, even in the absence of infection. In upper UTIs, the classic manifestations of flank pain and fever may be absent. Instead, the presenting signs and symptoms in older persons may be respiratory distress or gastrointestinal manifestations or delirium with severe dehydration[14]. Bacterial prostatitis is important to recognize because of its role in causing recurrent UTI in older men. Clinical clues include perineal pain, low back pain, difficulty urinating and low-grade fever[15,16].

Urinary tract infections in women are more common than in men until advanced age. UTIs are 25–30 times more common in younger women than in men, while in older women, they are only 2–3 times more common[17]. The risk factors for urinary tract infections differ in older women from those in the

Table 3 Factors contributing to recurrent urinary tract infections (UTIs) in women of different age groups. Adapted from reference 18

Younger women	Older women (community)	Older women (institutionalized)
Sexual intercourse	lack of estrogen	catheterization
Spermicide exposure	non-secretor status	incontinence
Maternal history of UTI	history of premenopausal UTI	antimicrobial exposure
History of childhood UTI	incontinence	functional status
?Non-secretor status	presence of cystocele	
	post-void residual urine	

young (Table 3). Bladder dysfunction and atrophic urethritis are more likely to be seen in the older female. The range of infecting organisms is also broader in this age group[18]. *Escherichia coli* and *Staphylococcus saprophyticus* comprise more than 95% of the uropathogens in the young. Older individuals living in the community have uropathogens that are largely similar to those seen in the younger age group. However, in older, institutionalized women, *E. coli*, *Proteus spp.*, *Klebsiella pneumoniae*, other Enterobacteriaciae, *Pseudomonas* spp., *Acinetobacter* and *Enterococcus* spp. constitute the organisms cultured.

Genetic predisposition to recurrent infections in both younger and older women has been the non-secretor genotype of the tissue–blood group antigens. Non-secretors synthesize specific *E. coli*-binding receptors on their vaginal epithelial cells[18,19].

In older, postmenopausal women, the absence of estrogen plays a central role in the pathogenesis of urinary tract infections. Estrogen promotes colonization of the vagina with normal flora, dominated by the presence of lactobacilli. This in turn lowers the vaginal pH, which inhibits growth of pathogenic organisms[19].

Among older, institutionalized women, urinary catheterization and declining functional status are the most important risk factors associated with UTIs[20]. Indwelling catheters allow introduction of bacteria into the bladder. Most patients with long-term catheters (present longer than 30 days) are bacteriuric, but only a small percentage

develop symptomatic infection. Fecal and urinary incontinence may also predispose the older woman to UTI. Exposure to an increased quantity of uropathogens around the urethra potentially increases the risk for UTI. Diagnosis of complicated UTI in older residents in the long-term care setting is difficult. A positive urine culture in a setting where there is no localized finding, but there is clinical deterioration, leads to an uncertain diagnosis of UTI. Management issues arise in these settings[18,20].

Asymptomatic bacteriuria is defined as $> 10^5$ organisms/ml urine in the absence of symptoms[21]. In both men and women, the prevalence of asymptomatic bacteriuria increases with advanced age, with women having double the rate. In residents of long-term care facilities or hospitals, the rates are similar in both groups. Numerous studies have shown that antibiotic treatment does not prolong survival in patients with asymptomatic bacteriuria[21,22]. Treatment may result in only transient clearing but is often complicated by adverse drug reactions.

Symptomatic urinary tract infections should be treated in both young and old persons. Antibiotic selection should be guided by a Gram-stained smear of the urine and the patient's history. Uncomplicated community-acquired infections can be treated effectively with oral agents that have adequate antibacterial levels in the urine; these include trimethoprim–sulfamethoxazole, quinolones and cephalosporins. Residence in a long-term care facility, recent hospital stays, repeated courses of antibiotics and use of indwelling

Table 4 Infectious complications of pressure ulcers

Localized wound infections
Cellulitis of surrounding tissues
Contiguous osteomyelitis
Bacteremia and sepsis
Remote infections (endocarditis)
Tetanus (rare)

bladder catheters are all associated with more resistant organisms. For the elderly patients with complicated urinary tract infections needing parenteral therapy, empiric antibiotics may be a third-generation cephalosporin or a penicillin inhibitor, trimethoprim–sulfamethoxazole or a quinolone. For Gram-positive infections, ampicillin or vancomycin may be used. Final antibiotic selection should be guided by antibiotic susceptibility studies[21,23].

SKIN AND SOFT TISSUE INFECTIONS

Pressure sores are a common source of morbidity among seriously disabled elderly patients, and are difficult to treat. After a 1-year stay in a long-term care facility, the prevalence of pressure sores was found to be 10.4% in one study[24]. For patients admitted to nursing homes with a pressure ulcer, the first-year mortality rate is over 50%. Although these patients are usually debilitated and have serious co-morbid illnesses, infections from ulcers are frequently the cause of death[25,26].

Pressure ulcers occur primarily in persons with impaired mobility. The interplay of pressure, shear friction and maceration gives rise to tissue necrosis[27]. Immobile persons in bed or chair can garner pressures over the greater trochanter and sacrum of over 150 mmHg, greatly exceeding the 35 mmHg which is enough to block capillary flow. The ulcer that develops may be associated with a number of infectious complications, some of which are serious (Table 4).

Pathogenic organisms from pressure ulcers causing bacteremia include *Proteus mirabilis*, *Staphylococcus aureus*, *E. coli* and anaerobes[28].

Mortality is high (over 50%) with polymicrobial sepsis common. Osteomyelitis is often the underlying cause of delayed or failed wound healing. Diagnostic clues include high sedimentation rate, leukocytosis, abnormal radiographs and abnormal computerized tomography (CT) scan; definitive diagnostic tests include bone biopsy and culture. If osteomyelitis is determined, a more prolonged course of antibiotic therapy is prescribed.

Most pressure ulcers in the elderly yield multiple organisms when cultured. Assessing the bacteriologic etiology of pressure ulcers is full of pitfalls. Wound swabs often yield organisms that are colonizers. Aspiration of material from the margin or base of the ulcer using a needle through intact skin might give a more accurate bacteriologic diagnosis, but is cumbersome. Cultures of wounds should not be performed unless evidence of purulence, deep infection or failure to heal is present. Bacteria in healing wounds can be misleading, resulting in inappropriate antibiotic therapy. Clean wounds do not need systemic or topical antibiotics (Table 5[29]).

The key to management of pressure ulcers is prevention. Guidelines for preventing development of pressure lesions have been published including clinical strategies for identifying patients at risk and early intervention.

Healing is impossible if pressure continues; therefore relief of pressure by change of position and use of pressure-relieving devices is vital. Debridement can be performed in several ways, depending on the necrosis. Adequate nutrition is important. Reducing bacterial concentration promotes healing. In the presence of clinical signs of fever, chills and hypotension, antibiotics (with Gram-negative and Gram-positive coverage) are indicated.

BACTERIAL MENINGITIS

The incidence of bacterial meningitis in the elderly is on the increase. Recognition of bacterial meningitis in the elderly is difficult, since the expected signs and symptoms may

Table 5 Common isolates recovered from biopsy cultures of pressure ulcers. From reference 29

Superficial ulcers without necrosis
Aerobes
    Pseudomonas aeruginosa

Deep ulcers without necrosis
Aerobes
    P. aeruginosa
    Staphylococcus aureus
    Morganella morganii
    Escherichia coli
    Providencia stuartii

Necrotic tissue
Aerobes
    E. coli
    S. aureus
    P. aeruginosa
    Proteus mirabilis
    Enterococcus spp.
    Staphylococcus epidermidis
Anaerobes
    Bacteroides fragilis
    Bacteroides asaccharolyticus
    Bacteroides melaninogenicus
    Clostridium spp.
    Peptostreptococcus prevotii
    Peptostreptococcus magnus

not be present. Fever, headache, nuchal rigidity and photophobia may be absent in the aged[30]. Nuchal rigidity may also be the result of cervical degenerative arthritis. On the other hand, the presentation of altered mental status may be secondary to other causes besides meningitis (Table 6).

The range of etiologic agents causing meningitis in older adults is broad, with infectious pathogens predominantly bacterial, as opposed to infections in younger adults, which are mostly viral. *Streptococcus pneumoniae* is still the most common etiologic bacterium. There is grave concern over the increasing incidence of penicillin-resistant *S. pneumoniae*. *Listeria monocytogenes*, which is usually associated with ingestion of soft cheese and other delicatessen products, is also seen in bacterial meningitis in the elderly. Gram-negative bacillary meningitis is fairly common and usually results from hematogenous spread from infections at distant sites,

such as from a urinary tract infection[31,32]. *Haemophilus influenzae* and *Neisseria meningitidis* are also found in meningitis in the elderly, although they are less common than in the younger population[30] (Table 6).

Bacterial meningitis has high case fatality rates in the aged. Complications related to this disease such as neurologic deficit, seizures, hydrocephalus and accompanying pneumonia, bacteremia and urinary tract infections are more frequent in the elderly than in younger patients[30,33]. Prompt initiation of antibiotics is the cornerstone of successful treatment of bacterial meningitis. In the elderly, empiric combination of ampicillin and a third-generation cephalosporin such as ceftriaxone or cefotaxime is recommended. In situations where drug-resistant *S. pneumoniae* is suspected, vancomycin is added to the regimen[30]. In other clinical scenarios where staphylococcal infection may be the etiology, nafcillin, oxacillin or vancomycin should be included.

GASTROINTESTINAL INFECTIONS

In addition to host factors in the elderly that predispose to increased risk for infections, certain factors are unique with respect to gastrointestinal infections. The elderly may not have the capability for proper preparation and adequate storage of food that is essential for prevention of food-borne infections.

Physiologically, in the gastrointestinal tract, a major barrier against pathogens is gastric acidity. A pH of 4 or less usually kills bacteria. With aging, hypochlorhydria or achlorhydria may develop. Thus, it will take a smaller concentration of ingested bacteria to establish intestinal infection. In addition, reduction of gastric acid may occur from medications that further reduce gastric pH, such as H_2 blockers and proton pump inhibitors[34].

Infectious pathogens have to attach to the mucosal surface of the intestines in order to colonize and cause disease. Intestinal mucus, made up of glycoproteins, traps these

Table 6   Meningitis in the elderly

Signs and symptoms	Common etiologic agents
Fever	Streptococcus pneumoniae
Lethargy, confusion or coma	Listeria monocytogenes
Headache	Neisseria meningitidis
Respiratory symptoms	Group B streptococci
Photophobia	Gram-negative organisms
Nuchal rigidity	(Escherichia coli, Haemophilus influenzae,
Altered level of consciousness	Enterobacteriaciae)
Seizures	

pathogens and prevents their adherence to the mucosa. The resultant package is then cleared by normal intestinal motility. In older subjects, there is a decrease in the production of mucus, rendering the intestines more susceptible to adherence and colonization by infectious agents. The decrease in intestinal motility may be explained by multiple factors: diet, drugs and physical activity. Low-fiber diets and limited physical activity diminish intestinal motility. Patients who are bed-bound or those with restricted activity are usually constipated. Narcotic analgesics administered for pain can further reduce motility.

The immune system in the intestines is made up of lymphoid follicles in Peyer's patches or in isolated lymphoid follicles in the mucosa. The macrophages and lymphocytes work together to produce cellular and antibody immune responses. The secretory antibodies play a major role in preventing bacterial attachment to the mucosa and in destroying the infectious organisms. Although the concentration levels of IgA in the elderly are the same as in the young, specific antibodies to new antigens are not produced as efficiently in the elderly.

Deterioration of personal hygiene increases hand-to-mouth transmission of infectious agents. Incontinence adds to this deterioration, and further contaminates the environment with fecal material[34].

Economic factors play a role in different living settings: in institutionalized patients such as those in long-term care facilities and rehabilitation units, in retirement communities with common eating facilities and even in the elderly patients living independently in the general community. As the density of the population in a certain unit increases, there is a higher likelihood of transmission of infections, as seen in hospitals and long-term care facilities. As the number of caregivers and support staff for facilities are reduced, infection control practices are not followed as rigorously, further increasing the possibility of spread of infection. Economic limitations may predispose to difficulty in proper preparation of food and adequate storage facilities. Reluctance to dispose of food and improper refrigeration of food contribute to contamination with bacteria and their associated toxins[35] (Table 7).

The clinical symptoms of nausea, vomiting and diarrhea are common in the elderly. However, diarrhea may manifest only as frequent soft stools in a patient who was previously constipated. Abdominal pain and leukocytosis may be milder. The only presentation of gastrointestinal infection may be dehydration, hypotension or confusion. Fever may or may not be present. Dehydration may have more severe consequences in the elderly. Fluid replacement, regardless of the etiologic agent, is of utmost importance.

Infectious agents that affect the general community also affect the aged. However, the infection may be more severe and prolonged in this age group. Some pathogens differ in the various age groups. Rotavirus, for example, is more commonly seen in infants

Table 7 Factors predisposing to gastrointestinal infections in the elderly

Physiologic factors
Reduction in gastric acid
Decreased intestinal motility (drugs, reduced physical activity)
Decreased production of specific antibodies
Incontinence and poor hygiene

Economic factors
Long-term care facilities
Improper food preparation/storage

Table 8 Common etiologic agents causing gastroenteritis in the elderly

Bacterial
  Shigella
  Salmonella
  Escherichia coli 0157:H7
  Campylobacter jejuni
  Aeromonas hydrophila
  Clostridium perfringens
  Staphylococcus aureus
  Clostridium difficile

Viral
  Norwalk virus
  other calicivirus
  astrovirus
  rotavirus

Parasitic
  Cryptosporidium
  Giardia lamblia

and young children. Outbreaks of rotavirus have occured in geriatric wards, in older adults in a cardiology ward and in nursing homes[36,37].

Norwalk and Norwalk-like viruses are the most common cause of viral infections in the elderly, occurring usually in the winter[38]. Symptoms of nausea, non-bloody diarrhea and abdominal cramps are present, but the most prominent symptom is vomiting. Prolonged constitutional symptoms are a particular problem in outbreaks in nursing homes. In institutions with an outbreak, strict infection control management, including restriction of visitors, cohorting of ill patients and rigorous handwashing, should be enforced[39,40]. Other caliciviruses besides the Norwalk virus have been seen in long-term care facilities. Outbreak management and treatment is the same as for the Norwalk virus, with provision for oral or intravenous rehydration if needed[40]. If calicivirus infection is identified in facilities, needless use of antibiotics may be avoided. Astrovirus is another viral pathogen that has been reported to cause outbreaks in nursing homes[40] (Table 8).

Although there have been reported outbreaks of *Salmonella*[41] and *Shigella*[42] infections, these are uncommon. These bacterial infections are a problem in the elderly, who tend to have underlying medical conditions that complicate the illness. In infections caused by *Shigella flexneri*, the severity of symptoms increases with age[43]. The very

young and the very old seem to be at particular risk for the new *E. coli* serotype, 0157:H7. Such infections are usually associated with undercooked bovine meat. In nursing homes, the highest attack rate occurs among the oldest patients. Deaths from *E. coli* 0157:H7 have been mostly in the elderly. Mortality rates of up to 35% have been reported in infected elderly nursing home residents[44]. Other bacterial causes of outbreaks in long-term care facilities are *Aeromonas hydrophila* (Bloom) and *Campylobacter jejuni*. The attack rate of *C. jejuni* in those older than 85 years was 75%. Bacteremia with *C. jejuni* is much more common in those over 65 years of age than in the younger age group (5.9 cases per 1000 *C. jejuni* infections)[45].

Clostridium difficile infections are a major problem in hospitalized geriatric patients, as well as in residents of long-term care facilities[34]. Patients given antibiotics have altered intestinal flora, which permit overgrowth of *C. difficile*. Infected individuals tend to be older, with dementia, low albumin and incontinence of stool[34,46]. They also tend to be co-infected with other resistant organisms such as vancomycin-resistant enterococcus, methicillin-resistant *S. aureus* and yeast infections[47].

PNEUMONIA

Pneumonia is an important cause of morbidity and mortality in the elderly, and its impact on health-care costs is staggering. Pneumonia is more dangerous in persons over 65; complications and hospitalizations are more common[48]. Once hospitalized, the older individual may require a longer hospital stay.

S. pneumoniae is the most likely causative organism in community-acquired pneumonia. The rapid emergence of drug-resistant strains precludes appropriate use of antibiotics[48]. Management of pneumonia has become more complicated because of drug resistance, not only in S. pneumoniae but in other pathogenic bacteria such as S. aureus and Gram-negative bacteria. Judicious use of antibiotics must be emphasized in treatment strategies of pneumonia and other infections[49].

A further discussion on pneumonia appears in Chapter 42.

HERPES ZOSTER

Varicella-zoster virus (VZV) is the etiologic agent of both varicella, more commonly known as chickenpox, and herpes zoster, or shingles. Reactivation of VZV leads to herpes zoster, a disease that occurs at all ages, especially in the older age group[50]. The highest incidence of disease varies between five and ten cases per 1000 for persons older than 60 years[51]. Herpes zoster is characterized by a unilateral vesicular eruption usually involving one dermatome. Common complications of herpes zoster include acute neuritis and post-herpetic neuralgia. Post-herpetic neuralgia is of utmost clinical significance in the older population. It may occur in up to 50% of patients older than 50 years[52] and may cause debilitating and incapacitating pain that may persist for longer than a month[53].

Antiviral medications for herpes zoster include acyclovir, valacylovir (the prodrug of acyclovir) and famciclovir. Oral therapy of

Table 9 Risk factors for endocarditis in the elderly

Degenerative heart disease
Valvular heart disease
Rheumatic or congenital heart disease
Nosocomial endocarditis
   central venous catheters
   hyperalimentation lines
   pacemakers
   dialysis catheters, shunts
Increased procedures and manipulations
   upper gastrointestinal endoscopy
   sigmoidoscopy/colonoscopy
   urethral dilatation/catheterization
   transurethral prostatectomy

herpes zoster accelerates cutaneous healing and reduces pain in acute neuritis. Concomitant use of steroids and antivirals is still controversial. However, a recent study[54] in patients more than 50 years of age demonstrated improvement in quality of life and in resolution of acute neuritis when steroids and antivirals were used together, without any added significant adverse effects.

ENDOCARDITIS

Infective endocarditis (IE) has been gaining in importance in the older population. In 1926, the median age of patients with IE was less than 30 years[55]. More recently, data suggested that more than 50% of cases were seen in patients over 50 years of age[56]. There are numerous reasons for causing this shift to an older age group (Table 9). Degenerative heart lesions which may include calcifications in the mitral annulus, nodular lesions secondary to arteriosclerotic heart disease and cardiac thrombi after myocardial infarcts[57] are underlying risk factors for IE. Rheumatic or congenital heart diseases are usually risk factors in younger patients. However, such patients are increasingly surviving longer. Prosthetic valve endocarditis is a distinct form of IE that carries a higher morbidity and mortality. Use of intravascular devices and presence of infections with implantable devices increase the risk for bacteremia, therefore increasing the risk for IE. As more invasive procedures are performed in the elderly, the chances of bacteremia and IE are higher.

The diagnosis of IE may be problematic in the elderly because of the non-specificity of signs and symptoms. More than 60% of IE was misdiagnosed on admission in one study in the older population[58]. The Duke criterion for endocarditis proposed in 1994[59] is well recognized as a sensitive tool in the clinical diagnosis of IE and is now increasingly used[60].

The microbiology of IE may also be different in the aged. Gram-positive organisms predominate. In addition to *S. aureus* and *Streptococcus viridans*, there are other prominent organisms causing IE in this age group, namely *Enterococcus* spp. (usually originating from the urinary tract) and *Streptococcus bovis* (usually from the gastrointestinal tract)[21]. *Enterococcus* spp. are also agents seen in prosthetic valve endocarditis. Therapy for IE is the same for all age groups. Due to the altered renal function in the older patient, care must be used in proper antibiotic dosing[61], especially for IE because of the longer duration of therapy.

INFLUENZA

Influenza virus infection is one of the most important communicable infections in the elderly. Outbreaks of influenza occur frequently in nursing facilities and other long-term care facilities. People 65 years of age or older account for at least 50% of hospitalizations and 75–80% of deaths attributed to influenza. Mortality ranges from 1/100 000 among those with low risk to 217/100 000 among patients with only one high-risk condition and 306/100 000 among those with two or more high-risk conditions[62]. High-risk conditions for complications from influenza infections include chronic cardiac disease, pulmonary disease and diabetes.

The diagnosis of influenza infection is usually based on the seasonal timing, clinical presentation and presence of outbreaks, usually presenting first in the community, then in the long-term care facility. If influenza A is suspected, nasopharyngeal swabs may be obtained within 24–48 h of the onset of symptoms, and sent for viral cultures and rapid diagnostic testing for influenza antigens.

Immunization with the influenza vaccine is a potent preventive measure for this viral infection as well as for possible subsequent bacterial pneumonia. The population of persons aged 65 years or older is a primary target for immunization. While some studies suggest that the immune response to the vaccine in older subjects is satisfactory, others state that the response is suboptimal because of nutritional or immunologic deficits[63].

TUBERCULOSIS

Tuberculosis (TB) is an important and frequent disease in the elderly. The incidence is twice that in the community, and even higher among the residents of nursing homes. Tuberculosis in the older population is usually a reactivation of the infection. The elderly are in the high-risk group for the development of TB due to numerous factors. Residence in nursing homes and other long-term care facilities means a high-exposure setting for these patients (Table 10).

The new guidelines for skin testing and treatment of TB target individuals at high risk for developing the infection, who would benefit by treatment of latent TB infection. Testing is widely carried out in the elderly, especially in residents of long-term care facilities. The two-step Mantoux test may be appropriate in the older person. The two-step test entails an initial step that involves placement of five tuberculin units intradermally on the patient's arm, with the results read within 48–72 hours. If the result is positive, the patient is presumed to have latent TB

Table 10   Risk factors for development of tuberculosis in the elderly

---

Decline in cellular immunity
Concurrent illnesses (diabetes mellitus, pulmonary disease, chronic renal failure)
Use of certain medications (steroids, other immunosuppressive agents)
Poor nutrition
Residence in long-term care facilities

---

infection and no further steps are necessary. If the result is negative, the second step is repeated in 2 weeks. If the second reading is also negative, the patient is deemed to be uninfected. On the other hand, if the second reading is positive, the patient truly has latent TB infection and therapy should be considered.

A change from prior recommendations in interpretation of tuberculin testing is the TB skin test conversion, which is a change in status within a 2-year span of time. A conversion is now defined as an increase of ≥ 10 mm of induration, regardless of age.

In the new guidelines, infected persons who are considered to be at high risk for developing active TB should be offered treatment for latent TB infection irrespective of age[64]. Therapy for latent TB infection is preferably isoniazid given for 9 months instead of 6 months. Another regimen is a combination of rifampin and pyrazinamide given for 2 months. Pyridoxine (vitamin B_6) may be added to isoniazid regimens, especially for the elderly or for patients who are malnourished. Therapy should be individualized and caution should be used in patients who are on other medications that may be hepatotoxic or who have underlying liver disease. Dutt and Stead reported a 4.5% incidence of non-fatal hepatitis in a group of 2000 elderly individuals given isoniazid prophylaxis[65]. Baseline testing is not routinely indicated in older persons. However, such testing may be considered on an individual basis, particularly for patients who are taking other medications for chronic medical conditions. Clinical monitoring is essential, but routine liver function tests are no longer recommended except in patients with HIV or chronic liver disease and those who use alcohol regularly.

References

1. Yoshikawa TT. Epidemiology and unique aspects of aging and infectious diseases. *Clin Infect Dis* 2000;30:931–3
2. Baker H, Frank O, Thind IS, *et al.* Vitamin profiles in elderly persons living at home or in nursing homes versus profiles in healthy young subjects. *J Am Geriatr Soc* 1979;27:444–50
3. Waldorf DS, Wilkens RF, Decker JI. Impaired delayed hypersensitivity in an aging population. *J Am Med Assoc* 1968;203:831–4
4. Ben-Yehuda A, Weksler ME. Host resistance and the immune system. *Clin Geriatr Med* 1992;8:701–11
5. Yoshikawa TT. Infectious diseases, immunity and aging: perspectives and prospects. In Powers DC, Morley JE, Coe RM, eds. *Aging, Immunity and Infection*. New York: Springer, 1994:1–11
6. Inkeles B, Innes JB, Kuntz, *et al.* Immunological studies of aging. III. Cytokinetic bases for impaired response of lymphocytes from aged humans to plan lectins. *J Exp Med* 1977;149:1029–141
7. Rivnay B, Bergman S, Shinitzky M, *et al.* Correlation between membrane viscosity, serum cholesterol, lymphocyte activation and aging in man. *Mech Aging Dev* 1980;12:119–26
8. Phair JP, Kauffman CA, Bjornson A, *et al.* Host defenses in the aged: evaluation of components of the inflammatory and immune responses. *J Infect Dis* 1978;138:67–73

9. Gardner I. The effect of aging on suscepti-bility to infection. *Rev Infect Dis* 1980;2:801–10

10. Norman DC. Fever in the elderly. *Clin Infect Dis* 2000;7:387–90

11. Downton JH, Andrews K, Puxty JAH. Silent pyrexia in the elderly. *Age Ageing* 1987;16:41–4

12. Bentley DW, Bradley S, High K, *et al.* Practice guidelines for evaluation of fever and infection in long-term care facilities. *Clin Infect Dis* 2000;31:640–53

13. Rockwood K. Acute confusion in elderly medical patients. *J Am Geriatr Soc* 1989; 37:150–4

14. Boscia JA, Kaye D. Asymptomatic bacteri-uria in the elderly. *Infect Dis Clin North Am* 1987;1:893–903

15. Stamm WE, Hooton TM. Management of urinary tract infections in adults. *N Engl J Med* 1993;329:1328–34

16. Nicolle LE. Asymptomatic bacteriuria in elderly institutionalized men. *N Engl J Med* 1983;309:1420–5

17. Kaye D. Urinary tract infections in the elderly. *Bull NY Acad Med* 1980;56:209–20

18. McCue JD. Urinary tract infection: treat-ment guidelines for older women. *Consultant* 1997;27:2135–42

19. Stamm WE, Raz R. Factors contributing to susceptibility of postmenopausal women to recurrent urinary tract infection. *Clin Inf Dis* 1999;28:723–5

20. Nicolle LE. Asymptomatic bacteriuria in the elderly. *Infec Dis Clin North Am* 1997;11: 647

21. Crossley KB, Peterson PK. Infections in the elderly. In Mandell GI, Bennett JE, Dolin R, eds. *Principles and Practice of Infectious Diseases*, 5th edn. Philadelphia: Churchill Livingstone, 2000:3164–9

22. Nicolle LE. Urinary tract infection in long-term-care facility residents. *Clin Infect Dis* 2000;31:757–61

23. McCue JD. Complicated UTI. Effective treatment in the long-term care setting. *Geriatrics* 2000;55:48–61

24. Brandeis GH, Morris JN, Nash DJ, *et al.* The epidemiology and natural history of pressure ulcers in elderly nursing home res-idents. *J Am Med Assoc* 1990;264:2905

25. Jahnigen DW. Infectious complications of pressure ulcers. *Geriatr Focus* 1992;2: 1–3,12

26. Allman RM. Pressure ulcers among the elderly. *N Engl J Med* 1989;320:850

27. Langemo DK, Olson B, Hunter S, *et al.* Incidence of pressure sores in acute care rehabilitation, extended care, home, health and hospice in one locale. *Decubitus* 1989;2:42

28. Bryan CS, Dew CE, Reynolds KL. Bacteremia associated with decubitus ulcers. *Arch Intern Med* 1983;143:2093

29. Sapico FL, Ginunas VJ, Thornhill-Joynes M, *et al.* Quantitative microbiology of pres-sure sores in different stages of health. *Diagn Microbiol Infect Dis* 1986;5:31

30. Choi C. Bacterial meningitis in the elderly. *Geriatr Focus* 1993;3:10–16

31. Gorse G, Thrupp L, Nudleman K, *et al.* Bacterial meningitis in the elderly. *Arch Intern Med* 1984;144:1603–7

32. Behrman RE, Meyers BR, Mendelson MH, *et al.* Central nervous system infections in the elderly. *Arch Intern Med* 1989;149: 1596–9

33. Roos K. Meningitis as it presents in the elderly: diagnosis and care. *Geriatrics* 1990; 45:3–75

34. Owen RL, Lew JF. Gastrointestinal infec-tions in the elderly. In Blaser MJ, Smith PD, Ravdin JI, Greenberg HB, Guerrant RL, eds. *Infections of the Gastrointestinal Tract.* New York: Raven Press, 1995:551–64

35. Schouten EG, Pelt FL, Reitsma W, *et al.* Food hygiene and the prevalence of diar-rhea and vomiting in independent elderly. *Tijdschr Gerontol Geriatr* 1988;19:7–10

36. Marrie TJ, Lee SHS, Faulkner RS, *et al.* Rotavirus infection in a geriatric popula-tion. *Arch Intern Med* 1982;142:313–16

37. Hardy DB. Epidemiology of rotaviral infec-tion in adults. *Rev Infect Dis* 1987;9:461–9

38. LeBaron CW, Furutan NP, Lew JF, *et al.* Viral agents of gastroenteritis: public health importance and outbreak manage-ment. *Morbid Mortal Weekly Rep* 1990; 39:1–24

39. Gellert GA, Waterman SH, Ewert D, *et al.* An outbreak of acute gastroenteritis caused by a small round structure virus in

a geriatric convalescent facility. *Infect Control Hosp Epidemiol* 1990;11:459–64

40. Gray JJ, Wreghitt TG, Cubitt WD, Elliot PR. An outbreak of gastroenteritis in a home for the elderly associated with astrovirus type 1 and human calicivirus. *J Med Virol* 1987;23: 377–81

41. Choi M, Yoshikawa TT, Bridge J, *et al. Salmonella* outbreak in a nursing home. *J Am Geriatr Soc* 1990;38:531–4

42. Horan MA, Gulati RS, Fox RA, *et al.* Outbreak of *Shigella sonnei* dysentery on a geriatric assessment ward. *J Hosp Infect* 1984;5:210–12

43. Halpern Z, Dan M, Giladi M, *et al.* Shigellosis in adults: epidemiologic, clinical, and laboratory features. *Medicine* 1989:68: 210–17

44. Griffin PM, Ostroff SM, Tauxe RV, *et al.* Illnesses associated with *Escherichia coli* 0157:H7 infections: a broad clinical spectrum. *Ann Intern Med* 1988;109:705–12

45. Bloom HG, Bottone EJ. *Aeromonas hydrophila* diarrhea in a long-term care setting. *J Am Geriatr Soc* 1990;38:804–6

46. Ramaswamy R, Grover H, Corpuz M, Daniels P Pitchumoni CS. Prognostic criteria in *Clostridium difficile* colitis. *Am J Geriatr* 1996;91:460–4

47. Poduval R, Kamath R, Corpuz M, *et al. Clostridium difficile* and vancomycin resistant enterococcus – the new nosocomial alliance. *Am J Geriatr* 2000;95:3513–15

48. Butler JC, Cetron MS. Pneumococcal drug resistance: the new 'special enemy of old age.' *Clin Infect Dis* 1999;28:730–5

49. Fein AM. Pneumonia in the elderly: overview of diagnostic and therapeutic approaches. *Clin Infect Dis* 1999;28:726–9

50. Ragozzino MW, Melton LJ III, Kurland LT, *et al.* Population-based study of herpes zoster and its sequelae. *Medicine (Baltimore)* 1982;5:310–16

51. Weller TH. Serial propagation *in vitro* of agents producing inclusion bodies derived from varicella and herpes zoster. *Proc Soc Exp Biol Med* 1954;83:340–6

52. Watson PN, Evans RJ. Postherpetic neuralgia; a review. *Arch Neurol* 1986;43:836–40

53. Kost RG, Straus SE. Drug therapy: postherpetic neuralgia – pathogenesis, treatment and prevention. *N Engl J Med* 1996;335:32

54. Whitley RJ, Gnann JW. Acyclovir: a decade later. *N Engl J Med* 1992;327:782–9

55. Thayer WS. Studies on bacterial (infective) endocarditis. *Johns Hopkins Hosp Rep* 1926;22:1

56. Garvey GJ, Neu HC. Infective endocarditis: an evolving disease. *Medicine* 1978;57:105

57. McKinsey DS, Ratts TE, Bisno AL. Underlying cardiac lesions in adults with infective endocarditis. The changing spectrum. *Am J Med* 1987;82:681–8

58. Terpenning MS, Buggy BP, Kauffman CA. Infective endocarditis: clinical features in young and elderly patients. *Am J Med* 1987;83:626

59. Durack DT, Lukes AS, Bright DK, *et al.* New criteria for diagnosis of infective endocarditis. *Am J Med* 1994;96:200–9

60. Bayer AS, Bolger AF, Taubert KA, *et al.* Diagnosis and management of infective endocarditis and its complications. *Circulation* 1998;25:2936–48

61. Dharmarajan TS, Ranganathan R, Corpuz M, Norkus EP. Is antibiotic dosing appropriate for renal function in older adults? *World J Med Today* 2000;1950:441–4

62. Bentley DW. Immunizations in the elderly. *Bull NY Acad Med* 1987;63:533–49

63. Ender PT, DeRussy PK, Caldwell MM, *et al.* The effect of multivitamin on the immunologic response to the influenza vaccine in the elderly. *IDCP* 2001;10:81–5

64. Targeted tuberculin testing and treatment of tuberculosis infection. *Morbid Mortal Weekly Rep* 2000;45:1–51

65. Dutt AK, Stead WW. Tuberculosis. *Clin Geriatr Med* 1992;8:761–75

44 Hematologic disorders in older adults

T.S. Dharmarajan, MD, FACP, AGSF,
May Luz F. Bullecer, MD, *and Niyati Bhagwati*, MD

RED CELL DISORDERS

Anemia

Introduction and definition

Anemia in older adults is not a disease, rather a sign of an underlying problem for which an etiology must be sought. In most instances, anemia is not a result of the aging process alone, with a principal cause demonstrated in more than half the cases. Thus it should not be considered a normal physiological response to aging[1,2]. The incidence of anemia increases with age, with males more affected than females in those over 65, and appears more common than suspected clinically[1].

While definitions of anemia are controversial, anemia as defined by the World Health Organization is present when the hemoglobin concentration is less than 13 g/dl in males and less than 12 g/dl in females. For clinical purposes, data suggest that a comprehensive evaluation in those with hemoglobin concentrations of ≥ 12 g/dl seldom yields an underlying etiology[3].

Does hemoglobin level decline with age? Surveys suggest that 12–25% of individuals over age 65 are anemic, with a lower hemoglobin level more likely in nursing home residents over age 75. Data also suggest a mild decline in hemoglobin value from age 70 to 81[4,5]. A specific cause, however, is not always demonstrated.

Erythropoiesis

The initial step involves commitment of the stem cell progeny to erythroid differentiation followed by formation of the burst-forming unit erythroid (BFU-E), which in early stages proliferates and differentiates independently of erythropoietin (EPO). From these units the colony-forming unit erythroid (CFU-E) forms in 6–8 days. These cells contain the most surface EPO receptors and are sensitive to and dependent on EPO for survival. As these cells proliferate and differentiate, proerythroblasts are formed[6]. Erythroblasts are nucleated red cells, normal (normoblasts) and pathologic (megaloblasts)[6]. Several stages of normoblastic differentiation occur, beginning with the proerythroblast and eventual extrusion of the nucleus, forming the reticulocyte.

Hemoglobin is composed of protein (globin), protophorphyrin and iron. Complex metabolic pathways form these structural components. Hemoglobin is a tetramer composed of two pairs of polypeptides while heme is a ferrous iron complex of protophorphyrin IX[6].

The role of erythropoietin EPO regulates the final stages of maturation of erythroid cells. EPO is a 165-amino-acid glycoprotein hormone with molecular weight 30 400 Da, mainly (90%) produced in the kidneys[7]. Its effect is mediated by interaction with a 508-amino-acid glycoprotein receptor. While the exact mechanism is not well understood, hypoxia and anemia clearly stimulate the production of EPO[6]. EPO maintains the viability of erythroid precursor cells by delaying DNA cleavage and programmed cell death (apoptosis), allowing them to mature and differentiate[6,7].

EPO levels can be measured by enzyme-linked immunosorbent assay (ELISA) or by bioassays. Normal serum levels differ with the methodology used, and usually range between 5 and 30 mU/ml. In the absence of renal failure, a low or normal value of EPO in the presence of anemia denotes an inappropriate response. However, elevated levels do not always mean that the response is adequate for the degree of anemia. While hypoxia increases the production of EPO, cytokines inhibit production; thus, inflammation limits the erythropoietic response[4,7,8].

Aging and erythropoiesis   Red cell survival, normally 120 days, mainly depends on the pliability of the cell membrane. With aging, a minimal increase in the red cell size and membrane viscosity are noted, along with a slight decline in enzyme content and metabolic activity, with the red cell span somewhat shortened[4,5]. The mild degree of subclinical hematopoietic hypofunction that is probably related to diminished reserve becomes manifest in the presence of stress or disease, demanding augmented hematopoiesis[9–11]. While the blunted response is not well understood, it is believed to be associated with age-related deficits in the bone marrow progenitor cell numbers, changes in the marrow microenvironment and decreased production of regulatory growth factors[12]. More recent observations include the role of cytokines; a reduction in the production of interleukin-2 and the increased levels of interleukin-6 may possibly be attributed to age-related changes in hematopoiesis[7,8,10] (Table 1). Despite these changes, it is worth

Table 1   Aging and erythropoiesis

Minimal degree of subclinical hematopoietic hypofunction
Slight increase in red cell size and membrane viscosity
Minimal decline in red cell lifespan
Decreased production of regulatory growth factors
Reduction in interleukin-2, increase in interleukin-6 production
Slight decline in enzyme content and metabolic activity
Deficit in bone marrow progenitor cell numbers

noting that the elderly respond well to purified hematopoietic stimulators[10,12].

Classification of anemia

Anemia may be classified on the basis of red blood cell characteristics or the functional defect of erythropoiesis (Table 2). The morphologic classification (based on size and hemoglobin content) of anemia is convenient for differential diagnosis of the underlying etiology and treatment. Mean cell volume (MCV) is helpful among the red blood cell indices. Anemia is macrocytic if the MCV is more than 100 fl, microcytic if less than 80 fl, and normocytic if between 80 and 90 fl[13]. Examples of macrocytic, normocytic and microcytic anemias are illustrated in Table 2.

Yet another classification resorted to by hematologists is anemia from blood loss, hypoproliferative, hemolytic and from ineffective erythropoiesis[14]. Hypoproliferative anemia is preponderant in the clinical setting, and due to iron deficiency, chronic disease or inflammation, renal and endocrine disease. Anemias from ineffective erythropoiesis result from maturation disorders, related to defective DNA synthesis as a result of vitamin deficiency (B_{12}, folate) and drugs. Anemias from ineffective erythropoiesis also result from sideroblastic anemias and abnormalities in globin synthesis such as thalassemias. Hemolytic anemia (red cell destruction) can occur in the elderly and results from collagen vascular disease,

Table 2 Anemia: classification. From references 3, 4, 10, 14

Physiologic

Hypoproliferative
   iron deficiency anemia
   anemia of chronic disease
   anemia of chronic inflammation
   thyroid disease
   nutritional

Ineffective erythropoiesis
   vitamin B_{12} deficiency
   folate deficiency
   myelodysplastic syndrome
   sideroblastic anemia

Blood loss*
   gastrointestinal
   genitourinary
   iatrogenic
   other

Hemolytic
   idiopathic
   drugs
   tumors
   metabolic
   mechanical

Morphologic

Microcytic anemia
   iron deficiency
   anemia of chronic disease
   Sideroblastic anemia

Normocytic anemia
   acute blood loss
   *anemia of chronic disease
      rheumatoid arthritis
      renal failure
      thyroid disorders
   sideroblastic anemia
   hemolytic anemia

Macrocytic anemia
   vitamin B_{12} deficiency
   folate deficiency
   hemolytic anemia
   sideroblastic anemia

*The list of conditions is for illustration and not all-inclusive

chronic lymphocytic leukemia, infection (with disseminated intravascular coagulation) and the use of medications. While iron deficiency is the most common etiology of anemia in the community setting, anemia of chronic disease is more common in hospitalized patients[4]. Less common, but pertinent,

are multiple myeloma and myelodysplastic syndromes as the underlying basis for anemia in the older age group.

There is debate regarding the overlap of the terms 'anemia of chronic disease' and 'anemia of chronic inflammation'[4]. In any case, an effort should be made to determine the underlying etiology of anemia. The following reviews the common types of anemia seen in older adults; the reader is encouraged to also refer to several excellent reviews for more detailed information on this subject[3,4,10].

Approach to anemia

Clinical The usual clinical manifestations classically seen in the young may not be evident in the elderly. Presentations include loss of stamina, easy fatigability or depression and day-to-day complaints[2]. Diminished quality of life may be evident. Alternatively, the presentation may be manifestations of end-organ dysfunction, such as angina, worsening heart failure, syncope or falls (Table 3). The usual reflex tachycardia seen in younger individuals with severe anemia may not manifest in older subjects. A small improvement in hemoglobin concentration nevertheless may provide dramatic symptomatic improvement.

History and physical examination should include a review of past medical problems (e.g. gastrointestinal bleed, malignancy, number of pregnancies, gynecologic blood loss), review of medications (prescribed and over-the-counter), nutritional intake and preferences (e.g. vegetarianism), lifestyle (e.g. alcoholism), alteration in bowel habits, anorexia and weight loss. The objective findings may substantiate features of the underlying etiology, e.g. rheumatoid arthritis, chronic liver disease or renal disease. Further, certain findings are characteristic of some anemias. Subacute combined degeneration, peripheral neuropathy or neuropsychiatric manifestations are classic for vitamin B_{12} deficiency. An aortic stenosis murmur may be associated with arteriovenous malformations and blood

Table 3 Approach to anemia

Clinical manifestations
Fatigue, weakness, pallor
Diminished quality of life
Manifestations of end-organ dysfunction
   cognitive decline, delirium
   congestive heart failure, angina
   pulmonary decompensation
   syncope
   falls

Evaluation
History and physical examination
   focused medical history, review of medications,
      dietary habits
   findings suggestive of arthritis, liver disease,
      malignancy, etc.
Laboratory tests
   routine
      complete blood count with peripheral smear
      stool for occult blood
      ferrokinetics, serum B_{12} and folic acid assays
      creatinine, blood urea nitrogen
   ancillary tests
      total protein and albumin
      reticulocyte count, indirect bilirubin, lactic
         dehydrogenase
      haptoglobin, Coombs' test
      thyroid function
      antinuclear antibody, rheumatoid factor,
         complement
      endoscopy
      serum and urine protein electrophoresis,
         erythrocyte sedimentation rate
      methylmalonic acid, homocysteine, intrinsic
         factor antibodies
      bone marrow evaluation including Prussian
         blue stain

loss in the gastrointestinal tract, while microangiopathic hemolytic anemia may result from an artificial (metallic) heart valve.

Diagnosis   The initial approach should include a complete blood count, to provide information on the severity of anemia and red cell indices, along with a review of the peripheral blood smear to delineate the morphology and associated findings involving the white cell and platelet counts. An absolute reticulocyte count may be computed to determine the functional capacity of the bone marrow (normal: 1–2%). In addition to a focused history and physical evaluation,

further tests may be requested to delineate an etiology (see Table 3).

Specific anemias in the elderly

Iron deficiency anemia   Dietary iron occurs in two forms: heme and non-heme. Heme iron is from hemoglobin and myoglobin of animal foods, while non-heme iron is found in cereals, fruits, vegetables and dairy products[15]. Dietary iron usually exists as ferric salts that form insoluble complexes at physiologic pH. Gastric acidity maintains iron in a soluble (ferrous) form. Iron in the ferrous form is absorbed mainly in the duodenum and upper jejunum. Under normal conditions, approximately 10% of the 10–20 mg dietary iron intake is absorbed; in the presence of augmented demand for iron in states of iron deficiency, absorption is increased. Dietary compounds that chelate iron, e.g. tannins found in tea, plant phytates, milk/soy proteins and phosphates, affect iron absorption. Zinc and antacids commonly used by the elderly interfere with iron absorption[16,17]. Rich sources of iron include green vegetables, legumes, beef and eggs, while milk products are poor sources.

Transferrin is the protein that transports iron to the tissues throughout the body, normal transferrin saturation being 20–45%. Iron absorption and loss are well balanced in physiologic states, with any loss pathologic. Iron storage occurs in two forms: ferritin (rapid exchanging pool) and hemosiderin (slow exchanging pool). Normal hemoglobin iron level is approximately 1 g and storage iron about 1 g[16].

An imbalance between intake, utilization and loss results in iron deficiency[17]. In the elderly, iron deficiency is overwhelmingly a result of blood loss, most often from the gastrointestinal tract. Commonly used medications, particularly non-steroidal anti-inflammatory agents and aspirin (prescribed and over-the-counter), predispose to painless gastrointestinal blood loss. Peptic ulcer disease, esophagitis, diverticulosis, angiodysplasia, polyps, arteriovenous malformations and hemorrhoids are other causes. Malignancies of the gastrointestinal tract, less frequent, should be excluded in the presence of iron deficiency anemia, particularly associated with guaiac-positive stools[3-5]. Less common sources of blood loss may be genitourinary, pulmonary or bleeding disorders[18]. In the hospitalized elderly, frequent blood tests are a contributory factor.

Iron deficiency is determined by ferrokinetics. Serum iron (SI) is the iron bound to transferrin (50–150 µg/dl) while total iron binding capacity (TIBC) is the total binding capacity of transferrrin. Transferrin saturation is calculated by using the formula: (SI/TIBC) × 100. Normal values are 25–45%, less than 20% suggesting iron deficiency. Normal ferritin values are 50–150 µg/l; below 18 µg/l is diagnostic of iron deficiency, while less than 50 µg/l is suggestive[4]. As ferritin is an acute phase reactant, its diagnostic utility is limited. In the presence of inflammation, infection, or malignancy, values may be falsely elevated. In normal individuals, ferritin correlates well with body iron stores. If ferritin assays are non-diagnostic, bone marrow evaluation can assess iron stores using Prussian blue stain. Further, this can differentiate iron deficiency anemia from sideroblastic anemia[19].

Iron replacement therapy in the elderly is limited by gastrointestinal side-effects (nausea, vomiting, taste disturbances, constipation and diarrhea). Gastric sensitivity may result in poor tolerance and low compliance. Rather than the usual replacement of 325 mg thrice daily, one tablet daily taken regularly may result in correction. The dose may be gradually titrated upwards if tolerated[5,20]. Slow-release and enteric-coated preparations are more expensive and not necessarily better absorbed[4].

For those unable to tolerate oral iron or with non-compliance, parenteral therapy is an alternative with one of several preparations: iron dextran, iron sucrose and ferric gluconate. Side-effects of parenteral iron include anaphylaxis, hypotension, myalgias, fever and urticaria. Blood transfusions are an option, especially with acute blood loss and compromised organ function, and should be used with caution in those with cardiac dysfunction to avoid precipitation of heart failure.

Anemia of chronic disease Anemia of chronic disease is common in older adults, particularly in association with malignancy, rheumatoid arthritis, renal failure, liver disease, thyroid disease and chronic systemic infections (tuberculosis, osteomyelitis, endocarditis, etc.)[10,21]. The underlying mechanisms may relate to decreased red cell life span, inappropriate marrow response, limited EPO production and impaired mobilization of iron from the reticuloendothelial system mediated by cytokines[7,8,22].

When hemoglobin values are lower than 8 g/dl, concomitant blood loss or other causes have to be excluded[21]. Red cells in anemia of chronic disease are usually normocytic and normochromic, but they can be microcytic[10,21]; iron deficiency can coexist[10,21]. Serum iron and TIBC are subnormal despite normal iron storage. Ferritin values may be normal or elevated as an acute phase reactant. Soluble transferrin receptor assay may differentiate anemia of chronic disease from iron deficiency, being normal in the former[10,23].

In patients with chronic renal failure, the etiology of anemia is multifactorial. While decreased EPO production is the predominant basis, coexisting iron deficiency, decreased red cell production, shortened red cell survival, hemolysis and blood loss may play additional roles[24]. Measurement of ferritin levels helps assess adequacy of iron stores and response to EPO therapy. Further iron depletion can result from the use of EPO and may account for a suboptimal response. Anemia in renal failure may be responsible for several manifestations related to other organ dysfunction.

Table 4 Erythropoietin

Properties
165-amino-acid glycoprotein
Molecular weight: 30 400 Da
Over 90% produced by the kidneys, small
    amounts by the liver and brain
Growth factor for red cell precursors
Most potent stimulus: hypoxia
Inhibited by cytokines

Benefits shown in:
Anemia due to renal insufficiency and failure
Cancer-related anemia
Anemia of rheumatoid arthritis
Perioperative anemia
Anemia of HIV infection
Anemia in the intensive care unit setting

Preparations
Recombinant human erythropoietin (rHuEPO)
    (Procrit®, Epogen®)
Darbepoetin-α (Aranesp®)

Dosage
rHuEPO: 50–100 U/kg thrice weekly parenterally
Darbepoetin-α: 0.45 μg/kg weekly parenterally
Titrate dose based on hemoglobin/hematocrit

Side-effects
Exacerbation of hypertension
Headache, arthralgia

Treatment of anemia of chronic disease is directed at the underlying etiology. Anemia due to chronic renal insufficiency or failure demonstrates a satisfactory response to recombinant human erythropoietin (rHuEPO) with improvement in hematocrit, organ function and, above all, the quality of life[25,26]. The gene for EPO was cloned in 1985. rHuEPO is immunogenetically and biologically indistinguishable from endogenous EPO (Table 4). Therapy with rHuEPO is initiated when the hematocrit is around 30% or less, with the target hematocrit 33–36% (hemoglobin level 11–12 g/dl) (National Kidney Foundation's Kidney Disease Outcomes Quality Initiative Guidelines). While dosages of rHuEPO vary, treatment is begun with 50–100 U/kg thrice a week parenterally. Larger doses can be administered once weekly; in the presence of inflammation, particularly in the intensive care unit setting, pharmacologic doses have been required to elicit a response. Studies have demonstrated the response of rHuEPO in other situations as well; these include anemia associated with HIV infection, cancer, rheumatoid arthritis and the perioperative setting.

Recombinant EPO is marketed as Epogen® for end-stage renal disease requiring dialysis and as Procrit® for all other indications. Further, a novel erythropoiesis-stimulating protein, darbepoetin-α (Aranesp®) is now available; it has a longer half-life and can be administered weekly or every other week in a dosage of 0.45 μg/kg parenterally[27]. Lack of response to recombinant EPO in renal failure along with the development of unexplained anemia have been described. This is due to pure red cell aplasia on the emergence of neutralizing antierythropoietin antibodies[28].

Megaloblastic anemia   Megaloblastic anemia results from defective DNA synthesis with compromised cell division but normal cytoplasmic development, with the large cells prone to destruction in the bone marrow (ineffective erythropoiesis). Folic acid and vitamin B_{12} (cobalamin) deficiencies are the common causes.

(1) *Vitamin B_{12} deficiency*   The prevalence of vitamin B_{12} deficiency is 3–40% in older adults with megaloblastic anemia and macro-ovalocytosis the characteristic findings. Hematologic manifestations (anemia, leukopenia, thrombocytopenia and pancytopenia) may be absent, or be coexistent with or present independent of neuropsychiatric manifestations. Although the body cobalamin stores are around 5 mg and the recommended dietary allowance is only 2.4 μg/day, a defect anywhere in the complex absorption pathway of cobalamin accounts for the development of deficiency[29–31]. A detailed discussion on vitamin B_{12} deficiency appears in Chapter 55.

(2) *Folic acid deficiency*   Folates are present in most natural foods, but are vulnerable to oxidation with protracted cooking, decreasing the content by 50–90%. Dietary folate is absorbed in the entire length of the small intestine, mainly the proximal jejunum. Folic acid is converted to the reduced form in the gut lumen and methylated or formylated[32]. Methyltetrahydrofolate, which comprises most of the serum folate, is the form efficiently absorbed across the intestine and transferred to the bone marrow, reticulocytes and liver. Total body folate content ranges from 5 to 10 mg, with 50% found in the liver. The WHO recommended daily allowance for adults is 3.1 µg/kg body weight, i.e. about 0.2 mg/day. Increased metabolic demand (e.g. infection, hyperthyroidism) or increased cell turnover (e.g. hemolysis, rapid tissue growth, malignancy) warrants higher intake. Folate deficiency results from insufficient ingestion, absorption and utilization or increased requirement, excretion and destruction[32].

As with cobalamin deficiency, hematologic manifestations result from defective DNA synthesis. Ineffective erythropoiesis occurs due to destruction of the cells in the bone marrow. A megaloblastic bone marrow may be associated with peripheral blood anemia, leukopenia, hypersegmentation and thrombocytopenia[32]. Besides, the defective DNA synthesis due to folate and B_{12} deficiencies augments the risk of cancer development[32].

Anemia need not be present to have sequelae of B_{12} deficiency. In particular, diagnosing cobalamin deficiency can be difficult, because serum levels do not always correlate with tissue status; low normal levels have even been associated with neurological disease[33–36]. Screening for vitamin B_{12} is recommended in older adults, especially in those at risk (see Chapter 55)[34–36]. While evaluation of serum folate level is usually adequate, tissue content is better estimated by red blood cell folate level[37]. Further testing to elucidate the etiology of either deficiency (e.g. malabsorption, role of medications, gastric or intestinal resection) may be indicated.

Treatment for vitamin B_{12} deficiency must be initiated for deficient individuals; it is discussed in Chapter 55. Replacement may be parenteral, oral, intranasal or sublingual[29,36,38,39]. As for folic acid deficiency, oral therapy is instituted with 1 mg daily for 4–6 months[4]. Therapy may be discontinued if the diet contains at least one fresh fruit or fresh vegetable daily, along with avoidance of alcohol[4,32]. Correction of anemia with folic acid alone in those with concomitant B_{12} deficiency may result in worsening of the neurologic manifestations[32,39].

Sideroblastic anemia   The condition may be sex linked or acquired; the former is common in the young while acquired sideroblastic anemia is a disorder of the older age group[3,40]. Ringed sideroblasts (mitochondrial iron inclusions within normoblasts) when present in at least 15% of marrow erythroid precursors suggest the diagnosis[41]. Serum iron, transferrin saturation and ferritin levels are elevated[4]. The condition results from defective heme synthesis from inherent marrow lesions, inflammation, neoplasia, alcohol, toxins (lead) and medications (isoniazid, phenytoin)[4,40]. Chromosomal pattern testing is recommended for older adults, as some are in transition into myelodysplasia[41]. Pyridoxine, 100–200 mg thrice daily, is effective in the hereditary group, while only a few of the elderly respond.

Miscellaneous causes   Hemolytic anemia should be excluded in high-risk individuals[3]. The presence of elevated reticulocyte count, lactate dehydrogenase and indirect bilirubin with a lower haptoglobin suggests destruction of red cells. Causes are outlined in Table 2. Medication review may delineate a basis. The

Coombs' test is positive in autoimmune hemolytic anemia[3].

Myelodysplastic syndrome, a preleukemic condition, is characterized by disorganized hematopoiesis[3,14,40,41] and is a cause of anemia, with median age of occurrence between 70 and 80 years[14]. Chronic lymphocytic leukemia (CLL) and multiple myeloma are causes of anemia in older adults, often deserving consideration as etiology[14,42] (see Chapter 45), especially when no other basis is apparent.

Erythrocytosis

Erythrocytosis is a condition characterized by increased red cell mass (25% higher than the normal predicted value for an individual) or packed cell volume that is greater than 0.51 for males and 0.48 for females[43,44]. The condition is not uncommon in older adults and is classified as primary (congenital or acquired), secondary (congenital or acquired) and idiopathic[44]. Polycythemia vera is an example of primary erythrocytosis which results from a clonal proliferation of primitive precursor cells with peak age of onset at 65 years. Differentiating primary from secondary erythrocytosis is important, as treatment differs. Secondary erythrocytosis may be due to: generalized or localized renal hypoxia with increased production of EPO (e.g. chronic obstructive lung disease (COPD) or hydronephrosis); a malignant process, e.g. hypernephroma, hepatoma and cerebellar hemangioblastomas[44]. Measurement of arterial oxygen saturation may support the presence of compensatory erythrocytosis from secondary causes. Other tests to delineate a secondary etiology will help. Low EPO levels suggest polycythemia vera, while levels are elevated in secondary causes. In view of the increased risk with hyperviscosity, cautious phlebotomy may be performed in those with hematocrit values greater than 55%[42].

Table 5   Causes of neutrophilia

Primary
Chronic idiopathic neutrophilia
Chronic myeloid leukemia and other
   myeloproliferative diseases
Down syndrome

Secondary
Asplenia and hyposplenism
Drug-induced
Generalized marrow stimulation (as in hemolysis)
Heatstroke
Infection
Myocardial infarction
Non-hematologic malignancy
Stress neutrophilia

WHITE CELL DISORDERS

Introduction and definitions

Leukocytosis is elevation of the white blood cell (WBC) count > 2 SD above the mean of one or more subsets of circulating WBCs. The usual explanation for leukocytosis is neutrophilia, which is calculated by multiplying the percentage of neutrophilic granulocytes by the total WBC count. The mean adult total leukocyte count is 7500/mm^3 (4500–11 000) and the mean neutrophil count is 4400/mm^3 (1800–7700).

The usual explanation of leukopenia is neutropenia, which is defined as a neutrophilic granulocyte count of < 1500/mm^3 [45]. This definition can be used for all ages and races except for certain populations of Blacks and Yemenite Jews, who normally have lower granulocyte counts. The absolute neutrophil count is calculated by multiplying the total WBC count by the percentage of bands and mature neutrophils.

Neutrophils are the principal phagocytes in the circulation and thus are key effector cells in host defenses against pathogenic bacteria and fungi. The peripheral neutrophil count reflects an equilibrium between the marrow pool, the circulating pool and the tissue pool. The largest pool of neutrophils exists in the bone marrow, a smaller number circulate in the peripheral blood and a similar number is present in the tissues.

Neutrophilia

The major causes of neutrophilia in the elderly are outlined in Table 5. Rapidly developing neutrophilias may be secondary to acute shifts from the marginated pool to the circulating pool caused by exercise, epinephrine, β-agonists, hypoxia as well as stress analogs of vigorous exercise such as convulsions (postictal state) and severe vomiting. Rapid egress from the marrow to the circulating pool can be caused by the administration of corticosteroids, endotoxins (sepsis) and chemical intoxicants.

Neutrophilia characterized by a large number of immature forms (myelocyte, metamyelocyte and bands) or 'left shift' is seen commonly with acute bacterial infections, especially those caused by pneumococcus or *Staphylococcus*. Specific conditions which may be associated with elevated numbers of mature neutrophils include various carcinomas (gastric, breast, lung, adrenal, Hodgkin's disease), acute alcoholic hepatitis, active rheumatoid arthritis and acute glomerulonephritis. Leukocytosis exceeding 50 000/mm^3 with a significant increase in neutrophil precursors is referred to as a leukemoid reaction. Leukemoid reactions to infections may be accompanied by toxic granulation, Döhle bodies and cytoplasmic vacuoles in the neutrophils. It is important to distinguish this from chronic myeloid leukemia (CML), which is a myeloproliferative disorder of the stem cell in which more than one cell line may be elevated (panmyelosis). There may be accompanying hepatomegaly or splenomegaly. CML can be distinguished from the leukemoid reaction by a low leukocyte alkaline phosphatase score. The presence of the Philadelphia chromosome (t (9; 22) (q34; q11)) on karyotype analysis of the bone marrow in CML further differentiates these two entities[46].

Table 6 Causes of neutropenia

Acquired
Autoimmune neutropenia
Benign familial neutropenia
Chronic idiopathic neutropenia
Drug-induced neutropenia
Neutropenia associated with metabolic diseases
Neutropenia due to increased margination
Neutropenia due to nutritional deficiency
Post-infectious neutropenia

Intrinsic
Neutropenia usually present in infancy and childhood

When the marrow is invaded by tumor cells, granulomas or fibrosis, the peripheral smear shows neutrophilia associated with immature forms, nucleated red cells, teardrop cells and often thrombocytopenia. This is called a leukoerythroblastic response; a bone marrow biopsy and marrow cultures help make the diagnosis.

Neutropenia

Common causes of neutropenia in the geriatric population are listed in Table 6. Like neutrophilia, neutropenia may be caused by shifts from the circulating to the marginated pool, as seen early during Gram-negative sepsis (effects of endotoxin and complement activation). Other causes of neutropenia in this age group are primary marrow disease as in myelodysplastic syndrome and leukemias, marrow infiltration by infection or metastasis, drugs and autoimmunity secondary to low-grade lymphoproliferative disorders. Severe neutropenia (0–500/μl) is associated with a demonstrable increase in risk of infections. If the patient is febrile, aggressive evaluation and prompt institution of broad-spectrum antibiotics is mandatory in order to prevent overwhelming sepsis[47].

Myelodysplastic syndrome is a clonal disorder of hematopoietic progenitor cells. The affected cells are unable to mature normally and also reduce the capacity of normal progenitors to differentiate. It occurs predominantly in the elderly, with > 80% of patients being over 60 years of age. The best documented etiologic factor is alkylating agent therapy for previous malignancies. Secondary myelodysplastic syndrome occurs 5–10 years after initial exposure to alkylating agents and is typically accompanied by cytogenetic abnormalities. In particular, these include loss of chromosomes 5 and/or 7 (–5, –7) or parts of their long arms (5q–, 7q–). Compared to the young, older patients have these cytogenetic abnormalities even if they present with *de novo* myelodysplastic syndrome. It has been proposed that these anomalies result from a long undocumented exposure to toxins[48].

Patients with myelodysplastic syndrome typically present with symptoms of refractory anemia or pancytopenia depending on disease severity. Blood and bone marrow studies reveal morphologic abnormalities in all three lineages. Dyserythropoiesis, including ringed sideroblasts, anisocytosis, poikilocytosis, bizarre nuclear shapes, dense chromatin and megaloblastoid precursors is seen in addition to white cell abnormalities such as hypolobulated (Pelger–Huët-like anomaly) and hypogranulated granulocytes. Morphologic abnormalities of platelets include giant platelets, micromegakaryocytes, mononuclear megakaryocytes and hypogranulation. A variable number of blasts may be present ranging from < 5% to > 30%. The transformation of myelodysplastic syndrome to acute leukemia occurs in patients with poor prognostic factors. Despite various therapeutic interventions, the outcome for this subset of patients is dismal.

Acute leukemias can be divided into two subtypes: acute myeloid leukemia (AML) and acute lymphocytic leukemia (ALL). AML is a disease of hematopoietic progenitor cells that reduces the ability of affected cells to differentiate morphologically and functionally into mature cells. This clonal proliferation eventually inhibits the production and differentiation of cells in the normal hematopoietic compartments. AML affects non-lymphoid marrow-derived lineages (granulocyte, monocyte, erythroid and megakaryocytic lineages), whereas ALL affects the lymphoid progenitor cell. AML accounts for 90% of all acute leukemias in adults. Age-specific incidence rises linearly after age 40 years and the median age is 62–65 years. Genetic predisposition, drug (alkylating agents), environmental (ionizing radiation) and occupational (benzene) factors have been implicated as possible leukemogenic agents[49].

The clinical manifestations primarily reflect bone marrow failure. Patients present with fatigue, infections and bleeding secondary to anemia, neutropenia and thrombocytopenia, respectively. In the elderly, AML typically presents with new cardiac symptoms or exacerbation of previous cardiac disease[50]. Fever may be a manifestation without an identifiable source of infection; in such cases, as most of the patients are neutropenic, it is imperative to begin broad-spectrum antibiotics at the earliest opportunity[50]. Tissue invasion (gum, skin, perianal, renal and most ominously lung and/or brain) occurs with a high blast count and monocytic component. The presence of disseminated intravascular coagulation is commonly seen in acute promyelocytic leukemia (APL). The diagnosis of acute leukemia is made by blood and bone marrow studies which reflect pancytopenia and the presence of circulating blasts. Immunophenotyping and cytogenetics help characterize the subsets and provide prognostic information, with combination chemotherapy being the standard of care. Therapy for APL is distinct and consists of all-*trans* retinoic acid (ATRA), a differentiating agent, combined with an anthracycline.

Further, older adults often have a history of another hematological disorder that progresses to AML; this is often myelodysplastic syndrome[50]. Elderly individuals are also known to progress to AML following courses of chemotherapy they receive for a different malignant disorder[50].

Table 7   Causes of thrombocytopenia

Pseudo-thrombocytopenia
Giant platelets
In vitro platelet clumping caused by EDTA-dependent
    agglutinins

True thrombocytopenia
Autoimmune diseases (lymphoproliferative disorders,
    systemic lupus erythematosus)
Disseminated intravascular coagulation
Drug-induced (quinine, quinidine, heparin, thiazides,
    sulfonamides, chemotherapy, sedatives,
    anticonvulsants, aspirin, digitoxin, chlorpropamide,
    ethanol, chloroquine, gold salts, methyldopa)
Hemolytic–uremic syndrome
Hypersplenism due to chronic liver disease
Myelodysplasia
Thrombotic thrombocytopenic purpura
Viral infections (hepatitis, cytomegalovirus, varicella,
    mumps, parvovirus)

Lymphocytosis

CLL is the most common cause of lymphocytosis in the elderly patient. It is a lymphoproliferative disorder manifested by a clonal expansion of mature but functionally deficient lymphocytes. It constitutes 30% of all leukemias in the Western hemisphere and is predominantly of B-cell origin (95% of cases). In Asia, CLL constitutes 5% of all leukemias, and the majority of cases are of T-cell phenotype. It is more prevalent in males, with a sex ratio of 2 : 1. The median age is 60–65 years, the incidence rising steadily with age. It is not associated with exposure to radiation, chemicals and alkylating agents, but has a tendency for familial aggregation.

Approximately 40% of patients are asymptomatic and are diagnosed on routine blood tests. Symptomatic disease presents as fever, weight loss, adenopathy, hepatosplenomegaly, recurrent bacterial and viral infections, and manifestations of anemia and thrombocytopenia. The diagnosis is confirmed by the demonstration of absolute lymphocytosis in the blood (5×10^9/l) of mature lymphocytes sustained over at least a 4-week period, 30% of lymphocytes in the bone marrow, and presence of monoclonality and CD5 positivity by immunophenotyping[51].

Some patients have an indolent form of CLL, with survival comparable to that of the normal population of the same age. Therefore, not all patients with CLL require therapy. Treatment is needed for those with advanced disease, worsening constitutional symptoms, recurrent infections, progressive lymphadenopathy or hepatosplenomegaly, and those with autoimmune hemolytic anemia or autoimmune thrombocytopenia.

PLATELET DISORDERS

Thrombocytopenia

Common causes of thrombocytopenia in the elderly population are listed in Table 7. Drug-related thrombocytopenia is extremely common in this age group and is usually secondary to an immune mechanism or production deficit. Examples of drugs implicated in the suppression of platelet production are provided in Table 7. Ingestion of large quantities of alcohol has a similar marrow-depressing effect. Most drugs induce thrombocytopenia by eliciting an immune response in which the platelet is an innocent bystander. The platelet is damaged by complement activation following the formation of drug–antibody complexes. The majority of patients recover in 7–10 days after cessation of the drug. Heparin is a common cause of thrombocytopenia in hospitalized patients. It deserves special mention, as it can cause paradoxical thrombosis which can often be fatal. Prompt discontinuation of heparin will reverse both thrombocytopenia and heparin-induced thrombosis[52].

Production disorders are also observed secondary to marrow infiltrative processes (metastatic cancer, lymphoma and leukemia), radiation therapy, viruses (cytomegalovirus, varicella, parvovirus, hepatitis and mumps), ineffective erythropoiesis secondary to nutritional deficiencies (vitamin B_{12} and folate) and myelodysplasia. Blood and bone marrow studies are essential to determine the cause of thrombocytopenia.

Patients usually present with petechiae, purpura and mucocutaneous bleeding (epistaxis, gingival bleeding, gastrointestinal bleeding, menorrhagia). Older patients, however, are more likely to develop intracranial bleeds. The risk of spontaneous hemorrhage increases with platelet counts of $< 20\,000/\mu l$. Therapeutic interventions focus on both prevention and management of bleeding complications as well as treatment of the underlying cause.

Thrombocytosis

Thrombocytosis can be subdivided into primary thrombocythemia and thrombocytosis due to secondary causes. Primary thrombocythemia is a myeloproliferative disorder characterized by a sustained proliferation of megakaryocytes which leads to platelet counts in excess of $600\,000/\mu l$. This disorder affects people aged 50–60 years and has a clinical course punctuated by hemorrhagic or thrombotic episodes or both. Splenomegaly is common and patients can occasionally suffer from constitutional symptoms. The diagnosis is made with the help of a bone marrow biopsy; therapy consists of the administration of a platelet-lowering agent[53,54].

The causes of secondary or reactive thrombocytosis are numerous. They include acute or chronic infections, rheumatoid arthritis, ankylosing spondylitis, chronic inflammatory bowel disease, iron deficiency anemia, non-hematologic malignancies, sickle cell anemia and postoperative after splenectomy. A thorough history and physical examination helps make the diagnosis and distinguishes between primary and secondary thrombocytosis. Treatment of the specific underlying illness usually leads to normalization of the platelet count.

References

1. Ania BJ, Suman VJ, Fairbanks VF, *et al.* Incidence of anemia in older people: an epidemiologic study in a well defined population. *Am Geriatr Soc* 1997;45:825–31

2. Murphy PT, Hutchinson RM. Identification and treatment of anaemia in older patients. *Drugs Aging* 1994;4:113–27

3. Chatta GS, Lipschitz DA. Anemia. In Hazzard WR, Blass JP, Ettinger WH, *et al.*, eds. *Principles of Geriatric Medicine and Gerontology*, 4th edn. New York: McGraw Hill, 1999:899–906

4. Walsh JR. Hematologic problems. In Cassel CK, Cohen HJ, Larson EB, *et al.*, eds. *Geriatric Medicine*, 3rd edn. New York: Spring Verlag, 1997:627–36

5. Gautier M, Crawford J, Cohen HJ. Hematologic disorders. In Duthie EH Jr, Katz PR, eds. *Practice of Geriatrics*, 3rd edn. Philadelphia, PA: WB Saunders, 1998;397–409

6. Dessypris EN. Erythropoiesis. In Lee GR, Lukens J, Foerster J, *et al.*, eds. *Wintrobe's Clinical Hematology*, 10th edn. New York: Lippincott Williams and Wilkins, 1999:169–92

7. Krantz SB. Pathogenesis and treatment of anemia of chronic disease. *Am J Med Sci* 1994;307:353–9

8. Means RT Jr, Krantz SB. Progress in understanding the pathogenesis of anemia of chronic disease. *Blood* 1992;80:1639–49

9. Dharmarajan TS, Ugalino JT. The aging process. In Dreger D, Krumm B, eds. *Geriatric Medicine Board Review Manual*. Wayne, PA: Turner White Communications, 2000;1:1–12

10. Carmel R. Anemia and aging: an overview of clinical diagnostic and biological issues. *Blood Rev* 2001;15:9–18

11. Baraldi-Junkins CA, Beck AC, Rothstein G. Hematopoiesis and cytokines. Relevance to

cancer and aging. *Hematol Oncol Clin North Am* 2000;14:45–61

12. Chatta GS, Dale DC. Aging and haemopoiesis. Implications for treatment with haemopoietic growth factors. *Drugs Aging* 1996;9:37–47

13. Lee GR. Anemia: a diagnostic strategy. In Lee GR, Lukens J, Foerster J, *et al.*, eds. *Wintrobe's Clinical Hematology*, 10th edn. New York: Lippincott Williams and Wilkins, 1999:908–40

14. Ershler W. Hematologic diseases and disorders. In Cobbs EL, Duthie EH Jr, Murphy J, eds. *Geriatrics Review Syllabus*, 4th edn. Dubuque, IA: Kendall/Hunt Publishing, 1999:274–9

15. Chanarin I. Nutritional aspects of hematologic disorders. In Shils ME, Olson JA, Shike M, *et al. Modern Nutrition in Health and Disease*, 9th edn. Baltimore, MD: Williams and Wilkins, 1999:1419–37

16. Fairbanks VF. Iron in medicine and nutrition. In Shils ME, Olson JA, Shike M, *et al. Modern Nutrition in Health and Disease*, 9th edn. Baltimore, MD: Williams and Wilkins, 1999:193–221

17. Duffy TP. Microcytic and hypochromic anemias. In Goldman L, Bennett JC, eds. *Cecil Textbook of Medicine*, 21st edn. New York: WB Saunders, 2000:855–9

18. Smith DL. Anemia in the elderly. *Am Fam Physician* 2000;62:1565–72

19. Hillman RS. Iron deficiency and other hypoproliferative anemias. In Fauci AS, Braunwald E, Isselbacher KJ, *et al.*, eds. *Harrison's Principles of Internal Medicine*, 14th edn. New York: McGraw Hill, 1998:638–45

20. Fulcher RA, Hyland CM. Effectiveness of once daily iron in the elderly. *Age Ageing* 1981;10:44–6

21. Bunn F. Anemia associated with chronic disorders. In Fauci AS, Braunwald E, Isselbacher KJ, *et al.*, eds. *Harrison's Principles of Internal Medicine*, 14th edn. New York: McGraw Hill, 1998:1732–4

22. Means RT Jr. Clinical application of recombinant erythropoietin in the anemia of chronic disease. *Hematol Oncol Clin North Am* 1994;8:933–44

23. Fitzsimons EJ, Brock JH. The anemia of chronic disease remains hard to distinguish from iron deficiency anemia in some cases. *Br Med J* 2001;322:811–12

24. Fernandez-Rodriguez A, Guindeo-Casasus M, Molero-Labarta T, *et al.* Diagnosis of iron deficiency in chronic renal failure. *Am J Kidney Dis* 1999;34:508–13

25. Soignet S. Management of cancer related anemia: epoietin alfa and quality of life. *Semin Hematol* 2000;37:9–13

26. Ludwig H, Strasser K. Symptomatology of anemia. *Semin Oncol* 2001;28:7–14

27. Locatelli F, Olivares J, Walker R, *et al.* Novel erythropoiesis stimulating protein for treatment of anemia in chronic renal insufficiency. *Kidney Int* 2001;60:741–7

28. Casadevall N, Nataf J, Viron B, *et al.* Pure red cell aplasia and antierythropoietin antibodies in patients treated with recombinant erythropoietin. *N Engl J Med* 2002; 346:469–75

29. Dharmarajan TS, Norkus EP. Approaches to vitamin B_{12} deficiency: early treatment may prevent devastating complications. *Postgrad Med* 2001;110:99–106

30. Stabler SP, Lindenbaum J, Allen RH. Vitamin B_{12} deficiency in the elderly: current dilemmas. *Am J Clin Nutr* 1997;66: 741–9

31. Herbert V. Vitamin B_{12}: an overview. In Herbert V, ed. *Vitamin B_{12} Deficiency*. London: Royal Society of Medicine Press, 1999:1–8

32. Herbert V. Folic acid. In Shils ME, Olson JA, Shike M, *et al.*, eds. *Modern Nutrition in Health and Disease*, 9th edn. Baltimore, MD: Williams and Wilkins, 1999:433–46

33. Smith D. Management and treatment of anemia in the elderly. *Clin Geriatr* 2002; 10:47–54

34. Snow CF. Laboratory diagnosis of vitamin B_{12} and folate deficiency. *Arch Intern Med* 1999;159:1289–98

35. Stabler SP. Screening the older population for cobalamin (vitamin B_{12}) deficiency. *J Am Geriatr Soc* 1995;43:1290–7

36. Dharmarajan TS, Norkus EP. An algorithmic approach to the screening of vitamin B_{12} status and the treatment of identified

deficiency. In Herbert V, ed. *Vitamin B₁₂ Deficiency*. London: Royal Society of Medicine Press, 1999:49–52

37. Johnson L. Malnutrition. In Cobbs EL, Duthie EH Jr, Murphy JB, eds. *Geriatrics Review Syllabus*, 4th edn. Dubuque, IA: Kendall/Hunt Publishing, 1999:130–5

38. Seal EC, Metz J, Flicker L, *et al.* A randomized double-blind, placebo-controlled study of oral vitamin B₁₂ supplementation in older patients with subnormal or borderline serum B₁₂ concentrations. *J Am Geriatr Soc* 2002;50:146–51

39. Smith RL. Evaluation of vitamin B₁₂ and folate status in the nursing home. *J Am Med Dir Assoc* 2001;2:230–8

40. Mansouri A, Lipschitz D. Anemia in the elderly patient. *Med Clin North Am* 1992; 76:619–30

41. Gardner FH. Refractory anemia in the elderly. *Adv Intern Med* 1987;32:155–76

42. Rothstein G. White cell disorders. In Hazzard WR, Blass JP, Ettinger W, *et al.* eds. *Principles of Geriatric Medicine and Gerontology*, 4th edn. New York: McGraw Hill, 1999:907–18

43. Hall R, Malia RG. Basic haematological practice. In Hall R, Malia RG, eds. *Medical Laboratory Haematology*. Oxford: Butterworth Heinemann, 1991:84–112

44. Messinezy M, Pearson TC. The classification and diagnostic criteria of the erythrocytoses (polycythemias). *Clin Lab Haematol* 1999:21:309–16

45. Coates TD, Baehner R. Leukocytosis and leukopenia. In Hoffman R, Benz EJ, Shattil SJ, *et al.*, eds. *Hematology Basic Principles and Practice*, 2nd edn. New York: Churchill Livingston, 1995:769–84

46. Sawyers CL. Chronic myeloid leukemia. *N Engl J Med* 1999;340:1330–40

47. Pizzo PA. Fever in immunocompromised patients. *N Engl J Med* 1999;341:893–900

48. Heaney ML, Golde DW. Myelodysplasia. *N Engl J Med* 1999;340:1649–60

49. Levine EG, Bloomfield CD. Leukemias and myelodysplastic syndromes secondary to drug, radiation and environmental exposure. *Semin Oncol* 1992;19:47–84

50. Seiter K. Treatment of acute myelogenous leukemia in the elderly patient. *Clinical Geriatrics* 2002;10:41–46

51. Rozman C, Montserrat E. Current concepts; chronic lymphocytic leukemia. *N Engl J Med* 1995;333:1052

52. Chong BH. Heparin-induced thrombocytopenia. *Br J Haematol* 1995;89:431–9

53. Anagrelide Study Group. Anagrelide, a therapy for thrombocythemic states: experience in 577 patients. *Am J Med* 1992; 92:69–76

54. Cortellazzo S, Finazzi G, Ruggeri M, *et al.* Hydroxyurea for patients with essential thrombocythemia and a high-risk for thrombosis. *N Engl J Med* 1995;332: 1132–6

45 Oncologic disorders in older adults

Janice P. Dutcher, MD, and Peter H. Wiernik, MD

CANCER AND AGING

Cancer is a disease process of the aging population, with more than half of cancers arising in people over the age of 65 years, and with more than 70% of cancer deaths occurring in the older population (Tables 1 and 2)[1]. Age remains the greatest risk factor for developing cancer. Some researchers state that understanding aging will help us better understand cancer. Although life expectancy differs in different countries, overall it is lengthening; thus, cancer is and will become increasingly a major health problem among the aging population.

AGE RELATED CHANGES: PHYSIOLOGY, CARCINOGENESIS AND TUMOR DEVELOPMENT

The process of carcinogenesis is believed to derive from a number of insults that impair cellular integrity and function. This is the multi-step carcinogenesis model. The human body has numerous repair mechanisms, but with age, the number of molecular changes which are part of intermediate carcinogenic steps increases[2]. This process of carcinogenesis takes considerable time, so that the clinical manifestation of cancer is more likely to be observed in an older person. In this process, mutations occur which activate proto-oncogenes and which inactivate suppressor genes[3]. Studies have indicated that,

when older individuals and younger individuals are exposed to similar carcinogens, there is more likelihood of the development of cancer in the older individual[4]. The theory to explain this suggests that, with aging, the slowing of cellular proliferation also renders the cells more susceptible to environmental carcinogens[5]. In contrast, it has also been demonstrated that cells with less proliferative capacity are less likely to develop a malignant phenotype[6]. Nevertheless, in the process of cellular senescence, there is more resistance to apoptosis and thus more risk of mutations that lead to immortalization of abnormal cells[5].

In a variety of tumors, the most frequently observed mutations are in the genes for p53 and Rb (retinoblastoma) – genes that normally help eliminate cells with malignant potential. With these mutations, cells lose the normal tumor suppressor function and become unstable and are perhaps immortalized as malignant cells[5,7,8].

Another theory regarding the aging of tissues and the development of cancer describes the ability of aging cells to affect and disrupt the microenvironment. An example cited is the loss of organization of the dermis with aging, with an age-dependent decline in dermal matrix and collagen. Fibroblasts that are characterized by markers of aging cells can be readily identified[9]. These cells carry a greater concentration of enzymes

Table I Risk factors and cancer

Age (increased incidence in most cancers with aging population)
Senescence of cells
Impaired repair mechanisms
Chronic exposure to carcinogens

Genetic predisposition (usually develop cancer at much younger age)
Specific gene abnormalities
BRCA-1; BRCA-2
Familial adenomatous polyposis
Hereditary non-polyposis colorectal cancer
Neurofibromatosis
Multiple endocrine neoplasia
Retinoblastoma
Von Hippel–Lindau disease

Exposure to carcinogens
Hormonal exposure or chronic hormonal enviroment – breast cancer, endometrial cancer, ovarian cancer,
   prostate cancer
High-fat diet – colorectal cancer
Low-selenium diet – adenocarcinoma of esophagus, cardia of stomach
Occupational exposures – asbestos – mesothelioma; vinyl chloride – angiosarcoma of liver; aniline
   dyes – bladder cancer; radium – watch dial painters – osteosarcoma of the jaw
Cigarette smoke – lung, head and neck, pancreas, bladder, kidney cancers, acute myeloid leukemia

Exposure to radiation
Ionizing radiation – leukemia, thyroid cancer, solid tumors following radiation for Hodgkin's disease; thymus
Ultraviolet radiation – cutaneous damage and cancers
Radon – lung cancer

Viruses
HTLV-1 – lymphoma
Epstein–Barr virus – Burkitt's lymphoma; AIDS-related lymphoma; nasopharyngeal carcinoma; cardiac
   transplant lymphoproliferative disorder
Herpes virus 8 – myeloma; Kaposi's sarcoma
Papillomavirus – cervical cancer; some types of head and neck cancer
Hepatitis virus – hepatoma

with the ability to degrade the extracellular matrix and release cytokines. Could this lead to greater susceptibility for skin cancers that are more prominent among the sun-exposed elderly? It is very possible.

Additionally, older cells generate substances that function as growth factors and preferentially stimulate cells that carry amplified oncogenes. Oncogenes such as erb B2 are over-expressed and functional in many breast cancer cells and are expressed in a number of other tumors[5].

Thus, events related to aging may also provide a predisposition for the development of malignancy. One recent, interesting study in transformed mice showed that, when the p53 gene was mutated and further altered, but with limited remaining p53 gene activity, the mice no longer developed cancer, but they prematurely aged![10]

CLINICAL BEHAVIOR OF CANCER IN THE ELDERLY

Malignant diseases which occur in both younger and older patients, although similar in presentation, may in fact behave differently in the two populations. This may reflect inherent differences in the malignancy in the younger and older populations as well as differences in the host's ability to confront the disease and its treatment.

Table 2   Reported deaths from five leading cancer sites by gender and age – USA, 1999

	All ages	40–59 years	60–79 years	> 80 years
Males				
Lung	89 401	15 457	57 263	16 242
Prostate	31 729	not in top 5	15 158	15 523
Colorectal	28 313	4 615	15 470	7 823
Pancreas	14 176	2 948	8 145	not in top 5
Non-Hodgkin's lymphoma	11 794	2 268	6 224	not in top 5
Leukemia				3 005
Females				
Lung	62 662	10 182	38 260	13 786
Breast	41 144	11 525	17 773	10 415
Colorectal	28 909	3 571	12 940	12 044
Pancreas	14 906	1 860	7 747	5 202
Ovary	13 627	2 964	7 100	not in top 5
Lymphoma				3 983

From US mortality public use data, 1999; and Center for Disease Control, 2001

An example of a biological difference that is age-related is apparent in acute leukemia. In acute myeloid leukemia (AML), specific chromosomal (cytogenetic) abnormalities are the most important prognostic factors associated with outcome, including remission duration and survival. The three cytogenetic alterations with better prognosis are almost exclusively seen in younger patients, less than age 40 years. These are translocations of chromosomes t(15;17) or t(8;21) and inversion of chromosome 16[11,12]. In contrast, the older population of patients who develop AML are much more likely to evolve the disease from a pre-existing hematologic disorder such as refractory anemia, suggesting prior marrow damage. When these leukemias in older patients are associated with chromosomal changes with a poor prognosis such as deletions of chromosomes 5 or 7 and/or a multitude of less specific abnormalities, they are much more difficult to treat and are associated with a poorer outcome[11,12]. These types of cytogenetic abnormalities are believed to reflect marrow damage from exposures leading to multiple chromosomal insults. The frequent occurrence of the pre-existing hematologic disorder again speaks for the process evolving over a considerable period of time.

Similarly, in acute lymphocytic leukemia (ALL), a disease primarily of younger individuals, a small subset of young patients have a specific chromosomal translocation, t(9;22), the Philadelphia chromosome, which confers a poor prognosis[12,13]. However, this cytogenetic abnormality is far more frequently observed among older adults who develop ALL.

On the other hand, those older patients who develop a leukemia without a poor prognostic chromosomal pattern have a similar disease-related prognosis as does a younger patient with the same chromosomal pattern. Their outcome then becomes a function of the co-morbid medical conditions, rather than being determined by the biology of the disease.

An example of a solid tumor with a different biology in younger and older populations is breast cancer. Whereas the median age at development of breast cancer is in the mid-fifties, the spectrum in age runs from the late twenties to the end of life[14]. Breast cancer in premenopausal women is, in general, an aggressive disease, and is associated with the absence of receptors for estrogen or progesterone. Hormonal therapy is not an option and these patients are treated with chemotherapy. These cancers are often associated with over-expression of an oncogene-defined growth factor receptor, HER-2/neu, which is also associated with aggressive biology[14]. In contrast, breast cancer that develops in postmenopausal women tends to be less aggressive, and the aggressiveness declines with the age of the patient[14]. Elderly patients with breast cancer almost always demonstrate receptors for estrogen and progesterone on the tumor and thus can be managed with hormonal therapy (antiestrogens and aromatase inhibitors). There is continued debate regarding the value of chemotherapy in the post-surgical management of women with breast cancer who are over the age of 65 years[15]. Studies in general show benefit from adjuvant chemotherapy in most postmenopausal women, but the discussion surrounds both the degree of benefit in a given age group, and the intensity of treatment required[16,17]. This approach is the subject of a major inter-group clinical trial being conducted in the USA.

Other solid tumors are more likely to occur as people age, particularly those related to cigarette smoking and other carcinogen exposures (Tables 1 and 2). Differences in clinical behavior between younger and older populations are not so well-defined in many of these.

CANCER SCREENING IN THE ELDERLY

The evaluation of a possible diagnosis of a malignancy is part of the general health evaluation of any individual. Elderly patients who maintain medical care are equally as likely to have a diagnosis of early cancer as is a younger patient, provided that the same criteria for medical evaluation are utilized. The diagnosis should be sought in the healthy older person, and once made, a series of evaluations are conducted. The positive predictive value is likely to be higher in older persons, given the increasing risk of cancer observed with increasing age. Once a diagnosis is made, part of the assessment and advice given is related to the functional status and life expectancy of the given individual.

Nevertheless, cancer screening in the elderly continues to be an area of controversy. The cost-effectiveness is likely to be dependent upon both age and functional level. However, if a healthy older person with an otherwise reasonable life expectancy is diagnosed with an early, surgically resectable cancer, the mortality of elective surgery does not greatly increase with age[18–20]. Colorectal cancer, for example, is a disease primarily of older patients, and when detected late, creates significant morbidity and mortality. Older patients are more likely to have proximal (right colonic) tumors and thus to present with bleeding. Fecal occult blood testing is a reasonable screening approach to detect earlier tumors in older patients. Surgery in an earlier stage of colorectal cancer has a similar morbidity and mortality to those in younger patients[19,20].

On the other hand, given that most women do not die of breast cancer, no study has been able to determine that mammography decreases breast cancer mortality in women aged 70 years or older[21,22]. Similarly, no survival benefit has been shown for colorectal cancer screening in persons over the age of 80 years[21].

Current recommendations suggest that it is reasonable to screen for breast and colorectal cancer in subjects with a life expectancy of 3 years or more[18–20]. Early detection will identify early tumors that can be treated with much less morbidity than would occur with detection of advanced disease. Balducci and colleagues recommend that, in older persons with a life expectancy of 3 or more years, examination of the stool for fecal occult blood annually is sufficient and effective. In older women with life expectancy of 3 or more years and with average risk for breast cancer, good medical practice includes annual breast examination and mammography every 2 years[18,22,23].

Screening recommendations for gynecologic malignancies are consistent whether in the younger or elderly population. For vulvar cancer, physical examination is the best method of evaluation to identify early disease. Vulvar cancer dramatically increases in incidence above age 60, and thus complete physical examination, including genitalia, remains important in the older population. If lesions are noted, a high index of suspicion and early biopsy will improve outcome[24]. Endometrial cancer is also a disease of postmenopausal women. The key to early detection of surgically curable disease is to impress on postmenopausal women the need to report the onset of new vaginal bleeding[23,25]. Cervical cancer screening has been demonstrated to save lives. Regular Pap smears must be strongly recommended to all postmenopausal women. There is no upper age limit in the American Cancer Society guidelines, but the frequency recommended differs among various medical societies[23]. Current American Cancer Society and Gynecologic Society recommendations are once every 3 years if there are three prior normal examinations. However, the American College of Physicians suggests a reduced frequency of cervical screening in women over age 65 years if there have been two negative Pap smears in recent years. Cervical screening becomes more difficult clinically in the very elderly, but should still be encouraged in appropriate patients. Ovarian cancer is the most lethal of the gynecologic malignancies, and thus early detection is desirable. Unfortunately, no new approach has yet improved on the pelvic examination when screening the general population. In high-risk populations, such as those with genetic mutations (BRCA-1 and BRCA-2), studies are evaluating the potential benefit of serial serum CA-125 levels and periodic transvaginal ultrasonography. The latter have not been additionally helpful in the general population[26].

Screening for early detection of lung cancer among those with a smoking history or significant exposure to secondhand smoke remains problematic. Initial studies evaluating serial chest radiographs and sputum cytology were disappointing in terms of detecting early, surgically curable lung cancers. Recently, the development of low-radiation, helical computerized tomography (CT) scans has been applied to screening for lung cancer. Several studies have demonstrated the ability to detect very early lung cancers, with potential for surgical cure[27,28]. However, there are many false-positive findings requiring subsequent serial scans. A large multicenter trial is ongoing to evaluate the positive yield of this approach in subjects with a 10-pack-year smoking history and over the age of 60 years. The American Cancer Society acknowledges the popularity of this approach, and recommends that physicians and patients clearly understand the limitations and potential pitfalls[23].

Early detection of prostate cancer has many issues, including a limited understanding of the actual aggressiveness or lack thereof of an individual cancer. The biology of prostate cancer continues to be a major area of clinical research. In attempting to provide guidelines, the American Cancer Society and the American Urologic Association recommend that men of average risk begin to be screened at age 50 years, as well as men with at least a 10-year life expectancy[23]. Screening consists of an annual blood test for prostate-specific antigen (PSA) and an annual digital rectal examination of the prostate gland. However, the American College of Physicians does not recommend aggressive screening in older men, and the entire screening approach remains highly controversial.

CANCER PREVENTION IN THE ELDERLY

Current cancer prevention strategies in general oncology include smoking cessation and chemoprevention of breast cancer. A series of large clinical trials of dietary supplements is ongoing. The best data exist for smoking cessation and breast cancer chemoprevention. The latter is of particular interest, since the median age of onset of breast cancer is in the mid-fifties and increases with age. Thus, older women may be candidates for anti-estrogen therapy. Two agents, tamoxifen and raloxifen, are being studied in an ongoing clinical trial of breast cancer prevention. The initial trial results with tamoxifen versus placebo were strongly in favor of a treatment effect in reducing breast cancer incidence by 40%[29]. However, the older the patient, the greater the risk of toxicity from tamoxifen. Raloxifen is currently approved for prevention of osteoporosis in older women, and appears also to have benefit in preventing breast cancer. It is hoped that it will have less toxicity than tamoxifen in this population.

Balducci and co-workers outlined a series of criteria for inclusion of older women in breast cancer prevention programs[18,22]. The following subjects might be included: women with a life expectancy of 10 or more years and normal risk of breast cancer, since the risk increases by age; and women with a life expectancy of 5 or more years and an increased risk of breast cancer (such as a personal history of ductal carcinoma *in situ* or atypical hyperplasia, or a family history of breast cancer). Considerations for not enrolling in an antiestrogen breast cancer prevention program would be a medical history of deep vein thrombosis or cerebrovascular disease, since there is an increase in these complications with the use of these agents.

ADJUVANT TREATMENT AS PREVENTION OF RECURRENT CANCER IN THE ELDERLY

Finally, between primary prevention and treatment of advanced disease with chemotherapy is adjuvant therapy to prevent recurrence of cancer. This approach, in which therapy is administered following surgical resection of the primary tumor, at a time when there is no metastatic disease, is accepted in the management of breast and colorectal cancer and is being studied in other diseases. Certainly, it is standard therapy in younger patients with high-risk breast or colorectal cancer. Determining the role of adjuvant therapy in older persons requires an analysis of benefit and the factoring of co-morbid conditions which will increase toxicity.

Several meta-analyses of adjuvant therapy in breast cancer patients have shown a benefit in reducing the incidence of recurrence, and this is particularly effective as the risk of recurrence rises, i.e. in those with positive lymph nodes or those with larger tumors at the time of initial surgery[16,17]. However, this approach remains controversial in older patients with primarily resected breast cancer, even with these disease-related features. The question is based on defining the risk of recurrence in a 10-year period versus the risk of death from other than cancer-related causes. Recently, Extermann and associates attempted to model an evaluation of risk reduction based on the age of the individual and the degree of co-morbidities in patients 65 years and older[30]. The authors analyzed recently published literature that studied adjuvant hormonal therapy and chemotherapy in those aged 65–85 years. They considered a risk reduction of recurrence or mortality of 1% at 10 years (or more) as signifying benefit of intervention. This is similar to the risk reduction of myocardial infarction with β-blockers[31] or of cerebrovascular accident with antiplatelet agents[32]. They also looked at the effect of three levels of co-morbidity – healthy, average, and sick – on survival in the following 5 or 10 years.

Older breast cancer patients have a reduction in relapse with the use of adjuvant therapy, very similar in magnitude to that seen in younger patients. Both hormonal therapy and chemotherapy offer benefit. In women aged 50–69 years, the reduction in relapse was 20.3% and in mortality was 11.3%[16]. In women aged 70 years or older, the reduction in relapse should be the same. However, the reduction in risk of death is confounded by other causes of death in this population. As has been found in other studies, co-morbidities, not just functional impairment (other medical problems), were independent predictors of survival, and when present, decreased the positive impact of adjuvant treatment[30,33,34].

Stage III colorectal cancer, with lymph node involvement at the time of initial surgery, is highly likely to recur, and adjuvant chemotherapy based on 5-fluorouracil has been demonstrated in numerous studies to reduce that risk, when compared with observation[35]. Meta-analyses of previously published studies have confirmed this and are used to evaluate the benefit in subgroups of patients. Sargent and colleagues evaluated the effect of adjuvant chemotherapy in colorectal cancer by age at diagnosis, examining decades < 50 years, 50–60 years, 60–70 years and > 70 years[36]. Overall, each treated group did better in terms of overall and disease-free survival[36]. Among all of these trials, older patients benefited from 5-fluorouracil-based therapy to the same degree as did younger patients, and with no greater toxicity. Age alone should not determine who receives adjuvant therapy, but again, functional status and co-morbidities will enter into the decision of whether to treat or not in the adjuvant setting[29].

TREATMENT OF CANCER IN THE ELDERLY

General modalities available

Modalities utilized for cancer treatment in the elderly are the same as in other cancer patients. The ability to utilize these modalities to their full extent depends largely on the overall medical condition of the older person. For example, elective surgery can be performed safely in older patients into their eighties, but emergency surgery is associated with high mortality, usually from sepsis, in patients over age 65 years[37]. Thus, early diagnosis is more likely to have a successful surgical outcome. Also, palliative surgery must be a consideration in cases of painful, disturbing exophytic tumors. Such approaches may improve the quality of life.

Radiation therapy at standard doses can be administered safely to patients in their eighties and may be utilized in certain cases in lieu of major surgery[38]. More intensive approaches such as combined modality therapy with radiation and chemotherapy may not be well tolerated by older patients. This approach in esophageal cancer, while yielding better results compared with either modality alone, is associated with considerable morbidity in middle-aged patients, and attention to nutritional support is paramount[39]. This approach in older patients must be applied selectively, based on functional and co-morbidity factors.

Chemotherapy remains a widely utilized approach for the treatment of advanced cancer. The modality is available to older patients and data suggest that outcome is dependent upon both disease and subject. The baseline functional level of the individual will dictate the likelihood of tolerance to aggressive therapy. Optimal but intensive therapy should not be denied on the basis of age, but may need modification if there are functional issues that will lead to increased morbidity. Data suggest, however, that older patients are more likely to be under-treated as a result of physician concern and fear of toxicity[40,41].

The pharmacology of antineoplastic agents in the elderly has become an area of intense interest in oncology. Current lack of knowledge regarding the processing of these drugs in patients well beyond the age of 65 years may limit treatment in this patient population[40,41]. Physiologic changes that occur with age include reductions in glomerular filtration rate, starting after the fourth decade, and have led to recommendations for dose adjustments for chemotherapeutic agents that are renally excreted[42,43]. Alterations in hepatic enzyme systems, such as cytochrome P450, may occur in healthy elderly subjects[44,45].

Less well known are the effects of changes in body composition and nutrition with aging on drug metabolism and storage. Currently there is major interest in the study of alterations in the pharmacokinetics and pharmacodynamics of drugs, including chemotherapeutic agents, in the aging population[46]. This information is likely to increase the safety and efficacy of cancer treatment in older persons.

Specific disease entities

Treatment approaches to cancer are outlined in Table 3.

Hematologic malignancies

Hematologic malignancies include leukemias, lymphomas and myeloma. Myelodysplasia will be discussed elsewhere. These are diseases in which a reasonable percentage of patients can be placed into prolonged remission with treatment and a subgroup can be cured. The diseases develop with increasing frequency among the elderly, and the biology of the disease, rather than strictly the age of the individual, determines the outcome. Data support the use of standard chemotherapy doses and regimens in the elderly to obtain the best opportunity for achieving remission. Reductions in dose, in attempts at 'sparing' patients, usually lead to a poorer response rate and greater morbidity. In general, overall outcome is poorer in the older than in younger patients, again based on a combination of disease- and patient-related factors. However, in patients equally 'healthy', the outcome is similar, regardless of age.

AML is the most common acute leukemia of adults and is rapidly fatal without treatment. Prognosis is dependent upon the cytogenetic abnormalities detected, since these imply the sensitivity of the disease to treatment with chemotherapy. In the chemosensitive subgroup, the elderly should be treated with standard dose and regimens, similar to younger patients. Lowering the dose of important drugs, such as the anthracyclines, leads to increased morbidity and mortality, because the lower doses have less anti-leukemic activity, but are likely to be as toxic to bone marrow and other tissues as at standard doses[47]. When standard doses are used in the elderly, although the overall response rate is lower than in younger patients, quality remissions are commonly achieved in patients with comparable risk factors (cytogenetics)[47–49]. Recently, the use of hematopoietic growth factors in elderly leukemic patients has been demonstrated to enhance outcome[50,51]. Post-remission therapy is also beneficial in elderly patients, and although they do not tolerate the intensification of agents used in younger patients for a short period of time[52], prolonged maintenance therapy has been shown to be efficacious and well tolerated in older patients, with long-term remissions frequently achieved[48].

Chronic lymphocytic leukemia is the most common leukemia in adults, with a median age of onset of 60 years, and often a very indolent course. The decision to initiate treatment is determined by the stage of disease, and whether the disease is impacting upon normal blood function, causing anemia, thrombocytopenia and neutropenia. With progression of disease, the patient suffers from the absence of normal blood cells and progressive immunosuppression. Treatment approaches range from low-dose oral medications to control the lymphocytosis and lymphadenopathy to more intensive intravenous medication which will eradicate the disease for a period of time. To date, no treatment has improved survival, however[53]. Therefore, treatment decisions are based on the need to control symptoms of the disease.

Lymphomas in adults range from low-grade, often indolent disease, with slowly progressive adenopathy, to highly aggressive, undifferentiated lymphomas demonstrating

Table 3 Standard treatment approaches

Breast cancer
Early stage: limited surgery; adjuvant hormonal therapy; possibly radiation
Advanced stage: hormonal therapy; chemotherapy

Colorectal cancer
Early stage: surgery; radiation if rectal cancer; adjuvant chemotherapy
Advanced stage: chemotherapy depending upon site of disease; radiation therapy depending upon site of
  disease

Lung cancer
Early stage non-small-cell cancer: surgery if possible; radiation therapy if no surgery
Advanced stage non-small-cell cancer: chemotherapy ± radiation
Limited small-cell cancer: chemotherapy + radiation
Advanced small-cell cancer: chemotherapy ± radiation

Prostate cancer
Initial diagnosis, depending upon rate of rise of PSA – surgery or radiation; older patients: monitor or
  hormonal therapy
Advanced disease – hormonal therapy, radiation to bony disease; chemotherapy if hormone refractory

Pancreatic cancer
Initial diagnosis: surgery if possible; if unresectable: chemotherapy or palliative care

Non-Hodgkin's lymphoma
Indolent: monitor extent and pace of disease; chemotherapy or biologic therapy with monoclonal antibody
Aggressive: chemotherapy plus monoclonal antibody; radiation to bulky disease

Leukemia
Chronic lymphocytic: monitor extent and pace of disease; chemotherapy as indicated by blood counts
Acute myeloid: chemotherapy; regimen dictated by cytogenetic evaluation
Acute lymphocytic: chemotherapy; Gleevec (tyrosine kinase inhibitor) if Philadelphia chromosome positive
Chronic myeloid: Gleevec; consider interferon, if possible to tolerate; consider stem cell transplant in younger
  patients

Multiple myeloma
MGUS: monitor level of M-spike and for evidence of bone disease, anemia or organ dysfunction
Smouldering leukemia: monitor level of M-spike, and for evidence of progression to myeloma, with bone
  disease, anemia, renal insufficiency or hypercalcemia
Myeloma: chemotherapy – with oral alkylating agents (melphalan, cyclophosphamide) plus corticosteroids
  (prednisone or dexamethasone) or with intravenous continuous infusion agents (doxorubicin and vinblastine).
  Bisphosphonates for improvement in bone disease. Irradiation of painful bone disease. Younger patients,
  consider stem cell transplantation

PSA, prostate-specific antigen; MGUS, monoclonal gammopathy of unknown significance

rapid growth and rapid demise. Aggressive non-Hodgkin's lymphoma appears, by several reports, to be a more aggressive disease in the elderly[54-56]. Elderly patients frequently have more adverse prognostic factors, according to the International Prognostic Index. Despite this, intensive therapy is often effective. Studies for the past 30 years have demonstrated the importance of anthracyclines in the treatment of this disease[57,58] and several studies, as well as a meta-analysis, have confirmed this in elderly patient populations[54-56,59]. These studies evaluated anthracycline-containing regimens, and once again, the importance of using the standard, aggressive approach was demonstrated, in that the benefit in terms of disease response and survival outweighed toxicity issues[54-56]. Other approaches to delivering anthracyclines to patients with cardiac compromise include the use of a cardioprotective agent[60] or, more appealing, a change in schedule to a continuous infusion approach[61].

Myeloma is another hematologic malignancy with clinical features at presentation that range from indolent to very advanced[62,63]. This may reflect early or late diagnosis, but it is clear that different patients have different rates of proliferation of the disease[64]. The disease spectrum ranges from a benign monoclonal gammopathy (monoclonal gammopathy of unknown significance; MGUS) and smouldering myeloma, both of which can be monitored for a period of time, to full-blown multiple myeloma requiring treatment. In the elderly, myeloma must be part of the differential diagnosis of new anemia or new renal insufficiency. Both of these features are prominent in this disease.

Treatment for myeloma includes both intravenous (vincristine, doxorubicin) and oral (melphalan, prednisone, cyclophosphamide, dexamethasone) medications, all of which are very well tolerated, even in elderly patients. Treatment outcome is palliative, however, with rarely prolonged survival beyond 5 years. The goal of treatment is to maintain function and to prevent or reduce bony events that lead to disability. The addition of bisphosphonates has been extremely helpful in bone disease and should be part of the treatment regimen[62].

Differentiating active myeloma from MGUS is important, since the former requires treatment and MGUS requires monitoring. The median age for both is similar, in the mid-sixties, and an elevation of protein is noted in the standard chemistry panel[62,63]. Both diseases are associated with a monoclonal protein spike, which is γ-globulin in the majority and IgG in more than 70% of either disease. The level of the M-protein is lower in MGUS, with a median of 1.7 g/dl compared to a median of 3–5 g/dl in overt myeloma in a Mayo Clinic series[62,63]. Other distinguishing features in those presenting with myeloma, include anemia, lytic bone lesions or osteoporosis, more than 10% plasma cells in the marrow and often renal insufficiency and/or hypercalcemia. Patients with MGUS are asymptomatic, without bone lesions or other organ dysfunction, and with less than 10% plasma cells in the marrow. Patients with MGUS are monitored for progression to myeloma, which occurred in 17% at 10 years and in 33% at 20 years in the Mayo Clinic series[63]. In between these two entities is smouldering myeloma, with an intermediate monoclonal protein value, more than 10% plasma cells in the marrow biopsy, but no organ dysfunction or anemia. The plasma cell labeling index is slow, suggesting a very indolent course of this disease. However, these patients may develop features of advanced myeloma and must be monitored.

Metastatic solid tumors

In metastatic solid tumors, beyond surgical cure the goal of treatment is to maintain function and activity, and to alleviate difficult symptoms, such as pain, bleeding, dyspnea and metabolic complications. Particularly in the elderly, the goal is to provide a treatment regimen that is not debilitating but can offer relief for a meaningful period of time. In this setting, radiation, chemotherapy and hormonal therapy are often intermixed. The identification of new agents with reduced toxicity is a major area of drug development in oncology. In addition, improved knowledge of pharmacology and drug metabolism with aging and of the impact of co-morbidity and functional capacity with treatment then enter into treatment decisions[65,66].

Metastatic breast cancer in elderly women expresses receptors for estrogen (ER) and/or progesterone (PR) in more than 80% of patients and the disease is frequently indolent in clinical behavior. This allows the use of hormonal therapy for a major part of the treatment period, an approach often successful for an extended period of time. Additionally, patients with ER/PR-positive breast cancer frequently have disease predominantly involving bone, and two additional modalities may be successful in palliating this disease. For painful or weight-bearing bone lesions, radiation therapy is generally successful in improving pain relief and function. The use of bisphosphonates has been demonstrated to reduce the frequency of bony events, such as pain and fracture. Chemotherapy can be utilized to treat more aggressive breast cancer in the elderly, and newer regimens involving weekly treatments at similar cumulative doses compared to older regimens appear to be efficacious and well tolerated. The outcome is determined by the degree of sensitivity to chemotherapy and by the sites of disease, with visceral disease being of poorer prognosis.

Colorectal cancer that recurs following surgery or that is locally advanced at diagnosis is treated with chemotherapy, including 5-fluorouracil and most recently the addition of irinotecan. Therapy is at best palliative, and the goal is to prevent decline in function which can be achieved with treatment. The major complication of treatment is diarrhea, and patients must be monitored for this to prevent dehydration. Radiation may be needed if obstructive symptoms or pain develop. The overall risk/benefit ratio must be discussed with patients and their families.

Pancreatic cancer is among the top five causes of cancer death (Table 2). At diagnosis, it is rarely surgically resectable. The new agent, gemcitabine, appears to improve quality of life by reducing pain for a finite period of time in patients with advanced disease. This drug is well tolerated, and elderly patients with reasonable performance status might benefit from treatment.

Small-cell lung cancer is treated initially with chemotherapy plus radiation, whereas non-small-cell lung cancer may be amenable to surgery, depending upon the stage at diagnosis. If surgery is not an option, then chemotherapy and/or radiation therapy should be considered. Small-cell lung cancer is a rapidly growing disease, with rapid onset of morbidity, and thus if the patient can tolerate chemotherapy he should be treated. The disease is chemosensitive and treatment is likely to achieve a remission for a period of time. If the disease is localized to the chest, there are long-term survivors of small-cell lung cancer. Treatment of non-small-cell lung cancer with chemotherapy in the elderly depends upon the degree of functional impairment caused by the disease. Newer chemotherapy agents such as vinorelbine and gemcitabine are very well tolerated and provide some relief of symptoms. However, responses are of limited duration (a matter of months) and the overall outcome should be carefully discussed with patients and their families prior to initiating treatment.

With the exception of cervical cancer, gynecologic tumors increase in frequency in postmenopausal women; these include ovarian, endometrial and vulvar cancer. Regular gynecologic examinations of postmenopausal women must be encouraged, since early diagnosis of either endometrial or vulvar cancer is likely to allow a surgical procedure of reduced extent and morbidity. The need for additional therapy is reduced if either of these diseases is detected early. Radiation therapy has a role in the treatment of more advanced cervical or endometrial cancer. Ovarian cancer is usually diagnosed as stage III, despite frequent pelvic examinations, and treatment at this stage includes both surgery and chemotherapy. Untreated ovarian cancer leads to early morbidity and mortality, and therefore, aggressive treatment is indicated in patients who are able to tolerate chemotherapy. Prolonged remissions can be achieved with modern chemotherapy. However, the chemotherapeutic agents used to treat ovarian cancer are not without morbidity, and this must be weighed with the functional status of the patients.

Management of prostate cancer in the elderly male is a subject of controversy, and is discussed in detail in Chapter 51. Suffice it to say that treatment is determined by the extent of disease and the rate of growth of the disease. Patients with indolent prostate cancer, or those with only elevated PSA, are often monitored for progression for extended periods of time.

Cutaneous malignancies also increase in frequency in older individuals, a result of cumulative sun exposure. These consist of basal cell carcinoma or squamous cell carcinoma. The onset of melanoma is less age related, and suggests a different biology.

Decisions regarding the aggressiveness of the treatment approach in a given older patient are based on the responsiveness of the disease, the risk of acute demise if untreated, the projected disease pace, and the current level of function and co-morbidities of the individual. Otherwise healthy patients with longer life expectancy should be offered standard therapy for treatment of cancer.

Characteristics that appear to impact on survival in older patients are: first, functional status, including strength, ability to perform simple exercises and the risk of falls[65]; second, the number of co-morbid conditions and the seriousness of these conditions[34]; and third, the level of cognitive function of the individual[66]. These three assessments appear to have independent predictive value on life expectancy, and may also enter into the development of a treatment plan for an elderly person who has developed cancer.

The oncologist is fully aware of the potential disease progression and the potential drug effects. The primary physician and geriatrician are aware of the functional status, emotional and physical support systems and co-morbidities which impact on initiating treatment. All of these should interplay to develop a treatment recommendation and plan. Therefore, ongoing communication and evaluation of all of these parameters are essential in the appropriate evaluation and management of elderly patients with malignancies.

References

1. Jemal A, Thomas A, Murray T, Thun M. Cancer statistics, 2002. *Cancer J Clin* 2002; 52:23–47

2. Anisimov I. Age as a risk factor in multistage carcinogenesis. In Balducci L, Lyman GH, Ershler W, eds. *Comprehensive Geriatric Oncology*. Newark, NJ: Harwood Academic Publishers, 1998:157–78

3. Bishop JM. Cancer – the rise of the genetic paradigm. *Genes Dev* 1995;9:1309–15

4. Barbone F, Bovenzi M, Cavallieri F, et al. Air pollution and lung cancer in Trieste, Italy. *Am J Epidemiol* 1995;141:1161–9

5. Campisi J. Aging and cancer: The double-edged sword of proliferative senescence. *J Am Geriatr Soc* 1997;45:482–90

6. Newbold RF, Overell RW, Connell JR. Induction of immortality is an early event in malignant transformation of mammalian cells by carcinogens. *Nature (London)* 1982;299:633–5

7. Shay JW, Wright WR. Defining the molecular mechanisms of human cell immortalization. *Biochim Biophys Acta* 1991;1071:1–7

8. Shay JW, Werbin H, Wright WE. You haven't heard the end of it: telomere loss may link human aging with cancer. *Can J Aging* 1995;14:511–14

9. Dimri GP, Lee X, Basile G, et al. A novel biomarker identifies senescent human cells in culture and aging skin *in vivo. Proc Natl Acad Sci USA* 1995;92:9363–7

10. Kaiser J. Cancer-stalling system accelerates aging. *Science* 2002;295:28–9

11. Wiernik PH. Diagnosis and treatment of acute myelocytic leukemia of adulthood. In Wiernik PH, Goldman J, Kyle R, Dutcher JP, eds. *Neoplastic Diseases of the Blood*, 4th edn. Cambridge: Cambridge University Press, 2002

12. DeWald G, Litzow M. Cytogenetics of acute leukemia. In Wiernik PH, Goldman J, Kyle R,

Dutcher JP, eds. *Neoplastic Diseases of the Blood, 4th edn.* Cambridge: Cambridge University Press, 2002

13. Hoelzer DF. Diagnosis and treatment of acute lymphocytic leukemia of adulthood. In Wiernik PH, Goldman J, Kyle R, Dutcher JP, eds. *Neoplastic Diseases of the Blood, 4th edn.* London: Cambridge University Press, 2002

14. Winer EP, Morrow M, Osborne CK, Harris JR. Malignant tumors of the breast. In DeVita VT, Hellman S, Rosenberg SA, eds. *Cancer: Principles and Practice of Oncology, 6th edn.* Philadelphia. PA: Lippincott, Williams and Wilkins. 2001:1651–17

15. Muss HB. Breast cancer in the elderly: The role of systemic adjuvant therapy. In Perry MC, ed. *American Society of Clinical Oncology Education Book 2001*. Baltimore, MD: ASCO/Lippincott Williams & Wilkins, 2001:106–10

16. Early Breast Cancer Trialists' Collaborative Group. Tamoxifen for early breast cancer: an overview of the randomised trials. *Lancet* 1998;351:1451–67

17. International Breast Cancer Study Group. Effectiveness of adjuvant chemotherapy in combination with tamoxifen for node-positive postmenopausal breast cancer patients. *J Clin Oncol* 1997;15:1385–94

18. Balducci L. Prevention and treatment of cancer in the elderly. *Oncol Issues* 2000;15:26–8

19. Colorectal Cancer Collaborative Group. Surgery for colorectal cancer in elderly patients: a systematic review. *Lancet* 2000; 356:968–74

20. Alley PG. Surgery for colorectal cancer in elderly patients. *Lancet* 2000;356:956

21. Robinson B, Beghe C. Cancer screening in the older patient. *Clin Geriatr Med* 1997;13: 97–118

22. Balducci L, Silliman RA, Baekey P. Breast cancer in the older woman: an oncologic perspective. In Balducci L, Lyman GH, Ershler W, eds. *Comprehensive Geriatric Oncology.* Newark, NJ: Harwood Academic Publishers. 1998:629–60

23. Smith RA, Cokkinides V, von Eschenbach AC, *et al*. American Cancer Society guidelines for the early detection of cancer. *Cancer J Clin* 2002;52:8–22

24. Rotmensch J, Herbst AL. Neoplasms of the vulva and vagina. In Holland JF, Frei E, eds.

Cancer Medicine, 5th edn. Hamilton, Ontario: BC Decker, Inc, 2000:1622–30

25. Cohen CJ, Thomas GM, Hagopian GS. Endometrial cancer. In Holland JF, Frei E, eds. *Cancer Medicine, 5th edn.* Hamilton, Ontario: BC Decker, 2000:1667–82

26. Berek JS, Thomas GM, Ozols RF. Ovarian cancer. In Holland JF, Frei E, eds. *Cancer Medicine, 5th edn.* Hamilton, Ontario: BC Decker, 2000;1687–720

27. Henschke CI, Yankelevitz DF, Libby DM, *et al*. Early lung cancer action project: annual screening using single-slice helical CT. *Ann NY Acad Sci* 2001;952:124–34

28. Sobue T, Moriyama N, Kaneko M, *et al*. Screening for lung cancer with low-dose helical computed tomography: anti-lung cancer association project. *J Clin Oncol* 2002;20: 911–20

29. Fisher B, Costantino JP, Wickerham DL, *et al*. Tamoxifen for prevention of breast cancer: report of the National Surgical Adjuvant Breast and Bowel Project P1 Study. *J Natl Cancer Inst* 1998;90:1371–88

30 Extermann M, Balducci L, Lyman GH. What threshold for adjuvant therapy in older breast cancer patients? *J Clin Oncol* 2000;18: 1709–17

31. Yusuf S, Wittes J, Friedman L. Overview of results of randomized clinical trials in heart disease. *J Am Med Assoc* 1988;260:2088–93

32. Antiplatelets Trialists' Collaboration. Collaborative overview of randomised trials of antiplatelet therapy: I. Prevention of death, myocardial infarction, and stroke by prolonged antiplatelet therapy in various categories of patients. *Br Med J* 1994;308:81–106

33. Satariano WA, Ragland DR. The effect of comorbidity on 3-year survival of women with primary breast cancer. *Ann Intern Med* 1994; 120:104–10

34 Extermann M, Overcash J, Lyman GH, *et al*. Comorbidity and functional status are independent in older cancer patients. *J Clin Oncol* 1998;16:1582–87

35. Kennedy BJ. Colon cancer in older persons: the role of adjuvant therapy. In Perry MC, ed. *American Society of Clinical Oncology Education Book 2001*. Baltimore, MD: ASCO/Lippincott Williams & Wilkins, 2001: 111–15

36. Sargent D, Goldberg R, MacDonald J, et al. Adjuvant chemotherapy for colon cancer is beneficial without significant increased toxicity in elderly patients. Results from a 3351 patient meta-analysis. *Proc Am Soc Clin Oncol* 2000;19:241a (abstr 933)

37. Berger DH, Roslyn JJ. Cancer surgery in the elderly. *Clin Geriatr Med* 1997;13:119–42

38. Olmi P, Ausili-Cefaro GP, Balzi M, et al. Radiotherapy in the aged. *Clin Geriatr Med* 1997;13:143–68

39. Cooper JS, Guo MD, Herskovic A, et al. Chemoradiotherapy of locally advanced esophageal cancer: long-term follow-up of a prospective randomized trial (RTOG 85-01). Radiation Therapy Oncology Group. *J Am Med Assoc* 1999;281:1623–7

40. Fentiman IS, Tirelli U, Mondfardini S, et al. Cancer in the elderly: why so badly treated? *Lancet* 1990;355:1020–2

41. Samet J, Hunt WC, Key C, et al. Choice of cancer therapy varies with age of patient. *J Am Med Assoc* 1986;255:3383–90

42. Balducci L, Extermann M. Cancer chemotherapy in the older patients: what the medical oncologist needs to know. *Cancer* 1997;80:1317–22

43. Balducci L, Extermann M. Management of cancer in the older person: a practical approach. *Oncologist* 2000;5:224–37

44 Sotaniemi EA, Arranto AJ, Pelkonen O, et al. Age and cytochrome P450-linked drug metabolism in humans: an analysis of 226 subjects with equal histopathologic conditions. *Clin Pharmacol Ther* 1997;61:331–9

44 Vestal RE. Aging and pharmacology. *Cancer* 1997;80:1302–10

45. Lichtman SM, Skirvin JA. Pharmacology of antineoplastic agents in older cancer patients. *Oncology* 2000;14:1743–59

46. Yates JG, Glidewell OH, Wiernik PH, et al. Cytosine arabinoside with daunorubicin or adriamycin for therapy of acute myelocytic leukemia. A CALGB study. *Blood* 1982;60:454–60

47. Dutcher JP, Wiernik PH, Markus S, et al. Intensive maintenance therapy improves survival in adult nonlymphocytic leukemia: an eight year follow-up. *Leukemia* 1988;2:413–18

48. Preisler H, Davis RB, Kirshner J, et al. Comparison of three remission induction regimens and two post-induction strategies for the treatment of acute non-lymphocytic leukemia: a Cancer and Acute Leukemia Group B study. *Blood* 1987;69:1441–9

49. Rowe JM, Andersen JW, Mazza JJ, et al. A randomized placebo-controlled phase III study of granulocyte-macrophage colony-stimulating factor in adult patients (> 55 to 70 years of age) with acute myelogenous leukemia: a study of the Eastern Cooperative Oncology Group (E1490). *Blood* 1995;86:457–63

50. Stone RM, Berg DT, George SL, et al. Granulocyte-macrophage colony-stimulating factor after initial chemotherapy for elderly patients with primary acute myelogenous leukemia. *N Engl J Med* 1995;332:1671–80

51. Bloomfield CD, Lawrence D, Byrd JC, et al. Frequency of prolonged remission duration after high dose cytarabine intensification in acute myeloid leukemia varies by cytogenetic subtype. *Cancer Res* 1998;58:4173–9

52. O'Brien S, Keating MJ: Diagnosis and treatment of chronic lymphocytic leukemia. In Wiernik PH, Goldman J, Kyle R, Dutcher JP, eds. *Neoplastic Diseases of the Blood*, 4th edn, Cambridge: Cambridge University Press, 2002

53. Bastion Y, Blay J-Y, Divine M, et al. Elderly patients with aggressive non-Hodgkin's lymphoma: disease presentation, response to treatment, and survival – a Groupe d'Etude des Lymphomes de l'Adulte study on 453 patients older than 69 years. *J Clin Oncol* 1997;15:2945–53

54 Tirelli U, Errante D, Van Glabbeke M, et al. CHOP is the standard regimen in patients ≥ 70 years of age with intermediate-grade and high-grade non-Hodgkin's lymphoma: results of a randomized study of the European Organization for Research and Treatment of Cancer Lymphoma Cooperative Study Group. *J Clin Oncol* 1998;16:27–34

55. Gomez H, Mas L, Casanova L, et al. Elderly patients with aggressive non-Hodgkin's lymphoma treated with CHOP chemotherapy plus granulocyte-macrophage colony-stimulating factor: identification of two age groups with differing hematologic toxicity. *J Clin Oncol* 1998;16:2352–8

56. Bishop JF, Wiernik PH, Wesley MN, *et al.* A randomized trial of high dose cyclophosphamide, vincristine, and prednisone plus or minus doxorubicin (CVP versus CAVP) with long-term follow-up in advanced non-Hodgkin's lymphoma. *Leukemia* 1987;1: 508–13

57. Fisher RI, Gaynor ER, Dahlberg S, *et al.* A phase III comparison of CHOP vs m-BACOD vs ProMACE-CytaBOM vs MACOP-B in patients with intermediate- or high-grade non-Hodgkin's lymphoma: results of SWOG-8516 (Intergroup 0067), the National High-Priority Lymphoma Study. *Ann Oncol* 1994;5 (Suppl 2):91–5

58. Kouroukis CT, Browman GP, Esmail R, Meyer RM. Chemotherapy for older patients with newly diagnosed, advanced-stage, aggressive-histology non-Hodgkin lymphoma: a systematic review. *Ann Intern Med* 2002;136:136–43

59. Speyer J, Wasserheit C. Strategies for reduction of anthracycline cardiac toxicity. *Semin Oncol* 1998;25:525–37

60. Sparano JA, Wiernik PH, Leaf A, Dutcher JP. Infusional cyclophosphamide, doxorubicin, and etoposide in patients with relapsed or resistant non-Hodgkin's lymphoma: evidence for a schedule dependent effect favoring infusional administration of chemotherapy. *J Clin Oncol* 1993;11:1071–9

61. Joshua DE, Gibson J. Diagnosis and treatment of multiple myeloma. In Wiernik PH, Goldman J, Kyle R, Dutcher JP, eds. *Neoplastic Diseases of the Blood, 4th edn,* Cambridge: Cambridge University Press, 2002

62. Griepp PR, Kyle RA. Staging, kinetics and prognosis of multiple myeloma. In Wiernik PH, Goldman J, Kyle R, Dutcher JP, eds. *Neoplastic Diseases of the Blood, 4th edn,* Cambridge: Cambridge University Press, 2002

63. Kyle RA, Rajkumar V. Monoclonal gammopathies of undetermined significance. In Wiernik PH, Goldman J, Kyle R, Dutcher JP, eds. *Neoplastic Diseases of the Blood, 4th edn.* Cambridge: Cambridge University Press, 2002

64 Siu AL, Moshita L, Blaustein J. Comprehensive geriatric assessment in a day hospital. *J Am Geriatr Soc* 1994;42:1094–9

65. Extermann M, Balducci L. Practical proposals for clinical protocols in elderly patients with cancer. In Balducci L, Lyman GH, Ershler WB, eds. *Comprehensive Geriatric Oncology.* Newark, NJ: Harwood Academic Publishers, 1998:263–70

66. Margolese RG, Fisher B, Hortobagyi GN, Bloomer WD. Neoplasms of the breast. In Holland JF, Frei E, eds. *Cancer Medicine, 5th edn.* Hamilton, Ontario: BC Decker, 2000: 1735–822

46 Musculoskeletal disorders

Barry Fomberstein, MD, FACP, FACR, *Dilip Unnikrishnan*, MD, *and T.S. Dharmarajan*, MD, FACP, AGSF

INTRODUCTION

Musculoskeletal disorders predominate in the older adult and are a major reason for chronic disability and health-care utilization in the geriatric age group[1,2]. Disorders of the musculoskeletal system impair mobility, interfering with activities of daily living (ADL) and function. The illnesses are usually chronic and not life threatening, but affect quality of life. Disability results in increased health-care utilization from medication use, appliances, home care requirements and institutionalization[3]. Due to their frequency, musculoskeletal disorders are often mistakenly attributed to normal aging rather than being recognized as disease processes[4]. Symptoms may be non-specific, suggesting a wide range of illnesses.

AGE-RELATED CHANGES

Aging is associated with a significant decline in functional status of all organ systems, decreasing the ability to respond to stress. Structurally, increased fibrillation occurs at the articular surface, especially at areas of increased stress. Biochemically, there is a decrease in hydration of the cartilage secondary to changes in proteoglycan structure, affecting water binding[5]. Cellularity is decreased, along with an increase in crystallization and calcification and a probable decrease in the response to growth factor stimulation[4]. These changes result in a tissue that is less able to handle mechanical stress.

Similar changes occur in the menisci, synovial membrane, tendons and ligaments, but in lesser proportions[4]. Sarcopenia or muscle loss results from a decrease in number and size of type II muscle fibers with a decline largely influenced by the activity level[6]. A decline in the range of motion occurs with most joints, influenced greatly by site, extent of use and disease. Osteoporosis, referring to a decrease in density of bone with aging, is described in detail elsewhere in the text.

EVALUATING THE PATIENT

History

The history should include onset and progression of illness, inquiry about an inflammatory process (swollen, hot, tender joints with constitutional symptoms), functional limitations, treatment response to initial therapy, co-morbid conditions and a comprehensive review of medications[7]. The presence or absence of morning stiffness is sometimes helpful; stiffness for less than 30 min is observed in osteoarthritis (OA), whereas longer duration (an hour or more) is commonly seen in the active phase of rheumatoid arthritis[1]. Musculoskeletal complaints may reflect an underlying disorder such as hypo- or hyperthyroidism, Paget's disease, infectious disease (hepatitis or HIV disease), inflammatory bowel disease or occult malignancy, warranting evaluation for such disorders.

The age of the subject is helpful in the differential diagnosis. OA is rarely a consideration under age 40; rheumatoid arthritis and gout can occur at any age and increase in frequency with aging. Polymyalgia rheumatica, giant cell arteritis and calcium pyrophosphate deposition disease are primarily seen in the geriatric age group[2].

Initial screening for cognitive status and depression helps formulate decisions on management. Complex drug regimens result in non-compliance, adverse drug events and treatment failures in the cognitively impaired. Functional status and social support systems influence decisions. Instruments to assess functional limitations such as the Health Assessment Questionnaire (HAQ) and Arthritis Impact Measurement Scales (AIMS 1 and 2) are predominantly for research purposes[7].

Physical examination

Physical examination should include focused evaluation of all joints for joint swelling, tenderness, effusion, deformities, synovial thickening, passive and active mobility, range of motion, strength of muscles and crepitus[8]. It is essential to observe the patient rising from the chair, ambulating and returning to the sitting position. Further, one should attempt to identify systemic involvement from rheumatic illness or the presence of another primary disorder with musculoskeletal manifestations. Characterizing the illness as acute or chronic (more than 6 weeks' duration), monoarticular, oligoarticular (2–3 joints) or polyarticular, axial or peripheral, symmetrical or asymmetrical is helpful[1]. Presence of rheumatoid nodules (rheumatoid arthritis), tophi (gout), malar rash, photosensitivity or pleurisy (systemic lupus erythematosus) may point to specific diagnoses.

Infection should be ruled out in any patient with acute mono- or oligoarthritis, since untreated septic arthritis carries high morbidity and mortality. Pre-existing joint disease

Table 1 Common laboratory tests for evaluation of musculoskeletal disease (all tests are not required in every case)

Initial routine tests
Complete blood count and differential
Erythrocyte sedimentation rate, C-reactive protein (quantitative)
Basic metabolic profile including renal function
Serum uric acid, calcium, phosphorus and alkaline phosphatase
Serum and urine protein electrophoresis
Antinuclear antibodies, rheumatoid factor assay, anti-double stranded DNA
Radiographs

Specific tests requested on an individual basis
Thyroid function tests
Serology for syphilis, Lyme disease
Antibodies (anti-Ro, anti-La, anti-RNP, anti-Sm), serum complement (C_H50, C_3, C_4)
Joint fluid analysis, synovial biopsy
Special imaging studies (ultrasound, computerized tomography scan, magnetic resonance imaging)

such as OA or rheumatoid arthritis, trauma, diabetes, immunosuppression, malignancies or infections elsewhere are risk factors for septic joint disease[1]. Swelling or inflammation of a joint that contains a prosthesis should heighten suspicion for infection.

Physical examination should help determine whether the symptoms are due to arthritis or to periarticular conditions such as bursitis or tendinitis. Acute exacerbations of an arthritic illness have to be differentiated from other conditions; e.g. a ruptured Baker's cyst in rheumatoid arthritis can present as acute knee and calf swelling, simulating deep vein thrombosis. Diagnosis is made using ultrasonography or magnetic resonance imaging (MRI).

Diagnostic evaluation

It is worth bearing in mind that some common test results have higher 'normal values' in the elderly. For example, erythrocyte sedimentation rate (ESR) of 30 mm/h is considered 'acceptable' in the older adult[2]. In general, because of co-morbidity in the elderly, one

Table 2 Aging versus osteoarthritis: articular changes. From references 4, 5 and 9

Changes	Normal aging	Osteoarthritis
Cartilage hydration	decreased	increased
Denatured type II collagen	present	more extensive
Degradative enzyme activity	normal	increased
Amount of proteoglycans	normal	decreased
Chondrocyte proliferation	normal or reduced	increased
Chondroitin sulfate	normal	decreased
Keratan sulfate	increased	decreased
Changes in underlying bone	thinning of bone	subchondral thickening

Table 3 Synovial fluid analysis in common joint disorders in the elderly. From references 1 and 8

	Normal	Osteoarthritis	Rheumatoid arthritis	Gout/ pseudogout	Septic
Appearance	clear	clear	clear/cloudy	inflammatory/ hemorrhagic	turbid
Cells/mm^3	< 200	< 5000	5000–25 000	10 000–20 000	> 100 000
Viscosity	normal	normal/low	low	low	low
Glucose*	normal	normal	low	normal/low	low
Crystals	absent	absent	absent	present[†]	Absent

*Compared to serum glucose. Normal ratio of synovial fluid to serum glucose is 0.8–1
[†]Needle shaped, negatively birefringent in gout; polymorphic, weakly positive birefringent in pseudogout

tends to request several laboratory and radiologic investigations. Some commonly used screening tests for the diagnosis of musculoskeletal disorders are listed in Table 1, from which selections may be individualized. Specific tests for hyperparathyroidism, multiple myeloma, connective tissue diseases or thyroid disease are obtained following initial clinical and laboratory evaluation. Serological tests help identify antibodies to various cellular components. Interpretation of results in older adults is also complicated by high rates of false positivity; assays for antinuclear antibody and rheumatoid factor may be positive, without clinical significance.

Radiologic tests may be requested to obtain diagnostic information, e.g. radiographs in the standing position to assess for osteoarthritis of the knee[2,8]. Radiographic changes consistent with OA are common in the older adult (Table 2); the prevalence of abnormalities increases with age to nearly half the individuals over 80 years[1]. The mere presence of radiological evidence of OA does

not necessarily indicate that symptoms are from OA; further, X-rays do not correlate with the extent of symptoms, especially with lumbar spinal disease[1]. Diffuse idiopathic skeletal hyperostosis (DISH) is an incidental finding resulting from excessive bone formation at the bony insertion of tendons in the spine[1]. Rarely, DISH can result in dysphagia or spinal stenosis from a pressure effect. Although plain radiographs are the initial choice, computerized tomography (CT) and/or MRI are useful in specific instances (e.g. compressive symptoms from spinal arthritis). CT scans delineate bone and joint abnormalities, while MRI offers better soft tissue imaging (intervertebral disc prolapse, rotator cuff tears). Joint fluid analysis helps evaluate acute mono- or oligoarticular inflammation and joint effusion. The characteristic synovial fluid analysis of common joint diseases is listed in Table 3. The mere presence of crystals does not rule out infection; a Gram stain and fluid culture should be obtained. A low glucose level (compared to blood glucose) usually signifies bacterial infection except in rheumatoid arthritis, where the synovial fluid glucose is usually low. Septic joints characteristically have white blood cell counts over 80 000[1]. The organism most commonly identified in septic joints in the elderly is *Staphylococcus aureus*; Gram-negative organisms might be responsible in joints with prosthetic material or in the immunocompromised[1].

OSTEOARTHRITIS

Clinical and pathologic features

OA or degenerative joint disease (DJD) is the most common articular disease in the elderly, with a steep rise in incidence after age 50 in men and age 40 in women. Clinically, the knee is the most affected joint, followed by the hip, although radiologically the distal and proximal interphalangeal joints are the most prevalent locations[9]. Symptomatic knee OA increases with age[4]. Polyarticular involvement appears more common in females[9].

Pathophysiologically, OA is a derangement in cartilage matrix degradation and repair. The chondrocytes are unable by proliferation and secretion of proteoglycans to match the degradative process; the result is fibrillation, erosion and cracking of the articular cartilage[4,5]. Normal aging and OA are compared in Table 2. Several risk factors are associated with the development of OA; age is consistently identified as a risk factor for all articular sites[4,9]. Other predisposing factors include joint damage on any basis (trauma, sepsis), occupation-related mechanical stress or repetitive injury (metacarpophalangeal, wrist), accumulation of crystals in articular cartilage (ochronosis, gout), congenital deformities imposing altered joint mechanics, endocrine disorders (acromegaly), avascular necrosis of bone and perhaps genetic factors. Obesity is associated with OA of the knee in older women and influences pain symptoms[4,9].

The diagnosis of OA is made on the basis of symptoms, physical examination and radiological changes. Commonly affected joints include the carpometacarpal joint of the thumb, distal interphalangeal joints, knees, hips, and the cervical and lumbar spine. Joint pain with OA is worsened with activity and relieved with rest in the early stages[10]. Rest pain and nocturnal pain characterize advanced disease. The etiology of pain in OA is complex; the sources may be synovitis, nerve involvement, muscle spasm, periostitis and subchondral bone ischemia or microfractures. Acute worsening of pain should prompt evaluation for septic arthritis, crystal-induced synovitis, stress fractures, osteonecrosis, ligament tears or bursitis. The 'gel phenomenon' refers to stiffness in the joints following inactivity, while 'locking' or 'buckling' is a result of internal derangement from advanced disease[9].

Physical examination evaluates the presence of joint tenderness, bony hypertrophy, synovial thickening or effusion, crepitus, mobility and deformities. In the hands, degenerative disease characteristically affects the interphalangeal joints or the carpometacarpal joint of the thumb; inflammatory involvement of the metacarpophalangeal joints suggests rheumatoid arthritis. Degenerative changes in the proximal interphalangeal joints are referred to as Bouchard's nodes and in the distal interphalangeal joints as Heberden's nodes. A focused physical examination is indicated in specific situations; e.g. DJD of the spine requires neurological examination for radiculopathy or gait disturbance.

Spinal arthritis can result in paresthesias or weakness, by affecting the neural foramen or from pressure effects. Symptoms may be referred to the shoulder, hand or wrist in cervical spine disease or to the buttocks and legs in lumbar spine involvement. The nerve roots in the cervical region are in close proximity to the apophyseal joints; hence radicular symptoms are common in the cervical region[11]. Moreover, the cervical neural canal is narrower, causing more myelocompressive symptoms compared to the rest of the spinal cord, including motor weakness, gait imbalance, incoordination or hyperreflexia.

Radiologically, early osteoarthritis is associated with narrowing of the joint space, resulting from thinning of the articular cartilage[8]. Late stages demonstrate subchondral thickening or sclerosis of bone, with osteophytes at joint margins, and possibly deformities. Cystic changes in the subchondral bone also appear in advanced cases. The extent of radiographic involvement in DJD does not correlate with severity of symptoms or functional impairment[8]. The ESR is normal, and synovial fluid analysis reveals a few white cells and normal viscosity (see Table 3).

Management

The primary goal in management of OA is relief of symptoms and maintenance of function[10,12]. Treatment is mostly symptomatic, since no agent reverses or slows the progression of OA. A judicious combination of non-pharmacologic and pharmacologic measures is the mainstay of treatment. In general, medications should be used with caution in the elderly, due to the risk of adverse drug reactions resulting from altered pharmacokinetics, polypharmacy and co-morbidity[13].

Non-pharmacologic measures

In addition to control of pain, management includes measures to improve joint mechanics, muscle strength and exercise capacity[3]. Weight loss is important in OA of the knees and hips and should be encouraged[8,14]. A relationship between weight loss and improvement in symptoms with OA has been shown[3,15]. The exercise prescription, beneficial for both weight loss and OA, includes strengthening exercises for the extremities (handgrip exercises, quadriceps exercises) and aerobic exercises (walking, jogging, swimming, cycling)[10,16]. Quadriceps weakness is common

with knee OA; isometric exercises are helpful here[3,15]. Long-term aerobic walking and weight training exercises improve balance in the older adult, and decrease the incidence of falls[4,17]. The patient's favorite exercise may be chosen, initiated at a low level and gradually stepped up in duration and intensity[4,13]. The exercise program may be designed and supervised by a physical or occupational therapist[13]. Optimal use of warm or cold applications helps relieve pain, with cold packs useful for acute flare-ups of the disease. Heating pads, hot water bottles or ice packs may be used, keeping in mind the impaired ability of the frail elderly to perceive heat and cold, and risk of thermal injury[13]. Appropriate use of orthotics helps maintain joint stability and gives relief of pain in those with gait abnormalities or angular deformities (e.g. heel pads, cushioned footwear, canes, etc.). Help is best sought from physical and occupational therapy in such instances[10]. The cane is held on the healthy (unaffected) side; special shoes help absorb shock or improve alignment[15]. Acupuncture, transcutaneous electrical nerve stimulation, T'ai Chi training and spa therapy have been utilized with varying results[3,9,13,18].

Medications

Medications are most effective when combined with one or more non-pharmacologic measures. The initial analgesic of choice for osteoarthritis is acetaminophen, based on efficacy, cost and safety profile[3,10,13,15]. Acetaminophen has been shown to be superior to placebo and as efficacious as non-steroidal anti-inflammatory drugs (NSAIDs) for the short-term treatment of knee OA[3,12]. Oral acetaminophen is well absorbed, has a plasma half-life of around 2 h, does not have significant protein binding, and is mainly metabolized in the liver[12]. Treatment is initiated with 500 mg twice a day and titrated up to 4 g/day in divided doses[13,19]. Acetaminophen is the drug of choice for pain in renal disease[10,12].

Caution should be exercised in prescribing acetaminophen to those who consume excessive amounts of alcohol. Prolongation of international normalized ratio (INR) may occur in those on warfarin and acetaminophen, requiring monitoring[15].

For those not responsive to acetaminophen and non-pharmacotherapeutic measures, NSAIDs are an alternative for pain control[3,20]. Anti-inflammatory medications are used by older individuals for a variety of complaints, sometimes poorly substantiated. Minimum doses should be used, titrated to optimum benefit and short duration to avoid complications from therapy[13]. Many NSAIDs are available without prescription in the USA. While NSAIDs provide relief, side-effects, including drug–drug and drug–disease interactions, are a concern. Bothersome adverse effects include gastrointestinal (bleeding, perforation) and renal toxicity (renal insufficiency, progression to renal failure, sodium and fluid retention and hyperkalemia); NSAIDs can also cause delirium, sleeplessness, paranoia and depression. There is no consensus on the choice of NSAIDs, although indomethacin is best avoided in older subjects in view of its higher toxicity, including central nervous system (CNS) effects and delirium, and progression of joint space narrowing noted in clinical trials[3]. One may initiate NSAIDs with a short half-life such as ibuprofen[13,15]. Increased side-effects occur with advanced age, congestive cardiac failure, peptic ulcer disease, diabetes mellitus, steroid and anticoagulant use, prior volume depletion from diuretics, hepatic dysfunction, pre-existing renal disease and smoking[3]. Adverse effects on the gut are dose dependent and minimized with the use of proton pump inhibitors or H_2 blockers, preferably the former. Unlike non-selective NSAIDs, non-acetylated salicylates (e.g. choline magnesium trisalicylate, salsalate) have no platelet or renal effects and may be useful in many patients[8,10]. Periodic monitoring of clinical status and laboratory parameters is required with chronic therapy using this class of medication. There is no proof that NSAIDs alter the course of OA.

As noted, NSAIDs are associated with drug–drug and drug–disease interactions. Hyperkalemia may occur in combination with angiotensin converting enzyme (ACE) inhibitors and potassium-sparing diuretics. They can reduce efficacy of antihypertensive agents, precipitate congestive heart failure, worsen renal function and potentiate the effect of anticoagulants.

NSAIDs act presumably by inhibiting the cyclo-oxygenase (COX) pathway of prostaglandin metabolism, blocking both the 'housekeeping' constitutive (COX-1) and inducible (COX-2) forms of the enzyme[21]. The COX-2 inhibitors carry the advantage of inhibiting only the inducible component, causing fewer gastrointestinal adverse effects[22]. However, they also inhibit renal and cerebral prostaglandin synthesis and hence are not devoid of nephrotoxicity or cerebral toxicity[10,23]. Currently available COX-2 inhibitors, celecoxib and rofecoxib, appear superior to placebo and comparable to other potent NSAIDs, with a lower incidence of gastrointestinal complications[10,22,24]. They are thus especially advantageous in the management of high-risk patients[10,25]. Additionally, the lack of antiplatelet action is beneficial in patients on anticoagulant therapy or in the perioperative stage[10]. Celecoxib is contraindicated in those allergic to sulphonamides[10]. However, certain physiological roles have been demonstrated for the COX-2 enzymes, such as synthesis of prostacyclins, which have vasodilatory and antithrombotic properties. Whether inhibition of prostacyclin production by COX-2 inhibitors increases thrombotic tendency in patients at increased cardiovascular risk, needs clarification pending further evaluation[26].

Codeine in small doses is often added to conventional medications for acute exacerbations; it can cause dependence and is best avoided for chronic musculoskeletal pain.

Tramadol is an oral synthetic opioid, and useful when NSAIDs or COX-2 inhibitors are ineffective or contraindicated[10]. Tramadol acts by binding to pre-opioid receptors or inhibiting serotonin and norepinephrine uptake by cells[15]. Opioids are generally avoided, except in severe end-stage OA and patients not suitable for surgery; adverse effects such as cognitive impairment, constipation and dependence are of concern in the elderly.

Topical agents are useful adjuncts to oral medications and at times used as monotherapy. NSAIDs and counterirritants such as capsaicin are available as topical preparations[3]. Capsaicin, a plant derivative from Cayenne pepper, is applied three to four times a day. As it is an irritant, precautions should be taken to avoid accidental application to eyes and mucous membranes[10]. Intra-articular injections of corticosteroids or hyaluronic acid of the affected joint can relieve symptoms; the effect lasts a few weeks and may require repeating. Triamcinolone hexacetonide (40 mg) is injected with 1% lidocaine after aspiration of fluid; methyl prednisolone and triamcinolone acetonide are alternatives[3,10]. Concerns with intra-articular steroid injections include infection, post-injection flare up and, in the long term, joint damage. Fewer than four glucocorticoid injections are recommended per year[15]. Hyaluronic acid contributes to improved lubrication and viscoelastic properties to the joint; weekly injections are required for 3–5 doses, and the regimen may be repeated up to twice a year[15]. Advanced stages of the disease, without response to measures, described may be an indication for surgery. Age by itself is not a contraindication for surgery; rather, the limiting factors are co-morbidity and life expectancy.

Alternative therapy

A series of compounds claimed to be beneficial in OA have emerged, the most common being glucosamine with or without chondroitin sulphate[4,27]. Glucosamine may benefit cartilage metabolism and chondrocyte biosynthesis[15,18]. Antioxidants (vitamins C and E or β-carotene) are claimed to decrease radiographic progression of the disease, although this has not been confirmed by controlled studies[3,28,29].

Surgery

Incapacitating disease of the lower extremities, failure of medical management and functional limitations are indications for surgical total joint replacement. Hip and knee replacements are common, followed by intense physical therapy to accelerate recovery[10,11]. In candidates not suitable for surgery, arthroscopy and tidal lavage with saline might alleviate symptoms, although efficacy of these procedures has not been conclusively demonstrated[3,28,29].

RHEUMATOID ARTHRITIS

New-onset rheumatoid arthritis is recognized with increasing frequency in older adults. Around 20–30% of rheumatoid arthritis patients present after age 60[21]. There is less gender variation in frequency, although a female preponderance exists[3]. The presentation varies from mild small joint disease to an acute illness with disabling symptoms. Involvement of the large, proximal joints such as the shoulder may be the initial presentation. Compared to onset at a younger age, rheumatoid arthritis in the older adult often involves fewer joints, with the rheumatoid factor absent in over half the patients[19]. Rheumatoid nodules, joint erosions, vasculitis, pulmonary disease and neuropathy are less evident than in younger adults. Remissions are less likely in the elderly with established disease, resulting in much discomfort and disability[30].

Seropositive disease is similar in all ages with symmetrical small joint involvement, bony erosions and rheumatoid nodules. However, seronegative disease is often oligoarticular in the old, affects the shoulder, knees or wrists, is not associated with nodules, is of acute onset, and with a lesser tendency for radiologic erosions[21]. In spite of an explosive onset with significant morning stiffness, seronegative disease has a better outcome in terms of joint involvement, radiologic disease and mortality[3,21,30]. Seronegative rheumatoid arthritis has to be distinguished from polymyalgia rheumatica, seronegative spondyloarthropathies, psoriatic arthritis, SLE, amyloidosis and hemochromatosis. Crystal-induced arthritis, atypical OA and paraneoplastic illness also enter the differential diagnosis.

Low titers of rheumatoid factor are common in 25–40% of the over-70 age group[21]. The mere presence of the antibody is not diagnostic of rheumatoid disease in the absence of characteristic signs and symptoms. Differentiation from OA may be difficult. Joint involvement in the older adult may not follow the classic patterns seen in younger patients. A subgroup of patients with rheumatoid arthritis resembles polymyalgia rheumatica, with symptoms in the neck and shoulders[19,26]. Both diseases can present with symmetrical joint involvement and morning stiffness, elevated ESR and negative rheumatoid factor. Resorptive lesions in the hands are rare in polymyalgia rheumatica. Both entities respond to steroid therapy[21].

Therapy for rheumatoid arthritis constitutes use of pharmacotherapy along with non-pharmacologic measures such as physical therapy, exercises and psychological support. The patient is likely to be sick and bed bound in the acute stages. Even so, enforced rest affects quality of life and is associated with complications. Appropriate use of heat or cold therapy, analgesic creams, immobilization with splints and passive exercises improves symptoms in the acute stages[21]. The prescription for strengthening and stretching exercises is designed to improve the strength of the specific muscle that maintains joint position[8,16]. NSAIDs are the agents of choice, due to the inflammatory nature of the disease. Acetaminophen is used to supplement the analgesic effect. Opioids are usually avoided, although they provide relief when painful disease is not responsive to conventional medications.

Low-dose corticosteroids help rapid control of symptoms, particularly in patients with restricted mobility. Steroid use requires monitoring for side-effects, including hypertension, hyperglycemia, fluid and electrolyte abnormalities, glaucoma and cataracts, weight gain, gastrointestinal bleeding and osteoporosis. Even so, the benefit from use of short-term low-dose steroids outweighs the complications resulting from a bedridden status in rheumatoid arthritis. The lowest possible dose for a short period of time may be used (e.g. 2.5–7.5 mg of prednisone or its equivalent for less than 6 months), after discussion of risks and benefits of therapy with the patient and/or caregiver. Steroid therapy should be supplemented with 1000–1500 mg calcium and 400–800 IU vitamin D daily, directed to minimize osteoporosis.

More recently, disease-modifying antirheumatic agents (DMARDs) have been used early in the disease, based on observations that accelerated erosive changes occur mostly in the initial phase of the illness[21]. Moreover, control of symptoms with DMARDs helps decrease the chronic use of NSAIDs and steroids, which cause significant adverse effects with long-term use. Hydroxychloroquine, methotrexate and sulfasalazine are commonly used medications in the group. Hydroxychloroquine is well tolerated and improves symptoms in nearly half the patients[21]. Ophthalmology evaluation is indicated pretreatment and every 6 months for early detection of eye complications from the medication[31]. Methotrexate has a dependable clinical response, rapid action and fewer long-term adverse effects compared to the other DMARDs. Older adults are usually maintained on lower doses of methotrexate

(7.5–15 mg/week) due to higher rates of abdominal discomfort, cytopenias, mucositis, megaloblastic anemia, hepatotoxicity and lung injury[2,21]. Monitoring of liver and renal function, as well as peripheral cell counts, is recommended. Sulfasalazine causes gastrointestinal side-effects, skin rashes and occasionally agranulocytosis, renal and hepatic damage.

Leflunomide (pyrimidine nucleotide synthesis inhibitor), infliximab and etanercept (tumor necrosis factor-α antagonists) are recently approved DMARDs, and clinical trials with these agents have shown encouraging results in the treatment of rheumatoid arthritis[32,33]. Leflunomide is used in a daily oral dose of 10–20 mg following a loading dose of 100 mg/day for 3 days; the loading dose is lowered or avoided in the elderly[34]. The medication may cause hepatic injury and must be avoided in those who consume alcohol or manifest abnormal liver function; frequent laboratory testing is therefore recommended. Etanercept is a bioengineered fusion product and administered in a dose of 25 mg subcutaneously twice weekly[34], as monotherapy or in combination with methotrexate. Infliximab is a chimeric antibody (human-murine) against TNF (tumor necrosis factor); use may be associated with the formation of human antibodies and hypotension, facial flushing and headaches. Pretreatment with antihistamines and acetaminophen is recommended; the drug is used only in conjunction with methotrexate, which decreases response to these antibodies. Infliximab has been studied in doses of 3 mg/kg and 10 mg/kg intravenously with additional doses at 2 and 6 weeks, and every 8 weeks thereafter[34]. Anakinra is a recombinant form of human interleukin-1 (IL-1) receptor antagonist, recently approved for the treatment of rheumatoid arthritis; the drug is used subcutaneously in a dose of 100 mg daily[35]. Patients on treatment with TNF antagonists and IL-1 inhibitors must be monitored for leucopenia and infections[34].

Permanent joint deformities with severe functional impairment can be helped by surgical interventions, including arthroscopic synovectomy, release of contractures, cartilage repair or joint stabilization, while advanced secondary osteoarthritis of the hips and knees can be treated with total joint replacement[3,8].

CRYSTAL ARTHROPATHIES

Monosodium urate and calcium pyrophosphate dihydrate crystals deposited in the joint result in gout and pseudogout, respectively. Presentation can be asymptomatic or alternatively, acute, chronic or destructive arthritis. Deposition of crystals activates cellular and immunologic response in the synovium, resulting in an acute inflammatory response mediated by cytokines.

Pseudogout

Deposition of calcium pyrophosphate in the articular cartilage increases with advancing age. This might be asymptomatic or result in acute inflammation, termed pseudogout. The crystals are radio-opaque and are visualized on radiographs as linear calcified opacification of the articular cartilage (chondrocalcinosis) in the knee, menisci, triangular cartilage of the wrist, the glenoid, acetabular labrum and intervertebral discs[36]. Rapidly destructive disease may resemble Charcot joints on radiographs. Both gout and pseudogout occur with increased frequency in patients with pre-existing joint disease, e.g. OA. The acute attack evolves over days, often accompanied by fever and constitutional symptoms. Synovial fluid analysis demonstrates the characteristic weakly positive birefringent rhomboid-shaped crystals.

Treatment of the acute attack includes rest and use of NSAIDs. Synovial fluid aspiration, intra-articular steroid injections and oral colchicine have also been used with success. Presently there are no measures to deplete calcium pyrophosphate-dihydrate (CPPD) crystals from the joint, as opposed to measures available in gout. Once the acute attack subsides, exercise programs are considered.

Gout

Gout is rare in premenopausal women, and should be considered in males beyond middle age and in older women with arthritis. Joints with pre-existing disease tend to get involved and hence gout should be suspected in any case of acute arthritis, including those with prior joint disease. Initial attacks may affect the first metatarsophalangeal joint of the great toe or other larger joints of the lower extremities, while recurrences tend to be polyarticular or tophaceous[36]. Polyarticular gout is the presentation in 3–14% of cases[37]. Alcohol, acute illness and stress, trauma, drugs or dietary excess often precipitate attacks. The acute stage lasts days; if untreated, recurrences occur at shorter intervals and are associated with chronicity. Subcutaneous tophi containing urate crystals may result after years of recurrent bouts, around the olecranon, the Achilles tendon or as secondary tophi in Heberden's and Bouchard's nodes[36]. While serum uric acid levels may be elevated, as many as 40% of acute attacks are associated with normal levels. Conversely, an elevated uric acid level in a patient with arthritis is not synonymous with a diagnosis of gout. The diagnosis is confirmed by demonstrating negatively birefringent needle-shaped crystals in synovial fluid analysis[36].

Treatment is aimed at alleviating acute symptoms and introducing measures to prevent future attacks. Alcohol and purine-rich foods are limited. Treatment of the acute attack includes rest and local therapy, usually cold applications. NSAIDs are effective in pain control, with the standard precautions observed[36]. Oral colchicine is helpful, 1.2 mg initially followed by 0.6 mg every 2 h until control of symptoms is achieved (maximum 5 mg/day). The significant adverse effect is diarrhea. Short-term systemic steroids and adrenocorticotropic hormone (ACTH) are alternatives when other medications fail to produce benefit or are contraindicated[36]. Therapy to some degree may be based on patient preferences. Systemic steroids are probably the drug of choice in those with co-morbidity and contraindications to NSAIDs. Local steroid injections are helpful in mono- or oligoarticular gout when infection is ruled out[2]. Initiation of urate-lowering therapy, e.g. allopurinol, is considered after the acute symptoms subside; however, patients already on allopurinol may continue therapy during an acute attack to avoid rapid fluctuations in uric acid level.

PAGET'S DISEASE

Paget's disease is a focal disorder of bone characterized by increased osteoclast resorption and subsequent osteoblastic formation of immature bone with disrupted lamellar structure. The new bone formed appears hyperdense on radiographs, but is nevertheless prone to fractures and bowing, due to inferior architecture. The illness is thought to arise from slow virus infection of bone cells, mainly affecting the osteoclasts[38]. The disease is more common in males older than 60 years. Approximately half the affected patients are asymptomatic; often the disease is incidentally diagnosed following laboratory or radiologic evaluation.

Bone pain in affected individuals results from increased vascularity of bone, stretching of periosteum or fractures; sometimes pain may result from secondary osteoarthritis or gouty arthritis. Bowing of long bones (tibia, femur), neurologic complications from pressure effects (deafness, blindness), skull deformities (frontal bossing) or high-output cardiac failure are other presenting features[2]. Hypercalcemia and hypercalciuria can develop when the patient with Paget's disease is bedridden for any reason; antiresorptive treatment should be utilized in such situations. Fractures in abnormal bones are often associated with non-union. Malignancies such as osteosarcoma can complicate Paget's disease, typically arising in a pre-existing lesion.

The diagnosis is suggested by an elevated alkaline phosphatase level, signifying osteoblastic activity. Radiographs showing increased diameter of affected bones or bone scans revealing hot spots help in diagnosis. Bisphosphonates and calcitonin are used to prevent resorption of bone and thus control remodeling rates[2]. Alendronate in a dose of 40 mg daily for 6 months is currently the preferred medication[38]. It may be restarted with recurrence of pain or evidence of increased bone turnover. Bone pain is controlled by use of acetaminophen or NSAIDs. Canes or shoes help correct impairments resulting from bony deformities. Intravenous pamidronate or subcutaneous calcitonin controls the remodeling process and hypercalcemia during emergency surgery[38].

MISCELLANEOUS CONDITIONS

Systemic lupus erythematosus and other connective tissue disorders

The incidence of SLE and other connective tissue disorders in the older population is less than in the young. 6–20% of all cases diagnosed in adults are in those over age 60, with a female preponderance for the disease maintained in late-onset disease[31,39]. Early SLE with insidious onset and constitutional features may mimic rheumatoid arthritis or polymyalgia. Interstitial pneumonitis, serositis, cytopenias and Sjögren's syndrome are more common in older adults, while nephritis, lymphadenopathy, alopecia, photosensitivity and neurologic changes are less apparent[31,39,40]. The serologic diagnosis of SLE in the elderly is complicated by the increased prevalence of autoantibodies with normal aging, with a positive titer noted in up to 36% of healthy older adults[1,31,39]. Titers less than 1 : 160 may not be significant; the positive predictive value increases with higher titers of antinuclear antibody (ANA)[2,31]. Anti-dsDNA autoantibodies are highly specific and sensitive for the disease, generally not increased with aging, and used to substantiate the diagnosis[31]. The disease runs a milder course, with the prognosis complicated by co-morbid illnesses[39].

Drug-induced lupus is increasingly recognized as a result of improved longevity and use of multiple medications. Clinically, the syndrome resembles idiopathic SLE. Medications implicated include hydralazine, procainamide, isoniazid, penicillin, sulphonamides and phenytoin, amongst others[2,40]. Antinuclear and antihistone antibodies are present, while antibodies to soluble antigens, Sm, Ro and La antibodies are absent. Treatment is directed at discontinuing the inciting medications[2].

Because of the milder illness, corticosteroids or immunosuppressants are usually not required[39]. Low-dose NSAIDs or non-acetylated salicylates control arthritic symptoms, and may be supplemented by acetaminophen. Rash and arthritis respond well to hydroxychloroquine, while pneumonitis, hemolytic disease or thrombocytopenia requires steroids[31]. Glomerulonephritis in late-onset SLE is rare, and is treated with corticosteroids and immunosuppressants, similar to young-onset disease[31]. Methotrexate and antimalarial compounds offer steroid-sparing benefits.

Sjögren's syndrome in the elderly can present as primary disease or secondary to other conditions such as rheumatoid arthritis or SLE[2]. Secondary Sjögren's syndrome is common, occurring in almost half the patients with late-onset rheumatoid arthritis[21]. Symptoms include dryness of the oral and ocular mucosa, resulting in grittiness, photophobia, dysphagia, altered taste, dental caries and fissuring of the mucosa[21,31]. Diagnosis is made by Schirmer's test (demonstrating lack of tear wetting), presence of anti-Ro and anti-La antibodies, or rarely by demonstrating lymphocyte infiltration in the minor salivary glands on inner lip biopsy[31]. Treatment

Table 4 Fibromyalgia. From references 2, 43–45

American College of Rheumatology classification criteria
(1) Widespread pain for more than 3 months
(2) Location: right and left sides of the body; above and below the waist; and axial
(3) Pain manually elicited with pressure of about 4 kg/cm² at defined tender points

Associated somatic complaints
Chronic fatigue, subjective morning stiffness, sleep disturbances
Regional pain: headache, chest, pelvic or myofascial pain, temporomandibular joint disorder
Skin sensitivity: hyperalgesia, paresthesia, heat and cold intolerance
Problems with memory and concentration
Rhinitis, auditory, vestibular and/or ocular complaints
Irritable bowel syndrome, dysphagia
Urinary frequency and urgency

Fibromyalgia differs from polymyalgia rheumatica in the following:
Symptoms are chronic
Pain is widespread
Sedimentation rate is not elevated
Response to steroids is not dramatic

includes the use of artificial tears and saliva and general measures to improve hydration. Use of pilocarpine and cevimeline, cholinergic agonists that stimulate salivary glands and relieve xerostomia, has facilitated management[41]. Hydroxychloroquine, systemic steroids and immunosuppressives have been used in severe systemic disease[31]. The commonest cause of mucosal dryness in older adults is medications, prompting a review of prescribed and other medications.

A recently described entity seen in older adults with a clinical presentation similar to rheumatoid arthritis is remitting seronegative symmetrical synovitis with pitting edema (RS3PE syndrome)[42]. More common in males, this is characterized by seronegative symmetric polyarthritis affecting the wrists and hands, with diffuse hand swelling, marked morning stiffness, significant synovitis and involvement of the flexor tendon sheaths[1,2]. The disease is often abrupt in onset, erosions are absent on hand radiographs and patients generally respond to steroids. The presence of the HLA-B7 antigen is associated with an increased risk of developing the disease.

Fibromyalgia

Fibromyalgia is a form of non-articular rheumatism characterized by diffuse musculoskeletal pain and tender points at characteristic sites on physical examination[2,43–45]. Numerous tender points are described, including the insertions of suboccipital and trapezius muscles, the lower cervical area, supraspinatus, costochondral regions, lateral epicondyles, gluteal, greater trochanters and medial knees[43]. Abnormalities in sleep pattern, fatigue, paresthesias, irritable bowel symptoms, generalized anxiety and subjective morning stiffness are common features (Table 4). Because of the non-specific nature of the complaints, systemic illnesses such as thyroid disease or malignancy should be excluded.

Symptoms of the disease might resemble polymyalgia rheumatica and cause difficulty in diagnosis. Onset of polymyalgia rheumatica, however, is usually acute with symptoms referred to the shoulder or hip girdle; unlike fibromyalgia, a high sedimentation rate and dramatic response to steroid therapy is characteristic. Soreness and stiffness are prominent complaints in polymyalgia rheumatica, while pain and tenderness predominate in fibromyalgia[1]. NSAIDs may help, but low-dose tricyclics or muscle relaxants may be more useful[31].

Shoulder pain

Shoulder pain in the older adult may arise from the joint or periarticular structures, or be referred from the heart, diaphragm, neck or lungs[8,43,44]. Rotator cuff disorders are a common cause of shoulder complaints in this age group. The rotator cuff muscles are essential in shoulder movements and maintain stability. In rotator cuff tendinitis, impingement of the supraspinatus tendon between the humeral head and the acromion results in pain when the arm is abducted to 90°. The patient presents with shoulder pain that is worse with activity, especially with maneuvers such as putting on a coat or reaching above the head. Calcific tendinitis is another entity causing shoulder pain in the older adult, and usually follows degenerative changes in the rotator cuff tendons. Rotator cuff tears, common with steroid therapy, should be suspected when painful abduction beyond 90° is accompanied by weakness on resisted abduction (supraspinatus tear) or external rotation (infraspinatus tear)[43,46]. Sustained elevation of the arm at 90° may not be possible in such situations (drop arm sign). Adhesive capsulitis or 'frozen shoulder' refers to loss of passive range of motion at the shoulder, in the absence of intrinsic disease of the bone or joint. It follows stroke, trauma or other painful conditions leading to prolonged disuse of the shoulder and responds well to stretching exercises[46].

Differential diagnosis includes rheumatoid arthritis and polymyalgia rheumatica, and also metastatic disease[46]. Plain radiographs, CT scan and MRI are imaging modalities helpful in diagnosis. MRI offers the advantage of soft tissue and bone images in multiple planes and is useful in rotator cuff tears to identify the site and extent of the tear, and the role for surgical repair. Management of rotator cuff problems includes a brief period of immobilization, analgesics, steroid injections and muscle strengthening exercises.

Back pain

Back pain is common in the elderly and can result from disorders of the spine or abdominal and pelvic pathology. Most common are degenerative disease of the spine (OA, disc disease, spondylolisthesis), lumbar spinal stenosis, osteoporotic fractures and metastatic disease. Degenerative processes are typical radiological findings in the older patient and their mere presence by itself does not indicate the basis for symptoms[1]. CT or MRI are more sensitive and specific for evaluation of disc disease, infections or metastases[47]. Prostatic disease, retroverted uterus, hip joint disease or abdominal aortic aneurysms are extraspinal disorders that may present with back pain. Evaluation for spine tenderness, motor or sensory deficits (straight leg raising test, knee and ankle jerk reflexes) and gait abnormalities is indicated. Absence of the ankle jerk reflex may occur in 10% of older adults and by itself is non-diagnostic[47].

Lumbar spinal stenosis causes compression of exiting nerve roots and the cauda equina, resulting in neurogenic claudication, and bowel and bladder dysfunction. The encroachment into the spinal canal can be bony or from soft tissues such as the ligamentum flavum or posterior longitudinal ligaments[47]. Neurogenic claudication refers to aching pain or paresthesia in the gluteal, thigh or calf region, precipitated by lumbar extension (walking downhill, standing) and is relieved by forward flexion of the spine (stooping, sitting, walking uphill). The flexed or 'simian' posture increases the neural canal space and improves symptoms[11]. The symptoms differ from those of vascular claudication where relief of symptoms occurs with resting (standing, lying). MRI or CT scans provide evidence of spinal stenosis; however, due to the high prevalence of degenerative disease of the spine in older adults, radiologic diagnosis must be correlated with history and clinical findings.

Treatment includes rest, analgesia with acetaminophen or short-term NSAIDs, thermal methods and exercise to improve strength and mobility. Corsets or braces offer symptomatic relief. Pressure effects on the nerves or spinal cord may require definitive therapy by surgical decompression.

Bursitis, tendinitis

In addition to subacromial bursitis or supraspinatus tendinitis described above, olecranon bursitis, medial and lateral epicondylitis, DeQuervain's disease (tenosynovitis of anatomical snuff box), trochanteric, iliopsoas and prepatellar bursitis might also be seen in the older adult[43]. Management includes analgesics, anti-inflammatory agents, judicious use of local steroids and exercises after the acute stage resolves.

Reflex sympathetic dystrophy

Reflex sympathetic dystrophy is a condition seen in the elderly following fractures or nerve injury, and also following trauma, myocardial infarction or cerebrovascular disease. The disease is characterized by pain, increased sensitivity to touch (hyperpathia), pain with repetitive touch (allodynia), vasomotor instability (color, temperature), dystrophic skin changes and sudomotor dysfunction (sweating) in the affected extremity[43]. Treatment includes physical therapy, sympathetic blockade and corticosteroids.

SUMMARY

The presentation of musculoskeletal disorders in the elderly may be different compared to those in the young. Treatment principles must keep in mind the differences in age-related physiology, altered pharmacokinetics and dynamics, and reduction in functional and cognitive abilities, widely prevalent in the older adult. The diagnosis is easily missed in older adults; aging changes, inflammation, malignancy-associated, crystal and sepsis-based musculoskeletal disorders result in dilemmas in diagnosis and management. Much can be done, however, for many musculoskeletal disorders, to help improve the older person's function and provide for a better quality of life[48].

References

1. Loeser RF Jr. Evaluation of musculoskeletal complaints in the older adult. *Clin Geriatr Med* 1998;14:401–15
2. Calkins E, Vladutiu AO. Musculoskeletal disorders. In Duthie EH Jr, Katz PR, eds. *Duthie: Practice of Geriatrics*, 3rd edn. Philadelphia: WB Saunders, 1998:421–35
3. Creamer P, Flores R, Hochberg MC. Management of osteoarthritis in older adults. *Clin Geriatr Med* 1998;14:435–54
4. Loeser RF Jr. Aging and the etiopathogenesis and treatment of osteoarthritis. *Rheum Dis Clin North Am* 2000;26: 547–67
5. Hamerman D. The biology of osteoarthritis. *N Engl J Med* 1989;320: 1322–30
6. Dharmarajan TS, Ugalino JT. The aging process. In Dreger D, Krumm B, eds. *Hospital Physician: Geriatric Medicine Board Review Manual*. Wayne, PA: Turner White Communications, 2000;1:2–12
7. McGann PE. Geriatric assessment for the rheumatologist. *Rheum Dis Clin North Am* 2000;26:415–32
8. Dearborn JT, Jergesen HE. The evaluation and initial management of arthritis. *Primary Care* 1996;23:215–40

9. Ling SM, Bathon JM. Osteoarthritis in older adults. *J Am Geriatr Soc* 1998;46:216–25

10. Recommendations for the medical management of osteoarthritis of the hip and knee: 2000 update. American College of Rheumatology Subcommittee on Osteoarthritis Guidelines. *Arthritis Rheum* 2000; 43:1905–15

11. Sculco TP. Orthopedic disorders. In Duthi EH Jr, Katz PR, eds. *Duthie: Practice of Geriatrics*, 3rd edn. Philadelphia: WB Saunders, 1998:436–47

12. Shamoon M, Hochberg MC. The role of acetaminophen in the management of patients with osteoarthritis. *Am J Med* 2001;110:46–9

13. American Geriatrics Society. The management of chronic pain in older persons: AGS Panel on Chronic Pain in Older Persons. *J Am Geriatr Soc* 1998;46:635–51

14. Messier SP, Loeser RF, Mitchell MN, *et al.* Exercise and weight loss in obese older adults with knee osteoarthritis: a preliminary study. *J Am Geriatr Soc* 2000;48: 1062–72

15. Manek NJ. Medical management of osteoarthritis. *Mayo Clin Proc* 2001;76: 533–9

16. Minor MA, Lane NE. Recreational exercise in arthritis. *Rheum Dis Clin North Am* 1996;22:563–77

17. Messier SP, Royer TD, Craven TE, O'Toole ML, Burns R, Ettinger WH Jr. Long-term exercise and its effect on balance in older, osteoarthritic adults: results from the Fitness, Arthritis, and Seniors Trial (FAST). *J Am Geriatr Soc* 2000;48:131–8

18. Conn DL, Arnold WJ, Hollister JR. Alternative treatments and rheumatic diseases. *Bull Rheum Dis* 1999;48:1–3

19. Hirsh MJ, Lozada CJ. Medical management of osteoarthritis. *Hosp Physic* 2002;38:57–66

20. Todd C. Meeting the therapeutic challenge of the patient with osteoarthritis. *J Am Pharm Assoc* 2002;42:74–82

21. Sewell KL. Rheumatoid arthritis in older adults. *Clin Geriatr Med* 1998;14:475–94

22. Silverstein FE, Faich G, Goldstein JL, *et al.* Gastrointestinal toxicity with celecoxib vs nonsteroidal anti-inflammatory drugs for osteoarthritis and rheumatoid arthritis: the CLASS study: a randomized controlled trial. Celecoxib Long-term Arthritis Safety Study. *J Am Med Assoc* 2000;284:1247–55

23. Whelton A. Renal aspects of treatment with conventional nonsteroidal anti-inflammatory drugs versus cyclooxygenase-2-specific inhibitors. *Am J Med* 2001;110 (3 suppl 1):33–42

24. Buttgereit F, Burmester GR, Simon LS. Gastrointestinal toxic side effects of nonsteroidal anti-inflammatory drugs and cyclooxygenase-2-specific inhibitors. *Am J Med* 2001;110(3 suppl 1):13–19

25. Lipsky PE. Recommendations for the clinical use of cyclooxygenase-2-specific inhibitors. *Am J Med* 2001;110(3 Suppl 1): 3–5

26. FitzGerald GA. Cardiovascular pharmacology of nonselective nonsteroidal anti-inflammatory drugs and coxibs: clinical considerations. *Am J Cardiol* 2002;89: 26D–32D

27. Towheed TE, Anastassiades TP. Glucosamine and chondroitin for treating symptoms of osteoarthritis: evidence is widely touted but incomplete. *J Am Med Assoc* 2000;283:1483–4

28. Moseley JB, O'Malley K, Petersen NJ, *et al.* A controlled trial of arthroscopic surgery for osteoarthritis of the knee. *New Engl J Med* 2002;347:81–8

29. Felson DT, Buckwalter J. Debridement and lavage for osteoarthritis of the knee. *New Engl J Med* 2002;347:132–3

30. Yazici Y, Paget SA. Elderly-onset rheumatoid arthritis. *Rheum Dis Clin North Am* 2000;26:517–26

31. Mishra N, Kammer GM. Clinical expression of autoimmune diseases in older adults. *Clin Geriatr Med* 1998;14:515–42

32. O'Dell JR. Combinations of conventional disease-modifying antirheumatic drugs. *Rheum Dis Clin North Am* 2001;27:415–26

33. Cohen S, Cannon GW, Schiff M, *et al.* Two-year, blinded, randomized, controlled trial of treatment of active rheumatoid arthritis with leflunomide compared with methotrexate. Utilization of Leflunomide in the Treatment of Rheumatoid Arthritis

Trial Investigator Group. *Arthritis Rheum* 2001;44:1984–92

34. Gonzalez FB. Management of rheumatoid arthritis in the elderly. *Clin Geriatr* 2002; 10:34–47

35. Breedveld FC. Current and future management approaches for rheumatoid arthritis. *Arthrit Res* 2002;4(Supplement 2):S16–21

36. Agudelo CA, Wise CM. Crystal-associated arthritis in the elderly. *Rheum Dis Clin North Am* 2000;26:527–46

37. Schumacher RH Jr. Crystal arthropathies in the elderly: gout (monosodium urate) and calcium pyrophosphate dihydrate disease. In Hazzard WR, Blass JP, Ettinger WH Jr, *et al.*, eds. *Principles of Geriatric Medicine and Gerontology*, 4th edn. New York: McGraw-Hill, 1998:1163–73

38. Lyles KW. Hyperparathyroidism and Paget's disease of bone. In Hazzard WR, Blass JP, Ettinger WH Jr, *et al.*, eds. *Principles of Geriatric Medicine and Gerontology*, 4th edn. New York: McGraw-Hill, 1998: 1085–96

39. Kammer GM, Mishra N. Systemic lupus erythematosus in the elderly. *Rheum Dis Clin North Am* 2000;26:475–92

40. Barkhuizen A, Campbell SM. Pulmonary involvement in common rheumatologic diseases in the elderly. *Immunol Allergy Clin North Am* 1997;17:727–44

41. al-Hashimi I. The management of Sjögren's syndrome in dental practice. *J Am Dent Assoc* 2001;132:1409–17

42. McCarty DJ, O'Duffy JD, Pearson L, Hunter JB. Remitting seronegative symmetrical synovitis with pitting edema. RS3PE syndrome. *J Am Med Assoc* 1985; 254:2763–7

43. Holland NW, Gonzalez EB. Soft tissue problems in older adults. *Clin Geriatr Med* 1998;14:601–11

44. Winfield JB. Pain in fibromyalgia. *Rheum Dis Clin North Am* 1999;25:55–79

45. Wolfe F, Smythe HA, Yunus MB, *et al.* The American College of Rheumatology 1990 criteria for the classification of fibromyalgia: report of the multicenter criteria committee. *Arthritis Rheum* 1990;33: 160–72

46. Daigneault J, Cooney LM Jr. Shoulder pain in older people. *J Am Geriatr Soc* 1998;46: 1144–51

47. O'Rourke KS. Bursitis, tendinitis, back pain, and related disorders. In Hazzard WR, Blass JP, Ettinger WH Jr, *et al.*, eds. *Principles of Geriatric Medicine and Gerontology*, 4th edn. New York: McGraw-Hill, 1998:1175–90

48. Erkan D, Yazici Y, Paget SA. Inflammatory musculoskeletal diseases in the elderly: part 2. *J Musculoskel Med* 2002;19:320–9

47 Geriatric oral health

Jonathan A. Ship, DMD

INTRODUCTION

The oral cavity serves three essential functions in human physiology: the production of speech; the initiation of alimentation; and protection of the host. In order to fulfill these functions, many specialized tissues have evolved in the oral–facial region (Table 1). The teeth, the periodontium and the muscles of mastication prepare food for deglutition. The tongue, besides occupying a central role in communication, is also a key participant in food bolus preparation and translocation. Salivary glands secrete a fluid that lubricaties and protects all oral mucosal tissues, and helps fashion the developing food bolus into a swallow-acceptable form.

The oral cavity is vulnerable to a limitless number of environmental insults, and therefore extensive mechanisms have evolved to protect the mouth and permit normal oral function. Robust sensory systems (taste, thermal, textural, tactile and pain discrimination) contribute to enjoyment of food and alert the host about potential problems. Saliva also has an important protective role and contains a broad spectrum of antimicrobial proteins that modulate oral microbial colonization and protect the functional integrity of the teeth.

All of these tissue activities are finely co-ordinated and a disturbance in any one function can significantly compromise speech, alimentation and protection of the host, and can diminish the quality of a person's life (Table 2). The passage of time (aging) has a moderate negative impact on some but not all of these functions. Importantly, however, numerous acute and chronic medical problems as well as their treatments (e.g. medications, radiation therapy, chemotherapy), particularly in the older adult, have a much greater deleterious impact on oral health and function[1,2]. This chapter provides a brief overview on the effects of aging and systemic diseases on the oral tissues (Table 3). It also briefly reviews the evaluation and management of dental, periodontal, oral mucosal and salivary gland disorders commonly observed in older adults.

THE DENTITION

National (USA) health surveys on adults aged 65+ years demonstrate an edentulous prevalence of 40%, and this group has, on average, 11 missing teeth[3]. Edentulousness has dramatically decreased over the past 40 years, due to advances in dental treatment, disease prevention, increased availability of dental care and improved awareness of dental needs[4]. However, partial and complete tooth loss still affects the vast majority of older adults, which can adversely affect phonation, mastication, deglutition and facial esthetics. Tooth loss is attributed to two major etiologic processes: dental caries and periodontal diseases (see below)[5]. Caries

Table 1 Tissues of the oral–facial region and their functions

Oral tissue	Function
Teeth	mastication, bone regeneration
Periodontium	mastication, bone regeneration, host defense
Salivary glands	lubrication, buffering acids, antimicrobial activity, mechanical cleansing, mediation of taste, remineralization of teeth, oral mucosal repair
Taste buds	taste, host defense
Oral mucosa	host defense, mastication, swallowing, speech
Muscles of mastication and facial expression, and the temporomandibular joint	mastication, swallowing, speech, posture

Table 2 Clinical manifestations of oral diseases

Disease	Oral manifestations
Dental and periodontal infections	
Dental caries	soft to hard discolored defect on tooth surface
Gingivitis and periodontitis	erythematous, edematous and hemorrhagic gingiva, which may be accompanied by gingival recession and tooth mobility
Viral infections	
Primary herpes simplex	clear to yellow vesicles rupture and form shallow, painful ulcers. Gingival tissues are inflamed, edematous and painful
Recurrent herpes simplex	burning or tingling prodrome in lesion sites (lip, hard palate, attached gingiva). Whitish-gray vesicles rupture to form painful ulcers which then develop a crust
Herpes zoster	vesicular eruptions (usually unilateral) in areas following the distribution of ophthalmic, maxillary or mandibular divisions of trigeminal sensory nerves
Cytomegalovirus	mononucleosis-like symptoms, petechial hemorrhages, enlarged salivary glands, pharyngotonsillitis
Fungal infections	
Pseudomembranous candidiasis	soft, white/yellow plaques can be wiped off to expose an underlying erythematous mucosa
Acute atrophic candidiasis	painful erythematous oral mucosal lesions. Tongue appears 'bald'
Chronic atrophic candidiasis	diffuse inflammation of denture-bearing areas
Angular cheilitis	erythematous cracked or fissured lesions at the lip commissures
Salivary gland infections	
Acute sialoadenitis	tender salivary gland swelling with purulent discharge upon palpation of the gland duct
Chronic sialoadenitis	recurrent, tender swellings of salivary gland progresses to firm and atrophic gland

affects the exposed dental surfaces, and periodontal diseases are confined to the supporting bony and ligamentous dental structures. With current trends of increasing tooth retention in aging populations, there is a correspondingly greater risk for the development of both of these disease entities[6].

There are two classifications of dental caries, depending upon the dental surface affected. Coronal caries, which is characteristic of caries in young adults and children, occurs when the enamel and dentin of the coronal portion of the tooth are affected (Figure 1). In older adults, if gingival recession or periodontal disease cause the root surfaces of the tooth to become exposed to the oral environment, root surface or cervical caries may occur[7]. *Streptococcus* (most commonly

Table 3 Oral–pharyngeal processes in older adults

Process	Healthy older adults	Medically compromised older adults
Taste	unaffected	diminished
Smell	diminished	diminished
Food enjoyment	unaffected	diminished
Salivary output	unaffected	diminished
Chewing efficiency	slightly diminished	diminished
Swallowing	slightly diminished	diminished

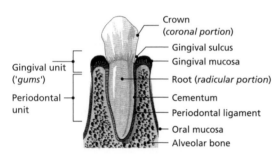

Crown (*coronal portion*)
Gingival sulcus
Gingival mucosa
Root (*radicular portion*)
Cementum
Periodontal ligament
Oral mucosa
Alveolar bone

Gingival unit ('*gums*')
Periodontal unit

Figure 1 Dental and periodontal anatomy

Streptococcus mutans), *Actinomyces* and *Lactobacillus* organisms are found in dental plaque and are the cause of dental caries. As the dentate individual ages, there is susceptibility to coronal caries due to recurrent decay around existing restored surfaces, and the prevalence of root surface caries increases due to greater gingival recession[8].

Dental caries appears as darkish lesions, frequently associated with dental plaque[9]. Caries may not be painful until the destructive process affects the neurovascular structures subserving the tooth. When detected early, caries can be debrided from a tooth and the missing tooth structure restored with a wear-resistant, insoluble dental material (e.g. silver amalgam, composite resin). Untreated dental caries, however, will in most circumstances progress to severe or even total loss of tooth structure, and possibly pain, abscess formation, cellulitis and bacteremia. Endodontic therapy or complete extraction is required if caries has extended into the dental neurovascular or alveolar bone-supporting tissues.

Prevention strategies are identical to those employed in younger individuals: fluoride, daily oral hygiene and regular dental examinations[10,11]. Continuous exposure to fluoride via water supplies, dentifrices and mouth rinses is necessary throughout a person's lifetime[12]. Older adults at greater risk for developing new and recurrent dental caries have: sensory and motor problems that inhibit adequate oral hygiene; gingival recession exposing tooth cementum to plaque and caries-causing microbes; salivary dysfunction secondary to medications, diseases, and head and neck radiotherapy; and inadequate access to preventive and interceptive professional oral health-care services.

THE PERIODONTIUM

The periodontium consists of those tissues that invest and support the tooth (Figure 1). Gingivitis occurs when the gingival unit is inflamed. Periodontitis (or periodontal disease) exists when there is inflammation and appreciable loss of the attachment apparatus due to the presence of pathogenic microorganisms. Microbial species, particularly Gram-negative anaerobes[13], cross the gingival epithelium and enter subepithelial tissues, where they activate specific host defense mechanisms[14]. Eventually this causes tissue destruction, including bone loss and tooth morbidity.

Gingivitis is identified by edematous and inflamed gingival tissues surrounding the tooth. It is frequently accompanied by dental plaque accumulations at the gingival–dental interface. Spontaneous bleeding from the gingival sulcus is a sign of severe gingivitis. Gingival recession appears as an apical migration of gingival tissues, exposing the root surface of the tooth. The tooth will appear longer, with enlarged interdental spaces. Periodontitis is frequently associated with gingivitis, and extensive gingival recession is a sign of significant attachment loss. Periodontal infections can produce a serous exudate from the gingival sulcus, and/or fistula tracts in the alveolar supporting bone. Bleeding gingival tissues are an early sign of gingivitis, and mobile teeth are late signs of periodontal diseases. Importantly, many cases of periodontitis remain asymptomatic until the development of severe periodontal and bone abscesses.

Older adults show a gradual increase in accumulation of dental plaque and calculus (calcified dental plaque), as well as in the frequency of bleeding gingival tissues[15]. The prevalence of gingival recession increases moderately with aging, and periodontal attachment loss occurs at small increments in all age cohorts[16]. Periodontitis is more prevalent and usually more extensive among African-Americans, adults with less education and those who have not seen a dentist recently, as well as those with gingivitis and certain pathogenic organisms[17]. However, many systemic diseases and therapeutic regimens common to older individuals adversely affect periodontal health[18]. Several classes of medication (calcium channel blockers, phenytoin and cyclosporin) have been associated with gingival overgrowth or gingival hyperplasia, a condition that, left untreated, predisposes to both caries and destructive periodontitis. Diabetes, particularly poorly controlled glycemia, has been associated with destructive periodontal disease[19]. Immunosuppression due to infectious diseases, medications for immune-mediated diseases and agents to prevent organ transplant rejection all predispose adults to rapidly progressing periodontal infections. Therefore, the older medically compromised adult is susceptible to developing periodontal diseases and is at risk for associated dental-alveolar infections, pain and tooth loss.

Periodontal diseases also have systemic effects on health[20,21]. Untreated periodontitis has been reported to interfere with blood glucose control in diabetics[22,23]. Associations have also been suggested between cardiovascular disease and periodontitis after controlling for such traditional risk factors as weight, gender, tobacco use, age and blood lipid levels[24,25]. Gram-negative bacteria are implicated in the pathogenesis of periodontal disease, and colonization of the oropharynx with Gram-negative bacilli predisposes to pneumonia[26]. Aspiration pneumonia can occur when oropharyngeal secretions are aspirated into the lungs, causing infection, a condition exacerbated by salivary hypofunction[27].

Treatment of gingivitis and periodontitis begins with tooth brushing and flossing after each meal. Electric tooth brushes and mechanical irrigation systems will assist older patients who have motor and/or cognitive disorders[28]. Antimicrobial oral rinses, such as chlorhexidine gluconate 0.12%, are helpful for gingivitis. Periodontal therapy ranges from conservative (e.g. dental prophylaxis) to surgical techniques (e.g. debridement, excision of hyperplastic tissue), depending upon the extent of periodontal infection and bony destruction. Topical and/or systemic antimicrobial therapy may be warranted to reduce microbial colonization of the periodontal attachment apparatus and to diminish the destructive process initiated by pathogens and propagated by the local immune system[29,30]. Periodontal healing following surgery tends to be slower in even healthy older persons, yet long-term results from periodontal therapy are indistinguishable from those of younger adults[31]. The decision either to save the dentition and restore periodontal health, or to extract teeth with moderate periodontal disease should be determined after all oral and systemic factors have been evaluated[32].

Table 4 Etiology of salivary dysfunction in older adults

Category	Examples
Medications	anticholinergics
	antidepressants
	antihistaminics
	antihypertensives
	anti-Parkinsonisms
	anxiolytics
	diuretics
Oncological therapy	cytotoxic chemotherapy
	head and neck radiotherapy
Oral diseases	acute and chronic bacterial and viral infections
	obstruction
	traumatic lesions
	neoplasms
Systemic diseases	Alzheimer's disease
	cerebrovascular accidents
	diabetes mellitus
	dehydration
	Parkinson's disease
	Sjögren's syndrome
	systemic lupus erythematosus

Therefore, the health of a person, rather than age *per se*, should be the determinant of the extent of periodontal treatment.

SALIVARY GLANDS

Three major pairs of salivary glands (parotid, submandibular, sublingual) and hundreds of minor glands (located in the lips, palate and buccal mucosa) have the principal function of salivary production. Saliva's most important functions are the lubrication of the oral mucosa, promoting remineralization of teeth, and protection against microbial infections. Although the role of saliva in digestion is limited, saliva helps prepare the food bolus for deglutition, and is responsible for dissolving tastants and delivering them to taste buds[33].

Many older individuals have a dry mouth and complain of xerostomia[34,35]. However, recent studies have revealed that, in general, there are no major changes in the quality or quantity of saliva produced from the salivary glands across the human life span in healthy adults[36,37]. Salivary hypofunction and complaints of a dry mouth should not be considered to be normal sequelae of aging, but rather are indicative of oral and systemic diseases and/or their treatment (Table 4). The most frequent etiology of salivary gland dysfunction is iatrogenic[38]. Many medications taken by older persons reduce or alter salivary gland performance[39]. Additionally, common forms of oncologic therapy, such as radiation for head and neck neoplasms and cytotoxic chemotherapy, can have direct and dramatic deleterious effects on salivary glands. The most common disease affecting salivary glands is Sjögren's syndrome, an autoimmune exocrinopathy predominantly occurring in postmenopausal women[40]. Alzheimer's and Parkinson's diseases, diabetes and dehydration have also been associated with salivary dysfunction. In addition, a variety of oral inflammatory and obstructive salivary gland disorders (e.g. acute and recurrent bacterial infections or sialadenitis, sialoliths, trauma, neoplasms) will result in reduced gland function.

The clinical appearance of salivary hypofunction is characterized by desiccated and cracked lips, tongue and other oral mucosal surfaces[33]. The tongue, hard palate and buccal mucosa may be erythemic, edematous and shiny. Masses due to obstruction, infections and neoplasms can be palpated in the lips, palate, floor of the mouth, buccal mucosa and parotid regions. Fungal infections are more likely to develop, and may appear as leukoplakic plaques that can be removed or erythemic regions beneath removable prostheses. Dental caries is more prevalent, and dental plaque is likely to be visible on tooth surfaces. Patients will complain of difficulty chewing, swallowing and tasting, and impaired retention of removable dental prostheses.

Treatment begins with identification of the etiology[33,38]. Microbial infections require appropriate antibiotic therapy (amoxicillin with or without clavulanate, cephalosporins). Tumors require diagnosis after tissue biopsy, and complete excision. Neoplasms may require post-surgical radiotherapy, particularly if regional lymph node and neurovascular spread has occurred. Medication-induced salivary problems may be eliminated by stopping drug use, modifying drug use and dosage, or substituting one drug with another that has fewer anticholinergic side-effects[39]. Even when no reduction in the daily dose is recommended, the splitting of a dose into several smaller and more frequently taken doses may alleviate or diminish the sensation of oral dryness.

Salivary stimulation is helpful in the patient who has remaining salivary function. Gustatory (sugarless mints, candies), masticatory (sugarless gums) and pharmacological (pilocarpine hydrochloride 5 mg four times a day or cevimeline hydrochloride 30 mg three times a day) therapies can be useful. Salivary substitutes, rinses and moisturizing gels will assist the patient who has little or no remaining function. Prevention of dry mouth problems is essential, with the frequent use of sugarless beverages, topical fluorides and regular oral hygiene after meals. Removable prostheses must be kept clean, and out of the mouth during sleeping hours. Frequent lubrication of the lips will help prevent lip cracking and infections. Finally, clinicians prescribing one or more medications that adversely affect salivary function should be cognizant of the potential oral sequelae from these agents.

THE ORAL MUCOSAL TISSUES

The primary function of the oral mucosa is to act as a barrier protecting the underlying structures from desiccation, noxious chemicals, trauma, thermal stress and infection. Aging has been frequently associated with changes in the oral mucosa, similar to those in the skin, with the epithelium becoming thinner, less hydrated and thus supposedly more susceptible to injury[41,42]. Clinical investigations have demonstrated that age *per se* has no effect on the clinical appearance of the oral mucosa[43]. However, there is considerable evidence to suggest that the utilization of removable prostheses has a potentially adverse effect on the health of the oral mucosa[44]. The denture-bearing mucosa of aged maxillary and mandibular ridges shows significant morphologic changes. Ill-fitting dentures can produce mechanical trauma to the oral tissues, as well as causing mucosal hyperplasia. Oral candidiasis is frequently found on denture-bearing areas in the edentulous individual, often occurring with angular cheilitis (deep fissuring and ulceration of the epithelium at the commissures of the mouth)[45]. Therefore, the clinician should ask the patient to remove all removable prostheses in order to conduct an adequate oral examination.

Oral mucosal alterations in the older person are often a result of multiple oral and systemic factors[46] (Table 5). Numerous medications have been associated with oral mucosal changes[46]. For example, long-term utilization of antibiotics will frequently result in oral

Table 5 Conditions associated with oral mucosal changes

Classification	Disease/disorder	Examples
Oral conditions	infections	candidiasis, herpes simplex, herpes zoster
	ulcerative conditions	recurrent aphthous stomatitis
	periodontal diseases	gingivitis, periodontitis
	prosthodontic problems	poorly fitting dentures
	salivary gland dysfunction	desiccated oral tissues
	food allergies	cinammon allergy
	social habits	tobacco and alcohol consumption
	trauma	traumatic fibroma, mucocele
Systemic diseases	dermatologic disorders	systemic lupus erythematosus, lichen planus, pemphigus vulgaris, cicatricial pemphigoid, erythema multiforme
	endocrine disorders	diabetes mellitus
	cancer	oral and pharyngeal cancers
	neurologic disorders	Alzheimer's disease, Parkinson's disease, CVA
	immunocompromising disorders	HIV, AIDS, rheumatoid arthritis
Medical therapies	medications	diuretics, antibiotics, immunomodulating drugs
	head and neck radiotherapy	head and neck radiotherapy
	cytotoxic chemotherapy	methotrexate, 5-FU, cyclosporin

CVA, cerebrovascular accident; 5-FU, 5-fluorouracil

Table 6 Treatment of common vesiculobullous and erosive diseases in older adults

Medication	Regimen
Topical treatments[*,†,‡]	
Fluocinonide gel 0.05%	
Triamcinolone acetonide in gel base 0.1%	Apply to affected regions three times a day and qhs
Clobetasol propionate gel 0.05%	
Oral rinses[†,‡,**]	
Dexamethasone elixir 0.5 mg/5 ml	Rinse and spit 10 ml four times a day for 5 min
Diphenhydramine elixir 12.5 mg/5 ml	
Dyclonine HCl 1%	
Systemic medications[†,††]	
Prednisone 5 mg	12 tabs qod for 2 days, decreasing by 2 tabs every other day
Azathioprine 50 mg	1 tab twice a day

[*] If extensive gingival lesions are present, use with a custom-fabricated tray
[†] Oral candidiasis may result and concomitant antifungal therapy may be necessary
[‡] Taper as indicated by clinical response
[**] Can be combined in a 1:1 mixture with sucralfate, kaopectate, or maalox
[††] Dose and duration depend on severity of disease and concomitant systemic diseases. Azathioprine in combination with prednisone permits use of lower doses of prednisone

candidal infections, while drugs with xerostomic side-effects (see above) will likewise increase the potential for mucosal injury[47]. Drugs commonly used in older patients for arthritic conditions, hypertension, cardiac arrhythmias, seizures and dementia have been associated with lichenoid reactions[48]. Withdrawal of a causative drug usually results in complete resolution of the lesion within 2–3 weeks, but if there is no clinical improvement, a tissue biopsy is required in order to obtain a definitive diagnosis.

Numerous oral mucosal disorders affect the elderly, ranging from benign (e.g. recurrent aphthous ulcers, traumatic lesions) to malignant (e.g. squamous cell carcinomas)[49]. The diagnosis of mucosal diseases requires a detailed history and a thorough head and neck and oral examination including all mucosal tissues[50]. Oral mucosal lesions present with diverse colors (red, white, blue, brown, black) and surface characteristics (ulcers, erosions, pedunculated or sessile masses, smooth, papillated or atrophic surfaces). For vesiculobullous and erosive diseases, a simple three-item classification is helpful: acute multiple lesions (e.g. erythema multiforme, herpetic gingivostomatitis, herpes zoster, allergic reaction); recurring oral ulcers (e.g., recurrent aphthous stomatitis, traumatic ulcer, herpes labialis); and chronic multiple lesions (e.g., pemphigus vulgaris, cicatricial pemphigoid, lupus, lichen planus, dysplasia, squamous cell carcinoma). If a lesion does not resolve after 2–3 weeks, then a tissue biopsy is required[51]. For lesions suspected of being oral manifestations of autoimmune connective tissue disorders (e.g. pemphigus, pemphigoid, lichen planus), biopsies should also include specimens for direct immunofluorescence. If trauma is suspected, due to an injury or an ill-fitting denture, removal of the etiology should allow the lesion to heal. Many of these conditions have an immunologic etiology, and therefore management strategies involve topical and/or systemic immunomodulating agents[52] (Table 6).

The oral mucosal disease with the greatest potential morbidity and mortality is cancer. Approximately 2.2% of all cancers are from the head and neck region. There are 30 000 newly diagnosed cases each year in the USA, and they account for over 8000 deaths/year[53]. The strongest risk factors for developing oral cancer are age, and alcohol and tobacco use, with 95% of all oral cancers occurring in persons over 50 years of age[54]. The average age at the time of diagnosis is about 60 years, and males are more than twice as likely to develop oral cancer than females. While attempts to diagnose and treat oral cancer have improved in the past 30 years, 5-year survival rates have not improved dramatically, and the average 5-year survival rate is only about 50%[55].

Neoplasms may arise in all oral soft and hard tissues, and oropharyngeal and salivary gland regions[54,55]. The clinical appearance of an oral carcinoma is quite diverse (ulcerative, erythematous, leukoplakic, papillary), and may be innocuous as well as asymptomatic. If a patient presents with an unusual and suspicious lesion, with no readily apparent etiology (such as with a denture sore), the patient should be referred to a specialist more familiar with the appearance of the oral mucosa. Carcinoma should be considered as part of the differential diagnosis of any oral lesion.

Oral cancer therapy involves surgery, radiotherapy, chemotherapy, or a combination of any of these three modalities, depending upon histological diagnosis, location and stage of the tumor[56]. Prior to oncologic therapy, the patient should receive a comprehensive oral examination so that focal areas of infection or potential infection (dental caries, periodontal disease, dental-alveolar infections, soft and hard tissue lesions) can be treated[57]. The patient must be educated about many potential risks: surgery-related sensory, aesthetic and functional problems; radiotherapy-induced mucositis, salivary gland dysfunction and osteoradionecrosis; chemotherapy-induced mucositis and immunosuppression.

THE TEMPOROMANDIBULAR JOINT AND MUSCLES OF MASTICATION

The oral motor apparatus is involved in several routine yet intricate functions (speech, posture, mastication and swallowing). Regulation of these activities may occur at three levels: the local neuromuscular unit, central neuronal pathways and systemic influences. In general, aging is associated with changes in neuromuscular systems, and investigations of oral motor function have shown that some alterations in performance (mastication, swallowing, oral muscular posture and tone) can be expected with increased age[58]. Neurologic disorders that can produce sensory and motor disturbances (e.g. strokes, Alzheimer's disease, Parkinson's disease) will adversely affect oral motor function[2]. Several medications have deleterious sequelae to the oral motor apparatus, such as the frequent association of tardive dyskinesia with phenothiazine therapy[6]. These dyskinesias may include diminished performance and speech pathoses as well as alteration in movement (chorea, athetosis).

Edentulousness has been implicated in oral motor disorders, and the most common manifestation is diminished masticatory efficiency[59]. Older persons are more likely to be partially or completely edentulous than other age groups, and therefore the geriatric population is susceptible to altered chewing[6]. It has also been reported that older persons tend to swallow larger-sized food particles than do younger adults[60]. Therefore, older and particularly edentulous adults are more likely to experience chewing and swallowing problems, which can predispose this population to aspiration pneumonia. In summary, the majority of research findings suggest that dentition, not age *per se*, has a direct influence on mastication.

The temporomandibular joint (TMJ) is located between the glenoid fossa of the temporal bone and the condylar process of the mandible. The TMJ exhibits a unique gliding and hinge-like movement, and is the focus of a variety of craniofacial pain disorders. Several joint components undergo mild age-related degenerative alterations. However, TMJ disorders are more likely related to oral and systemic conditions commonly seen in the elderly[61]. In general, two types of pathology are associated with the TMJ: articular, related to the joint itself, and non-articular, pathology occurring in structures unrelated to the joint but causing similar or referred symptomatology[62]. Many types of articular abnormalities, common to all joints, affect the TMJ, including trauma, ankylosis, dislocation and arthritis. Non-articular disorders may result from a variety of clinical entities including trigeminal neuralgia, dental pulpitis, otitis and masticatory myalgia. Orofacial habits (e.g. jaw clenching and tooth grinding) and poor head and neck posture can produce muscle fatigue and subsequent spasm. Moreover, psychological conditions (stress, depression) can exacerbate underlying articular or non-articular disorders.

Patients will present with pain in the TMJ, temporal, cervical, or neck region, masticatory muscles and oral cavity[63]. Limited jaw opening and pain upon mastication or during jaw movements may be indicative of TMJ disorders. Treatment, as with other arthritic or muscular disorders, requires establishment of an appropriate diagnosis. Therapy ranges from conservative and reversible (anti-inflammatory medications, skeletal muscle relaxants, physical therapy, oral bite splints) to more invasive procedures for unresolved painful conditions (e.g. TMJ surgery).

SUMMARY

The health of the oral cavity and its ability to fulfill its function of communication, nutritional intake and host protection can be impaired in older adults. Age alone does not appear to play a strong role in the impairments. Rather, oral and systemic diseases and the treatment of medical problems compromise oral health and function. This will predispose an older person to develop oral microbial infections, pain, altered chemosensation, dysphagia, difficulty chewing and speaking, greater risk for disseminated systemic infections and, importantly, a diminished quality of life. All health-care providers should attempt to identify older persons at risk for developing oral diseases, be able to recognize existing oral diseases and either treat or refer patients who have stomatological disorders.

References

1. Ghezzi EM, Ship JA. Systemic diseases and their treatments in the elderly: impact on oral health. *J Pub Health Dent* 2000;60: 289–96

2. Chavez EM, Ship JA. Sensory and motor deficits in the elderly: impact on oral health. *J Pub Health Dent* 2000;60:297–303

3. Miller AJ, Brunelle JA, Carlos JP, *et al. Oral Health of United States Adults.* Washington, DC: US Department of Health and Human Services, National Institutes of Health, Public Health Service, 1987

4. Heft MW, Gilbert GH. Tooth loss and caries prevalence in older Floridians attending senior activity centers. *Comm Dent Oral Epidemiol* 1991;19:228–32

5. Burt BA. Epidemiology of dental diseases in the elderly. *Clin Geriatr Med* 1992;8:447–59

6. Shay K, Ship JA. The importance of oral health in the older patient. *J Am Geriatr Soc* 1995;43:1414–22

7. Shay K. Root caries in the older patient: significance, prevention, and treatment. *Dent Clin North Am* 1997;41:763–94

8. Berkey DB, Shay K. General dental care for the elderly. *Clin Geriatr Med* 1992;8: 579–97

9. Ship JA, Kerr HR. Extrinsic and intrinsic causes of tooth discoloration. *eMed J* (serial online) 2001;http://www.emedicine.com/derm/contents.htm

10. Heifetz SB. Fluorides for the elderly. *J Calif Dent Assoc* 1994;22:49–54

11. Winston AE, Bhaskar SN. Caries prevention in the 21st century. *J Am Dent Assoc* 1998;129:1579–87

12. Erickson L. Oral health promotion and prevention for older adults. *Dent Clin North Am* 1997;41:727–50

13. Socransky SS, Haffajee AD, Cugini MA, *et al.* Microbial complexes in subgingival plaque. *J Clin Periodonotol* 1998;25: 134–44

14. Ximenez-Fyvie LA, Haffajee AD, Socransky SS. Comparison of the microbiota of supra and subgingival plaque in subjects in health and periodontitis. *J Clin Periodontol* 2000;27:648–57

15. Burt BA. Periodontitis and aging: reviewing recent evidence. *J Am Dent Assoc* 1994; 125:273–9

16. Ship JA, Beck JD. A ten year longitudinal study of periodontal attachment loss in healthy adults. *Oral Surg Oral Med Oral Pathol Oral Radiol Endo* 1996;81:281–90

17. Beck JD, Slade GD. Epidemiology of periodontal diseases. *Curr Opin Periodontol* 1996;3:3–9

18. Ship JA, Crow HC. Diseases of periodonal tissues in the elderly. Description, epidemiology, aetiology, and drug therapy. *Drugs Aging* 1994;5:346–57

19. Taylor GW. Periodontal treatment and its effects on glycemic control: a review of the evidence. *Oral Surg Oral Med Oral Pathol Oral Radiol Endo* 1999;87:311–16

20. Beck JD, Offendacher S. Oral health and systemic disease: periodontitis and cardiovascular disease. *J Dent Educ* 1998;62: 859–70

21. Garcia RI, Krall EA, Vokonas PS. Periodontal disease and mortality from all causes in the VA Dental Longitudinal Study. *Ann Periodontol* 1998;3:339–49

22. Grossi SG, Genco RJ. Periodontal disease and diabetes mellitus: a two-way relationship. *Ann Periodontol* 1998;3:51–61

23. Taylor GW, Burt BA, Becker MP, *et al.* Severe periodontitis and risk for poor glycemic control in patients with non-insulin-dependent diabetes mellitus. *J Periodontol* 1996;67(10 suppl):1085–93

24. Elter JR, Beck JD, Slade GD, Offenbacher S. Etiologic models for incident periodontal attachment loss in older adults. *J Clin Periodontol* 1999;26:113–23

25. Beck JD, Offenbacher S, Williams R, *et al.* Periodontitis: a risk factor for coronary heart disease? *Ann Periodontol* 1998;3:127–41

26. Loesche WJ, Lopatin DE. Interactions between periodontal disease, medical diseases and immunity in the older individual. *Periodontol 2000* 1998;16:80–105

27. Gibson G, Barrett E. The role of salivary function on oropharyngeal colonization. *Spec Care Dent* 1992;12:153–6

28. Ettinger RL. The unique oral health needs of an aging population. *Dent Clin North Am* 1997;41:633–49

29. Feres M, Haffajee AD, Goncalves C, et al. Systemic doxycycline administration in the treatment of periodontal infections (I). Effect on the subgingival microbiota. *J Clin Periodontol* 1999;26:775–83

30. van Winkelhoff AJ, Rams TE, Slots J. Systemic antibiotic therapy in periodontics. *Periodontol 2000* 1996;10:45–78

31. Lindhe J, Socransky S, Nyman S, et al. Effect of age on healing following periodontal therapy. *J Clin Periodontol* 1985; 12:774–87

32. Berkey DB, Berg RG, Ettinger RL, et al. The old-old dental patient: the challenge of clinical decision-making. *J Am Dent Assoc* 1996;127:321–32

33. Atkinson JC, Wu A. Salivary gland dysfunction: causes, symptoms, treatment. *J Am Dent Assoc* 1994;125:409–16

34. Narhi TO. Prevalence of subjective feelings of dry mouth in the elderly. *J Dent Res* 1994;73:20–5

35. Thomson WM, Chalmers JM, Spencer AJ, Ketabi M. The occurrence of xerostomia and salivary gland hypofunction in a population-based sample of older South Australians. *Spec Care Dent* 1999;19:20–3

36. Ship JA, Nolan N, Puckett S. Longitudinal analysis of parotid and submandibular salivary flow rates in healthy, different aged adults. *J Gerontol Med Sci* 1995;50A: M285–9

37. Wu AJ, Atkinson JC, Fox PC, et al. Cross-sectional and longitudinal analyses of stimulated parotid salivary constituents in healthy different aged subjects. *J Gerontol Med Sci* 1993;48:M219–24

38. Fox PC. Management of dry mouth. *Dent Clin North Am* 1997;41:863–76

39. Sreebny LM, Schwartz SS. A reference guide to drugs and dry mouth – 2nd edition. *Gerodontology* 1997;14:33–47

40. Fox RI, Stern M, Michelson P. Update in Sjögren syndrome. *Curr Opin Rheum* 2000;12:391–8

41. Hill MW, Karthigasan J, Berg JH, Squier CA. Influence of age on the response of oral mucosa to injury. In: Squier CA, Hill MW, eds. *The Effect of Aging in Oral Mucosa and Skin*. Boca Raton, FL: CRC Press, 1994:129–42

42. Williams DM, Cruchley AT. Structural aspects of aging in the oral mucosa. In Squier CA, Hill MW, eds. *The Effect of Aging in Oral Mucosa and Skin*. Boca Raton, FL: CRC Press, 1994:65–74

43. Wolff A, Ship JA, Tylenda CA, et al. Oral mucosal appearance is unchanged in healthy, different-aged individuals. *Oral Surg Oral Med Oral Path* 1991;71: 569–72

44. Nevalainen MJ, Narhi TO, Ainamo A. Oral mucosal lesions and oral hygiene habits in the home-living elderly. *J Oral Rehab* 1997;24:332–7

45. Epstein JB, Polsky B. Oropharyngeal candidiasis: a review of its clinical spectrum and current therapies. *Clin Ther* 1998;20: 40–57

46. Fantasia JE. Diagnosis and treatment of common oral lesions found in the elderly. *Dent Clin North Am* 1997;41:877–90

47. Chaushu G, Bercovici M, Dori S, et al. Salivary flow and its relation with oral symptoms in terminally ill patients. *Cancer* 2000;88:984–7

48. Scully C, Beyli M, Ferreiro MC, et al. Update on oral lichen planus: etiopathogenesis and management. *Crit Rev Oral Biol Med* 1998;9:86–122

49. Ship JA. Geriatric oral medicine. *Alpha Omegan* 2001;94:44–51

50. Scully C, Porter S. ABC of oral health. Swellings and red, white, and pigmented lesions. *Br Med J* 2000;321:225–8

51. Golden DP, Hooley JR. Oral mucosal biopsy procedures. Excisional and incisional. *Dent Clin North Am* 1994;38:279–300

52. Ship JA, Mohammad AR. *Clinician's Guide to Oral Health in Geriatric Patients*, 1st edn. Baltimore, MD: American Academy of Oral Medicine, 1999

53. Greenlee RT, Murray T, Bolden S, Wingo PA. Cancer statistics, 2000. *Cancer J Clin* 2000;50:7–33

54. Ship JA, Chavez EM, Gould KL, et al. Evaluation and management of oral cancer. *Home Health Care Consult* 1999;6: 2–12

55. Silverman SJ. *Oral Cancer*, 4th edn. Hamilton, Canada: The American Cancer Society, 1998

56. Scully C, Epstein JB. Oral health care for the cancer patient. *Oral Oncol* 1996;32B: 281–92

57. Silverman S, Jr. Oral cancer: complications of therapy. *Oral Surg Oral Med Oral Pathol Oral Radiol Endo* 1999;88:122–6

58. Fucile S, Wright PM, Chan I, *et al.* Functional oral-motor skills: do they change with age? *Dysphagia* 1998;13:195–201

59. Gunne HS. Masticatory efficiency and dental state. A comparison between two methods. *Acta Odont Scand* 1985;43: 139–46

60. Feldman RS, Kapur KK, Alman JE, Chauncey HH. Aging and mastication: changes in performance and in the swallowing threshold with natural dentition. *J Am Geriatr Soc* 1980;28:97–103

61. Akerman S, Jonsson K, Kopp S, *et al.* Radiologic changes in temporomandibular, hand, and foot joints of patients with rheumatoid arthritis. *Oral Surg Oral Med Oral Pathol* 1991;72:245–50

62. Kamelchuk LS, Major PW. Degenerative disease of the temporomandibular joint. *J Orofac Pain* 1995;9:168–80

63. Ship JA, Heft M, Harkins S. Oral facial pain in the elderly. In Lomranz J, Mostofsky DI, eds. *Handbook of Pain and Aging*, 1st edn. New York: Plenum Publishing, 1997:321–46

48 Geriatric hypertension

T.S. Dharmarajan, MD, FACP, AGSF, and Lekshmi Dharmarajan, MD, FACP, FACC

INTRODUCTION

Hypertension is amongst the most common medical disorders, afflicting over 60% of those above the age of 60 years and affecting African-Americans, Caucasians and Mexican-Americans alike. In the USA the prevalence of hypertension over the age of 60 is double that of the population as a whole. The Third National and Nutritional Examination Survey (NHANES III) revealed that the prevalence of hypertension in the USA is 71% and 74% for African-American males and females, respectively, and 51% and 50% for male and female Caucasians, in the 60–74 age group. Isolated systolic hypertension is almost entirely a syndrome of the elderly, with a prevalence of less than 1% around age 50 rising to nearly a quarter of the over-80 age group. High blood pressure is associated with considerable morbidity and mortality, as a result of cardiac, cerebral and renal damage. Adequate control of blood pressure has been consistently associated with a reduction of complications particularly with regards to the heart and brain. In spite of data from trials suggesting that blood pressure control is clearly beneficial and cost effective, only 25% of the elderly appear to be well controlled. This is particularly apparent over the age of 70 irrespective of gender. The following discussion supplements several excellent reviews on the subject[1-7].

Recommendations have been put forth periodically by the Joint National Committee (JNC) for prevention, evaluation, detection and treatment of high blood pressure and the National High Blood Pressure Education Program Coordinating Committee, with the last recommendations of JNC VI released in 1997. Other guidelines include the 1999 Canadian Recommendations for the Management of Hypertension and the 1999 World Health Organization–International Society of Hypertension Guidelines for the Management of Hypertension[3]. JNC VI stressed several areas: the importance of risk stratification as part of a treatment strategy, the relevance of risks associated with systolic hypertension and the need for treatment, continued endorsement of lifestyle modification measures and the need to consider specific medications for compelling situations[1].

We have come a long way in the diagnosis and management of hypertension since the stunning news of the death of Franklin D. Roosevelt, President of the USA, in 1945; the blood pressure was around 300 systolic and 190 diastolic prior to his demise, with the final event described as 'a terrific occipital headache and lost consciousness'[8]. Although it is recognized that hypertension is amongst the leading causes for physician visits, that morbidity and mortality from cardiac, renal and cerebral complications are associated with untreated hypertension, and further that treatment substantially lowers this morbidity and mortality, our health-care system

Table 1 Classification of blood pressure (BP) in adults* (JNC VI guidelines; reference 1)

Category	Systolic BP (mmHg)		Diastolic BP (mmHg)
Optimal	< 120	and	< 80
Normal	< 130	and	< 85
High-normal	130–139	or	85–89
Hypertension: stage 1	140–159	or	90–99
Hypertension: stage 2	160–179	or	100–109
Hypertension: stage 3	> 180	or	> 110
Isolated systolic hypertension	> 140	and	< 90

*Not on antihypertensive drugs and not acutely ill

has failed to recognize and treat the disorder adequately. It is time for the health provider to recognize these facts and develop clear strategies and goals.

BLOOD PRESSURE READINGS: NORMAL AND ABNORMAL

Blood pressure readings at the initial visit are recorded in both arms after a rest of 5 min; supine and standing readings are measured. If only a single reading is taken, it may be in the sitting position; the British Hypertension Society recommends this position[7]. Coffee and smoking are avoided in the 30 min prior to measurements. Two readings are taken 2 min apart; if they differ by more than 5 mmHg, a third reading is warranted. An appropriate-sized cuff, based on the arm circumference, should be used. Systolic and diastolic readings are represented by phase I (appearance) and phase V (disappearance) of the Korotkoff sounds[9].

Normal blood pressure in adults is below 130 mmHg for systolic and 85 mmHg diastolic. Additional categories include optimal (below 120/80), high normal and stages 1, 2 and 3 (Table 1). The earlier four-stage JNC recommendations are no longer valid. Normal and abnormal values, including staging, are no different for younger and older adults. Isolated systolic hypertension, particularly common in the geriatric population, is defined as a systolic blood pressure over 140 mmHg with a diastolic blood pressure below 90 mmHg[1].

Blood pressure fluctuates during a 24-h period with readings lower at night and highest in the morning. There is a reduction of 10–20 mmHg in the blood pressure during sleep. Meals and exercise also influence the levels[10].

In addition to the blood pressure readings, an effort should be made to look for the presence or absence of risk factors and target organ damage (Table 2). This enables one to stratify the risk for cardiovascular disease. Initial investigations include complete blood count, serum creatinine, sodium, potassium, glucose and lipids in addition to urinalysis and an electrocardiogram[1,3]. The presence of diabetes places an individual at a higher risk[1].

AGING AND BLOOD PRESSURE

Systolic blood pressure goes up gradually with age because of degenerative changes contributing to vascular stiffening along with diminished ability to excrete salt and reduced baroceptor sensitivity; diastolic pressure, on the other hand plateaus around the fifth decade and may even drop thereafter[11]. In short, the mean systolic blood pressure increases while the mean diastolic pressure decreases with aging[5]. This results in a widening of pulse pressure with aging. The previous definition of isolated systolic hypertension as equal to 100 plus age is no longer valid. Values above 140 mmHg systolic are abnormal in adults at any age.

Orthostatic drop in blood pressure is frequently observed in older adults and may be

Table 2 Components of cardiovascular risk stratification in patients with hypertension

---

Major risk factors
Smoking
Dyslipidemia
Diabetes mellitus
Age > 60 years
Sex (men and postmenopausal women)
Family history of cardiovascular disease:
   women < 65 years or men < 55 years

Target organ damage/clinical cardiovascular disease
Heart diseases
   left ventricular hypertrophy
   angina or prior myocardial infarction
   prior coronary revascularization
   heart failure
Stroke or transient ischemic attack
Nephropathy
Peripheral arterial disease
Retinopathy

Reproduced with permission from: The sixth report of the Joint National Committee on prevention, evaluation, detection, and treatment of high blood pressure. *Arch Intern Med* 1997;157:2419 (Table 4)

a side-effect of medications or a result of illnesses common in the elderly (such as diabetes mellitus, Parkinson's disease or volume depletion). Orthostatic hypotension may be associated with falls, emphasizing the importance of recording standing blood pressure readings before and during therapy[4].

Erratic readings may be obtained because of faulty equipment, observer bias or faulty technique. On the other hand, conditions such as atrial fibrillation, a common arrhythmia in the elderly, leads to variability in both systolic and diastolic readings and consequent difficulty in management[9,12].

PATHOPHYSIOLOGY OF HYPERTENSION IN THE ELDERLY

The pathophysiology of hypertension is complex, and can be variable in each individual. The hallmark is stiffening of blood vessels with increase in peripheral vascular resistance. As a result, it is not unusual to see isolated systolic hypertension with readings of 180/70 mmHg. The renin–angiotensin system may be activated by disease of the renal vasculature (and influenced by medications). Renovascular hypertension is a recognized basis for secondary hypertension in the elderly. However, based on renin measurements, the activity of the renin–angiotensin system in general appears to decline with age. Physiologically, kidney function is altered with greater salt sensitivity and a diminished ability to excrete a sodium load. Insulin resistance and altered calcium metabolism may be contributory[5]. Vasoactive substances implicated include catecholamines (norepinephrine, epinephrine, dopamine), arachidonic acid products (prostaglandins, lipoxygenase enzyme products: leukotrienes), endothelium-derived factors, the kallikrein–kinin system (bradykinin), natriuretic peptides (atrial, brain and C-type) and others such as acetylcholine, serotonin, sex hormones, glucocorticoids, mineralocorticoids, substance P and vasopressin[13].

Hypertension and left ventricular hypertrophy

Even before the blood pressure is elevated, target organ damage occurs. Echocardiographic studies have demonstrated greater interventricular septum and posterior wall thickness, left ventricular mass and cross-sectional area in normotensive boys when the parents were hypertensive. Thus, left ventricular hypertrophy (LVH) occurs early and precedes the development of hypertension; however, LVH does not correlate with the extent of blood pressure elevation. Myocardial remodeling in the form of LVH is a predictor of cardiovascular events, with the severity of hypertrophy correlating with risk of adverse cardiovascular events[14]. Vascular remodeling includes increase in muscle mass (hypertrophy) and dilatation to improve blood flow. Cellular and non-cellular alterations take place with accelerated atherogenesis. All these result in alteration of arterial wall compliance, a function of distensibility or elasticity[15]. LVH is a cardiac adaptation to counter the increase in afterload from hypertension. Antihypertensives (except vasodilators), reduction in body weight and sodium restriction all help lower the blood pressure and achieve a reduction in ventricular mass and thickness. Regression of LVH in the electrocardiogram has been correlated with a lower cardiovascular risk[1].

IS CONTROL OF HYPERTENSION BENEFICIAL IN THE ELDERLY?

Myths and facts

There is plenty of evidence that blood pressure reduction in the elderly, up to age 80, is associated with benefit. The British Hypertension Society (BHS) guidelines stated that 'the absolute benefit from treatment in the elderly is much larger than for younger hypertensives'[16]. Several myths have clouded the management of hypertension in the past few decades. It was believed that control of hypertension in the oldest age group was not indicated and possibly even harmful. Poor perfusion and organ dysfunction (cardiac and cerebral) was feared a consequence. This turned out to be a myth. The fact is that control of hypertension as shown in numerous studies is beneficial, even in the very old. Another unproved myth in the past century was that the diastolic blood pressure is more dangerous to health than systolic blood pressure; the fact is the reverse, in that systolic hypertension is a more powerful risk factor than the diastolic[5].

Trials in the elderly

In the past, meta-analyses of trials in hypertension did not focus on isolated systolic hypertension. A follow-up of 15 693 patients with isolated systolic hypertension from eight trials followed for 3.8 years suggested that the benefit was greater for those aged over 70 years, and that treatment effectively prevented strokes more than cardiovascular events. The conclusion was that treatment for isolated systolic hypertension with a systolic pressure over 160 mmHg was justified[17]. A summary of several select trials on treatment of hypertension in older adults is provided in Table 3[18-23].

SPECIAL CONSIDERATIONS IN THE ELDERLY

Pseudoresistance

Pseudoresistance refers to white coat hypertension, pseudohypertension and elevated readings because of the use of an inadequately sized cuff for an obese arm[1]. It is essential that cuff size be tailored to arm size.

White coat hypertension

White coat hypertension is the elevation of blood pressure readings above usual values in an individual, encountered during clinic visits; ambulatory blood pressure measurements are lower in this situation. Whether organ damage is a consequence in white coat hypertension as in essential hypertension is uncertain. The entity is noted in a quarter or more of hypertensives[24]. A recent British study suggested that white coat hypertension may not be totally benign and that underlying central sympathetic overactivity could result in target organ damage[25].

Pseudohypertension

Pseudohypertension is the falsely elevated readings of blood pressure with indirect standard methods of measurement. Pseudohypertension is suggested by the presence of a positive Osler's maneuver, i.e. a palpable radial or brachial pulse in spite of occlusion by the blood pressure cuff. While the clinical significance of the Osler sign continues to be debated, pseudohypertension appears to exist in the elderly and poses problems in management. Suggestive signs are the absence of target organ damage in spite of poor control of

Table 3 Treatment of hypertension in older patients: data from select trials

---

European Working Party on High Blood Pressure in the Elderly trial (EWPHE)[18]
1972–84, 840 patients, mean age > 60 years
1, Thiazide (and/or triamterene); 2, α-methyl dopa
Reduction in fatal and non-fatal stroke and cardiovascular events

Systolic Hypertension in the Elderly Program (SHEP)[19]
1984–89, 4736 patients, mean age 72 years
1, Chlorthalidone; 2, atenolol
Reduction in stroke in patients with isolated systolic hypertension

Swedish Trial in Old Patients with Hypertension (STOP)[20]
1985–91, 1627 patients, mean age 76 years
1, Atenolol; 2, thiazide + amiloride or metoprolol or pindolol
Reduction in stroke (fatal and non-fatal), myocardial infarction and cardiac deaths

Medical Research Council Trial (MRC)[21]
1987–92, 4396 patients, mean age 70 years
1, Atenolol; 2, thiazide + amiloride; 3, nifedipine
Reduction in stroke

Systolic Hypertension in Elderly in Europe (Syst-Eur)[22]
1990–97, 4695 patients, mean age 70 years
1, Nitrendipine; 2, enalapril; 3, thiazide
Reduction in fatal and non-fatal strokes, and cardiac events

Systolic Hypertension in Elderly Chinese (Syst-China)[23]
1991–96, 2394 patients, mean age 67 years
1, Nitrendipine; 2, captopril; 3, thiazide
Reduction in cardiovascular morbidity and mortality

---

hypertension, orthostatic hypotension with small doses of drug therapy, and a wide pulse pressure. Diagnosis is confirmed by use of simultaneous measurements of cuff pressures and intra-arterial pressure readings[1,4,26]. Recently, brachial oscillometric recordings or finger cuff methods have been found helpful in the diagnosis of pseudohypertension.

Resistant hypertension

While the above causes (pseudohypertension, white coat hypertension) should be considered, resistance or inadequate response to therapy can arise from several causes. These include the ingestion of excess salt, volume overload related to medication or illness, poor compliance, cognitive impairment resulting in failure to take medications as recommended, simultaneous use of other medications that cause drug–drug interactions and/or the presence of a secondary cause (perhaps

unsuspected) for hypertension. Examples of drug interactions playing a role include non-steroidal anti-inflammatory agents (NSAIDs) which may be prescribed and are also available over the counter; they cause salt and fluid retention with worsening of blood pressure control[27]. Cold remedies and decongestants can cause substantial elevation of blood pressure by vascular reactivity. Excessive consumption of alcohol, smoking or illicit drugs may also be contributory. Table 4 offers some of the causes for resistance to treatment.

Blood pressure dysregulation

Blood pressure dysregulation includes swings in blood pressure with posture, meals, exercise and sleep. In the elderly, orthostatic hypotension and postprandial hypotension are particularly problematic and a frequent association with falls and syncope. On standing, the normal response entails a drop in

Table 4 Resistance to pharmacotherapy: possible factors. From reference 1

Pseudohypertension
White coat hypertension
Excessive sodium consumption
Alcoholism
Smoking
Volume overload (due to renal or cardiac disease)
Secondary hypertension, undetected

Drug related
Inadequate dosing of medications
Ineffective doses of diuretics
Adverse drug effect
   sympathomimetics (e.g. cold remedies,
     decongestants)
   non-steroidal anti-inflammatory drugs (NSAIDs)
   cyclosporine
   erythopoietin
   corticosteroids
   licorice
Drug–drug interaction
   angiotensin converting enzyme inhibitors
     and NSAIDs
   diuretics and NSAIDs

systolic blood pressure of less than 10 mmHg and a mild rise in diastolic blood pressure, usually less than 2.5 mmHg. The term orthostatic or postural hypotension is used for a drop in systolic blood pressure of > 20 mmHg and/or a decline in diastolic blood pressure of > 10 mmHg within 3 min of standing[10,28]. Orthostatic hypotension is common in the elderly. Causes vary and include volume depletion, medications, impaired homeostasis and changes in the autonomic nervous system including inappropriate catecholamine responses[10,28]. A Japanese study suggests that orthostatic hypotension is mediated by altered α-adrenergic activity in the elderly; the disorder may be a risk factor for cerebrovascular disease[29].

On the other hand, postprandial hypotension, with a fall in standing systolic blood pressure of over 20 mmHg, typically occurs within 2 h of a large meal. The pathogenesis may be splanchnic pooling of blood associated with impaired baroceptor reflexes. Dizziness, falls and syncope following meals are a consequence here[30].

Orthostatic and postprandial hypotension are associated with falls in any setting, including nursing homes. Revision of medication regimens, timing and content of meals and alteration of activities are measures to address the problem. Pharmacologic agents (midodrine, fludrocortisone, clonidine, octreotide) are available for the treatment of orthostatic and postprandial hypotension, when non-pharmacologic measures are of no avail[30].

The J-curve hypothesis

Concerns have been raised that excessive lowering of blood pressure may compromise diastolic perfusion in the coronaries, increasing the risk of cardiac ischemia. This so-called 'J point', or level at which a risk occurs with drop in blood pressure, has not been substantiated by data from trials; the likelihood is that, in those instances where a morbid event occurred, pre-existing coronary disease existed with hypertension. The increase in adverse events with low blood pressure does not appear to be primarily related to antihypertensive therapy[31]. The current consensus is that the reduction of blood pressure is best achieved to values below 140 mmHg systolic and 90 mmHg diastolic[1,32].

Hypertension, cognition and prevention of dementia

The prevalence and incidence of vascular dementia rises exponentially with age; a history of hypertension appears to be one factor clearly linked with this observation. Hypertension predisposes to the development of cognitive impairment over a period of years to decades. Antihypertensive therapy reduces the development of cerebrovascular events. While the data on control of hypertension and decline in vascular dementia are not consistent in all studies, the Systolic Hypertension in Elderly in Europe (Syst-Eur) trial demonstrated a reduction in the development of dementia by half. There is even a suggestion to incorporate formal cognitive assessment with the Mini-Mental State Examination in the evaluation and treatment of hypertension[33].

Hypertension and surgery

A blood pressure of 180/110 mmHg or higher increases perioperative cardiac risk, warranting reduction in blood pressure and possibly delaying elective surgery. Medications may be administered on the morning of surgery with sips of water. Beta blockers are particularly helpful in the perioperative period and help counter the hyperadrenergic state and may reduce cardiovascular complications[34]. Titration of beta blockers to a resting heart rate of 60 beats/ min is suggested if time permits. Sudden withdrawal of beta blockers or clonidine should be avoided prior to surgery. Calcium channel blockers have been associated with a risk of bleeding[1,34].

Compliance

Failure to take medications appropriately may be dependent on several factors in older adults. Besides financial hardship, other considerations include cognitive impairment, difficulty in swallowing large formulations (because of dysphagia from neurologic causes) and the inability to open (child proof) containers because of diminished dexterity from musculoskeletal impairment. Sometimes one encounters difficulties with the inability to administer long-acting, time-release preparations (that should not be crushed) through feeding tubes. Ensuring the correct timing of medication in relation to meals to avoid drug–nutrient interactions may not be easy, especially for those on tube feeding. Finally, the dependency on caregiver support may pose a problem. These factors should be borne in mind and may influence the antihypertensive prescription to enhance compliance in older adults[35–37].

GERIATRIC HYPERTENSION: SECONDARY CAUSES

While the most common form of hypertension in the elderly is primary or essential hypertension, secondary hypertension should be suspected in the presence of clinical signs or symptoms, abnormal laboratory tests (e.g. unprovoked hypokalemia), sudden onset of hypertension or unexplained change in blood pressure control and resistance to therapy[7]. Common etiologies for secondary hypertension in the elderly include renovascular disease and endocrine causes such as primary aldosteronism[1]. Renovascular hypertension in older adults results from atheroembolic renal disease secondary to atherosclerois or embolic occlusion of renal arteries and arterioles[38,39]. Renovascular disease is also unmasked with worsening of renal function with the use of angiotensin converting enzyme (ACE) inhibitors, when there is more than 70% occlusion of both renal arteries or of a single renal artery (single functioning kidney). This is the basis for the captopril challenge test for the diagnosis of hypertension due to renal artery stenosis[39]. Diminished renal perfusion increases production of renin, which elevates angiotensin II levels. This causes elevation of blood pressure and damages the heart and kidneys. Angiotensin II predisposes to vascular oxidative stress and vasoconstriction[40].

In the presence of unprovoked hypokalemia with hypertension, an adrenal basis must be suspected; an alternative explanation would be the surreptitious use of diuretics or laxatives. Adrenal causes for hypertension include primary aldosteronism, Cushing's syndrome and pheochromocytoma. Hyper- and hypothyroidism can cause secondary hypertension. Medications may play a role in the development of hypertension or lack of response to therapy; several of these are available without a prescription and should be sought for with a focused history[13].

Based on the clues obtained from the history and initial evaluation, further selective

Table 5 Renal hypertension: causes and features

Renal parenchymal disease
Clinical evidence of proteinuria and/or hematuria
Volume excess usually evident
Blood pressure response to salt restriction or diuretics
Renal biopsy to determine etiology

Renovascular disease
Usual cause atheromatous disease or embolism
Less commonly from aneurysm, compression of the renal artery
Unilateral or bilateral
Worsening renal function following administration of angiotensin converting enzyme inhibitors
Onset before age 30 or after 55 years
History of hyperlipidemia, smoking
Evidence of vascular disease elsewhere (cardiac, cerebral, peripheral)
Presence of abdominal (flank) bruit; often bruit not of renal origin
Abnormal renal function, unexplained; hypokalemia may be present
Diagnostic tests using one or more of:
   captopril administration test
   radioisotope scans, with captopril or furosemide challenge
   angiography (gold standard, invasive)
   magnetic resonance angiography
   color Doppler ultrasound
   digital subtraction angiography
   spiral computed tomography
   intravenous pyelogram (falling out of favor)

Miscellaneous renal causes
Obstructive uropathy
Polycystic kidney disease

testing may be indicated for secondary causes of hypertension as described above. Table 5 provides a summary of the clinical features and diagnosis of renal hypertension.

MANAGEMENT

Management of hypertension consists of non-pharmacologic measures and drug therapy; the two approaches should be complementary. Non-pharmacologic measures enhance the benefits of drug treatment, are cost effective and entail little risk. Most important, they also help modify other cardiovascular risk factors. In practice, many older adults find it difficult to make adequate lifestyle changes and may need to resort to drug therapy. There also appear to be substantial variations between physicians in the initial approach to management[3]. Patient and provider preferences may influence decision making.

LIFESTYLE MODIFICATION

While non-pharmacologic measures have been proved to be effective, in most instances the health provider appears to spend very little time counseling patients on this form of therapy. Education regarding lifestyle measures is important, for all subjects, including the geriatric age group. In older adults, this form of therapy has to be coupled with an intent to preserve or improve the quality of life. Table 6 from the JNC VI guidelines offers recommendations for lifestyle modification.

Diet in hypertension

The DASH diet (Dietary Approaches to Stop Hypertension) emphasizes the use of fruits, vegetables, low-fat dairy products, whole grains, poultry, fish and nuts and low

Table 6   Lifestyle modifications for hypertension prevention and management. From reference 1

Lose weight if overweight
Limit alcohol intake to no more than 1 oz (30 ml) of ethanol (eg. 24 oz (720 ml)) of beer, 10 oz (300 ml) of
  wine, or 2 oz (60 ml) of 100-proof whiskey) per day or 0.5 oz (15 ml) of ethanol per day for women and
  lighter-weight people
Increase aerobic physical activity (30–45 min most days of the week)
Reduce sodium intake to no more than 100 mmol/day (2.4 g of sodium or 6 g of sodium chloride)
Maintain adequate intake of dietary potassium (approximately 90 mmol/day)
Maintain adequate intake of dietary calcium and magnesium for general health
Stop smoking and reduce intake of dietary saturated fat and cholesterol for overall cardiovascular health

Reproduced with permission from: The sixth report of the Joint National Committee on prevention, evaluation, detection, and treatment of high blood pressure. *Arch Intern Med* 1997;157:2422 (Table 7)

amounts of red meat and sweets. The diet is low in saturated fat and cholesterol, but high in fiber, calcium, magnesium and potassium. In trials, the diet appeared effective in lowering blood pressure substantially; much of the beneficial effect was from the fruits and vegetables (including nuts). The DASH diet is also low in cost and is compatible with treatment of hyperlipidemia and coronary heart disease[41]. When the DASH diet was combined with a lowered sodium intake, the result was superior to that achieved by either alone; therefore, the combined approach is the best recommendation[42].

There is evidence that high salt (sodium chloride) intake is associated with worsening of blood pressure control. A reduction in sodium intake helps lower the blood pressure and even negate the age-related rise in pressure. Typical US diets contain far more than the recommended limit of 100 mmol sodium/day. Most (75%) of the sodium is a result of processing of foods, approximately 10% is inherent in the food prior to processing and about 15% is added while cooking or prior to eating[43]. Older individuals and many with renal disease are salt sensitive, with sodium intake clearly impacting on the blood pressure.

Weight reduction and physical activity

Weight loss and increased physical activity are both helpful. The prevalence of overweight and obesity is high in the USA; data are consistent in that a reduction in weight is associated with a reduction in blood pressure. More than half the Americans find it difficult to find time to exercise; exercise of moderate intensity (40–60% of maximum oxygen consumption) appears to decrease the blood pressure as well as exercise of high intensity. Aerobic exercise decreases blood pressure in both normotensives and hypertensives, and thus helps in the prevention and treatment of high blood pressure[44]. Aerobic exercises are recommended for 30–45 min most days a week; brisk walking is an ideal activity, although one may encourage the preferred activity for each individual. Those with heart disease may require evaluation and a cardiac stress test prior to beginning an exercise program[1,43]. It should be realized that the elderly often suffer from musculoskeletal disorders preventing them from exercising optimally; activity is always encouraged and some exercise is preferred to none.

Other considerations

Reduction in alcohol consumption in heavy drinkers can lower blood pressure in both normotensives and hypertensives. Women absorb alcohol better and light-weight individuals are more sensitive to the effects of alcohol, warranting a reduction in intake. Limits of alcohol consumption are provided in Table 6[1,43]. Smoking should be discouraged at all cost; smoking is associated with a rise in blood pressure, but the lower nicotine content of aids to quit smoking is not associated with risk[45]. Other non-pharmacologic considerations include an adequate intake of potassium, calcium and magnesium recommended as diet rather than as medications. While caffeine may cause an acute rise in blood pressure, a sustained effect does not appear to be evident. Data from trials on effects of garlic and onion on blood pressure are inconsistent[1].

PHARMACOLOGIC TREATMENT

In general, most older individuals require more than one drug for optimal control of blood pressure. This leads to the issue of polypharmacy, as most geriatric patients have co-morbid processes necessitating the use of several medications. In such situations, every effort must be made to simplify the regimen to achieve compliance. It may be possible to treat more than one disorder with the same agent. The agent should be appropriate and effective for hypertension and the co-morbid disorders. Examples include the use of β-blockers for hypertension with angina, or an ACE inhibitor for hypertension and congestive heart failure or diabetes, and calcium channel blockers for hypertension and peripheral vascular disease[46]. Long-acting preparations with a 24-h action are preferred, to improve compliance. Older adults depend on simple regimens and caregiver help for reminders.

The cost of drug treatment must be a consideration. The elderly often have financial constraints and it may become a choice between medication or food, with cost-based preferences for drugs. The choice may have to be between a generic and a brand preparation. When efficacy is equal, a generic choice is acceptable. Where one is considered more effective, cost becomes a secondary consideration[1].

While there are several classes of antihypertensives and numerous medications in each class, JNC VI recommends typically starting with a diuretic or a β-blocker. Either of these two agents may be added or substituted to improve the response. Several diuretics in the thiazide (with normal renal function) or the loop diuretic group (for renal insufficiency or failure) are available. The use of β-blockers is on the increase, especially for co-existing coronary artery disease and congestive heart failure; a variety of long-acting preparations are available. Failure to achieve optimum results may indicate the need for addition of one of several drugs; these include ACE inhibitors, calcium channel blockers and other choices.

A list of medications with dosages, select side-effects and comments is provided in Table 7. New medications continue to be made available; examples include ACE inhibitors such as perindopril (Aceon®, 4–8 mg/day), angiotensin receptor blockers (ARBs) such as candesartan (Atacand®, 8–32 mg/day), telmisartan (Micardis®, 20–80 mg/day), eprosartan (Teveten®, 400–800 mg/day) and lercanidipine, a new calcium antagonist, while others have been taken off the market, e.g. mibefradil (Posicor®). In most instances, the eventual choice of medication appears to be determined by the presence of co-morbidity, specific side-effects and preferences of the patient and health provider.

In the presence of certain disorders associated with hypertension, termed 'compelling' indications, the JNC VI guidelines have recommended the use of specific agents for control of elevated blood pressure. Examples include the use of ACE inhibitors in the presence of systolic dysfunction, β-blockers for coronary artery disease and ACE inhibitors with diabetes and proteinuria[1]. Tight control of blood pressure is recommended in older hypertensive diabetics to minimize complications such as myocardial infarction, cerebrovascular accident and renal failure; the target blood pressure here is below 130/85 mmHg. An ACE inhibitor or ARB is recommended as initial therapy along with lifestyle modification measures[47]. Other situations in the elderly which call for the consideration

Table 7 Oral antihypertensive drugs. From reference 1

Drug	Trade name	Usual dose range, total mg/day* (frequency per day)	Selected side-effects and comments*
Diuretics (partial list)			short term: increases cholesterol and glucose levels; biochemical abnormalities: decreases potassium, sodium, and magnesium levels, increases uric acid and calcium levels; rare: blood dyscrasias, photosensitivity, pancreatitis, hyponatremia
Chlorthalidone (G)†	Hygroton	12.5–50 (1)	
Hydrochlorothiazide (G)	Hydrodiuril, Microzide, Esidrix	12.5–50 (1)	
Indapamide	Lozol	1.25–5 (1)	(less or no hypercholesterolemia)
Metolazone	Mykrox	0.5–1.0 (1)	
	Zaroxolyn	2.5–10 (1)	
Loop diuretics			
Bumetanide (G)	Bumex	0.5–4 (2–3)	(short duration of action, no hypercalcemia)
Ethacrynic acid	Edecrin	25–100 (2–3)	(only non-sulfonamide diuretic, ototoxicity)
Furosemide (G)	Lasix	40–240 (2–3)	(short duration of action, no hypercalcemia)
Torsemide	Demadex	5–100 (1–2)	
Potassium-sparing agents			hyperkalemia
Amiloride hydrochloride (G)	Midamor	5–10 (1)	
Spironolactone (G)	Aldactone	25–100 (1)	(gynecomastia)
Triamterene (G)	Dyrenium	25–100 (1)	
Adrenergic inhibitors			
Peripheral agents			
Guanadrel sulfate	Hylorel	10–75 (2)	(postural hypotension, diarrhea)
Guanethidine monosulfate	Ismelin	10–150 (1)	(postural hypotension, diarrhea)
Reserpine (G)‡	Serpasil	0.05–0.25 (1)	(nasal congestion, sedation, depression, activation of peptic ulcer)
Central α-agonists			sedation, dry mouth, bradycardia, withdrawal hypertension
Clonidine hydrochloride (G)	Catapres	0.2–1.2 (2–3)	(more withdrawal)
Guanabenz acetate (G)	Wytensin	8–32 (2)	
Guanfacine hydrochloride (G)	Tenex	1–3 (1)	(less withdrawal)
Methyldopa (G)	Aldomet	500–3000 (2)	(hepatic and 'autoimmune' disorders)
α-Blockers			postural hypotension
Doxazosin mesylate	Cardura	1–16 (1)	
Prazosin hydrochloride (G)	Minipress	2–30 (2–3)	
Terazosin hydrochloride	Hytrin	1–20 (1)	
β-Blockers			bronchospasm, bradycardia, heart failure, may mask insulin-induced hypoglycemia; less serious: impaired peripheral circulation, insomnia,

(Continued)

Table 7   (Continued)

Drug	Trade name	Usual dose range, total mg/day* (frequency per day)	Selected side-effects and comments*
			fatigue, decreased exercise tolerance, hypertriglyceridemia (except agents with intrinsic sympathomimetic activity)
Acebutolol	Sectral	200–800 (1)	
Atenolol (G)[§¶]	Tenormin	25–100 (1–2)	
Betaxolol hydrochloride[§]	Kerlone	5–20 (1)	
Bisoprolol fumarate[§]	Zebeta	2.5–10 (1)	
Carteolol hydrochloride[‖]	Cartrol	2.5–10 (1)	
Metoprolol tartrate (G)[§]	Lopressor	50–300 (2)	
Metoprolol succinate[§]	Toprol-XL	50–300 (1)	
Nadolol (G)	Corgard	40–320 (1)	
Penbutolol sulfate[‖]	Levatol	10–20 (1)	
Pindolol (G)[‖]	Visken	10–60 (2)	
Propranolol hydrochloride (G)	Inderal	40–480 (2)	
	Inderal LA	40–480 (1)	
Timolol maleate (G)	Blocadren	20–60 (2)	
Combined α- and β-blockers			postural hypotension, bronchospasm
Carvedilol	Coreg	12.5–50 (2)	
Labetalol hydrochloride (G)	Normodyne, Trandate	200–1200 (2)	
Direct vasodilators Hydralazine hydrochloride (G)	Apresoline	50–300 (2)	headaches, fluid retention, tachycardia (lupus syndrome)
Minoxidil (G)	Loniten	5–100 (1)	(hirsutism)
Calcium antagonists Non-dihydropyridines			conduction defects, worsening of systolic dysfunction, gingival hyperplasia
Diltiazem hydrochloride	Cardizem SR	120–360 (2)	(nausea, headache)
	Cardizem CD, Dilacor XR, Tiazac	120–360 (1)	
Mibefradil dihydrochloride (T-channel calcium antagonist)	Posicor	50–100 (1)	(no worsening of systolic dysfunction; contraindicated with terfenadine (Seldane), astemizole (Hismanal), and cisapride (Propulsid))
Verapamil hydrochloride	Isoptin SR, Calan SR	90–480 (2)	(constipation)
	Verelan, Covera HS	120–480 (1)	
Dihydropyridines			edema of the ankle, flushing, headache, gingival hypertrophy
Amlodipine besylate	Norvasc	2.5–10 (1)	
Felodipine	Plendil	2.5–20 (1)	
Isradipine	DynaCirc	5–20 (2)	
	DynaCirc CR	5–20 (1)	
Nicardipine hydrochloride	Cardene SR	60–90 (2)	
Nifedipine	Procardia XL, Adalat CC	30–120 (1)	
Nisoldipine	Sular	20–60 (1)	

(Continued)

Table 7   (Continued)

Drug	Trade name	Usual dose range, total mg/day* (frequency per day)	Selected side-effects and comments*
Angiotensin converting enzyme inhibitors			common: cough; rare: angioedema, hyerkalemia, rash, loss of taste, leukopenia
Benazepril hydrochloride	Lotensin	5–40 (1–2)	
Captopril (G)	Capoten	25–150 (2–3)	
Enalapril maleate	Vasotec	5–40 (1–2)	
Fosinopril sodium	Monopril	10–40 (1–2)	
Lisinopril	Prinivil, Zestril	5–40 (1)	
Moexipril	Univasc	7.5–15 (2)	
Quinapril hydrochloride	Accupril	5–80 (1–2)	
Ramipril	Altace	1.25–20 (1–2)	
Trandolapril	Mavik	1–4 (1)	
Angiotensin II receptor blockers			angioedema (very rare), hyperkalemia
Losartan potassium	Cozaar	25–100 (1–2)	
Valsartan	Diovan	80–320 (1)	
Irbesartan	Avapro	150–300 (1)	

*These dosages may vary from those listed in the Physicians' Desk Reference 51st edn which may be consulted for additional infromation. The listing of side-effects is not all-inclusive, and side-effects are for the class of drugs except where noted for individual drug (in parentheses); clinicians are urged to refer to the package insert for a more detailed listing

†G indicates generic available. ‡Also acts centrally. §Cardioselective. ‖Has intrinsic sympathomimetic activity.
Reproduced with permission from: The Sixth report of the Joint National Committee on prevention, evaluation, detection, and treatment of high blood pressure. *Arch Intern Med* 1997;157:2425–26 (Table 8)

for specific medications include the use of α-blockers in the presence of hypertension and benign prostatic hyperplasia (in the absence of heart failure)[48], calcium channel blockers for co-existing peripheral vascular disease and thiazides for hypertension with osteoporosis (for its calcium-retaining property). Most agents other than α-blockers can be used as first-line therapy; the sole use of α-blockers did not appear beneficial in one study, where the doxazosin arm was terminated because of an increase in cardiac events[48,49].

Although JNC VI has stated that the newer agents have no advantage over β-blockers and thiazides, recent data from the Losartan Intervention For Endpoint reduction in hypertension study (LIFE) suggests that losartan, an ARB, was associated with greater reduction in cardiovascular morbidity and mortality from blood pressure control than atenolol[50,51]. ACE inhibitors and ARBs have become popular agents, with a major difference in that the latter is seldom associated with a common adverse effect, dry cough. The benefits of ACE inhibitors appear to be duplicated by ARBs[50]. However, until long-term data are available, the initial choice may be an ACE inhibitor with the ARB reserved for those unable to tolerate the former[1].

For older subjects with isolated systolic hypertension, a diuretic or long-acting dihydropyridine has been deemed appropriate. Short acting calcium channel blockers (including sublingual nifedipine) are currently not preferred therapy. In the mid 1990s an increased risk of coronary events was reported with calcium antagonist therapy, particularly short-acting preparations, such as immediate-acting nifedipine[52]. There

Table 8 Prescribing anti-hypertensives in older adults: considerations

Ensure proper blood pressure measurement technique
Start with small doses, titrate gradually
Avoid rapid reduction in blood pressure
Consider choice of drug based on co-morbid illness
Combine with counseling regarding life style modification measures
Keep cost of formulation in mind
Simplify dosing to enhance compliance (if possible, once or twice a day)
Long-acting preparations are preferred
Follow-up for side-effects, in particular orthostasis
Be on the alert for drug–drug, drug–disease and drug–nutrient interactions

were flaws in some of these studies and more recently the initial reports have been questioned. While calcium antagonists are effective antihypertensive agents regardless of age or race, well tolerated and antianginal, and reduce the risk of stroke, some may be pro-ischemic, and increase heart rate and sympathetic nervous system activity[53]. Risk reduction of stroke seems consistent. One view is to use calcium antagonists as supportive therapy for ACE inhibitors, ARB, β-blockers and diuretics with fewer candidates for monotherapy with calcium antagonists[53].

Quality of life must be considered while prescribing medications. The literature in this regard is somewhat conflicting. Thiazides and atenolol, commonly used in several trials, appear to have no effect on global quality of life[7]. Limited data claim benefits with ACE inhibitors. Sometimes the presence of a problem such as constipation may limit the use of a calcium channel blocker; or the tendency to hyperkalemia from renal tubular acidosis or obstructive uropathy may call for caution with ACE inhibitors.

If evaluation for hypertension reveals an underlying secondary etiology, corrective measures deserve consideration. As an example, widespread availability of percutaneous transluminal angioplasty offers the possibility for treatment and cure of atheromatous renal artery stenosis[39]. A diagnosis of primary aldosteronism from hyperplasia may benefit from the use of aldosterone antagonists (spironolactone).

Currently, hypertensive patients are undertreated[1,3]. Adequate control of hypertension requires the detection of elevated blood pressure, diagnostic evaluation and implementation of a suitable regimen with consideration for both lifestyle measures and pharmacologic therapy. It is essential to focus on the diagnosis and treatment of systolic hypertension, especially in the geriatric population; systolic blood pressure may become the primary variable in future[54]. The eventual regimen is individualized and often includes more than one drug. As therapy is long term, follow-up is recommended to minimize drug interactions and adverse drug events. Finally, cost of therapy and that of monitoring should be factored in, as many older adults face economic burdens (Table 8).

In the future, ambulatory blood pressure monitoring may play a role in earlier identification of hypertension in type 1 diabetes at risk for nephropathy, and predict risk for decline[55]. White coat hypertension needs to be better defined as also levels for initiating treatment; 24 hour ambulatory recordings may be utilized for reliably establishing the diagnosis of this entity[56]. Cognitive benefits will be an additional reason (besides the prevention of cardiovascular and cerebrovascular disease) for treatment of hypertension in older adults[57]. New JNC guidelines may need to elaborate further on several situations warranting unique considerations in management of hypertension in the elderly[58].

References

1. Joint National Committee on Prevention, Evaluation, Detection, and Treatment of High Blood Pressure. The sixth report. *Arch Intern Med* 1997;157:2413–46

2. National High Blood Pressure Education Program Working Group. Report on hypertension in diabetes. *Hypertension* 1994;23: 145–8

3. McAlister FA, Campbell NRC, Zarnke K, *et al*. The management of hypertension in Canada: a review of current guidelines, their shortcomings and implications for the future. *Can Med Assoc J* 2001;164:517–22

4. Hajjar IM. Concepts in geriatric hypertension. *Fam Pract Recertif* 2002;24:51–63

5. Butler RN, August P, Ferdinand KC, *et al*. Hypertension: setting new goals for lower readings. *Geriatrics* 1999;54:20–36

6. Burt VL, Whelton P, Rocella EJ, *et al*. Prevalence of hypertension in the US adult population: results of the Third National and Nutritional Examination Survey, 1988–91. *Hypertension* 1995;25:305–13

7. Scott AK. Hypertension. In Tallis RC, Fillit HM, Brocklehurst JC, eds. *Geriatric Medicine and Gerontology*, 5th edn. London: Churchill Livingstone, 1998:321–35

8. Messerli FH. This day 50 years ago. *N Engl J Med* 1995;332:1038–9

9. Karnath B. Sources of error in blood pressure measurement. *Hosp Physician* 2002;38:33–7

10. Alagiakrishnan K, Masaki K, Schatz I, *et al*. Blood pressure dysregulation syndrome: the case for control throughout the circadian cycle. *Geriatrics* 2001;56:50–60

11. Hajjar IM, Grim CE, George V, *et al*. Impact of diet on blood pressure and age-related changes in blood pressure in the U.S. population: analysis of NHANES III. *Arch Intern Med* 2001;161:589–93

12. Sykes D, Dewar R, Mohanaruban K, *et al*. Measuring blood pressure in the elderly: does atrial fibrillation increase observer variability? *Br Med J* 1990;300:162–3

13. Lawton WJ, DiBona GF. Normal blood pressure control and the evaluation of hypertension. In Johnson RJ, Feehally J, eds. *Comprehensive Clinical Nephrology*, 1st edn. New York: Mosby, 2000;37.1–37.12

14. Kannel WB. Blood pressure as a cardiovascular risk factor: prevention and treatment. *J Am Med Assoc* 1996;275:1571–6

15. Glasser SP. Hypertension syndrome and cardiovascular events: high blood pressure is only one risk factor. *Postgrad Med* 2001; 110:29–33

16. Guidelines for management of hypertension: report of the third working party of the British Hypertension Society. *J Hum Hypertens* 1999;13:569–92

17. Staessen JA, Gasowski J, Wang JG, *et al*. Risks of untreated and treated isolated systolic hypertension in the elderly: meta-analysis of outcome trials. *Lancet* 2000;355:865–72

18. Amery A, Brixko P, Clement D, *et al*. Mortality and morbidity results from the European Working Party on High Blood Pressure in the Elderly trial. *Lancet* 1985;1:1349–54

19. SHEP Cooperative Research Group. Prevention of stroke by antihypertensive drug treatment in older patients with isolated systolic hypertension: final results of the Systolic Hypertension in the Elderly program (SHEP). *J Am Med Assoc* 1991; 265:3255–64

20. Dahlof B, Lindholm L, Hansson L, *et al*. Morbidity and mortality in the Swedish Trial in Old Patients with Hypertension (STOP) Hypertension). *Lancet* 1991;338:1281–5

21. MRC Working Party. Medical Research Council trial of treatment of hypertension in older adults. *Br Med J* 1992;303:405–12

22. Staessen JA, Fagard R, Thijs L, *et al*. Systolic Hypertension in Europe (Syst-Eur) Trial Investigators. Randomized double-blind comparison of placebo and active treatment for old patients with isolated systolic hypertension. *Lancet* 1997;350: 757–64

23. Liu L, Wang JG, Gong L, *et al*. Comparison of active treatment and placebo in older Chinese patients with isolated systolic hypertension. *J Hypertens* 1998;16:1823–9

24. Pickering TG, James GD, Boddie C, *et al*. How common is white coat hypertension? *J Am Med Assoc* 1988;259:225–8

25. Smith PA, Graham LN, Mackintosh AF, *et al*. Sympathetic neural mechanisms in white-coat hypertension. *J Am Coll Cardiol* 2002;40:126–32

26. Spence JD. Pseudohypertension in the elderly: still hazy, after all these years. *J Hum Hypertens* 1997;11:621–3

27. Frishman WH. Effects of nonsteroidal anti-inflammatory drug therapy on blood pressure and peripheral edema. *Am J Cardiol* 2002;89(Suppl 1):18–25

28. Lipsitz LA. Orthostatic hypotension in the elderly. *N Engl J Med* 1989;321:952–7

29. Kario K, Eguchi K, Hoshide S, *et al*. U-curve relationship between orthostatic blood pressure change and silent cerebrovascular disease in elderly hypertensives. *J Am Coll Cardiol* 2001;40:133–41

30. Jansen RW, Lipsitz LA. Postprandial hypotension: epidemiology, pathophysiology, and clinical management. *Ann Intern Med* 1995;122:268–95

31. Boutitie F, Gueyffier F, Pocock S, *et al*. J-shaped relationship between blood pressure and mortality in hypertensive patients: new insights from a meta-analysis of individual patient data. *Ann Intern Med* 2002;136:438–48

32. Vaitkevicius PV, Niranjan BS. Hypertension. *Clin Geriatr* 2001;9:18–23

33. Birkenhager WH, Forette F, Seux M-L, *et al*. Blood pressure, cognitive functions, and prevention of dementias in older patients with hypertension. *Arch Intern Med* 2001;161:152–6

34. Fleisher LA. Preoperative evaluation of the patient with hypertension. *J Am Med Assoc* 2002;287:2043–6

35. Dharmarajan TS, Ugalino JT. Understanding the pharmacology of aging. In Dreger D, Krumm B, eds. *Geriatric Medicine Hospital Physician Board Review Manual*. Wayne, PA: Turner White Communications, 2001;1:1–12

36. Jayadevan R, Pitchumoni CS, Dharmarajan TS. Dysphagia in the elderly. *Pract Gastroenterol* 2001;25:75–88

37. Dharmarajan TS, Kumar A, Pitchumoni CS. Drug–nutrient interactions in older adults. *Pract Gastroenterol* 2002;26:37–55

38. Modi KS, Rao VK. Atheroembolic renal disease. *J Am Soc Nephrol* 2002;12:1781–7

39. Henrich WL. Renal artery disease in the elderly. In Oreopoulos DG, Hazzard WR, Luke R, eds. *Nephrology and Geriatrics Integrated*. London: Kluwer Academic Publishers, 2000:67–75

40. Sowers JR. Hypertension, angiotensin II and oxidative stress. *N Engl J Med* 2002;346:1999–2001

41. Sachs FM, Appel AJ, Moore TJ, *et al*. A dietary approach to prevent hypertension: a review of the Dietary Approaches to Stop Hypertension (DASH) Study. *Clin Cardiol* 1999;22(Suppl):III–6 to III–10

42. Sachs FM, Svetkey LP, Vollmer WM, *et al*. Effects on blood pressure of reduced dietary sodium and the Dietary Approaches to Stop Hypertension (DASH). *N Engl J Med* 2001;344:3–10

43. Appel LJ. Non pharmacologic therapies that reduce blood pressure: a fresh perspective. *Clin Cardiol* 1999;22(Suppl):III–1 to III–5

44. Whelton SP, Chin A, Xin X, He J. Effect of aerobic exercise on blood pressure: a meta-analysis of randomized, controlled trials. *Ann Intern Med* 2002;136:493–503

45. Greenberg G, Thompson SG, Brennan PJ. The relationship between smoking and the response to antihypertensive treatment in mild hypertensives in the Medical Research Council's trial of treatment. *Int J Epidemiol* 1987;16:25–30

46. McIntyre H. Treating hypertension: are we meeting the challenge? *Geriatr Med* 2002;32:59–64

47. Sadurska K, Prisant M. The older hypertensive patient with diabetes: the need for tight blood pressure control. *Clin Geriatr* 2002;10:18–25

48. Messerli FH. Implications of discontinuation of doxazosin arm of AALHAT. *Lancet* 2000;355:863

49. ALLHAT Collaborative Research Group. Major cardiovascular events in hypertensive patients randomized to doxazosin

vs. chlorthalidone: the antihypertensive and lipid-lowering treatment to prevent heart attack trial (ALLHAT). *J Am Med Assoc* 2000;283:1967–75

50. Brunner HR, Gavras H. Angiotensin blockade for hypertension: a promise fulfilled. *Lancet* 2002;359:990–1

51. Dahlof B, Desvereux RB, Kjeldsen SE, *et al.* Cardiovascular morbidity and mortality in the Losartan Intervention For Endpoint reduction in hypertension study (LIFE): a randomized trial against atenolol. *Lancet* 2002;359:995–1003

52. Furberg CD, Psaty BM, Meyer JV. Nifedipine: dose related increase in mortality in patients with coronary artery disease. *Circulation* 1995;92:1326–31

53. Weir MR. Appropriate use of calcium antagonists in hypertension. *Hosp Pract* 2001;36:47–55

54. Deedwania PC. The changing face of hypertension: is systolic blood pressure the final answer? *Arch Intern Med* 2002;162:506–8

55. Ingelfinger JR. Ambulatory blood pressure monitoring as a predictive tool. *New Engl J Med* 2002;347:778–9

56. Pickering T. White coat hypertension: should it be treated or not? *Cleveland Clin J Med* 2002;69:584–5

57. Jawde RA, Messinger-Rapport BJ. Is there a relationship between hypertension and cognitive decline in older adults? *Cleveland Clin J Med* 2002;69:664–9

58. Dharmarajan TS. JNC-VI Guidelines and long-term care: A misfit? *Ann Long-Term Care* 2001;9:78

49 Gynecologic disorders

Kevin D. Reilly, MD

INTRODUCTION

The issue of gynecologic care of the geriatric patient is relatively new to the field of medicine. The life expectancy of women exceeds that of men across all racial lines[1], a phenomenon so pronounced that the residents of nursing homes and retirement communities are overwhelmingly female. The life expectancy of women in the USA has increased from 50 in 1900 to around 80 today[2]. Yesterday's older woman resigned herself to a sedentary lifestyle. Today's older women are healthier than their mothers and grandmothers, and expect to continue to lead an active lifestyle. Gynecology must meet the challenge to keep its geriatric patients not just healthy, but active and productive.

RELEVANT PHYSIOLOGY

Many changes that occur with the aging process are hormonally dependent. The most dramatic hormonal change in the latter half of a woman's life is menopause. Menopause is defined as the permanent cessation of menses after 12 months of amenorrhea. It is a defined moment in time as opposed to a phase of life or extended period of time. The phase of life that precedes the defined point of menopause is referred to as the perimenopausal period. The median age for perimenopause is 47.5 years and for menopause is 51.3 years[3]. The period of time after menopause is called the postmenopausal period.

It is in the perimenopausal period that women may begin to experience the effects of fluctuating or declining estrogen levels. These effects comprise the menopausal syndrome and include irregular uterine bleeding, hot flushes, night sweats, mood swings and depression.

The occurrence, duration and severity of menopausal symptoms vary significantly from patient to patient. Some never experience any while others are greatly distressed by these symptoms and seek medical relief. Many others tolerate them and feel no need for intervention. The symptoms usually last for 1 or 2 years and gradually subside, but may occasionally persist for 5 or 6 years[4].

The geriatric patient at age 65 or above is postmenopausal and long past this 'menopausal syndrome'. What persists is the low estrogen level and the multi-organ system consequences attributable to the low level. Organ systems affected include the genital tract, connective tissue, bone, heart and nervous system, as depicted in Figure 1. Long-term organ effects may persist for 30 or more years after the menopause.

THE GYNECOLOGIC EXAMINATION

The elderly woman requires a complete gynecologic examination, including breast and pelvic examination, on an annual basis. Consideration should be given to the patient's emotional reluctance to have this examination as well as to the physical discomfort she may experience due to hypoestrogenic changes.

Age (years)

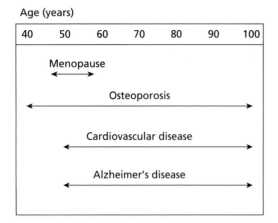

Figure 1 Time line for development of abnormalities of organ systems after the menopause

Gentleness, thorough explanation of what to expect with the examination, and appropriate lubrication will facilitate compliance. Use of a small or pediatric speculum may be necessary. Dorsal lithotomy or lateral Sims position of the patient facilitates the examination. Pap smears and mammograms should be performed according to American Cancer Society guidelines[4]. Bimanual and rectovaginal examinations should be performed annually even if Pap smears are not indicated, since they are the most cost-effective screen for ovarian cancer[5].

SYSTEMS AFFECTED BY MENOPAUSE

The female genital tract includes the lower genital tract, comprising the vulva and vagina, and upper genital tract, comprising the uterus, Fallopian tubes and ovaries. Both areas, along with their attendant connective tissue supports, undergo changes in postmenopausal patients.

Lower genital tract changes include a loss of connective tissue perineal support and atrophy of the introital epithelium. This frequently leads to a narrowing of the introitus and vaginal hymeneal ring. Similar atrophic changes may occur in the connective tissues supporting the urethra and rectum, resulting

in prolapse of these organs. The vaginal mucosa undergoes significant atrophic change resulting in loss of mucosal rugae and thinning of the mucosal epithelium. There is a concomitant loss of lubrication, due to decreased vascularity in these atrophic tissues. The changes result in discomfort on examination and coital activity and susceptibility to trauma and infection. Trauma may result in bleeding and lacerations, severe enough at times to require surgical intervention. Infection of the lower genital tract results from altered vaginal pH combined with mucosal atrophy, allowing bacterial or yeast overgrowth. The inflamed atrophic epithelium of the vulva frequently causes severe symptoms of itching or burning with vulvovaginitis. These infections may be precipitated by the presence of diabetes mellitus and fecal or urinary incontinence.

Management of these conditions may be simple, such as using a water-based lubricant for vulvovaginal atrophy. Appropriate antibiotic or antifungal agents should be used for infections. Genital hygiene may be needed for incontinence-related contamination. Estrogen replacement therapy can improve the atrophic changes that underlie these conditions. This therapy can be accomplished via topical, oral or transdermal routes.

The loss of connective tissue support frequently results in a prolapse or herniation of genital tract structures into the vagina or through the introitus, and termed as follows: urethra, urethrocele; urinary bladder, cystocele; small bowel, enterocele; rectum, rectocele; uterus, uterine prolapse. Combinations of any or all of these changes are common. Symptoms relate to the organs involved. Urinary incontinence, frequency, dribbling, urinary retention and urinary infection may relate to urinary bladder and urethral prolapse. Constipation may be associated with rectal changes. Pelvic pressure and back pain may be associated with uterine prolapse or enterocele. Also present may be a sensation of a mass protruding through the vagina.

Symptoms related to prolapse may be initially addressed with estrogen replacement therapy to improve connective tissue tone. Kegel exercises combined with biofeedback interventions help to ameliorate symptoms, especially in milder cases. Severe changes and symptoms may require additional interventions such as pessaries or surgical correction.

Pessaries in various shapes help support the affected structure. They come in various sizes, so that they are not extruded through the introitus or so large as to obstruct or erode the supported tissue. Knowledge of the design of each pessary type and experience in fitting will determine the success of this treatment modality. They may be especially useful in the elderly with multiple co-morbidities considered too high a risk for surgical correction or the patient who prefers not to have surgical corrections. Pessary wearers must have periodic examinations to remove and clean their pessaries and to confirm that the pessary is not overly compressing supported tissue. If this is not done at least three to four times per year the pessary may become adherent to the vagina and require surgical removal. The need for surgical correction for defects in pelvic organ support is determined by severity of symptoms, involvement of other organ systems, medical stability and desire for a surgical cure.

Urinary tract symptoms relate to pelvic support defects. It is imperative to determine the etiology of the urinary symptoms prior to recommending surgery. Not all urinary symptoms are amenable to surgical correction, even in the face of obvious support defects. Urinary tract infection should be ruled out. Urinary bladder function is ascertained by a thorough history that should include a voiding diary, dietary and fluid intake assessment, medication history and review of diseases. Demonstration of a large residual urine (more than 100 ml) on bladder catheterization or ultrasound examination performed immediately after voiding may point to pathology other than surgically correctable urinary stress incontinence. Demonstration of correction of urinary loss upon cough or strain (by the Bonney or Marshall test) indicates surgically correctable urinary stress incontinence. Surgical repair in the presence of other bladder abnormalities causing incontinence will result in almost certain failure or worsening of symptoms. For urinary stress incontinence, surgical repair by the retropubic or vaginal approach or a combined approach has been shown to be successful in up to 80% in restoring continence. Failures or recurrence of urinary stress incontinence are more likely in patients who do not have pure (genuine) stress incontinence, or who have chronic pulmonary disease or significant obesity.

The upper genital tract also undergoes atrophic changes with aging. The uterus reverts to a more infantile status resulting from lack of estrogen. The corpus becomes involuted due to a decrease in size of myometrial cells. The cervix eventually becomes proportionately larger than the corpus, a ratio similar to that in the prepubertal female. The endometrium becomes atrophic and inactive and is no longer shed as menses, and amenorrhea results. Any bleeding that occurs more than 12 months after the last menstrual period is abnormal and should be investigated to rule out endometrial carcinoma. Investigation includes a pelvic examination, Pap smear, endometrial biopsy and sonogram of the uterus for endometrial thickening of more than 6 mm. If this investigation is negative and no further bleeding occurs, the patient may be followed clinically. A dilatation and curettage or a hysteroscopy with biopsy should be performed when there is suspicion for malignancy, atypical complex hyperplasia, thickened endometrium or persistent bleeding.

GYNECOLOGIC MALIGNANT DISEASE

Malignant disease of the female genital tract encompasses both lower and upper genital

Table 1   Estimated new cancer cases and cancer deaths in the USA in 2002

	Estimated new cases	Estimated deaths
Uterine corpus	39 300	6 600
Ovary	23 300	13 900
Uterine cervix	13 000	4 100
Vulva	3 800	800
Vagina and other genital areas	2,000	800

tract malignanices. The most common genital malignancies in the geriatric age group in the USA are endometrial and ovarian carcinomas. The estimated new cancer cases and deaths for common gynecologic malignancies in 2002 in the USA are depicted in Table 1[6].

Lower genital tract malignancies

Vulvar carcinoma

Vulvar carcinoma comprises 4.7% of genital tract malignancies, and commonly occurs in the geriatric age group. Many patients are over 80 years old. Approximately 80% of the conditions are squamous cell carcinoma. They appear as an ulcerative process which may be secondarily infected. The lesion is usually non-tender. This lack of discomfort undoubtedly causes delay in seeking evaluation of such lesions. Vulvar carcinoma is more likely to occur in individuals who have had condyloma accuminata, vulvar dystrophy or cervical carcinoma in the past.

Treatment is primarily surgical. If detected in a pre-invasive or *in situ* stage, treatment is wide surgical excision. Multifocal or bilateral carcinoma may require a simple vulvectomy. If the disease is invasive a radical vulvectomy is indicated. In addition ipsilateral inguinal lymph node dissection is indicated. If Cloquet's node (the highest femoral node) is positive for carcinoma then treatment of the pelvic nodes with lymphadenectomy or external beam radiation is indicated. Surgery can be performed in stages to minimize operative morbidity. In spite of the magnitude of these dissections, these procedures are well tolerated by even the older geriatric patient. Because of restricted mobility postoperatively, anticoagulation is recommended.

Less common is Paget's disease of the vulva. The lesion is less ulcerated and with a velvety appearance. Key to successful treatment is early diagnosis with biopsy and wide local excision. Bartholin gland adenocarcinoma comprises only a small percentage of vulvar carcinomas. Treatment is primarily surgical.

Vaginal carcinoma

Less than 2% of genital malignancies are primary vaginal carcinomas, mostly of the squamous cell type. Vaginal carcinoma is more likely to occur in patients who have previously had squamous cell carcinoma of the cervix. Symptoms include vaginal bleeding or discharge. Diagnosis of vaginal carcinoma is by an abnormal Pap smear and confirmed by biopsy of suspicious vaginal lesions.

Treatment is determined by stage of the disease. *In situ* disease can be treated with wide excision, laser ablation or topical 5-fluorouracil. Invasive disease must be treated with radical surgery or radiation, determined by the older individual's general medical status and ability to withstand radical surgery.

Metastatic carcinoma to the vagina is common and should be suspected when vaginal bleeding occurs in patients with other primary carcinomas, especially those of the endometrium or ovary.

Cervical carcinoma

With increased Pap smear screening for cervical carcinoma in developed countries the predominance of cervical carcinoma as the most common genital tract malignancy has been supplanted by endometrial and ovarian carcinoma. This, however, does not preclude the occurrence of cervical carcinoma. The number of geriatric patients who do not avail themselves of regular screening combined with the influx of immigrants from underdeveloped countries who have not had access to screening results in a large reservoir of patients in whom cervical carcinoma is common. The American Cancer Society recommends Pap smear screening annually until three consecutive Pap smears have been obtained, then every 3 years until age 65 and at the discretion of the physician thereafter. High-risk patients should be screened annually[7].

Unlike in the younger population, in whom this disease is found in a preinvasive or premalignant stage, the geriatric patient is often found with invasive disease. Ninety per cent of cervical carcinomas are of the squamous cell type and usually arise at the transformation zone between the squamous cells of the exocervix and the glandular cells of the endocervical canal. Ten per cent are adenocarcinomas arising in the endocervical canal. Usual symptoms include vaginal bleeding, post-coital bleeding or vaginal discharge.

Key to diagnosis is the performance of a vaginal speculum examination, Pap smear and punch biopsy of suspicious lesions. Abnormal Pap smears require further evaluation with colposcopy, cervical punch biopsies and endocervical curettage. Invasive cervical carcinoma must be treated with radical hysterectomy and pelvic lymphadenectomy or by radiation. Modality of treatment, as with vaginal carcinoma, is determined by extent of disease of the lower third of the vagina, by attachment to the pelvic sidewall, by the patient's general medical condition and by the availability of a gynecologic oncology surgeon and radiotherapist. Generally, the older patient is treated by radiation rather than radical surgery.

Upper genital tract malignancies

Uterine corpus malignancy

Endometrial carcinoma This is commonly encountered in developed countries, a fact that may be related to dietary factors including a high-fat diet, alcohol consumption and estrogen replacement therapy. It comprises 48% of gynecologic malignancies in the USA. In undeveloped countries where dietary fat content is lower, the incidence of endometrial carcinoma is less than in the USA and Western Europe.

In women who take estrogen replacement therapy for treatment of menopausal symptoms such as hot flushes and vaginal dryness, or as prophylaxis for osteoporosis, it has been shown that the addition of a progestin to estrogen therapy can reverse the increased incidence of endometrial carcinoma caused by estrogen therapy alone[8]. For this reason it is recommended that women who receive estrogen replacement therapy and have their uterus present should receive combined estrogen–progestin therapy. A number of regimens enable combined hormone replacement therapy, from sequential to daily combined pills to combination skin patches. All of these regimens appear to achieve the desired effect of decreased incidence of endometrial carcinoma. The occurrences of withdrawal uterine bleeding, less likely with daily low-dose combination regimens, is an important consideration in deciding which regimen to employ.

The most common symptom of endometrial carcinoma is postmenopausal bleeding other than when expected as withdrawal from hormone replacement therapy. The development of bleeding requires evaluation of the endometrium by endometrial biopsy, dilatation and curettage, or hysteroscopy. Additional means of evaluation may include sonographic measurement of endometrial

Table 2   Common causes of postmenopausal bleeding

Local
Vulva
    abrasions or lacerations
    varicose veins
    ulcers – benign or malignant
    urethral caruncle
Vagina
    lacerations
    malignancy
Cervix
    carcinoma
    polyp
Endometrium
    carcinoma
    polyp
    atrophic endometrium

Other
Medications
    hormone therapy
    anticoagulants
Systemic disease
    coagulopathy
    hepatic disease

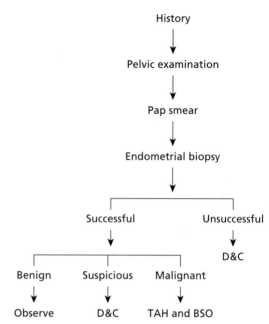

Figure 2   Evaluation of postmenopausal bleeding. D&C, dilatation and curettage; TAH, total abdominal hysterectomy; BSO, bilateral salpingo-oophorectomy

thickness or sonohysterography as adjunctive measures to direct endometrial sampling.

Other causes of postmenopausal bleeding are listed in Table 2. A sequential evaluation of postmenopausal bleeding is shown in Figure 2. Treatment of endometrial carcinoma centers on a staging procedure comprising total abdominal hysterectomy and bilateral salpingo-oophorectomy, pelvic and paraortic lymph node sampling, peritoneal and omental biopsies and peritoneal cytology. Adjunctive radiotherapy and/or chemotherapy are added based on depth of uterine wall invasion, cellular and nuclear differentiation and evidence of extrauterine or lymphovascular invasion. Radiotherapy may consist of brachytherapy (internal applications) and/or external beam therapy tailored to the patient's condition.

Because endometrial carcinoma usually presents early in its course with bleeding, it is frequently diagnosed at an early stage. It is thus amenable to therapy and results in cure in most cases with up to 90% 5-year survival noted in stage I disease.

Uterine sarcomas   Less common than endometrial adenocarcinomas are sarcomas of the uterus. Leiomyosarcoma occurs in less than 1% of patients thought to have fibroids or leiomyomas. It is no longer believed that leiomyomas 'degenerate' into sarcomas but rather that they originate *de novo* as malignant tumors. Suspicion of leiomyosarcoma should occur in postmenopausal patients who have enlargement of 'existing leiomyomas' or enlargement of a previously normal-sized uterus after the menopause. Intraoperative findings of soft, hemorrhagic or necrotic 'fibroids' are suspicious of malignancy. These findings and frozen sections suspicious for malignancy should prompt the surgeon to perform a 'staging procedure' so that appropriate therapy and adjunctive chemotherapy can be employed.

Ovarian carcinoma

Ovarian carcinoma is the second most prevalent gynecological malignancy. Unlike endometrial carcinoma, which usually presents in stage I with bleeding as an alarming symptom, ovarian carcinoma usually presents late with vague gastrointestinal symptomatology (75% detected in stage III or IV disease). Thus, the mortality is quite high, overall 5-year survival rates being approximately 40%.

Common symptoms are abdominal bloating and pain, early satiety and increased abdominal girth. Consequently patients may undergo extensive gastrointestinal evaluation. A pelvic examination should detect a pelvic mass, the presence of which should redirect the evaluation toward an ovarian neoplasm.

Sonography of the pelvis, computerized tomography (CT) or magnetic resonance imaging (MRI) may give further information about the extent of disease, but the mainstays of staging and treatment are exploratory laparotomy, peritoneal cytology, peritoneal biopsies, omental biopsy, subdiaphragmatic biopsy, biopsy of suspicious lesions and retroperitoneal lymph node sampling. The procedure includes total abdominal hysterectomy and bilateral salpingo-oophorectomy if possible, and debulking of the gross tumor mass. *En bloc* resection of involved structures such as large and small bowel is performed if necessary.

In the geriatric age group one should always suspect that a pelvic mass is malignant. Fibroids and physiologic cysts should not be enlarging after menopause. One should always be prepared for malignant disease when operating for a pelvic mass in the postmenopausal patient.

The geriatric ovarian cancer patient will usually be a candidate for adjuvant chemotherapy following the staging and debulking laparotomy. Chemotherapy will usually consist of a combination regimen appropriate for the cell type and chemotherapy response of the particular tumor tailored to the patient's disease and general medical status.

Mass screening for ovarian malignancy has met with frustrating results. Disappointing results have been obtained using sonography and tumor markers as a means of detecting ovarian carcinoma in the early stage. The usual aggressive nature of the disease and the high cost of screening have exasperated the clinician. To date, the mainstay of screening and early detection has remained the bimanual pelvic examination performed on an annual basis. Tumor markers have proved more successful in evaluating patients for persistent or recurrent disease.

The most common cell types and respective tumor markers are: for epithelial cell tumors, CA125; for sex cord tumors, testosterone; and for germ cell tumors, human chorionic gonadotropin and α-fetoprotein.

Carcinoma of the Fallopian tube

Carcinoma of the Fallopian tube is the least prevalent gynecologic malignancy. It comprises less than 1% of all gynecologic malignancies. The classic symptom of this disease is a watery bloody vaginal discharge that persists despite a negative evaluation of the endometrial cavity for malignancy. The tumor mass may be too small to feel on bimanual examination. In the face of this type of discharge a sonogram, a CT or MRI scan may be helpful in defining a mass. If no mass is noted and the bloody watery discharge persists, a laparoscopy or laparotomy should be performed. Like ovarian carcinoma, this tumor, usually of an epithelioid cell type, is very aggressive. The staging and therapy are identical to those of ovarian carcinoma. Debulking is the mainstay of treatment. Adjuvant chemotherapy is usually required.

Breast cancer

Breast cancer is the most common malignancy in the geriatric woman. The prevalence rises with age. The use of estrogen replacement therapy in the postmenopausal woman has been extensively evaluated regarding the impact on breast cancer. Meta-analysis and collaborative epidemiologic data[9,10] suggest a small increase in breast cancer risk.

OSTEOPOROSIS

Osteoporosis affects more than 25 million Americans with women comprising nearly 80% of these cases[11]. The incidence and severity increases as a woman lives three decades after menopause. The use of estrogen replacement therapy, selective estrogen receptor modulators (SERMs), bisphosphonates, calcitonin, calcium and behavior modification with weight-bearing exercise all improve the strength of medullary bone and decrease the morbidity and mortality in women from fractures.

CARDIOVASCULAR DISEASE AND ESTROGEN THERAPY

The number one cause of death in geriatric women is heart disease[12]. It has been well documented in the PEPI trial that estrogen replacement therapy improves the cardio-lipid profile in women[13]. It was inferred from this finding that there would be a significant decrease in cardiovascular deaths in women taking estrogen replacement therapy. Epidemiologic studies have supported this premise.

The recent report of data from the HERS research group[14], however, showed that women with pre-existing heart disease who newly start taking estrogen have an increased incidence of heart attacks in their first year of estrogen therapy. This observation, however, does not persist beyond the first year of therapy and indeed this same study has shown that, after the first year of therapy, the incidence of heart attacks decreased for women on estrogen therapy. The study did not address the issue in women who do not have pre-existing heart disease. This issue is being addressed in the ongoing Woman's Health Initiative study, the results of which will not be available until the year 2006 for the estrogen-only treatment group. However, the group receiving combined estrogen and progestogen was discontinued because of an increased risk of breast cancer and adverse cardiovascular and thrombovascular events[15]. Further evaluation of this issue is awaited.

ALZHEIMER'S DISEASE AND ESTROGEN THERAPY

Alzheimer's disease is common in older adults. It is expressed earlier in women than in men. It was suggested by observational studies that estrogen replacement therapy may play a role in decreasing the incidence of Alzheimer's disease. These studies were supported by a decreased incidence of myelin inflammatory plaques in the brains of deceased women who had been on estrogen replacement therapy. Counter arguments to this observation have centered on the concept that healthier, better motivated women take and continue to take estrogen and that these patients are less likely to have early Alzheimer's disease. Recent research reports that estrogen therapy may not prevent Alzheimer's disease from occurring, but rather may delay its onset and slow its progress[16].

CONCLUSION

Women are expected to live about a third of their life after the menopause. Some of the changes related to menopause such as vasomotor changes are short lived and easily managed with estrogen replacement therapy. Other changes are progressive and may seriously affect the quality and length of life in the geriatric patient. These changes include connective tissue disorders affecting pelvic support structures, osteoporosis, cardiovascular disease and neurodegenerative disorders. Modern medicine has developed many approaches to managing these processes. One central theme to all of these degenerative processes is a lack of estrogen. Estrogen replacement therapy can be a benefit to many women in the geriatric age group. This recognition must be tempered by the knowledge that some diseases such as endometrial carcinoma and thromboembolic disease are contraindications for estrogen therapy. Other diseases such as breast cancer require ongoing study to determine the relative risk of estrogen therapy in the larger picture of total health benefit for the geriatric female patient. Modern medicine has enabled women to live longer. Now we must explore ways to make them live better.

References

1. Evans WJ, Evans MI, Hajj SN. The aging population. In Hajj SN, Evans WJ, eds. *Clinical Postreproductive Gynecology*. East Norwalk, CT: Appleton and Lange, 1993:3
2. United States Bureau of the Census. Projections of the populations of the United States: 1977 to 2050. *Curr Pop Rep Serv* 1978;704:25
3. McKinlay SM, Brambillo DJ, Posner JG. The normal menopause transition. *Maturitas* 1992;14:103–15
4. Aksel S, Schomber DW, Tyrey L, Hammond CB. Vasomotor symptoms, serum estrogens and gonadotropin levels in surgical menopause. *Am J Obstet Gynecol* 1976;126:165–9
5. NIH Consensus Conference. Ovarian cancer. Screening, treatment and follow-up. NIH Consensus Development Panel on Ovarian Cancer. *J Am Med Assoc* 1995; 273:491–7
6. Jemel A, Thomas A, Murray T, Thun M. Cancer statistics, 2002. *CA Cancer J Clin* 2002;52:1, 23–47
7. Smith RA, Mettlin CJ, Davis KJ, *et al.* American Cancer Society guidelines for the early detection of cancer. *CA Cancer J Clin* 2000;50:34–49
8. Gambell RD Jr, Massey RM, Castaneda TA, *et al.* Use of the progestogen challenge test to reduce the risk of endometrial cancer. *Obstet Gynecol* 1980;55:732–8
9. Steinberg KK, Thacher SB, Smith SJ, *et al.* A meta-analysis of the effect of estrogen replacement therapy on the risk of breast cancer. *J Am Med Assoc* 1991;265:1985–90
10. Collaborative Group on Hormonal Factors in Breast Cancer. Breast cancer and hormone replacement therapy: collaborative reanalysis of data from 51 epidemidogical studies of 52,705 women with breast cancer and 108,411 women without breast cancer. *Lancet* 1997;350:1047–59
11. Ray NF, Can JK, Thamer M, *et al.* Medical expenditures for the treatment of osteoporotic fractures in the United States in 1995: report for the National Osteoporosis Foundation. *J Bone Miner Res* 1997;12: 24–35
12. US Department of Health and Human Services, Centers for Disease Control and Prevention. *Chronic Diseases and their Risk Factors: the Nation's Leading Causes of Death*. Washington, DC: National Center for Chronic Disease Preventions and Health Promotion, 1999
13. The Writing Group for the PEPI Trial. Effects of estrogen or estrogen–progestin regimens on heart disease risk factors in postmenopausal women. *J Am Med Assoc* 1995;273:199–208
14. Hulley S, Grady D, Bush T, *et al.*, for the Heart and Estrogen/Progestin Replacement Study (HERS) Research Group. Randomized trial of estrogen plus progestin for secondary prevention of coronary heart disease in postmenopausal women. *J Am Med Assoc* 1998;280:605–13
15. Writing Group for the Women's Health Initiative Investigators. Risks and benefits of estrogen plus progestin in healthy postmenopausal women. *JAMA* 2002;288: 321–33
16. Brenner DE, Kukell WA, Stergachis A, *et al.* Postmenopausal estrogen replacement therapy on the risk of Alzheimer's disease: a population based case–control study. *Am J Epidemiol* 1994;140:262–7

50 Sexuality and aging

Upinder Singh, MD

INTRODUCTION

Sexuality has been a focus since the inception of mankind. It undoubtedly has been the basic need for the procreation of race, for carnal pleasures and for a multitude of other reasons. Aging and sexuality are two fields beset by anxiety and erroneous folklore, with many of the problems originating from misinformation. We forget that the need for physical intimacy does not disappear when the hair turns gray or one is edentulous and the posture stooped from osteoporosis. As universal as the phenomenon may be, sadly sexual dysfunction has been an under-discussed and overlooked entity.

To understand sexual function, knowledge of relevant anatomy and physiology is worthwhile.

ANATOMY AND PHYSIOLOGY

The penis consists of three cylindrical columns of tissue surrounded by a sturdy fascia layer (Buck's fascia), subcutaneous tissue and skin[1]. The two paired cylinders of erectile tissue, the corpora cavernosa, run the length of the penis dorsally and are surrounded by a thick, non-expansible fibrous envelope, the tunica albuginea. The erectile tissue itself is composed of a distensible lattice of blood sinusoids surrounded by trabeculae of smooth muscle, which control the sinusoidal blood capacity. The third cylinder, the corpus spongiosum, lying ventrally, contains the urethra and forms the glans penis[1].

The arterial blood flow to the penis originates from the internal iliac arteries via the internal pudendal arteries. The venous drainage system collects blood from the sinusoids that run obliquely under the tunica albuginea[2].

Parasympathetic nerves from S2–4 are the principle mediators of erection, while sympathetic nerves from T11–L2 control ejaculation and detumescence[2]. The pelvic nerves contain sensory and motor elements that form a reflex arc through the spinal cord, and involve a spinal erection center. A 'reflex' erection therefore occurs as a direct result of stimulation of the penis, and can even occur in patients who have suffered a suprasacral spinal cord transection.

Mechanism of erection

Initiation

Neuroendocrine messages from the brain (due to either audio-visual stimuli or fantasy), either with or without tactile stimulation of the penis, activate the autonomic nuclei of the spinal erection center, sending messages to the erectile tissue of the corpora cavernosa via the cavernosal nerves. These result in:

(1) Dilatation of the cavernosal and helicine arteries, increasing blood flow into the lacunar spaces;

(2) Relaxation of cavernosal smooth muscle, opening the vascular lacunar space;

(3) Expansion of the lacunar spaces against the tunica albuginea, and compression of the obliquely running subtunical venous drainage channels, decreasing venous outflow and producing a rigid erection (also called the veno-occlusive mechanism).

Detumescence   Reversal of these events causes a flaccid state of the penis called detumescence, from increased sympathetic vasoconstrictor activity[1,2] and the enzymatic breakdown of cyclic guanosine monophosphate (cGMP) by phosphodiesterase type 5. This occurs naturally after orgasm and ejaculation, both of which are also mediated by the sympathetic nervous system.

SEXUAL DYSFUNCTION IN OLDER ADULTS

There is a decreased frequency of intercourse in older adult men[3,4], but many stay sexually active. It is clear that the frequency of this activity is swayed by cultural acceptance[5]. As expected, sexual dysfunction increases with age. About 7.5% of women under age 20 complain of sexual dysfunction, but 28% of those over the age of 50 do so[6]. Sexual activity in the elderly may be affected by multiple factors (Table 1). The aging process affects all the five phases of human sexual response, as originally described by Masters and Johnson[7]. The changes have been summarized in Table 2.

SEXUAL DYSFUNCTION IN MEN

Apart from expected physiologic changes, there may be additional basis for sexual dysfunction. Depending upon the component of the complex sexual cycle affected, sexual dysfunction could be of different types (Table 3).

Decreased libido

This is defined as the decreased desire to have sexual intimacy, and may be a result of

Table 1 Factors affecting sexual activity in older adults

Non-availability of a partner
Poor physical health
Poor mental health
Lack of privacy
Adverse effects of medicines
The individual's perception of sexuality
Social influences

unpleasant experiences in earlier life or because of decreased testosterone[8]. Diagnosis is based on obtaining a good history and checking free testosterone levels. Treatment is targeted to replacing androgen, via the intramuscular route or via dermal patches. The oral route is hepatotoxic and not recommended.

Erectile dysfunction

This is defined as the inability of the male to attain and maintain an erection of the penis sufficient to permit satisfactory sexual intercourse[9].

Pathophysiology

Erection is a highly complex mechanism with the interplay of many factors[2]. It is a neurovascular event modulated by psychological factors and hormonal status. On sexual stimulation, nerve impulses cause the release of neurotransmitters from the cavernous nerve terminals and of relaxing factors from the endothelial cells of the penis, resulting in the relaxation of smooth muscle in the arteries and arterioles supplying the erectile tissue and a several fold increase in penile blood flow. At the same time, relaxation of the trabecular smooth muscle increases the compliance of the sinusoids, facilitating rapid filling and expansion of the sinusoidal system. The subtunical venular plexuses are thus compressed between the trabeculae and the tunica albuginea, resulting in almost total occlusion of venous outflow. These events trap the blood within the corpora cavernosa

Table 2 Physiological changes with aging. From reference 7

Phase	In men	In women
Excitement	delay in erection	requires more stimulation
	scrotal vasocongestion decreases	vaginal lubrication decreases
	tensing of scrotal sac decreases	
Plateau	prolonged duration	less vaginal vasocongestion
	pre-ejaculatory secretions decrease	
Orgasm	shorter duration	fewer uterine contractions
	decreased ejaculatory force	
	decreased urethral contractions	
Resolution	rapid detumescence	rapid clitoral detumescence
	rapid testicular descent	
Refractory	prolonged	prolonged

Table 3 Types of sexual dysfunction in men

Sexual desire
Decreased libido
Hyperactive sexual drive

Arousal
Erectile dysfunction
Priapism

Orgasm
Premature ejaculation
Anorgasmia

Table 4 Risk factors for erectile dysfunction

Age
Hypertension
Diabetes mellitus
Alcohol
Smoking
Hypercholesterolemia

and raise the penis from a dependent position to an erect position, with an intracavernous pressure of approximately 100 mmHg[9]. Any disruption in the complex pathway can lead to erectile dysfunction.

Prevalence

It is appalling that very little is known about the exact prevalence of erectile dysfunction in the elderly. Data suggest that erectile dysfunction affects 20 million to 30 million men in the USA. It increases with age from around 5% below 40 years to about 50% by the age of 75[10,11].

Risk factors

Factors associated with increased risk for erectile dysfunction may either directly or indirectly decrease blood supply to the penis by increased atherogenesis. The common ones are listed in Table 4.

Etiology

Erectile dysfunction can result from involvement of any step required for normal erection. A disturbance at any level of the complex neurologic–endocrinologic–vascular phenomenon of erection can lead to erectile dysfunction. In older men, erectile dysfunction is usually organic in etiology, mostly due to vascular and/or neurologic disease[12]. The commonest reasons are listed in Table 5.

Sexual history

As is true with other medical problems, obtaining a good history is crucial to the success of any therapeutic doctor–patient interaction[2]. When the topic is a sensitive and a personal one like sexuality, patients and providers alike find open communication to be difficult. There may be many obstacles to overcome in obtaining a good sexual history.

Table 5 Causes of erectile dysfunction

Vascular
Coronary artery disease
Peripheral vascular disease
Impairment of veno-occlusive mechanism

Neurogenic
Trauma
Multiple sclerosis
Spina bifida

Endocrinologic
Low testosterone
High prolactin
Diabetes mellitus

Psychiatric
Depression

Medications
Antihypertensives
Antidepressants
Anticholinergics
Antihistaminics
LHRH analogs

Psychogenic

Other
Alcohol
Recreational drugs
Smoking
Pelvic surgery

LHRH, luteinizing hormone releasing hormone

Agism has infiltrated so deeply into the belief system of our society that many seniors see themselves as too old for sex. The elderly today have a relative lack of formal knowledge about sexual function and physiology, because they were raised during a time when scientific information on sex was not readily available or widely discussed. Their beliefs and sexual language are frequently different from those of the current culture[13].

The history should be taken in a comfortable and private setting. The patient may not volunteer the information, so the physician has to ask specifically about the problem, and be sensitive to cultural and ethnic aspects of the patient. Appropriate vocabulary[13] and a non-judgemental attitude should be maintained. The questions should be directed to:

(1) Confirm that the patient is suffering from sexual dysfunction;

(2) Assess the severity of the condition;

(3) Identify a possible underlying etiology;

(4) Determine whether the problem is psychogenic or organic in origin (Table 6);

(5) Identify any clinical symptoms from the known risk factors.

A good history should include information on marital history (married or not, availability of partner), place of residence (home, nursing home), drugs (recreational, prescription medicines, over-the-counter preparations), alcohol consumption, genitourinary surgery (prostate, hysterectomy, urinary bladder) and injuries (spinal cord, bicycle induced)[13]. It should also pursue personal, moral, cultural and religious views.

Physical examination should be performed to collaborate the leads obtained through history, and should include specifically peripheral pulses, blood pressure (arms and legs to assess brachial–femoral index), presence or absence of abdominal bruit, secondary sex characteristics (to look for hormonal etiology), examination of external genitalia and digital rectal examination (including the prostate)[2,13].

Investigations

A good history and physical examination helps in limiting the number of investigations. Those routinely required are urine analysis and serum glucose, essentially to rule out urinary tract infection and diabetes mellitus. Other tests should be guided by the history, such as thyroid stimulating hormone, free testosterone to rule out hypogonadism (diminished libido is likely as well), prolactin levels (history of headaches), prostate-specific antigen (prostatism) and lipid profile (hypercholesterolemia)[2,9,13]. Other advanced tests are required on an individual basis (Table 7).

Table 6 Psychogenic versus organic causes of sexual dysfunction in men. From reference 2

Feature	Psychogenic	Organic
Onset	abrupt	insidious
Course	episodic	persistent
Nocturnal erections	present	absent
Erections with other partner	present	absent
Erections with erotic stimulation	present	absent
Problems during sexual development	present	absent

Nocturnal penile tumescence testing

The presence of nocturnal erections, which is used to differentiate psychogenic from organic impotence, can be detected using devices placed around the penis during sleep. This is known as nocturnal penile tumescence testing[2]. The Snap-Gauge® band and Rigiscan® device are designed to be used at home and record the occurrence of nocturnal erections. Determining the presence or absence of nocturnal erections can also help treatment decisions.

Color Doppler imaging

This provides information about penile hemodynamics after maximal smooth muscle relaxation has been induced with a vasoactive agent. Its aim is to distinguish arterial insufficiency from other causes of erectile failure[2]. The velocity of blood in the cavernosal artery in the dynamic state can be measured during systole and diastole, and organic impotence can be differentiated from psychogenic impotence. It can also suggest the presence of a venous leak, although further studies are necessary to confirm this.

Pharmacocavernosography

Failure of the veno-occlusive mechanism to provide adequate venous outflow resistance can be demonstrated by pharmacocavernosography. This measures the blood flow required to maintain a pharmacologically stimulated erection[2]. Contrast medium injected into the corpora will identify the location of any leak, which often originates in the deep dorsal vein

Table 7 Investigations in men

Routine laboratory tests
Urinalysis
Serum glucose

Selective laboratory tests
Thyroid stimulating hormone
Serum creatinine
Blood urea nitrogen
Prostate-specific antigen
Lipid profile
Free testosterone
Prolactin

Specialized tests
Duplex ultrasonography
Cavernosography
Pelvic arteriography
Nocturnal penile tumescence

of the penis, but may also be present in less accessible cavernosal veins.

Pharmacoarteriography

In young men with erectile dysfunction caused by pelvic or perineal trauma, pudendal arteriography before and after a pharmacologically stimulated erection will identify those requiring arterial bypass[2].

Management

Various modalities are available to treat erectile dysfunction in men (Table 8).

Psychotherapy

Psychotherapeutic assessment and management are indicated for three clinical presentations:

Table 8 Treatment of erectile dysfunction

Psychotherapy
Vacuum devices
Hormonal therapy
Pharmacotherapy
 intracavernosal injections
 intraurethral injections
 transdermal applications
 oral preparations
Surgery
 arterial revascularizations
 venous leak repair
 penile implants
Herbal and unconventional therapies

(1) Where significant psychologic issues can be identified, e.g. depression, work-related stress and trauma;

(2) As an adjunct to other modalities of treatment;

(3) Where the patient requires help in coming to terms with absent or limited sexual functioning, which cannot be helped by further medical therapy.

Vacuum devices

The vacuum constriction device is very successful in producing an erection[14]. It involves placing a cylinder over an unerect penis, aspirating air to produce an erection, and then applying a wide rubber band at the base to maintain the erection. The vacuum is then released via a valve and the cylinder removed. The time taken to achieve an erection is generally around 2–3 min. The band should not be left in place for more than 30 min. Drawbacks to the vacuum device include pain, petechiae, obstruction of ejaculation, penile pivoting and coolness. Almost all patients with erectile dysfunction can use the device. However, it is not recommended for patients with severe Peyronie's curvature, severe phimosis and in the presence of bleeding disorders or when on anticoagulants.

Hormonal therapy

Historically, androgens were touted as enhancing male sexual function. Today, more effective treatments are available, and testosterone therapy should be discouraged in men in whom erectile dysfunction is not associated with hypogonadism.

In men with hypogonadism, oral testosterone preparations are less effective than intramuscular and transdermal testosterone preparations[15,16] and may be hepatotoxic (causing cholestasis, hepatitis and benign or malignant tumors). Testosterone cypionate and testosterone enanthate are often used for replacement therapy; the usual dosage is 200 mg intramuscularly every 2–3 weeks. The chief drawback is their roller-coaster effect: they have high activity the first week after injection, with a decrease thereafter. Transdermal administration has been developed recently. One to two patches containing 2.5–5.0 mg of testosterone applied daily to the abdomen, back or thighs have been shown to produce normal testosterone levels.

The most common adverse effects are skin irritation and contact dermatitis. Because it stimulates growth of the prostate, androgen therapy is contraindicated in men with prostate cancer or obstruction of the bladder neck caused by prostatic hypertrophy. In men receiving long-term testosterone therapy, the hematocrit, serum testosterone, lipids and prostate-specific antigen should be measured every 6 months.

Pharmacotherapy

Intracavernosal route Inracavernosal injection of vasodilator substances such as papaverine hydrochloride (smooth muscle relaxant)[17], phenoxybenzamine hydrochloride and phentolamine (β-adrenergic blockers), or prostaglandin E (alprostadil)[18] has become an important non-surgical technique for treating organically caused arousal disorder. It may also be helpful as adjunctive treatment for men with psychogenic impotence. Patients can be taught, with supervision, to inject themselves painlessly with 28-gauge needles. The amount of substance necessary to cause erection may vary from person to person and must be determined by the physician (usually a consulting urologist) with a challenge injection, which also serves the function of initiating instruction of the patient. This method of treatment has been more effective for men with neurogenic impotence than for those with vascular or other causes. Erection occurs 8–10 min after injection and lasts 2–4 h, with partial detumescence after ejaculation. Priapism and orthostatic hypotension have been the major untoward effects of treatment with papaverine or β-blockers[17]; penile pain after injection is more common with prostaglandin E. Fibrosis at injection sites leading to deformity of the penis is an uncommon late complication[17,18].

Intrauretheral route Alprostadil (prostaglandin E)[19,20] can now be administered through a novel transurethral drug delivery system (medicated urethral system for erection, or MUSE). The advantage of this method is substitution of a small pellet inserted via an applicator into the urethra rather than injection into the corpora. Some men experience urethral burning, but adherence to proper techniques of administration will minimize any discomfort. In controlled trials, 65% of men reported successful intercourse with MUSE compared with 19% using a placebo pellet.

Transdermal route Administration of vasoactive substances across the skin of the penis has the benefit in being a less invasive option. Agents used with limited efficacy through this route are minoxidil, papaverine and prostaglandin E_1 (PGE$_1$). Soft enhanced percutaneous absorption technology (SEPA) using PGE$_1$ has the highest efficacy.

Oral therapies The goal for the patient, the physician and the pharmaceutical industry alike has been the identification of an effective and safe oral agent. A plethora of drugs with differing mechanistic profiles have been used with varying degrees of success.

Sildenafil is a selective inhibitor of phosphodiesterase type 5, which inactivates GMP[9]. When sexual stimulation releases nitric oxide into the penile smooth muscle, inhibition of phosphodiesterase type 5 by sildenafil causes a marked elevation of GMP concentrations in the glans penis, corpus cavernosum and corpus spongiosum, resulting in increased smooth-muscle relaxation and better erection. Sildenafil has no effect on the penis in the absence of sexual stimulation, when the concentrations of nitric oxide and GMP are low. Sildenafil has little effect on libido, but is effective for practically all etiologic types of erectile dysfunction[9]. It is absorbed well during fasting, and the plasma concentrations are maximal within 30–120 min (mean 60). It is eliminated predominantly by hepatic metabolism, with a terminal half-life of about 4 h. The recommended starting dose is 50 mg taken 1 h before sexual activity, and the maximal recommended frequency is once per day. On the basis of effectiveness and side-effects, the dose may be increased to 100 mg or decreased to 25 mg.

Common side effects[9] include headache, flushing, nasal congestion and dyspepsia. Rarely it may cause a mild and transient bluish color tinge and increased sensitivity to light (probably related to inhibition of phosphodiestrase type 6 in the retina). Serious side-effects though rare include precipitation of angina and acute myocardial infarction. The use of nitrates in any form is a contraindication to use of sildenafil.

Yohimbine is an α_2-adrenergic-receptor antagonist produced in the bark of yohimbe trees. It presumably acts at the adrenergic receptors in brain centers associated with libido and penile erection. Its effects were most noticeable with respect to non-organic erectile dysfunction[21]. The most frequently reported side-effects are palpitation, fine tremor, elevation of blood pressure and anxiety. Yohimbine is not recommended for men with organic erectile dysfunction because its effect is marginal in such cases.

Apomorphine is a potent emetic that acts on central dopaminergic (D1 or D2) receptors. A dose–response effect has been apparent between 2 and 6 mg, although side-effects were more common at higher doses. The drug needs to be taken on a regular basis[22].

The observation that certain patients developed priapism after taking the antidepressant *trazadone* led to its evaluation as a treatment for erectile dysfunction[9]. It may act as a serotonin-receptor antagonist, although it is known to have some α-adrenoreceptor antagonist activity. Side-effects include drowsiness and nausea.

Surgical treatment

Arterial revascularization Candidates should be neurologically intact and have vasculogenic erectile dysfunction because of trauma (e.g. previous pelvic fracture), not systemic disease[2]. After a pelvic angiogram to confirm pathology, an anastomosis is established between the inferior epigastric artery and the penile dorsal arteries. Generally, good results are obtained in young men only.

Venous leakage Patients with veno-occlusive dysfunction typically complain of firm erections for short periods of time. Surgical procedures for venous incompetence are designed to increase venous outflow resistance in the sinusoidal spaces of the corpora cavernosa[2]. Prior to the procedure, patients are evaluated using cavernosography and cavernosometry to confirm venous leakage. Surgical treatment involves crural plication or deep penile dorsal vein excision or ligation.

Penile implants Since their introduction some 25 years ago, penile implants are still a widely chosen treatment option, mostly after failure of other forms of therapy for erectile dysfunction. The overall satisfaction rate is high. There are semi-rigid (two types – mechanical and malleable) and inflatable penile prostheses. Inflatable implants are more practical and popular. These involve a cylinder in the penis, a pump in the scrotum and a reservoir under the rectus sheath. When erection is required, the pump can be inflated. Contraindications include psychiatric disorders[2].

Herbal and unconventional therapies

Several folk remedies and alternative therapies enjoy considerable market share thanks to aggressive media campaigns and because of the universality of the problem. Most agents include ingredients such as arginine, yohimbine, damiana, ginseng, maca, zinc, *Gingko biloba*, *Avena sativa*, *Muira puama* etc. in different combinations. There has been no scientific controlled study to show their efficacy.

SEXUAL DYSFUNCTION IN WOMEN

As compared to men the epidemiology of female sexual dysfunction is even less known. Sexual dysfunction is more prevalent in women (43%) than men (31%) and is associated with various demographic characteristics, including age and educational attainment[23]. Women of different racial groups demonstrate different patterns of sexual dysfunction. Experience of sexual dysfunction is more likely among women with poor physical and emotional health. The prevalence of sexual problems also varies significantly across marital status. Premarital and postmarital (divorced, widowed, or separated) status is associated with elevated risk of experiencing sexual problems. Unmarried women are roughly 1.5 times more likely to have orgasm problems and sexual anxiety than married women. Afro-American women tend to have higher rates of low sexual desire and experience less pleasure compared with

White women, while the latter are more likely to have sexual pain than the former. Hispanic women, in contrast, consistently report lower rates of sexual dysfunction[23].

Sexual dysfunction in women can be divided into three major groups: low sexual desire, arousal disorder (anorgasmia) and sexual pain disorder.

Low sexual desire

Numerous epidemiologic studies have demonstrated a decline in sexual activity in females at the time of the menopause. The peak in loss of interest in sexual relations occurs between 45 and 50 years of age and is related to an increase in psychologic symptoms that occurred just prior to the menopause. In another study, 50% of women complained of a decline in sexual desire at the time of the menopause[24]. A Swedish study also found declining sexual interest at the time of the menopause[25]. This decline in sexual activity was not associated with total urinary estrogens, but rather with psycho-social factors.

The effect of estrogen replacement on libido in the years following the menopause has been poorly studied. Estrogens have been reported either to have no effect on sexual drive[26] or to produce a mild decrease in libido[27]. In 1943 testosterone was first suggested to improve libido in women[28]. A combination of estrogen and testosterone implants has been used to treat problems related to libido[29].

Anorgasmia

This is defined as persistent or recurrent delay in, or absence of, orgasm following a normal sexual arousal phase. It results in marked distress or interpersonal difficulty. Diabetic autonomic neuropathy is probably the most common organic cause of inhibited orgasm in women[30].

Apart from managing local vaginal conditions and discontinuing possible causal drugs, there is no other treatment for this dysfunction in women. Therefore, in women with known neuronal damage, including diabetic neuropathy, the goal of therapy should be to help patients adjust to the permanent loss of their sexual responsiveness.

Transient forms of anorgasmia caused by psychogenic factors are amenable to treatment with counseling. A history of previous orgasmic response is a good prognostic indicator. Counseling for married women and women who have a regular sexual partner should include the partner, provided it is agreeable to the patient. Counseling should be aimed primarily at resolving the dominant problems, usually life stress or interpersonal strife.

Women with anorgasmia of long duration can be given a trial of counseling. If counseling does not result in substantial improvement, additional evaluation may be needed.

Sexual pain disorder

Sexual pain disorder includes dyspareunia and vaginismus.

Dyspareunia

Dyspareunia is pain during intercourse. This pain may be of three types: superficial, vaginal or deep. Superficial dyspareunia occurs with penetration, and is usually caused by an anatomic or irritative condition, or vaginismus. Vaginal dyspareunia includes pain related to friction (e.g. lack of lubrication) or arousal disorders. Deep dyspareunia is pain resulting from thrusting during intercourse, and is usually associated with pelvic disease[31].

Vaginismus

This condition is characterized by uncontrollable spasms of the muscles in the outer third of the vagina, which can make intercourse very painful. It is often caused by sexual phobia, or a prior negative experience. It can also be induced by endometriosis. Management is targeted towards the cause.

EDUCATION

The role of the physician is not over with treating the sexual dysfunction. The physician needs to educate the patient about sexually transmitted diseases, as they are not confined to the young. As one resumes and enjoys sexual activity, necessary precautions must be taken.

Intimacy between two individuals is life affirming and valid throughout the life span. Youth is a time for exciting exploration and self-discovery, middle age a time for gaining skill and confidence and old age a time for bringing the experience of a lifetime and the unique perspective of the final years to the art of loving another person. Indeed, younger generations have much to learn from older adults who over the years have personally mastered this aspect of life.

References

1. Melman A, Gingell JC. The epidemiology and pathophysiology of erectile dysfunction. *J Urol* 1999;161:5–11
2. Kirby R, Holmes S, Carson C, eds. *Fast Facts – Erectile Dysfunction*, 2nd edn. Oxford: Health Press, 1998:7–58
3. Masters WH. Sex and aging – expectations and reality. *Hosp Pract* 1986;15:175–98
4. Pfeiffer E, Verwoerdt A, Wang HS. Sexual behavior in aged men and women. *Arch Gen Psychiatry* 1968;19:753–8
5. Comfort A, Dial LK. Sexuality and aging. *Clin Geriatr Med* 1991;7:1–7
6. Barsky AJ. Approach to the patient with sexual dysfunction. In Goroll AH, May LA, Mulley AG, eds. *Primary Care Medicine*, 2nd edn. Philadelphia: JB Lippincott, 1987:804–7
7. Kamel HK. Sexuality in aging: focus on institutionalized elderly. *Ann Long-term Care* 2001;9:64–72
8. Gray A, Feldman HA, McKinlay J, Longcope C. Age, disease, and changing sex hormone levels in middle-aged men: results of the Massachusetts Male Aging Study. *J Clin Endocrinol Metab* 1991;73:1016–25
9. Lue TF. Eerectile dysfunction. *N Engl J Med* 2000;342:1802–13
10. Benet AE, Melman A. The epidemiology of erectile dysfunction. *Urol Clin North Am* 1995;22:699–709
11. Feldman HA, Goldstein I, Hatzichristou DG, *et al*. Impotence and its medical and psychosocial correlates: results of the Massachusetts Male Aging Study. *J Urol* 1994;151:54–61
12. Mulligan T, Katz G. Why aged men become impotent. *Arch Intern Med* 1989; 149:1365
13. Sadovsky R, Dunn M, Grobe BM. Erectile dysfunction: the primary care practitioner's view. *Am J Managed Care* 1999; 5:333–41
14. Bodansky HJ. Treatment of male erectile dysfunction using the active vacuum assist device. *Diabet Med* 1994;11:410–12
15. Morles A, Johnston B, Heaton JW, Clark A. Oral androgens in the treatment of hypogonadal impotent men. *J Urol* 1994;152: 1115–18
16. Arver S, Dobs AS, Meikle AW, *et al*. Improvement of sexual function in testosterone deficient men treated for 1 year with permeation enhanced testosterone transdermal system. *J Urol* 1996;155: 1604–8
17. Virag R. Intracavernous injection of papaverine for erectile failure. *Lancet* 1982;2:938
18. Linet OI, Ogrinc FG. The Alprostadil Study Group. Efficacy and safety of intracavernosal alprostadil in men with erectile

dysfunction. *N Engl J Med* 1996;334: 873–87

19. Padma-Nathan H, Hellstrom WJG, Kaiser FE, *et al*. Treatment of men with erectile dysfunction with transuretral alprostadil. *N Engl J Med* 1997;336:1–7

20. Werthman P, Rajfer J. MUSE therapy: preliminary clinical observations. *Urology* 1997;50:809–11

21. Ernst E, Pittler MH. Yohimbine for erectile dysfunction: a systematic review and meta-analysis of randomized clinical trials. *J Urol* 1998;159:433–6

22. Heaton JP, Morales A, Adams A, *et al*. Recovery of erectile dysfunction by the oral administration of apomorphine. *Urology* 1995;45:200–6

23. Laumann EO, Paik A, Rosen RC. Sexual dysfunction in the United States. *J Am Med Assoc* 1999;281:537–44

24. Bachman GA, Leiblum SR, Sandler B, *et al*. Correlates of sexual desire in post-menopausal women. *Maturitas* 1985;7: 211–16

25. Person G. Sexuality in a 70-year-old urban population. *J Psychosom Res* 1980;24: 335–42

26. Morley JE. Endocrine factors in geriatric sexuality. *Clin Geriatr Med* 1991;7:85–93

27. Dennerstein L, Burrows GD. Hormone replacement therapy and sexuality in women. *Clin Endocrinol Metab* 1976;3: 661–8

28. Salmon TJ, Gast SH. Effect of androgens in libido in women. *J Clin Endocrinol Metab* 1943;3:235–8

29. Studd JWW, Collins WP, Charkrvate S. Oestradiol and testosterone implants in the treatment of psychosexual problems in the postmenopausal woman. *Br J Obstet Gynaecol* 1977;84:314–16

30. Mooradian AD. Geriatric sexuality and chronic diseases. *Clin Geriatr Med* 1991;7: 113–31

31. Bachman GA, Leiblum S, Grill J. Brief sexual inquiry in gynecologic practice. *Obstet Gynecol* 1989;73:425–7

51 Disorders of the prostate

Shahrad Aynehchi, MD, Albert A. Samadi, MD, and
Majid Eshghi, MD, FACS

INTRODUCTION

In the current practice of medicine, primary care providers have assumed a prominent role in the treatment of prostatic diseases in the elderly. This market trend has been primarily dictated by an increased awareness of the various pathologic conditions of the prostate among an aging population. Advancements in early diagnosis, enhanced delivery of care and a constellation of safe and effective treatment modalities have transformed this field in recent years. Emphasized here are basic pathology, clinical presentation and initial management strategies of prostatic disorders.

ANATOMIC CONSIDERATIONS

The prostate is a 20-g glandular organ that encircles the urethra as it emerges from the bladder neck (Figure 1). The base of the prostate is intimately adjacent to the bladder trigone. The major segments of the prostate are the peripheral zone, transition zone, central zone and anterior fibromuscular stroma (Figure 2). The peripheral zone is the portion that is palpated during digital rectal examination (DRE) for prostate cancer screening. The transition zone, on the other hand, may occlude the urethra and urine flow as a consequence of benign prostatic hyperplasia (BPH). Two seminal vesicles converge at the posterior aspect of the prostate, where each is joined by the vasa deferentia. These form the ejaculatory ducts that perforate the prostate and pass obliquely to enter the prostatic urethra at the verumontanum.

PROSTATE-SPECIFIC ANTIGEN

Prostate specific antigen (PSA), introduced in the past two decades as a tumor marker, denotes an important advance in early detection and management of prostate cancer. PSA is a serine protease, secreted in the cytoplasm of the prostatic endothelium and lining of the periurethral glands[1]. It primarily aids in the liquefaction of the ejaculate and release of motile spermatozoa. Although variations exist, it is generally accepted that PSA values range between 0 and 4 ng/ml in healthy adults. Normal PSA levels are expected to rise gradually with increasing age and differ among various ethnic groups. Although controversial, estimated normal age-dependent PSA levels by ethnic groups[2-4] have been proposed (Table 1)[5].

Various pathologic conditions of the prostate may cause an abnormal rise in PSA. In BPH, an enlarged transition zone may account for increases in PSA production. Elevated PSA levels may also occur as a result of prostate cancer, prostatitis, prostatic abscess, acute urinary retention, instrumentation, and trauma. Therefore, PSA levels should be measured approximately 4 weeks after resolution of the aforementioned

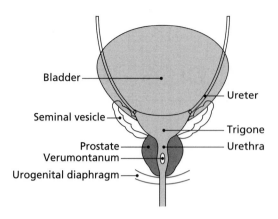

Figure 1 Anatomic relation of prostate to adjacent organs. (Illustration courtesy of Shirin Raban)

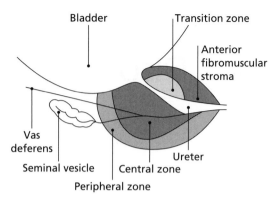

Figure 2 Lateral view of prostatic zones. (Illustration courtesy of Shirin Raban)

conditions. Further, a number of medications used in the treatment of BPH and prostate cancer can decrease PSA levels (Table 2). Although PSA elevation may occur after DRE, the effect is clinically insignificant[6].

Currently, PSA is used in conjunction with DRE as the primary screening tool for cancer of the prostate. PSA and DRE should be offered annually to all men after the age of 50 with an expected lifespan of more than 10 years and after age 40 in high-risk groups[7]. Men at high risk are those with first-degree relatives with prostate cancer and African-Americans. In patients who have an abnormal DRE or an elevated PSA, a prostate biopsy is indicated.

Assessing PSA velocity, defined as the rate of rise of PSA per year, has been proposed in an effort to improve diagnostic accuracy. The rate of increase is based on three separate PSA measurements, taken at least 6 months apart, over a 1.5–2 year period. An increase in PSA by 0.75 ng/ml over a 1-year period may indicate the presence of prostate cancer and prompt a prostate biopsy[8].

In serum, PSA exists in either bound (complexed) or unbound (free) form. The percentage of free PSA represents the total proportion of PSA in the unbound form. When PSA lies between 4 and 10 ng/ml in patients with a normal DRE, free PSA can help further define the risk of cancer. As the percentage of free PSA decreases, the risk for having prostate cancer increases. Although there is no clear consensus for a cut-off value, free PSA level less than 25% is associated with a higher probability of prostate cancer[9].

Prior to the PSA era, prostatic acid phosphatase was a widely utilized marker for metastatic prostate cancer. However, PSA is currently the standard marker in monitoring the progression of the disease in these patients. PSA levels reach a nadir after definitive treatment for cancer. Post-treatment elevations in PSA may indicate local recurrence or metastatic disease and warrant further investigation.

PROSTATITIS

Pathophysiology

Prostatic inflammatory conditions, termed prostatitis, commonly arise from bacterial infection of the gland. Possible routes of prostatic infection include:

(1) Retrograde ascent of bacteria from the urethra

(2) Retrograde ascent of infected urine

(3) Direct extension of infection from the rectum

(4) Hematogenous seeding

Table 1 Age-adjusted prostate-specific antigen (PSA) values by ethnic group. (Adapted with permission from WB Saunders[5])

Age (years)	PSA levels (ng/ml)		
	Asians[2]	Blacks[3]	Caucasians[4]
40–49	0–2.0	0–2.0	0–2.5
50–59	0–3.0	0–4.0	0–3.5
60–69	0–4.0	0–4.5	0–4.5
70–79	0–5.0	0–5.5	0–6.5

Table 2 Medications that decrease serum prostate-specific antigen

Agent class	Medication
Estrogens	diethylstilbestrol
	estradiol
LHRH agonists	goserelin (Zoladex®)
	leuprolide (Lupron®)
Pure antiandrogens	flutamide (Eulexin®)
	bicalutamide (Casodex®)
	nilutamide (Nilandron®)
Steroidal antiandrogens	cyproterone acetate
	megesterol acetate (Megace®)
Androgen synthesis inhibitors	ketoconazole (Nizoral®)
	aminoglutethimide (Cytadren®)
5α-reductase inhibitors	finasteride (Proscar®)
	epristeride
Alternative therapy	saw palmetto berry

LHRH, luteinizing hormone releasing hormone

Furthermore, chemical irritation from refluxing urine can cause an aseptic form of prostatitis. A number of defensive mechanisms are inherent to the prostate and sustain its resistance to infection.

(1) Rich blood supply protects against infection

(2) Forward flow of secretions retards retrograde invasion of the gland

(3) Prostatic secretions (zinc, citric acid, magnesium, etc.) have bactericidal properties

(4) Spermatozoa have antibacterial activity

(5) Immunoglobulins A and G provide local regulation of pathogens.

In spite of these protective means, prostatitis still accounts for one of the most common ailments affecting men of all ages. In older men, urinary obstruction from BPH is the primary causative factor. As a result, a pressure chamber is created within the posterior urethra which can force urine in a retrograde manner into the ejaculatory ducts leading to prostatitis[10]. Treatment, depending on the type, is often frustrating for both patient and clinician. Clinically, several categories have been recognized.

Acute bacterial prostatitis

Acute bacterial prostatitis, mostly encountered in young sexually active men, is commonly due to retrograde invasion of the gland by reflux of infected urine or periurethral pathogens. In the older population, more likely routes of acute infection include catheterization and instrumentation, as well

Table 3 Symptoms of acute bacterial prostatitis

Constitutional symptoms
fever
chills
fatigue
flank pain
perineal pain
testicular pain
muscle and joint aches
pain with bowel movement
painful ejaculation

Urinary symptoms
frequency
urgency
hesitancy
painful urination
urinary retention

as lymphatic and hematogenous spread. Symptoms are sudden and severe, and thus easily diagnosed (Table 3). The sensation has been described as 'sitting on a piece of hot charcoal'.

DRE reveals a warm, tense and boggy prostate. Aggressive DRE and prostatic massage are generally contraindicated, because of the severe pain and the possibility of spreading the infection into the bloodstream. Urinalysis usually shows pyuria, microhematuria and bacteriuria. Offending pathogens, as identified on urine culture, commonly include *Escherichia coli*, *Klebsiella* and *Pseudomonas* species[11].

In the presence of fever, a tender prostate and infected urine, antibiotics should be started immediately. In order to prevent disseminated infection, generally 4–6 weeks of treatment with a fluoroquinolone (i.e. ciprofloxacin or ofloxacin) is recommended. The recommended oral dosage is ciprofloxacin (Cipro®) 500 mg twice per day or ofloxacin (Floxin®) 300–400 mg twice per day. The dose must be adjusted for renal function. If the patient appears septic, immediate hospitalization for intravenous antibiotics and hydration is indicated.

Prostatic abscess is a possible complication of acute bacterial prostatitis. Most cases occur in the fifth or sixth decades of life, with *E. coli* being the most common causative organism. Immunocompromised patients, however, may present at a younger age with chronic infections associated with unusual organisms. An abscess must be suspected when the patient's clinical condition fails to improve or worsens despite appropriate antibiotic therapy[12]. Fluctuance within the prostate on examination frequently indicates an abscess and may be better visualized with a transrectal ultrasound or pelvic computerized tomography (CT) scan. Intravenous ampicillin (1–2 g every 6 h) and gentamicin (3–5 mg/kg per day divided into three doses) are appropriate initial treatments until culture results become available. Upon diagnosis, the abscess is drained via transurethral unroofing of the prostate. If the patient is unable to urinate, a suprapubic tube may be necessary for bladder drainage.

Serum PSA measurement in acute bacterial prostatitis is inappropriate, as it will be invariably elevated. The clinician should wait 4–6 weeks after treatment before obtaining a serum PSA level.

Chronic bacterial prostatitis

Unlike its acute counterpart, chronic bacterial prostatitis has a more variable presentation. Although at times it may emerge from an unresolved acute event, many patients do not recall a previous episode. Irritative voiding symptoms may be present accompanied with occasional low back or perineal pain, myalgia and arthralgia. Others may be only incidentally diagnosed because of asymptomatic bacteriuria. On DRE, the prostate may feel normal, boggy or indurated. Urinalysis typically reveals more than ten white blood cells per high power field. However, when urine cultures do not reveal an infecting organism, sequential urine collection accompanied by prostatic massage and collection of prostatic secretions can assist in making the diagnosis (Table 4)[11].

Table 4 Meares–Stamey Four Glass Test[11]

Sample	Method of collection	Localization
VB1	collect first voided urine (5–10 ml)	urethral flora
VB2	collect midstream urine	bladder flora
EPS	perform prostatic massage and collect secretions	prostatic flora
VB3	collect first voided 10 ml urine after massage	prostatic flora

VB, voided bladder; EPS, expressed prostatic secretion

This technique aids in localization of infection to the urethra, bladder or prostate. Once the presence of infection is established, appropriate culture-sensitive antibiotics are started. As in acute bacterial prostatitis, a minimum antibiotic course of 4–6 weeks is essential. Concomitant use of α-blockers to provide symptomatic relief is also conventional. In some men it is difficult to completely eradicate the infection, and longer periods (12 weeks or longer) of antibiotics are necessary[12]. Relief from symptoms and prevention of future acute infections is possible with continuous administration of low-dose oral antibiotics. In refractory cases, operative resection of infected prostatic calculi may be appropriate.

Non-bacterial prostatitis

Non-bacterial prostatitis is the most common and possibly the least understood form of prostatic inflammatory disease. Symptoms are similar to those of chronic bacterial prostatitis; however, patients typically do not have any history of previous urinary tract infections. Abnormal levels of inflammatory cells are evident on urinalysis and prostate secretions. Nonetheless, none of the studies have revealed any evidence of an infectious agent. This diagnosis, subclassified as a form of chronic pelvic pain syndrome[13], is one of exclusion. Several proposed etiologies include infection, neuropathy, pelvic floor dysfunction and autoimmune disease, with symptoms attributed to chemical irritation of refluxing urine into the prostate. Most patients are initially treated with a trial of antibiotics (at least 4 weeks) with minimal response. At that stage, further empiric use of antibiotics is not warranted. α-Blockers, typically used in the treatment of BPH, have yielded good results. Alternative treatments may alleviate symptoms and expedite recovery:

(1) Anti-inflammatory medications (e.g. ibuprofen 400–600 mg three times daily or Vioxx® 25–50 mg daily)

(2) Pentosanpolysulfate sodium (Elmiron® 100 mg three times per day)[14]

(3) Warm tub baths (sitz baths)

(4) Stool softeners

(5) Increased fluid consumption

(6) Avoidance of hot and spicy foods, caffeine, alcohol, citrus juices

(7) Alternating hot and cold compresses to perineal area

(8) Zinc supplements

(9) Yoga, relaxation therapy and biofeedback[15]

(10) Normal physical and sexual activity.

Prostatodynia

As in non-bacterial prostatitis, patients with prostatodynia present with irritative voiding symptoms as well. Prostatodynia, also a form of pelvic pain syndrome, is associated with a completely normal physical and laboratory examination. Expressed prostatic secretion and voided bladder specimen show no signs of inflammatory cells or infection. Instead, it has been proposed that a neuromuscular dysfunction of the pelvic floor musculature may cause a functional obstruction at the bladder neck or prostatic urethra. This in turn can cause reflux of sterile urine into the prostate with its untoward effects.

Treatment is similar to that for non-bacterial prostatitis. α_1-Blocking agents (terazosin 1–10 mg/day, doxazosin 1–4 mg/day, or tamsulosin 0.4 mg/day) have been effective. In cases of pelvic floor myalgia, muscle relaxants, new anti-inflammatory agents, physiotherapy and anticholinergic medications may be tried. Other proposed relevant factors include stress and depression, warranting psychiatric evaluation.

BENIGN PROSTATIC HYPERPLASIA

Pathophysiology

Although no clear etiology for BPH has been identified, it is apparent that growth of the prostate is directly related to age and the presence of dihydrotestosterone (DHT). The prostate undergoes a bimodal growth spurt, initially at about puberty and again around the fifth decade of life. The basis for the latter phase, which continues for the rest of the man's life, is BPH. This process involves a heterogeneous stromal and glandular hyperplasia of the prostate. Primarily affected are the transition and central zones, which encircle the proximal urethra and bladder neck area.

Due to its unique location, the enlarging prostate bulk may sequentially increase the resistance of the proximal urethra to the outflow of urine. This, in turn, results in higher pressures generated by the bladder to overcome the obstruction. Progressively, the bladder musculature de-compensates, resulting in a weak and flabby bladder with diverticuli. This stasis of urine harbors an environment ripe for infection and bladder stone formation. The most serious complication, however, is the transmission of high bladder pressures to the kidneys, resulting in hydronephrosis and gradual loss of renal function.

Symptoms

The constellation of voiding symptoms attributed to BPH is commonly referred to as lower urinary tract symptoms (LUTS). In BPH, the inability to empty the bladder completely is prevalent. This chronic retention of urine leads to more frequent filling of the bladder, resulting in shorter voiding intervals (frequency) and urinating at night (nocturia). Other symptoms may include difficulty initiating a urinary stream (hesitancy), straining to void, an intermittent urinary stream (intermittency), a weak urinary stream and dribbling. Urinary urgency and urge incontinence may develop secondary to the obstruction.

In order to facilitate obtaining a pertinent history and to monitor treatment progress, the International Prostate Symptom Score (I-PSS) has been widely adopted (Figure 3)[16]. This questionnaire is based on seven questions, each scored from zero to five, for a maximum symptom score of 35 points. It is generally accepted that overall scores below 7, in the absence of complications, warrant only watchful waiting. Scores ranging from 8 to 19 are generally indicative of moderate symptoms and scores between 20 and 35 indicate severe symptoms[17].

Evaluation

A thorough initial physical examination is important. Suprapubic distention indicates urinary retention. Flank tenderness may indicate pyelonephritis as the result of infected urine refluxing up to the kidney. Inguinal or abdominal wall hernias may serve as a clue to the presence of obstruction and straining. The penis must be examined for penile carcinoma, phimosis, meatal stenosis and urethral stricture, conditions that may also cause obstructive symptoms. DRE usually reveals

International Prostate Symptom Score (I-PSS)						
Urinary Symptoms	Not at all	Less than 1 time in 5	Less than half the time	About half the time	More than half the time	Almost always
1. Over the past month, how often have you had a sensation of not emptying your bladder completely after you finished urinating?	0	1	2	3	4	5
2. Over the past month, how often have you had to urinate again less than two hours after you finished urinating?	0	1	2	3	4	5
3. Over the past month, how often have you found you stopped and started again several times when you urinated?	0	1	2	3	4	5
4. Over the past month, how often have you found it difficult to postpone urination?	0	1	2	3	4	5
5. Over the past month, how often have you had a weak urinary stream?	0	1	2	3	4	5
6. Over the past month, how often have you had to push or strain to begin urination?	0	1	2	3	4	5
	None	1 time	2 times	3 times	4 times	5 or more
7. Over the past month or so, how many times did you most typically get up to urinate from the time you went to bed at night until the time you got up in the morning?	0	1	2	3	4	5
I-PSS = sum of questions 1-7						
QUALITY OF LIFE DUE TO URINARY SYMPTOMS						
	Delighted	Pleased	Mostly satisfied	Mixed	Mostly dissatisfied	Unhappy	Terrible
If you were to spend the rest of your life with your urinary condition just the way it is now, how would you feel about that?	0	1	2	3	4	5	6

Figure 3 International prostate symptom score for benign prostatic hyperplasia[16]

an enlarged, smooth prostate. Presence of nodularity raises the suspicion of cancer of the prostate. A neurologic examination is important for manifestations of advanced urinary obstruction and uremia.

Baseline serum creatinine and urinalysis should be obtained prior to initiation of treatment. The presence of white blood cells or bacteria in the urine specimen may indicate infection and warrant antibiotic treatment.

Proteinuria may signify already deteriorating renal function. Microhematuria should prompt a search for other pathology such as stones, tumors or infection. If serum PSA level is elevated on initial examination in a symptomatic patient, a repeat level should be obtained about 4 weeks after initiation of therapy.

Further investigation with uroflowmetry and post-void residual (PVR) measurements may be obtained in select cases in consultation with a urologist. Poor urine flow rates, as demonstrated on uroflowmetry, cannot differentiate between outflow obstruction and poor bladder contraction. However, when coupled with PVR, the values can be compared to pre-treatment levels to monitor therapeutic efficacy. In longstanding cases of BPH, renal ultrasound is useful to investigate the presence of hydronephrosis. Complex urodynamics have little role in the routine management of BPH.

Treatment

Medical

The advent of pharmacologic agents for the treatment of BPH has led to a significant decline in its surgical management. Currently, two classes of medication are widely used: α_1-blockers and antiandrogens.

The mechanism of action of α_1-blockers is to relax the muscular fibers surrounding the bladder neck and prostate, thus facilitating urethral opening during voiding. Currently available oral agents are terazosin (Hytrin® 1–10 mg/day), doxazosin (Cardura® 1–4 mg/day) and tamsulosin (Flomax® 0.4 mg/day). Their side-effect profile is related to their antihypertensive mode of action: dizziness, lightheadedness, tachycardia and palpitations. Nasal congestion and retrograde ejaculation are also reported.

Antiandrogens, in general, are utilized in the treatment of prostate cancer. Finasteride (Proscar® 5 mg/day) is the only antiandrogen currently in common use for the treatment of

Table 5 Phytotherapeutic agents tried for therapy for benign prostatic hyperplasia[21]

Phytotherapy agents
African plum
purple cone flower
pumpkin seeds
saw palmetto berry
South African star grass
stinging nettle

BPH. It blocks the transformation of testosterone to DHT by inhibiting the enzyme 5-α-reductase. By decreasing DHT, it reduces the main growth factor for prostatic tissue. Finasteride has been shown to decrease prostate size, improve urinary flow rates and decrease the risk of acute urinary retention[18]. These observations are significant primarily when finasteride is administered for at least 6 months. Finasteride is also an effective agent in controlling prostatic bleeding secondary to BPH[19]. Side-effects include headache, minimal loss of libido and lowering of PSA levels to about half the original value. Thus, PSA values should be doubled when evaluating a patient beyond 6 months of treatment with finasteride[20].

In recent years, there has been a rapid increase in the use of alternative medical treatments. Commonly used agents include zinc, selenium, vitamin E and 'health pills'. A number of phytotherapeutic agents are also widely purchased by patients for BPH (Table 5)[21]. Long-term, controlled, double-blind trials of these agents are lacking and their efficacy is debatable.

Surgical

Surgical therapy is reserved for those who have severe symptoms despite medical therapy, urinary retention, renal deterioration, bladder stones, recurrent infections, refractory prostatic bleeding and acquired bladder diverticuli. Over many decades, transurethral resection of the prostate (TURP) has been

Table 6 Minimally invasive modalities for the management of benign prostatic hyperplasia

Abbreviation	Procedure
HoLEP	holmium laser enucleation of the prostate[24]
S-TURP	saline transurethral resection of the prostate[47]
WIT	water-induced thermotherapy[48]
ILC	interstitial laser coagulation
TUIP	transurethral incision of the prostate
TULIP	transurethral laser induced prostatectomy
VLAP	non-contact visual laser ablation of the prostate
TUEP	transurethral evaporation of the prostate
TUMT	transurethral microwave thermotherapy
HIFU	high-intensity focused ultrasound
TUNA	transurethral needle ablation
TUEVP	transurethral electrovaporization of the prostate
TUBD	transurethral balloon dilatation

the gold standard in surgical treatment. TURP is regarded as a highly effective procedure. However, its potential morbidities include bleeding, transurethral resection (TUR) syndrome, bladder perforation, retrograde ejaculation, urethral stricture, impotence, infection and incontinence. TUR syndrome is characterized by a rapid change in intravascular volume and plasma concentrations of solutes. This is secondary to the absorption of hypo-osmolar irrigating fluid through the prostatic sinuses, resulting in marked postoperative hyponatremia and neurologic symptoms[22].

In the minimally invasive era, a number of alternative novel procedures have been developed (Table 6), although some have already fallen out of favor. Most of these therapies use heat to destroy prostatic tissue. The ensuing evaporation or sloughing of tissue, depending on the rate of energy deposition, results in an increased lumen size[23]. Flexible prostatic urethral stents have also been utilized with varying success. Open surgical treatment for BPH, referred to as simple prostatectomy, is traditionally reserved for very large glands. More recently, holmium laser enucleation of the prostate (HoLEP) has made it possible endoscopically to enucleate these larger glands with minimal morbidity[24].

CANCER OF THE PROSTATE

Risk factors

Prostate cancer is the most common cancer and the second leading cause of cancer-related death in men in the USA. Although its etiology is still poorly understood, several risk factors for the development and progression of this disease have been defined. The risk of cancer rises dramatically with age. The probability of developing cancer of the prostate rises from 1 in 103 for men aged 40–59 years to 1 in 8 for men aged 60–79 years[25]. Other contributing factors include Black race[26], history of prostate cancer in a first-degree relative[27], high fat consumption[28], exposure to androgens[29] and cadmium[30]. If prostate cancer is diagnosed and treated early, cure is the rule. Therefore, screening is essential.

Symptoms

Prostate cancer is a silent disease, often diagnosed on routine annual evaluation. LUTS may indicate the presence of local invasion into the prostatic urethra and bladder neck. Bone pain must raise suspicion of metastatic disease. If associated with spinal pain and lower extremity neurologic deficits, the patient must be promptly evaluated for spinal cord compression.

Evaluation

All men above age 50, African-Americans, or those with a family history of prostate cancer above age 40, should undergo annual screening. Annual evaluation consists of history, comprehensive physical examination, and serum PSA determination. The peripheral zone of the prostate, the portion that is palpated during DRE, harbors the cancerous tissue in approximately 70% of cases. Thus, induration or nodularity of the prostate on DRE is an indication for referral to a urologist for prostate biopsy. Furthermore, an elevated PSA, high PSA velocity (> 0.75 ng/ml per year) or low free PSA (< 25%) also warrant biopsy.

Transrectal ultrasound (TRUS)-guided biopsy of the prostate has emerged as the gold standard for diagnosis. The number of biopsies usually varies from six to 12 cores, although higher numbers have been advocated to ensure adequate sampling of all suspect areas[31]. The biopsy cores are assigned a histologic type and a Gleason score. Adenocarcinoma is by far the most common histologic type of prostate cancer. In determining a Gleason score, a primary grade is assigned to the most common pattern of cancer and a secondary grade is assigned to the second most common pattern of cancer observed. The grades range from 1 to 5. The Gleason score is the sum of the grades assigned to the two most predominant patterns, and thus, can range from 2 to 10. Higher Gleason scores are associated with higher malignant potential (Table 7).

Occasionally, prostatic intraepithelial neoplasia (PIN) is diagnosed. Although not considered malignant, high-grade PIN is considered as a precursor to invasive prostate cancer. Therefore, these lesions warrant a repeat biopsy every 6 months.

Once the diagnosis of prostate cancer has been established, the possibility of local invasion and metastatic disease must be investigated in order to formulate a treatment plan. Bones are the most common metastatic site

Table 7 Gleason scores and histologic pattern

Gleason score	Histologic pattern
2 – 4	well differentiated
5 – 6	moderately differentiated
7 – 10	poorly differentiated

for prostate cancer. A baseline bone scan is indicated for skeletal pain or when the PSA level is > 10 ng/ml[32]. Computed tomographic (CT) scan is performed to assess pelvic lymphadenopathy in high-risk patients (PSA > 25 ng/ml) who are considering definitive local therapy[33]. In some centers, endorectal coil magnetic resonance imaging (MRI) is used to assess local invasion of the tumor.

Nomograms (Partin tables) have been developed in recent years which take into account preoperative PSA level, biopsy Gleason score and clinical stage of the tumor[34]. These tables help determine the likelihood of organ-confined disease versus extraprostatic invasion, seminal vesicle invasion or lymph node invasion. They are invaluable in formulating a treatment plan.

Treatment

Watchful waiting

Although in progress, no randomized trials have yet been concluded regarding the benefit of observation versus definitive treatment for low-grade cancer. Older patients who have small, well-differentiated, slowly progressive cancers may be good candidates for watchful waiting. In the older patient with a slow-growing tumor and other illnesses, radical treatment for prostate cancer is associated with significant morbidity, while unlikely to prolong life. The age of the patient is critical in assessing outcome. In one study, only 25% of men over age 85 who deferred curative treatment for prostate cancer died of the disease. However, the cancer specific mortality rate for those under 55 years of age was 100%[35]. The decision to proceed with potentially curative treatment or to observe depends on the age of the patient, other associated illnesses and the patient's general life expectancy. The observation period may reach an end with rapidly rising PSA levels, newly found pelvic lymphadenopathy or new onset of symptoms. At this stage, some form of treatment may be warranted.

Radical prostatectomy

The best candidates for radical prostatectomy (retropubic or perineal approach) are those with organ-confined disease, low operative risk and a general life expectancy of at least 10 years. Radical prostatectomies are infrequently performed in men over 70 years of age. The risk of life-threatening complications of radical prostatectomy in the old is comparable to that in younger patients[36,37]. However, older adults are more likely to suffer from other diseases that would preclude them from having surgery altogether. Ten-year survival rates for patients with organ-confined disease who undergo radical prostatectomy have been reported as high as 85%[38]. Although neoadjuvant hormonal therapy and radiation may have a role in more aggressive tumors, firm indications are still under debate.

Occasionally, a patient may undergo salvage radical prostatectomy for local recurrence after primary radiation therapy. In these patients, morbidity and recurrence rates are significant.

Brachytherapy

Brachytherapy has become increasingly popular in the past decade as a primary form of definitive therapy for prostate cancer. It involves implantation of radioactive iodine-125 or palladium-103 seeds into the prostate under TRUS guidance. This treatment has been advocated for less aggressive cancers (PSA < 10 ng/ml, Gleason score < 6) and prostates with a smaller volume. Patients

with significant irritative and obstructive voiding symptoms prior to treatment tend to fare poorly. Post-treatment complications may include lower urinary tract symptoms as well as passage of sloughed tissue and seeds per urethra. Five-year biochemical relapse-free rates in patients with PSA ≤ 4 ng/ml have been reported as high as 83%[39]. This procedure may be the choice in patients with low-volume disease who may not be able to tolerate extensive radical surgery.

External-beam radiation

External-beam radiation therapy (XRT) has been traditionally reserved for patients who are candidates for curative therapy but not fit to undergo radical prostatectomy. Although a large proportion of these patients now opt for brachytherapy, recent reports have shown significant long-term survival rates with XRT[40]. The advent of three-dimensional conformal radiotherapy has allowed accurate delivery of higher doses of radiation to the prostate. In patients who have biochemical failure (i.e. elevated PSA) following XRT, consideration should be given to salvage radical prostatectomy, cryosurgery or androgen blockade.

Patients with locally invasive cancer are often treated with neoadjuvant hormonal therapy and XRT. Results of this combination are superior to those of XRT alone[41]. Salvage XRT also has a role in patients with local recurrence after radical prostatectomy.

Cryosurgery

In this age of minimally invasive surgery, there has been a resurrection of cryosurgical techniques in the treatment of localized prostate cancer. In this process, multiple probes are inserted transperineally into the prostate under TRUS guidance. The urethra is warmed via a catheter while the prostate undergoes freeze–thaw cycles, resulting in destruction of tissue[42]. In carefully selected patients with localized disease, cryotherapy has been proposed as a viable option for primary treatment[43]. Salvage cryotherapy after radiation has also been advocated in patients with PSA levels of < 10 ng/ml (prior to cryotherapy), clinical stage < T3 and a low Gleason score[44]. Postoperative irritative and obstructive voiding symptoms have been reported. More trials are needed to evaluate long-term morbidity and survival with this treatment.

Hormonal therapy

Most prostate cancers are hormone dependent, i.e. they respond to testosterone for growth and proliferation[45]. Most (95%) of the circulating testosterone is produced in the testes by Leydig cells, with the remainder coming from the adrenal cortex. The stimulus for the release of testosterone is provided from the pulsatile release of luteinizing hormone releasing hormone (LHRH) from the hypothalamus to the anterior pituitary. In response, the anterior pituitary releases LH systemically, which stimulates the production of testosterone in the Leydig cells. Subsequently, free testosterone can be converted to DHT via the enzyme 5α-reductase within the prostatic stroma. Disruption of different parts of this pituitary–gonadal cascade has been utilized to achieve androgen blockade. For a listing of the main agents, refer to Table 2.

Medical castration is achieved by LHRH analogs and is equivalent to surgical castration (bilateral orchiectomy). When castration is coupled with the oral administration of pure antiandrogens, total androgen blockade is achieved. Steroidal antiandrogens, although used in Europe, have not yet been approved for use in the USA. Side-effects of androgen deprivation may be significant, especially in older men. They include decreased libido, muscle wasting, osteoporosis, hot flashes, fatigue, psychologic changes and anemia.

The timing of hormonal therapy as well as the efficacy of partial versus complete androgen blockade have been the subject of debate for many years. It is generally agreed that, in cases of metastatic disease, hormonal therapy is appropriate. Hormonal therapy may be beneficial as neoadjuvant therapy, prior to radical prostatectomy or radiation in selected patients. Furthermore, when faced with recurrence after definitive therapy, hormonal therapy is widely utilized.

A patient is said to have progressed to a hormone refractory state when PSA levels continue to rise despite androgen blockade. It has been shown that withdrawal of antiandrogens in hormone refractory prostate cancer can result in temporary downward shifts in PSA levels[46]. Chemotherapy is reserved as a last resort for hormone refractory prostate cancer and its role is palliative.

PC-SPES, an over-the-counter herbal medication, had gained popularity in the treatment of hormone refractory prostate cancer. However, in early 2002, the US Food and Drug Administration issued a warning and this medication was discontinued in the US market.

References

1. Pollen JJ, Dreilinger A. Immunohistochemical identification of prostatic acid phosphatase and prostate specific antigen in female periurethral glands. *Urology* 1984; 23:303–4
2. Oesterling JE, Kumamoto Y, Tsukamoto T, *et al*. Serum prostate-specific antigen in a community-based population of healthy Japanese men: lower values than for similarly aged white men. *Br J Urol* 1995;75:347–53
3. Morgan TO, Jacobsen SJ, McCarthy WF, *et al*. Age-specific reference ranges for serum prostate-specific antigen in black men. *N Engl J Med* 1996;335:304–10

4. Oesterling JE, Jacobsen SJ, Chute CG, *et al*. Serum prostate-specific antigen in a community-based population of healthy men. Establishment of age-specific reference ranges. *J Am Med Assoc* 1993;270: 860–4

5. Richardson TD, Oesterling JE. Age-specific reference ranges for serum prostate-specific antigen. *Urol Clin North Am* 1997;24:339–51

6. Chybowski FM, Bergstralh EJ, Oesterling JE. The effect of digital rectal examination on the serum prostate specific antigen concentration: results of a randomized study. *J Urol* 1992;148:83–6

7. Carroll P, Coley C, McLeod D, *et al*. Prostate-specific antigen best practice policy – Part I: early detection and diagnosis of prostate cancer. *Urology* 2001;57:217–24

8. Carter HB, Pearson JD. Prostate-specific antigen velocity and repeated measures of prostate-specific antigen. *Urol Clin North Am* 1997;24:333–8

9. Catalona WJ, Partin AW, Slawin KM, *et al*. Use of the percentage of free prostate-specific antigen to enhance differentiation of prostate cancer from benign prostatic disease: a prospective multicenter clinical trial. *J Am Med Assoc* 1998;279:1542–7

10. Blacklock NJ. Anatomical factors in prostatitis. *Br J Urol* 1974;46:47–54

11. Meares EM, Stamey TA. Bacteriologic localization patterns in bacterial prostatitis and urethritis. *Invest Urol* 1968;5:492–518

12. Nickel JC. Prostatitis: evolving management strategies. *Urol Clin North Am* 1999; 26:737–51

13. Krieger JN, Byberg L Jr, Nickel JC. NIH consensus definition and classification of prostatitis. *J Am Med Assoc* 1999;282: 236–7

14. Nickel JC, Johnston B, Downey J, *et al*. Pentosan polysulfate therapy for chronic nonbacterial prostatitis (chronic pelvic pain syndrome category IIIA): a prospective multicenter clinical trial. *Urology* 2000;56: 413–17

15. Hellstrom WJ, Schmidt RA, Lue TF, Tanagho EA. Neuromuscular dysfunction in nonbacterial prostatitis. *Urology* 1987; 30:183–8

16. Denis L, McConnell J, Yoshida O, *et al*. Recommendations of the International Scientific Committee: the evaluation and treatment of lower urinary tract symptoms (LUTS) suggestive of benign prostatic obstruction. In Denis L, Griffiths K, Khoury S, *et al*., eds. *Proceedings of the 4th International Consultation on Benign Prostatic Hyperplasia (BPH)*. Plymouth, UK: Health Publication Ltd., 1998:672

17. Barry MJ, Fowler FJ Jr, O'Leary MP, *et al*. The American Urological Association symptom index for benign prostatic hyperplasia. *J Urol* 1992;148:1549–57

18. McConnell JD, Bruskewitz R, Walsh P, *et al*. The effect of finasteride on the risk of acute urinary retention and the need for surgical treatment among men with benign prostatic hyperplasia. Finasteride Long-Term Efficacy and Safety Study Group. *N Engl J Med* 1998;338:557–63

19. Sieber PR, Rommel FM, Huffnagle HW, *et al*. The treatment of gross hematuria secondary to prostatic bleeding with finasteride. *J Urol* 1998;159:1232–3

20. Gormley GJ, Ng J, Cook T, *et al*. Effect of finasteride on prostate-specific antigen density. *Urology* 1994;43:53–9

21. Lowe FC, Fagelman E. Phytotherapy in the treatment of benign prostatic hyperplasia: an update. *Urology* 1999;53:671–8

22. Balzarro M, Ficarra V, Bartoloni A, *et al*. The pathophysiology, diagnosis and therapy of the transurethral resection of the prostate syndrome. *Urol Int* 2001;66:121–6

23. Tewari A, Oleksa J, Johnson C, *et al*. Minimally invasive therapy of benign prostatic hypertrophy. *Hosp Phys* 1999;68: 29–43

24. Hettiarachchi J, Samadi AA, Konno S, *et al*. Holmium laser enucleation for large (greater than 100 ml) prostate glands. *Int J Urol* 2002;9:233–6

25. Wingo PA, Tong T, Bolden S. Cancer statistics. *Cancer J Clin* 1995;45:8–30

26. Moul JW, Douglas TH, McCarthy WF, McLeod DG. Black race is an adverse prognostic factor for prostate cancer recurrence following radical prostatectomy in an equal access health care setting. *J Urol* 1996;155:1667–73

27. Carter HB, Bova GS, Beaty TH, *et al.* Hereditary prostate cancer: epidemiologic and clinical features. *J Urol* 1993;150: 797–802

28. Zhou JR, Blackburn GL. Bridging animal and human studies: what are the missing segments in dietary fat and prostate cancer? *Am J Clin Nutr* 1997:66(suppl 6):1572–80

29. Shaneyfelt T, Husein R, Bubley G, Mantzoros CS. Hormonal predictors of prostate cancer: a meta-analysis. *J Clin Oncol* 2000;18:847–53

30. Elghany NA, Schumacher MC, Slattery ML, *et al.* Occupation, cadmium exposure and prostate cancer. *Epidemiology* 1990;1: 107–15

31. Eskew LA, Bare RL, McCullough DL. Systematic 5 region prostate biopsy is superior to sextant method for diagnosing carcinoma of the prostate. *J Urol* 1997; 157:199–203

32. Oesterling JE, Martin SK, Bergstralh EJ, Lowe FC. The use of prostate-specific antigen in staging patients with newly diagnosed prostate cancer. *J Am Med Assoc* 1993;269:57–60

33. Flanigan RC, McKay TC, Olson M, *et al.* Limited efficacy of preoperative computed tomographic scanning for the evaluation of lymph node metastasis in patients before radical prostatectomy. *Urology* 1996;48: 428–32

34. Partin AW, Mangold LA, Lamm DM, *et al.* Contemporary update of prostate cancer staging nomograms (Partin Tables) for the new millennium. *Urology* 2001;58: 843–8

35. Aus G. Prostate cancer. Mortality and morbidity after non-curative treatment with aspects on diagnosis and treatment. *Scand J Urol Nephrol Suppl* 1994;167:1–41

36. Dreicer R, Cooper CS, Williams RD. Management of prostate and bladder cancer in the elderly. *Urol Clin North Am* 1996;23:87–97

37. Kerr LA, Zincke H. Radical retropubic prostatectomy for prostate cancer in the elderly and the young: complications and prognosis. *Eur Urol* 1994;25:305–12

38. Walsh PC, Partin AW, Epstein JI. Cancer control and quality of life following anatomical radical retropubic prostatectomy: results at 10 years. *J Urol* 1994;152:1831–6

39. Storey MR, Landgren RC, Cottone JL, *et al.* Transperineal iodine-125 implantation for treatment of clinically localized prostate cancer: 5-year tumor control and morbidity. *Int J Radiat Oncol Biol Phys* 1999;43:565–70

40. Hanks GE, Hanlon A, Owen JB, Schultheiss TE. Patterns of radiation treatment of elderly patients with prostate cancer. *Cancer* 1994;74(suppl 7):2174–7

41. Pilepich MV, Krall JM, Al-Sarraf M, *et al.* Androgen deprivation with radiation therapy compared with radiation therapy alone for locally advanced prostatic carcinoma: a randomized comparative trial of the Radiation Therapy Oncology Group. *Urology* 1995;45:616–23

42. Onik GM, Cohen JK, Reyes GD, *et al.* Transrectal ultrasound-guided percutaneous radical cryosurgical ablation of the prostate. *Cancer* 1993;72:1291–9

43. Long JP, Bahn D, Lee F, *et al.* Five-year retrospective, multi-institutional pooled analysis of cancer-related outcomes after cryosurgical ablation of the prostate. *Urology* 2001;57:518–23

44. Chin JL, Pautler SE, Mouraviev V, *et al.* Results of salvage cryoablation of the prostate after radiation: identifying predictors of treatment failure and complications. *J Urol* 2001;165:1937–42

45. Huggins C, Hodges CV. Studies on prostatic cancer: I. The effect of castration, estrogen, and of androgen injection on serum phosphatases in metastatic carcinoma of the prostate. *Cancer Res* 1941;1:293–7

46. Figg WD, Sartor O, Cooper MR, *et al.* Prostate specific antigen decline following the discontinuation of flutamide in patients with stage D2 prostate cancer. *Am J Med* 1995;98:412–14

47. Botto H, Lebret T, Barre P, *et al.* Electrovaporization of the prostate with the Gyrus device. *J Endourol* 2001;15:313–16

48. Muschter R, Schorsch I, Danielli L, *et al.* Transurethral water-induced thermotherapy for the treatment of benign prostatic hyperplasia: a prospective multicenter clinical trial. *J Urol* 2000;164:1565–9

52 Foot disorders in the elderly

Harvey Strauss, DPM, FACFAS, and
William D. Spielfogel, DPM, FACFAS

INTRODUCTION

According to the American Podiatric Medical Association, since 1900 life expectancy of the average American has increased by approximately 30 years; in the year 2000, older people outnumbered children for the first time in the history of this country. By 2030, approximately 20% of the United States population will be aged 65 and older.

Approximately 75% of active older Americans complain of painful feet. The most common complaints are keratotic lesions (more than 50%), toenails (more than 30%) and bunions (25%). Twenty-six per cent of older adults complain of cold feet[1]. It has been estimated that 80% of people over the age of 50 will suffer, at some point during the course of their lives, from at least one significant foot problem[2]. A study to investigate the prevalence of foot problems in non-diabetic individuals compared with those in a diabetic population concluded that older individuals without diabetes are at high risk for foot-related disease and should receive the same foot care screening, education and follow-up as those with diabetes[3].

Despite the high incidence of foot problems, most health-care professionals give little attention to disorders involving the feet[4]. The role of the primary care physician is to evaluate, diagnose and treat the patient, and make appropriate referrals to the podiatrist. Over the span of an individual's life, the foot undergoes a significant amount of trauma, misuse and neglect. The stress of normal activity, heredity, systemic diseases and environmental factors associated with ambulation results in pathology, altering the individual's ability to function independently.

Treatment of foot disorders should be geared to providing relief of symptoms while preserving mobility as much as possible. Operative treatment should be considered only for those who fail to respond to conservative management. Along with treatment failures to non-surgical care, there are those conditions for which there is no conservative management. Surgical treatment should not be denied on the basis of age alone. Today's technology, in most cases of foot and ankle surgery, obviates the need for general anesthesia and permits procedures to be performed under local anesthesia and intravenous sedation. Depending on the pathology, the mechanics of the foot may need to be altered for the patient to function at an optimum level and without pain. The mechanics of the foot may be affected by many methods, ranging from conservative to surgical (Table 1).

The patient should be evaluated with and without shoes, and the gait evaluated. This will aid in determining whether the problem is related to shoe gear imbalance or general lower extremity weakness[5]. Prevention is important in minimizing foot problems. It is the role of the health-care provider to educate their patients. Some foot health tips that can be used are listed in Table 2.

Table 1   Order of efficiency of methods affecting the mechanics of the foot

Efficiency	Method	Location
Excellent	surgical	in the foot
Very good	padding	on the foot
Good	orthotic devices	in the shoe
Fair	shoe alteration	example:shoe wedging

Table 2   Health tips for the feet that can be used by a geriatrician

Shoes should fit properly
Shoes should have firm soles and soft uppers
Be aware that feet swell at the end of the day
Do not wear constricting socks and stockings
Do not self treat
Advise inspection of the feet daily
Over-the-counter products should be used only with the advice of a primary care physician or podiatrist

A common myth is that it is normal for the feet to hurt as one ages. Foot pain is not normal and should be treated. Another myth is that shoes cause foot problems; they do not. Most often pathomechanics (faulty skeletal structure), usually inherited, or less often disease states cause foot problems. Shoes may, however, aggravate pre-existing conditions and precipitate symptoms. Determining proper shoe fit in patients who have not lost protective sensation may best be achieved by relying on the level of patient comfort. A general rule of thumb may be 'If it feels good, wear it; if it doesn't feel good, don't wear it'. A higher price for a shoe does not ensure appropriateness or a better fit for the individual.

COMMON FOOT PROBLEMS

Heel and arch pain

Heel and arch pain are frequent presentations [6]. The pain can be due to mechanics or other etiology such as stress fracture, nerve entrapment, infection and many systemic diseases. Focus will be on three common causes of heel and arch pain: plantar fasciitis, heel spur and posterior tibial tendon dysfunction.

Plantar fasciitis and heel spur

Plantar fasciitis is commonly associated with heel spur formation, but heel spurs are also detected with no symptoms. Typically, there is strain or microtearing of the plantar aponeurosis at its attachment of the medial calcaneal tubercle. Overuse and chronic fatigue of the plantar fascia can lead to failure of the fascia. The patient will classically complain of medial heel pain after rest, especially when first awakening in the morning. Abnormal biomechanics can influence the stresses on the plantar fascia. These biomechanical factors include a cavus foot type, excessive pronation and ankle equinus [7].

Conservative management of heel pain/plantar fasciitis usually alleviates symptoms. Used in combination or individually, the following modalities are effective: heel cups, biomechanical strapping of the foot, stretching exercises, over-the-counter arch support, custom-molded orthotic devices, physical therapy, cortisone injections and non-steroidal anti-inflammatory medications. Recommendations for orthotic devices vary from the use of rigid devices to soft pliable devices [8]. The use of night splints for the treatment of chronic plantar fasciitis has been shown to be effective [9]. Surgical treatment is reserved as a last resort and should not be performed until a complete course of conservative management has been exhausted over a 6–9-month period [10].

Posterior tibial tendon dysfunction

The posterior tibial tendon is a powerful tendon in the function of the foot and ankle. Posterior tibial tendon dysfunction can cause an acquired adult flatfoot deformity. Severe arch pain, ankle swelling and loss of function can seriously alter a patient's lifestyle[11]. Chronic rupture of the posterior tibial tendon is seen commonly in middle-aged and elderly women who present with an acquired, progressive and painful flatfoot deformity. Patients usually present with a unilateral progressive flatfoot deformity with hind-foot valgus[12–14]. Swelling is usually seen medially with loss of the tendon, with inability to perform a single heel raise test (unable to rise up on the ball of the foot)[14].

Magnetic resonance imaging (MRI) is the modality of choice to diagnose posterior tibial tendon rupture and assess the dysfunction of the tendon. Conservative treatment consists of in-shoe orthotic devices to control the pronatory forces and the hind-foot valgus causing stress on the tendon. Footwear is another option. Functional shoes constructed with a firm heel counter and steel shanks can provide rear-foot control[15]. If conservative measures fail and/or there is rupture of the tendon, surgical management should be considered[13,14].

Toe deformities

The common lesser toe deformities are hammertoes, claw toes and mallet toes. The etiology for these deformities may be biomechanical, resulting in a weakness of the extrinsic or intrinsic musculature, or neuromuscular disease, causing a weakness in the musculature[16,17].

Hammertoe

A hammertoe is a common digital deformity and occurs on the sagittal plane. The proximal phalanx is dorsiflexed, and the middle and distal phalanges are plantar flexed[18,19]. Symptoms develop at the metatarsophalangeal joint, secondary to the retrograde pressure of the proximal phalanx. As the deformity progresses, a painful keratotic lesion may develop on the dorsal aspect of the toe as a result of continuous rubbing against the top of the shoe.

Claw toe

A claw toe is a distal deformity with a contracture present at the proximal and distal interphalangeal joints as well as at the metatarsophalangeal joint[20]. They are commonly seen in cavus foot deformities.

Mallet toe

A mallet toe is a sagittal plane deformity in which the distal phalanx is flexed on the middle phalanx. It does not necessarily involve the proximal interphalangeal joint or the metatarsophalangeal joint. A keratotic lesion may be evident on the distal aspect of the digit in addition to the dorsal aspect of the toe. Early on in most digital deformities, the contractures are reducible. As the deformities progress, they become fixed. Conservative treatment, consisting of shoe modification, padding and debridement of the keratotic lesions, will hopefully keep the patient comfortable and ambulatory. If conservative measures fail, surgical management may be indicated, consisting of soft tissue procedures such as tendon transfers, tenotomies and/or capsulotomies. Osseous procedures may also be indicated, consisting of joint arthroplasty or arthrodesis procedures.

Bunions

The first metatarsophalangeal joint is one of the most complex in the forefoot, because of the sesamoid apparatus. The joint connects the hallux with the first metatarsal. The range of motion at this joint is greater than at any other joint in the foot, and it bears the body weight at the end of propulsion. Its stability is important for normal gait[21,22]. The characteristic features of hallux abducto valgus (bunion) include lateral deviation and rotation of the hallux, lateral displacement of the sesamoids, medial deviation of the first metatarsal and deviation of the tendon-surrounding joint affecting their pull on the hallux[23].

The most common cause of hallux abducto valgus is hypermobility of the first ray (consisting of the first metatarsal and medial cuneiform). Abnormal pronation of the tarsal joints leads to a hypermobile first ray. Persons with a forefoot adductus (forefoot deviated toward the midline of the body) foot type go on to develop the classic stages of hallux abducto valgus and instability of the first metatarsophalangeal joint[21,24,25]. They will typically complain of pain over the medial eminence at the first metatarsophalangeal joint and have difficulty wearing shoes. Due to the medial deviation of the first metatarsal, pain may occur in the area of the second metatarsophalangeal joint. Conservative treatment includes modification of shoe gear, with use of a shoe with a wide and high toe box to accommodate the bunion deformity. In addition, padding and strapping may alleviate some discomfort. For those unresponsive to conservative measures, surgical management is a viable option. Hallux abducto valgus surgery requires the foot surgeon to be able to perform and interpret a static and dynamic examination of the individual along with radiographs. Bunion procedures have been modified over the years with no one specific procedure for all hallux abducto valgus deformities. Surgical procedures for hallux abducto valgus deformities range from joint destructive procedures to joint preservation procedures that include osteotomies of the distal midshaft and proximal ends of the first metatarsal[26].

Hallux limitus

Hallux limitus is a term commonly applied to a condition where dorsiflexion of the great toe on the first metatarsal is restricted or totally limited[27,28]. During the gait cycle, 65–75° of first metatarsophalangeal joint dorsiflexion is required[29]. In individuals with this condition, the lack of first metatarsophalangeal joint dorsiflexion causes pain and significant problems during ambulation. Hallux limitus or rigidus is a degenerative joint disease of the first metatarsophalangeal joint[30]. There are six specific causes of hallux limitus: a long first metatarsal; hypermobility of the first ray; immobilization of the first ray; metatarsus primus elevatus; degenerative joint disease; and trauma[16]. It most commonly affects middle-aged and older adults, males more than females. Symptoms are usually gradual in onset and occur with prolonged weightbearing. Conservative measures include shoe modification consisting of a rocker bottom sole, injection therapy and the use of non-steroidal anti-inflammatory medications in order to alleviate symptomatology. Surgical procedures range from a cheilectomy (removal of the osteophytic proliferation at the first metatarsophalangeal joint) to create more of a gliding motion at the joint, to osteotomies of the first metatarsals, arthroplasty procedures, implants and arthrodesis procedures of the first metatarsophalangeal joint[31].

Toenail disorders

Approximately one-third of the geriatric age group complains about painful toenails[2]. It is difficult for the elderly to care adequately for their toenails. Poor vision, loss of flexibility, arthritis of joints such as the knee and the hip, and obesity prevent them from taking proper care of their nails[32]. Many entities contribute to nail changes. These include infections from bacteria, fungi, yeast and viruses, local and systemic diseases, skin conditions, trauma caused by mechanical, chemical and physical agents, and congenital and idiopathic causes[33]. Table 3 identifies common entities that affect the nails[33,34]. A discussion on a common nail pathology, onychomycosis, follows.

Table 3 Entities affecting the nails

Common
Bacterial infection
Calluses and corns
Fungal infections
Granuloma pyogenicum
Ingrown nails
Onychauxis
Onychogryphosis
Onycholysis
Psoriasis
Subungual exostosis
Trauma

Less Common
Beau's lines
Clubbed digit
Eczematous conditions
Herpes
Koilonychia
Leukonychia
Lichen planus
Malignant melanoma
Pterygium unguium
Squamous cell carcinoma

Onychomycosis is highly prevalent among the aging population. The fungi attack the undersurface of the plate and nail bed and the nail usually thickens and degenerates over time into a caseous, disintegrating consistency[35]. As other entities that affect the nails may mimic the appearance of onychomycosis, the diagnosis should not be made clinically, but microscopically. Several tests that can help include a dermatophyte test media culture, potassium hydroxide (KOH) preparation and periodic acid Schiff (PAS) staining test. In our experience, the PAS stain detects the presence of viable and degenerating fungal organisms. The PAS stain has a higher sensitivity than the KOH test, and the turnaround time is faster than a dermatophyte test media culture. The treatment of onychomycosis consists of nail debridement, topical antifungal therapy (not very effective)[33] and oral antifungal agents. Treatment of other nail disorders, depending on the etiology and symptomatology, may consist of topical and oral medications and surgical removal of the nail or portion of the nail (total or partial matrixectomy).

Metatarsalgia

Metatarsalgia is defined as pain in the forefoot. The pain is typically diffuse and plantar to the metatarsal heads[36]. The common feature is pain on standing and walking, which tends to progress from occasional discomfort to constant pain. The primary complaint is a feeling of walking on the bones of the feet. Many times this is viewed as the normal process of aging; it is not. Metatarsalgia may be due to many factors. A differential diagnosis of metatarsalgia may include but is not limited to the following[37]: a rheumatologic, biomechanical, traumatic and/or neurologic basis. Some pathomechanical causes may include hypermobility of the first ray, previous bunion surgery or prior trauma to the foot. These conditions and many others may prevent the first ray from bearing its share of weight and causing an increase of weight transfer to the lesser metatarsals[16]. This may cause a chronic anterior metatarsal bursitis, tendinitis, tenosynovitis and capsulitis of the lesser metatarsophalangeal joints. When a patient presents with this symptom, it is important to have a radiograph taken in order to rule out the possibility of a stress fracture. If the radiographs do not yield a definite diagnosis, a bone scan may be in order. In the case of a stress fracture, treatment consisting of immobilization and a surgical shoe or stiff-soled shoe is effective. In other cases of metatarsalgia, modification of shoe gear, in-shoe orthotic devices, injection therapy, non-steroidal anti-inflammatory medications and physical therapy are helpful.

Plantar calluses

A callus is a hyperkeratotic lesion and may also be known as a keratoma, tyloma or tylosis. Callosities are acquired, superficial and circumscribed, yellowish-white or darker, flattened, thickened and horny patches of epidermis that are dense in structure, usually insensitive, and occur in areas of pressure and friction on the plantar surface of the foot.

Direct pressure evokes pain. If pared under unsterile conditions they may form a route of entry of infection in individuals with diabetes[38].

Plantar calluses commonly occur in those with metatarsalgia where there is a prominent metatarsal head and the plantar fat pad has atrophied. External factors, excessive standing or improper footwear resulting in excessive pressure and friction cause callosities. If left untreated, especially in the older individual, who is susceptible to an increased incidence of infection and ulceration, the loss of a limb may occur[39].

Conservative treatment, consisting of debridement of the lesions by a podiatrist and modification of shoe gear, padding and accommodative orthotic devices will usually maintain comfort and allow ambulation and mobility. If conservative measures fail, surgical management should be considered to address the bony abnormalities[40].

SURGICAL CONSIDERATIONS IN THE GERIATRIC PATIENT

Older individuals need to stay active in order to lead productive lives. The burden falls on the physician to help maintain or improve the quality of life. Painful disorders such as hallux abducto valgus, hammertoes and heel spurs are common. Keratotic lesions secondary to deformities may lead to pain and ulcerations. As a result, ambulation becomes difficult and the older patient becomes trapped in a downward spiral wherein limited ambulation leads to increased functional loss. Surgery is a viable alternative to keep the patient functioning at optimum level and should not be denied on the basis of age. In the authors' opinion, the primary goal for elective surgery is to reduce pain and improve function. Prior to a surgical procedure, the elderly patient should undergo comprehensive assessment, including the availability of an adequate support system for a successful postoperative course.

Wound care

There has been a recent proliferation of wound care products. Some of these products have been on the market for years without value in wound management or are not worth their considerable cost. In order to assess a wound, the senior author developed the acronym 'LIMP' which stands for loading, infection, malignancy and poor perfusion. If these factors are not present, a wound will heal with or without the use of a wound healing product. Conversely, if any one of these factors is present, a wound will not heal despite the use of any wound care product.

Loading

A wound under pressure will not heal. At present, there is no mechanism to quantify the amount of pressure that will impair wound healing. It is the physician's experience that will determine the necessary degree of off-loading. Off-loading must be provided for the bed-bound as well as the ambulatory patient.

Infection

An open lesion does not automatically imply infection. Diagnosing an infected open lesion is a clinical assessment, not a laboratory assessment. Laboratory studies may or may not be consistent with the clinical presentation. A normal white cell count does not rule out an infection in a diabetic ulcer. Cultures of wounds should not be employed unless there has been a deep surgical debridement of the wound. A bone scan to rule out osteomyelitis in the presence of an open lesion too often yields a false-positive result and should not be employed. Better imaging methods to rule out osteomyelitis in the presence of a wound are serial X-rays and MRI. If neuropathic osteoarthropathy is a consideration, then indium and/or hexamethyl propylene amine oxime scanning is appropriate.

Malignancy

Any wound failing to respond to appropriate care should undergo biopsy to exclude malignancy.

Poor perfusion

A limb wound must be perfused for healing to take place. If the limb is not adequately perfused, vascular reconstruction must be performed. If revascularization is not feasible and infection is not present, the status quo should be maintained as long as possible. If infection or pain is present without the possibility of vascular reconstruction, then amputation is indicated.

SUMMARY

Many older individuals complain of painful feet from a variety of causes, ranging from diabetes to vascular and biomechanical problems. The primary care physician should evaluate, diagnose, treat when able to, and make an appropriate referral to a podiatrist. It is important to evaluate and educate the patient and consider surgical management of a deformity if conservative options fail. Surgery is a viable alternative to keep the patient functioning at an optimum level. The goal is to provide relief of symptoms and keep the patient as mobile as possible.

References

1. Helfand AE. At the Foot of South Mountain, a five-year longitudinal study of foot problems and screening in an elderly population. *J Am Podiatry Assoc* 1973;63:512–21
2. Helfand AE. Guide to methodological approach for a community health foot study for the chronically ill and the aged. *J Am Podiatry Assoc* 1964;54:465–73
3. Plummer ES, Albert SG. Focused assessment of foot care in older adults. *J Am Geriatr Soc* 1996;44:310–13
4. Elwood TW. Older person's concerns about foot care. *J Am Podiatry Assoc* 1975;65:490–4
5. Karpman RR. Foot problems in the geriatric patient. *Clin Orthop Rel Res* 1995;316:59–62
6. McCarthy D. Gorecki G. The anatomical basis of inferior calcaneal lesions – a cryomicrotomy study. *J Am Podiatry Assoc* 1979;69:527–36
7. Contompasis JP. Surgical treatment of calcaneal spurs, a three-year post surgical study. *J Am Podiatry Assoc* 1974;12:987–8
8. Mizel MS, Marymount JV, Trepmon E. Treatment of plantar fascitis with a night splint and shoe modification consisting of a steel shank and anterior rocker bottom. *Foot Ankle Int* 1996;17:732–5
9. Perry JE, Ulbrecht JS, Derr JA, *et al*. The use of running shoes to reduce plantar pressures in patients who have diabetes. *J Bone Joint Surg* 1995;77A:1819–28
10. Ferkel RD. Arthroscopy of the foot and ankle. In. Coughlin MJ, Mann RA, eds. *Surgery of the Foot and Ankle*, 7th edn., vol 2. St Louis, MI: Mosby, 1999:1257–97
11. Baumhauer JF. Pathologic anatomy. *Foot Ankle Clin* 1997;2:217–26
12. Funk DA, Cass JR, Johnson KA. Acquired adult flatfoot secondary to posterior tibial tendon pathology. *J Bone Joint Surg* 1986;68A:95–102
13. Jahss MH. Spontaneous rupture of the tibialis posterior tendon: clinical findings, tenographic studies, and a new technique of repair. *Foot Ankle* 1982;3:158–66
14. Johnson KA. Tibialis posterior tendon rupture. *Clin Orthop Rel Res* 1983;177:140–7
15. Steb HS, *et al*. Conservative management of posterior tibial tendon dysfunction, subtalar joint complex, and pes planus deformity. *Clin Podiatr Med Surg* 1999;16:439–51
16. Root MC, O'Brien WP, Weed JH. Forefoot deformity caused by abnormal subtalar joint pronation. In. Root S, ed. *Normal and Abnormal Function of the Foot – Clinical*

Biomechanics, vol 2. Los Angeles: Clinical Biomechanics, 1977:442–61

17. Sarrafian SE, Topouzian LK. Anatomy and physiology of the extensor apparatus of the toes. *J Bone Joint Surg* 1969;51A:669–79

18. Kelikian H. Deformities of the lesser toes. In *Hallux Valgus, Allied Deformities of the Forefoot and Metatarsalgia*. Philadelphia: WB Saunders,1965:292–9

19. Myerson MS. The pathological anatomy of claw and hammertoes. *J Bone Joint Surg* 1989;71A:45–9

20. McGlamry ED. Lesser ray deformities. In McGlamry ED, Banks AS, Downey MS, eds. *Comprehensive Textbook of Foot Surgery*, 2nd edn. Baltimore: Williams & Wilkins, 1992:336–7

21. Root ML, Orien WP, Weed JH. Forefoot deformity caused by abnormal subtalar joint pronation. In Root S, ed. *Normal and Abnormal Function of the Foot – Clinical Biomechanics*, vol. II. Los Angeles: Clinical Biomechanics, 1977:376–435

22. Shereff MJ, Bejjani FJ, Kummer FJ. Kinematics of the first metatarsophalangeal joint. *J Bone Joint Surg* 1986;68A:392–8

23. Mann RA, Coughlin MJ. Hallux valgus and complications of hallux valgus. In Mann RA, ed. *Surgery of the Foot*. St Louis: Mosby, 1986:65–131

24. D'Amico JC, Schuster RO. Motion of the first ray. *J Am Podiatr Assoc* 1979;69:17–23

25. Haas M. Radiographic and biomechanical considerations of bunion surgery. In Gerbert J, Sokoloff TH, eds. *Textbook of Bunion Surgery*. Mount Kisco, NY: Futura, 1981:23–62

26. Clark JR, Gerbert J, Todd WF, *et al.* Surgical procedures. In Gerbert J, Sokoloff TH, eds. *Textbook of Bunion Surgery*. Mount Kisco, NY: Futura, 1981:103–277

27. Lapidus PW. Dorsal bunion: its mechanics and operative correction. *J Bone Joint Surg* 1940;22:627–37

28. Rzonca E, Levitz S. Hallux equinus: the stages of hallux limitus and hallux rigidus. *J Am Podiatr Assoc* 1984;74:390–3

29. Joseph J. Ranges of motion of the great toe in men. *J Bone Joint Surg* 1954;36B:450–7

30. Hawkins BJ, Haddad BJ. Hallux rigidus. *Clin Sports Med* 1988;7:37–49

31. Delauro TM, Positano RG. Surgical management of hallux limitus and rigidus in the young patient: *Clin Podiatr Med Surg* 1989;6: 83–92

32. Riccitelli ML. Foot problems of the aged and infirm. *Am Geriatr Stand Care* 1966;14:1058–66

33. Hay RJ. Infections affecting the nails. In Samman PD, Fenton DA, eds. *Samman's the Nails in Disease*, 5th edn. Oxford: Butterworth-Heinemann, 1995:32–55

34. Samitz MH. Toenail disorders. In Barry B, ed. *Cutaneous Disorders of the Lower Extremities*. Philadelphia: Lippincott, 1981: 235–41

35. Krausz C. Onychopathy. In McCarthy DJ, Montgomery R, eds. *Podiatric Dermatology*. Baltimore: Williams & Wilkins, 1986: 74–95

36. Jahss, MH. Examination. In Jahss M, ed. *Disorders of the Foot and Ankle*, 2nd edn. Philadelphia: WB Saunders, 1991:35–51

37. Pack L, Julien PH. Differential diagnosis of lesser metatarsalgia. *Clin Podiatr Med Surg* 1990;7:573–7

38. Wilkinson DS. Cutaneous reactions to mechanical and thermal injury. In. Rook A, Wilkinson DS, Ebling FJG, *et al.*, eds. *Textbook of Dermatology*, 4th edn. Boston: Blackwell Scientific Publications, 1986: 587–90

39. Jiminez AL, McGlamry ED, Green D. Lesser ray deformities. In McGlamry ED, ed. *Comprehensive Textbook of Foot Surgery*, vol 1. Baltimore: Williams & Wilkins, 1987:57–113

40. Myerson M. Principles of foot and ankle surgery. In. Myerson M, ed. *Foot and Ankle Disorders*, vol 1. Philadelphia: WB Saunders, 2000:1–24

41. Joseph, WS. Treatment of lower extremity infections in diabetics. *J Am Podiatr Med Assoc* 1992;82:361–70

53 Orthopedic disorders in the elderly

Kenneth J. Koval, MD, Frank A. Liporace, MD, and Joseph D. Zuckerman, MD

INTRODUCTION

Injuries to the musculoskeletal system in the elderly can be devastating. Many factors specific to older patients require special consideration when dealing with these injuries both acutely and throughout their rehabilitation. The geriatric segment of the population is rapidly growing and sustains a disproportionate number of fractures compared to others. The specific goal of all orthopedic care is to restore patient function to a pre-injury level. Decreased bone stock, muscular weakness, systemic disease, etc. make it difficult to attain an independent living status after sustaining an injury. Immobilization and the use of devices to assist in ambulation (crutches, walkers, wheelchairs, etc.) may require an elderly patient to be subjected to institutional care for a protracted course. The following is an overview of the etiology, pathophysiology and treatment considerations in treating geriatric patients with orthopedic injuries, with an emphasis on fractures.

THE PRE-INJURY STATUS

Orthopedic intervention attempts to restore or even improve a patient's pre-injury level of functioning. Medical and cognitive histories have significant impact on whether and how these goals can be reached. Pre-injury ambulatory status can specifically

Table 1 American Society of Anesthesiologists (ASA) preoperative risk rating

ASA rating	Health status
I	normal, healthy
II	mild systemic disease
III	severe systemic disease, not incapacitating
IV	severe incapacitating disease, constant threat to life
V	moribund patient

affect the type of operative intervention undertaken, or whether an intervention is needed at all.

Systemic diseases can impact on injury management. Specifically, cardiac and pulmonary compromise can diminish a patient's ability to tolerate recumbency, surgery and rehabilitation. The American Society of Anesthesiologists (ASA) has developed a rating system for determining preoperative risks (Table 1). Medical diseases can affect the intraoperative response during surgery (e.g. hypotensive response to cemented hip arthroplasty). The elderly may not tolerate such stresses, resulting in further cardiac and even cerebrovascular insults. Many orthopedic procedures can be performed with either general or spinal anesthesia. Recent reports have shown no difference in mortality with either one[1,2].

603

Diabetes has been shown to increase the risk of wound complications (dehiscence, infection) and cause delayed fracture union[3]. Peripheral vascular disease can also contribute to wound complications. Friability and changes in skin turgor, common in the elderly, can result in soft tissue complications when patients become sedentary or need to be immobilized in a cast, even if it is well padded. Thromboembolic disease is a significant threat, especially with lower extremity injury and surgery, and devastating with additional cardiopulmonary co-morbidities.

The importance of a patient's cognitive status pre- and post-injury cannot be overstressed. Since orthopedic injuries and treatments usually require protracted physical therapy and rehabilitation, it is necessary for patients to comprehend instructions, clearly communicate and perform multiple tasks. Individuals with Alzheimer's disease, cognitive deficits from cerebrovascular insults, Parkinson's disease and other forms of dementia will have difficulty participating in the therapy required to attain pre-injury functional status, resulting in increased mortality rates. Such considerations may be important in the determination of whether operative intervention should be conducted at all. One must not get lost in the idea that a 'good looking' radiograph is the goal of treatment. For example, a comminuted distal radius fracture may be served better by non-operative treatment and a suboptimal radiographic reduction if the patient is unable to co-operate with lengthy and specific therapy after surgical intervention. In contrast, a patient with pre-injury hemiplegia suffering from a proximal humerus fracture may not tolerate long-term immobilization of the functional upper extremity (the standard treatment) and may benefit from surgical intervention to allow earlier weightbearing, with use of the extremity for transfers and ambulation with assistive devices.

Decreased bone mass (osteopenia) is often seen in older subjects, resulting from osteoporosis or osteomalacia. Osteoporosis is a decrease in bone density that does not affect mineralization, while osteomalacia results from decreased bone mineralization, with or without changes in bone density. In either situation, less loading is required to cause fracture, as opposed to the loading sustained by normal bone. Factors affecting bone density such as sedentary lifestyle, excessive consumption of alcohol, smoking and co-morbid conditions (e.g. renal disease, malnutrition) should be factored in[4,5].

Osteopenia presents a problem with fracture stabilization and healing. It is difficult to attain stable fixation in fracture fragments that have decreased bone mass. Stable internal fixation is imperative to allow for early range of motion, weightbearing and therapy without risking fracture displacement. Osteopenia increases the risk for non-union, since fracture callus in these patients is less dense and not as well organized. If only tenuous fixation is attained and protracted immobilization is needed, further 'disuse' osteopenia can result. Bone remodels according to Wolff's law: removal of external stresses can lead to significant bone loss, but this situation can be reversed to varying degrees upon remobilization and reloading. Ways to compensate for these problems include use of methylmethacrylate (cement) to augment screw fixation, use of an allograft and use of a synthetic bone graft[6,7].

A fracture in an older patient is not just trauma to the musculoskeletal system. Understanding the pre-injury level of function and co-morbid status is imperative for working toward the goal of re-establishing the patient's functionality. A multidisciplinary approach must be taken with input from the orthopedic surgeon, geriatrician, anesthesiologist, physiatrist, therapist and caregiver.

HIP FRACTURES

General principles

Hip fractures in the elderly can be devastating or fatal, and affect functional and psychological status. Currently 250 000 hip fractures, at a total medical expenditure of almost 9 billion dollars, occur annually in the USA. The incidence is expected to double by the year 2050, because of aging trends[8-10].

As individuals age, their chance of sustaining a hip fracture greatly increases, doubling every decade after 50 years, and occurring twice as often in females. Hip fractures occur most frequently in Caucasian women, followed by Caucasian men, Afro-American women and Afro-American men. This may be due to differences in bone density between different ethnic groups[11-13]. Institutionalized patients are also more likely to sustain hip fractures[14-16].

Usually hip fractures occur from low-energy trauma (e.g. a fall while walking on a flat surface) in the elderly. They can be intracapsular (femoral neck) or extracapsular (intertrochanteric or subtrochanteric), with impact on healing potential. Vascularity is more significantly compromised with intracapsular fractures. More than 90% of hip fractures in patients over 65 are femoral neck or intertrochanteric in origin, with a slight predominance for intertrochanteric fractures in very old patients[17].

Presentation and management

Patients usually complain of hip and groin pain with an inability to bear weight on the affected extremity after sustaining relatively minor trauma. The supine patient will hold the affected extremity externally rotated with slight flexion at the hip; a leg length discrepancy is noticeable. This is the position of maximal capsular volume when there is a fracture hematoma, thus providing the most comfort. Evaluation should include a neurovascular examination of the affected extremity, examination of each extremity and the spine for other injuries, documentation of any loss of consciousness, a mental status examination and assessment of skin integrity in appropriate areas. Medical consultation should be obtained to prepare the patient for

possible surgery. Injury films, baseline laboratory investigations, chest radiograph and electrocardiogram (ECG) should be attained at the time of presentation. It may be prudent to acquire a baseline arterial blood gas (ABG), since hip fractures carry an inherent risk of deep venous thrombosis (DVT) and pulmonary embolus (PE). Placement of a Foley catheter will eliminate the need for a patient to transfer to a bedpan, thereby reducing potential discomfort and further fracture displacement. Care should be taken when acquiring injury films to obtain a true anteroposterior and cross-table lateral view of the hip. Obtaining a frog-leg lateral view could prove detrimental by further displacing fracture fragments and damaging vascular channels (Figure 1).

When a diagnosis of hip fracture is suspected clinically but not clear with routine radiography, other studies are indicated. For instance, a traction/internal rotation view will help visualize the entire length of the femoral neck. This view is conducted by obtaining an anteroposterior hip radiograph as the physician pulls traction at the ankle while internally rotating the hip 15° (the average amount of anteversion seen in the adult femoral neck). Care must be taken to avoid shearing the skin of the lower extremity while performing the maneuver. If question remains, a technetium bone scan or magnetic resonance image (MRI) may clarify whether an occult hip fracture is present. Both are sensitive but the bone scan may require 2–3 days post-injury to be positive, while the MRI can give an accurate reading in less than 24 h post-injury[18].

Ultimately, the preferred treatment of a hip fracture is surgery. This will decrease the period of non-weightbearing, risk of malunion/non-union, cardiopulmonary complications and eventually mortality. Additionally, operative treatment is the most economic management[19].

The risk of DVT or PE is a concern requiring preventive measures. Historically, warfarin has been considered the standard for prophylaxis. Currently, low molecular weight

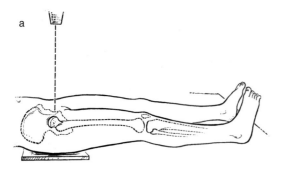

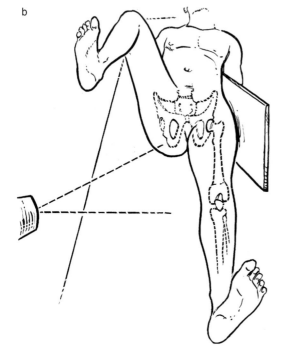

Figure 1 Diagramatic representation on patient positioning for anteroposterior (a) and cross-table lateral (b) X-rays of the hip

heparin (LMWH) has been used subcutaneously with good results, without the need for the constant laboratory monitoring required for warfarin. LMWH can be administered within 12–24 h post-surgically. In situations that will not permit the use of pharmacologic prophylaxis, an inferior vena cava filter may be used. Subcutaneous unfractionated heparin is not typically used for prophylaxis in orthopedic patients, since

it has been shown to be less effective than warfarin and LMWH in DVT prophylaxis, although continuous intravenous infusion of unfractionated heparin has been shown to provide adequate prophylaxis while waiting for warfarin to become therapeutic in patients[20–23]. Preoperatively, patients should be given pharmacologic and mechanical prophylaxis (e.g. venodyne boots, pneumatic compression stockings). Twelve hours prior to surgery, pharmacologic prophylaxis should be withheld, although mechanical prophylaxis may continue. This can decrease intraoperative and immediate postoperative bleeding complications.

Outcomes

As previously mentioned, the goal of surgery is to restore the patient's functional outcome. A study showed that, at 1-year follow-up, 41% of patients regained their pre-injury level of ambulatory function, 40% remained community or household ambulators but required assistive devices, 12% became solely household ambulators and 8% became non-ambulatory. The factors shown to improve the possibility of attaining the pre-injury ambulatory status are outlined in Table 2[24].

Initial mortality rates are increased in patients with hip fracture compared to age-matched controls. One-year mortality can be as high as 25%[25,26]. The highest rate is seen in the first 6 months, progressively declining to the same rate as in age-matched controls by 1 year. Factors shown to negatively affect 1-year mortality rates are outlined in Table 2[27].

Timing from injury to surgical stabilization has been a subject of debate, with studies citing both increased and decreased mortality with delaying surgery from 1 to several days following injury to allow medical stabilization. Many studies were based on heterogeneous populations and variables were not well controlled[25,26,28]. A prospective study from our institution, controlling for age, sex

Table 2   Hip fractures: factors influencing outcome

Factors favorable to regaining pre-injury ambulatory status
Age below 85 years
Preoperative ASA rating of I or II
Intertrochanteric fracture
Male sex
Absence of dementia

Factors contributing to 1-year mortality
Age over 85 years
Preoperative ASA rating of III or IV
Pre-injury dependency in activities of daily living
History of malignancy (excluding skin cancer)
Development of one or more complications during hospitalization

ASA, American Society of Anesthesiologists

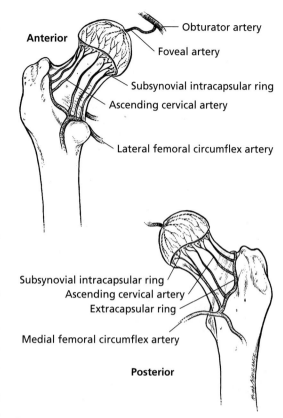

Figure 2   Contributing vessels to the major sources of blood supply to the proximal femur

and co-morbidities, comprised 367 hip fracture patients not suffering from dementia, capable of activities of daily living and ambulatory prior to injury. We demonstrated that a delay to surgical stabilization of more than 2 calendar days doubled mortality[29].

Postoperatively there is disparity in terms of therapy. Protocols range from non-weightbearing to immediate weightbearing as tolerated. Biomechanically, it has been shown that joint-reactive forces are greater across the hip when comparing non-weightbearing to toe-touch weightbearing[30]. Additionally, balance and upper extremity strength are important issues to consider when asking the older adult to be limited in their weightbearing. When patients are allowed weightbearing as tolerated immediately postoperatively, they self-regulate the amount of weight on the injured extremity and gradually increase the amount of weightbearing over time[31,32].

Femoral neck fractures

Femoral neck fractures occur between the base of the femoral head and the intertrochanteric line. These are considered intracapsular and have significant bearing on blood supply to the femoral head, treatment options and success of given treatments. The main blood supply to the femoral head comes from branches off the medial and lateral femoral circumflex arteries (medial with much greater contribution); these form an extracapsular ring at the base of the neck with ascending branches that are intracapsular, forming a network ending in bony perforators to the femoral head. The intracapsular extensions represent terminal vessels of the extracapsular ring; the ascending vessels are at significant risk during femoral neck fracture, especially when displaced. A minimal contribution to the femoral head also comes from the ligamentum teres (Figure 2).

Many classifications have been used to describe femoral neck fractures. The most common classification is that derived by Garden, in which types I and II are non-displaced while types III and IV represent displaced femoral neck fractures[33] (Figure 3).

Non-displaced

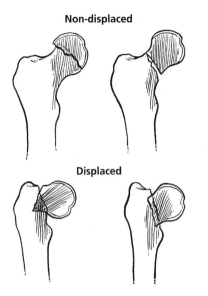

Displaced

Figure 3 Modification of Garden classification of femoral neck fractures into displaced and non-displaced categories

Rates for future osteonecrosis of the femoral head or non-union of the femoral neck fracture have ranged between 5 and 35% with significantly higher rates in displaced fractures (5–10% for minimally displaced and 20–35% for displaced)[33–37]. Non-union requires operation in up to 75% of cases while osteonecrosis requires revision surgery in only up to 30% of cases.

Surgery is the treatment of choice for this injury. Attempts at closed reductions and pinning for minimally displaced/impacted fractures should be made. Although these are inherently stable, they do have an 8–15% chance of displacement without operative stabilization[38]. Postoperatively, weightbearing status is surgeon dependent. We allow weightbearing as tolerated with assistive devices, since the elderly have difficulty following weightbearing guidelines, especially with problems concerning gait and balance. We believe patients will regulate their weightbearing based on pain[32].

In displaced fractures, obtaining and maintaining an adequate reduction with pinning is

not always possible. In a physiologically younger patient all efforts should be made for closed reduction and pinning, but in a physiologically older patient there is a lower threshold for arthroplasty. Preserving the femoral head is always preferred, but many factors influence this decision. In frail, old patients with pre-existing degenerative joint disease and significant medical risk for a time-consuming open reduction, a hemi- or total hip arthroplasty might be preferred. Primary total hip arthroplasty (prosthetic replacement of the femoral head and femoral neck, and resurfacing of the acetabulum) needs a longer operative time, needs a greater surgical exposure and results in a greater mortality rate than hemi-hip arthroplasty (prosthetic replacement of the femoral head and neck). There is also a greater risk of dislocation for primary total hip arthroplasty when performed for fractures as opposed to degenerative joint disease[21,39]. Before entertaining the option of hip arthroplasty, one must ascertain whether the patient can follow postoperative arthroplasty precautions to avoid dislocation. Neurologically impaired or cognitively impaired patients are suboptimal candidates.

Rarely, non-operative treatment is undertaken in non-ambulatory or morbidly ill patients. This comprises early mobilization to a wheelchair, adequate anesthesia, decubitus precautions and physical therapy as tolerated.

Intertrochanteric fractures

The intertrochanteric region is extracapsular, lying in the area distal to the femoral neck between the greater and lesser trochanters. Since there is metaphyseal bone with an abundant blood supply in this region, there is less danger of healing complications than is seen with femoral neck fractures. Postero-medially in this region is the calcar femorale. This is an area of dense cortical bone that acts as an internal strut to the significant forces

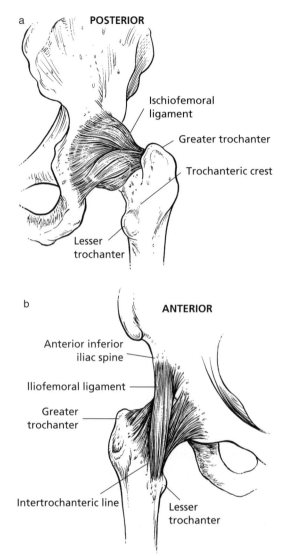

Figure 4 Hip joint with significant structures and capsule. Posterior (a) and anterior (b)

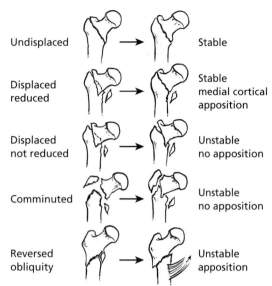

Figure 5 Stable vs. unstable and displaced vs. non-displaced intertrochanteric hip fractures based on a modified Evan's classification

transmitted across this region. The greater trochanter lies superolaterally and is the insertion site to the hip abductors and short external rotators. The lesser trochanter lies posteromedially and is the insertion site to the iliopsoas (Figure 4).

It is important to determine radiographically whether these fractures are stable. The ability to obtain stability is based on cortical continuity of the posteromedial cortex and calcar femorale. On plain radiographs, this is gauged by the lesser trochanter's position. If it is non-displaced without comminution, then the fracture is termed stable, while displacement and comminution represent an unstable fracture. Reduction attempts to establish stability[40] (Figure 5).

Surgery is the treatment of choice for intertrochanteric fractures. Closed reduction is attempted following the initiation of spinal or general anesthesia. If reduction is unobtainable by closed means, an open reduction is performed. Commonly, a device incorporating a telescoping screw and barrel inserted into the femoral neck with an accompanying sideplate or intramedullary component is used. The telescoping nature of the implant supplies stability and facilitates compression across the fracture site to stimulate bony healing. Currently, lesser trochanteric fractures are not reduced and stabilized with hardware[41].

Rarely, primary prosthetic replacement is indicated in cases of severe comminution. This implant differs from traditional arthroplasty since it is calcar replacing, due to the

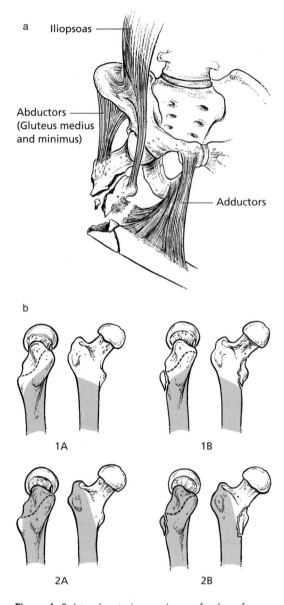

a

Iliopsoas

Abductors
(Gluteus medius
and minimus)

Adductors

b

1A

1B

2A

2B

Figure 6 Subtrochanteric region of the femur. Contributing muscle forces to displacement of fracture fragments (a). Shaded areas (b) represent location and extension of common subtrochanteric fracture patterns

location of this fracture. Implanting these prostheses is associated with prolonged operative time, increased blood loss and higher rates of dislocation than with elective total hip arthroplasties[41].

Indications and goals for non-operative treatment are similar to those mentioned for femoral neck fractures.

Subtrochanteric fractures

The subtrochanteric region of the femur lies in the first 5 cm of the femur distal to the lesser trochanter. Fractures in this area are less frequent in the elderly than femoral neck or intertrochanteric fractures. Although these occur with high-energy situations in the young, they may follow a simple fall in aged individuals[12,42].

Stability in these fractures is also based on the integrity of the posteromedial cortex[43]. Usually, these injuries are treated with an intramedullary nail or fixed angle plate and screw implant. Osteonecrosis is rarely a concern with these fractures[44,45]. Difficulty lies in obtaining an anatomic reduction prior to implant insertion, since there are numerous deforming muscle forces in this region of the femur[46] (Figure 6).

ANKLE FRACTURES

Ankle fractures are common in the geriatric population. The ankle joint consists of the distal aspects of the tibia and fibula (medial and lateral malleoli) and their articulation with the talar dome. The medial malleolus is connected to the navicular, calcaneus and talus by the superficial and deep layers of the deltoid ligament. The lateral malleolus is connected to the talus and calcaneus by a three-ligament complex. The tibia and fibula maintain their relationship via a ligamentous complex known as the syndesmosis (Figure 7).

Injuries to the ankle can occur by many mechanisms[47,48]. Frequently, ligamentous and bony injury can result from a twisting injury after a patient missteps or falls. Injuries can be bony, ligamentous or a combination; all affect ankle stability. Negative radiographs do not imply that there is only a minor injury, since a ligamentous disruption can result in substantial disability. If ligamentous injury is suspected, stress radiographs should be considered[49].

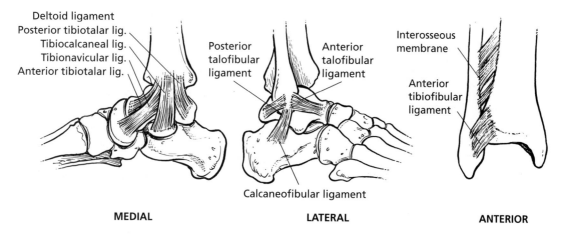

Figure 7 Ankle joint with ligamentous restraints (medial, lateral, syndesmosis)

Patients with ankle injuries often complain of an inability to ambulate along with tenderness around the ankle joint. Frequently, swelling and ecchymosis are present. Patients must undergo a full four-extremity and spine examination, since acute ankle pain can mask other injuries. The circumstances of the injury must be illicited to help establish the mechanism of injury to aid in treatment. Many injuries that mask ankle fractures should be excluded through a screening examination. These include fractures of the proximal fibula, lateral talus, anterior calcaneus and proximal fifth metatarsal[50]. A typical radiographic series includes three views of the ankle joint (anteroposterior, lateral and mortise (15° internal rotation view)) and full-length tibia/fibula films to exclude syndesmotic injury if the patient complains of medial malleolar tenderness. Foot films may also be considered.

Treatment of ankle fractures depends on the mechanism of injury and stability of the fracture. Isolated fibula fracture occurring at or below the level of the tibia–talar articulation are considered stable and may be treated in a short leg cast or air cast with early weightbearing. Fractures that are considered unstable are bi-malleolar or signify a disruption of the syndesmosis (i.e. high fibula fracture with medial joint line tenderness,

widening of the medial clear space of the tibia–talar articulation, or dissociation of the tibia–talar or tibia–fibula articulations). Slight malreduction can result in future arthritis[49]. Surgery provides a stable reduction and allows the patient to begin early joint range of motion to help avoid later stiffness and risk of malreduction. In contrast to non-operatively treated patients, surgically treated patients do not require long-leg immobilization and can be more easily mobilized with assistive devices. Operative intervention has been shown to achieve better fracture position and better patient satisfaction, although complications with hardware loosening have been seen in women with osteoporosis[51,52]. The presence of diabetes, vasculopathy or history of smoking increases the risk for soft-tissue complications (e.g. infection, wound dehiscence, etc.) with surgery. The ankle has a very tenuous blood supply. Preoperative ankle–brachial index (ABI), transcutaneous oxygen measurements, or toe pressures should be considered in such patients.

PROXIMAL HUMERUS FRACTURES

Proximal humerus fractures are frequently encountered in the geriatric population, four times more commonly in women[53]. Usually these occur from low-energy falls, frequently

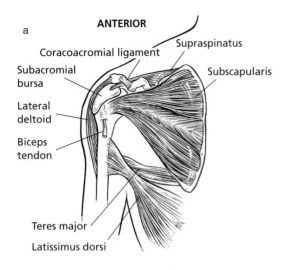

a

ANTERIOR

Coracoacromial ligament — Supraspinatus

Subacromial bursa — Subscapularis

Lateral deltoid

Biceps tendon

Teres major

Latissimus dorsi

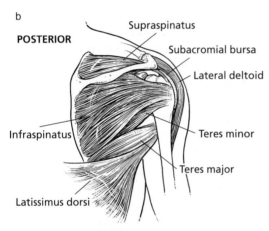

b

POSTERIOR

Supraspinatus

Subacromial bursa

Lateral deltoid

Infraspinatus — Teres minor

Teres major

Latissimus dorsi

Figure 8 Shoulder joint with representation of dynamic (rotator cuff and superfical musculature) restraints. Anterior (a) and posterior (b). Note: capsule lies deep to the rotator cuff (not shown)

minor and subscapularis (Figure 8). These four muscles, with the help of the deltoid and scapular rotators, provide dynamic stability to the shoulder throughout its active range of motion. The pull of these muscles causes predictable directional displacement of fracture fragments. Concomitant injury to the rotator cuff can negatively affect patient outcome.

Patients with proximal humerus fractures complain of an inability to move the arm because of pain. A radiographic series including anteroposterior, scapular 'Y' and axillary views is imperative to rule out concomitant fracture/dislocation. Minimally displaced fractures represent 80–85% of proximal humerus fractures in the elderly. Provided that the humerus/shoulder moves as 'a unit' on examination, it can be assumed that the surrounding soft tissues and periosteum provide stability. These injuries can be treated with a brief period of sling immobilization (1 week) and range of motion exercises (progressing from passive to active-assisted over 4–6 weeks). Minimally displaced proximal humerus fractures usually result in pain-free union[54,55]. Multi-part displaced fractures, which do not 'move as a unit' on examination, and fracture/dislocations may require hemi-arthroplasty (replacing the proximal humerus with an implant and leaving the native glenoid intact) or surgical stabilization, if possible. Acute hemi-arthroplasty is superior to attempting surgical stabilization and conducting delayed hemi-arthorplasty[56,57].

The ultimate goal in treatment of these injuries is to return the patient to a pain-free state with optimum capacity to perform activities of daily living. In summary, low-energy minimally displaced fractures exhibit better functional outcome compared to high-energy three- and four-part fractures with associated rotator cuff injuries. Prosthetic replacement results in predictable pain relief, but decreased range of motion compared to pre-injury.

require immobilization and thus interfere with activities of daily living. The goal is to restore pre-injury function with minimal loss of shoulder range of motion.

The shoulder joint has a complex bony and soft tissue relationship. The proximal humerus articulates with the glenoid to form a ball-and-socket joint. The shoulder capsule envelops this ball-and-socket joint to provide static stability. Superficial to the capsule lies the rotator cuff. The rotator cuff is composed of the supraspinatus, infraspinatus, teres

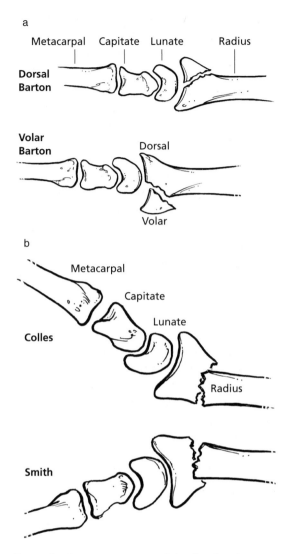

Figure 9 Common patterns of distal radius fracture: Barton's (a) and Colles' and Smith's (b)

DISTAL RADIUS FRACTURES

Fractures of the distal radius are frequently seen in elderly individuals, particularly women, who fall on an outstretched hand. Predisposing factors are osteoporosis, increased incidence of falls in the elderly, dementia, poor eyesight, decreased co-ordination, medications and possible history of strokes or transient ischemic attacks[58].

The wrist is composed of eight carpal bones and the distal radius and distal ulna.

The articulations are maintained via a complex ligamentous network on both the dorsal and volar aspects of the wrist. Important factors in predicting the need for surgery and ultimate outcome include angulation, comminution, shortening, articular surface involvement and pre-injury level of function[59]. A non-reduced articular surface can result in degenerative changes that lead to chronic pain. If the patient is physiologically active and the injury involves the dominant extremity, treatment should be guided toward an anatomic reduction.

The presentation of distal radius fractures is pain, swelling and wrist deformity. The force responsible for a distal radius injury can be transmitted proximally and result in elbow injury. Radiographic examination consists of posteroanterior, lateral and oblique views of both wrists. Views of the contralateral wrist help with evaluating the adequacy of reduction.

Common fracture patterns include: Colles' (dorsally displaced articular surface with apex–volar angulation); Smith's (volarly displaced articular surface with apex–dorsal angulation); Barton's (volar or dorsal shear); non-displaced; and concomitant fracture of the distal ulna[60] (Figure 9). The goal of treatment is to restore normal anatomy, enable painless range of motion and maintain grip strength. Whether cast immobilization or surgery is conducted, finger range of motion is encouraged from the onset of injury, since finger stiffness can adversely affect outcome.

Acutely, distal radius fractures should be treated with splint immobilization to grossly maintain alignment, protect neurovascular structures and allow for swelling. Non-displaced or stable, reduced fractures can ultimately be treated with a short arm cast for 4–6 weeks. When anatomic reduction cannot be obtained or maintained, surgery, with external fixation or open reduction and internal fixation, is required. If an adequate reduction is not obtained and if range of motion exercises are not encouraged, the incidence of pain, stiffness and decreased grip strength greatly increases. Anatomic reduction combined with early therapy results in excellent outcomes for up to 90% of patients[61].

PATHOLOGIC FRACTURES

As neoplasms are prevalent in the elderly, pathologic or impending fractures are relatively common. With higher rates of survival for patients with cancer, we see more skeletal metastases than in the past. The most common cancer found in bone is a result of metastases.

Metastases usually arise from primary neoplasms in the prostate, breast, lung, kidney and thyroid[62]. Prostate, adenocarcinoma, Hodgkin's lymphoma and some breast cancers can be osteoblastic ('bone forming', radio-opaque lesions on X-ray). Lung, kidney, thyroid and some breast cancers are osteolytic ('bone destroying', radiolucent lesions on X-ray). Both osteoblastic and osteolytic tumors disrupt normal bony architecture and promote fractures. Most metastases affect the axial skeleton and the appendicular skeleton proximal to the knee and elbow. An exception is lung cancer since it may metastasize distally. Multiple myeloma and lymphoma are common primary malignancies in older adults[63].

Non-operative intervention includes casting and immobilization of the affected bone. Risks of immobilization include pneumonia, decubiti and thromoembolic phenomena. Thromboembolism is especially a concern with malignancies that cause a hypercoagulable state. Non-operative treatment of patients with metastases is associated with higher rates of non-union.

Operative treatment is preferable in patients with pathologic fractures. Internal fixation with intramedullary rods is frequently used in these instances. The literature suggests a minimum life expectancy (between 1 and 3 months) for operative intervention[63,64]. Most importantly, the goal of operative stabilization is to improve the quality of remaining life, following discussion among the surgeon, oncologist, patient and caregiver. Upper-extremity surgery can potentially improve independence with activities of daily living by relieving pain and providing stability. Lower-extremity surgery can promote ambulation or transferring in the remainder of life. Most importantly, surgical stabilization, with or without adjunctive chemotherapy and radiotherapy, can alleviate pain.

Prior to undergoing surgery, a full body bone scan and selected radiographs help determine sites of other metastases. Many authors advocate prophylactic internal fixation of impending pathologic fractures based on size and location of lesions[63].

CONCLUSION

Orthopedic injuries are responsible for significant morbidity and mortality in the geriatric population. With increasing life expectancy trends, orthopedic problems are likely to increase. Ideally, treatment should focus on prevention of falls and management of osteoporosis. The primary goals of treatment are to decrease pain, allow mobilization and return the patient to the prior level of functioning. Treatment must include patient education and rehabilitation. This improves functional outcomes and has been shown to result in decreased long-term cost to the health-care system[65].

References

1. Davis FM , Woolner DF, Frampton C, *et al.* Prospective, multi-centre trial of mortality following general or spinal anaesthesia for hip fracture surgery in the elderly. *Br J Anaesth* 1987;59:1080–8

2. Valentin N, Lomholt B, Jensen JS, *et al.* Spinal or general anaesthesia for surgery of the fractured hip? *Br J Anaesth* 1986;58: 284–91

3. Loder RT. The influence of diabetes on the healing of closed fractures. *Clin Orthop* 1988;232:210–16

4. Aaron JE, Gallagher JC, Anderson J, *et al.* Frequency of osteomalacia and osteoporosis in fractures of the proximal femur. *Lancet* 1974;1:229–33

5. Lane JM, Vigorita VJ. Osteoporosis. *J Bone Joint Surg* 1983;65A:274–8

6. Jenkins DHR, Roberts JG, Webster D, Williams EO. Osteomalacia in elderly patients with fracture of the femoral neck: a clinico-pathological study. *J Bone Joint Surg* 1973;55B:575–80

7. Wilton TJ, Hosking DJ, Pawley E, *et al.* Osteomalacia and femoral neck fractures in the elderly. *J Bone Joint Surg* 1987;69B: 388–90

8. Brody JA. Commentary: prospects for an ageing population. *Nature (London)* 1985; 315:463–6

9. Frandsen PA, Kruse T. Hip fractures in the county of Funen, Denmark. Implications of demographic aging and changes in incidence rates. *Acta Orthop Scand* 1983;54: 681–6

10. Praemer A, Furner S, Rice DP, eds. *Musculoskeletal Conditions in the United States 1992.* Park Ridge, IL: The American Association of Orthopaedic Surgeons, 1992

11. Greenspan SL, Myers ER, Kiel DP, *et al.* Fall severity and bone mineral density as risk factors for hip fractures in ambulatory elderly. *J Am Med Assoc* 1994;271:128–33

12. Hinton RY, Lennox DW, Ebert FR, *et al.* Relative rates of fracture of the hip in the United States: geographic, sex, and age variations. *J Bone Joint Surg* 1995;77A: 695–702

13. Hinton RY, Smith GS. The association of age, race, and sex with the location of proximal femoral fractures in the elderly. *J Bone Joint Surg* 1993;75A:752–9

14. Garraway WM, Stauffer RN, Kurland LT, O'Falba WM. Limb fractures in a defined population. I: frequency and distribution. *Mayo Clin Proc* 1979;54:701–7

15. Johnell O, Sernbo I. Health and social status in patients with hip fractures and controls. *Age Ageing* 1986;15:285–91

16. Uden G, Nilsson B. Hip fracture frequent in hospital. *Acta Orthop Scand* 1986;57: 428–30

17. Gallagher JC, Melton LJ, Riggs BL, Bergtrath E. Epidemiology of fractures of the proximal femur in Rochester Minnesota. *Clin Orthop* 1980;150:163–7

18. Rizzo PF, Gould ES, Lyden JP, Asnis SE. Diagnosis of occult fractures about the hip. Magnetic resonance imaging compared with bone-scanning. *J Bone Joint Surg* 1993;75A:395–401

19. Parker MJ, Myles JW, Anand JK, *et al.* Cost–benefit analysis of hip fracture treatment. *J Bone Joint Surg* 1992;74B:261–4

20. Colwell CW, Spiro TE, Trowbridge AA, *et al.* Use of enoxaparin, a low-molecular-weight heparin, for the prevention of deep venous thrombosis after elective hip replacement. A clinical trial comparing efficacy and safety. Enoxaparin Clinical Trial Group. *J Bone Joint Surg* 1994;76A: 3–14

21. Geerts WH, Jay RM, Code KI, *et al.* A comparison of low-dose heparin with low-molecular-weight heparin as prophylaxis against venous thromboembolism after major trauma. *N Engl J Med* 1996;335: 701–7

22. Hull R, Delmore T, Genotn E, *et al.* Warfarin sodium versus low-dose heparin in the long-term treatment of venous thrombosis. *N Engl J Med* 1979;301:855–8

23. Merli GJ. Update deep venous thrombosis and pulmonary embolism prophylaxis in orthopaedic surgery. *Med Clin North Am* 1993;77:397–412

24. Koval KJ, Skovron ML, Aharonoff GB, *et al.* Ambulatory ability after hip fracture: a prospective study in geriatric patients. *Clin Orthop* 1995;310:150–9

25. Sexson SB, Lehner JT. Factors affecting hip fracture mortality. *J Orthop Trauma* 1988;1:298–305

26. White BL, Fischer WD, Lauren C. Rates of mortality for elderly patients after fracture of the hip in the 1980s. *J Bone Joint Surg* 1987;69A:1335–40

27. Aharonoff GB, Koval KJ, Skovron ML, Zuckerman JD. Hip fractures in the elderly: predictors of one year mortality. *J Orthop Trauma* 1997;11:162–5

28. Kenzora JE, McCarthy RE, Lowell JD, Sledge CB. Hip fracture mortality: relation to age, treatment, preoperative illness, time of surgery and complications. *Clin Orthop* 1984;186:45–56

29. Zuckerman JD, Skovron ML, Koval KJ, *et al.* Postoperative complications and mortality associated with operative delay in older patients who have a fracture of the hip. *J Bone Joint Surg* 1995;77A:1551–6

30. Frankel VH, Burstein AH, Lygre L, Brown RH. The telltale nail. *J Bone Joint Surg* 1971;53A:1232

31. Koval K, Friend KD, Aharanoff GB, Zuckerman JD. Weightbearing after hip fracture: a prospective series of 596 geriatric hip fracture patients. *J Orthop Trauma* 1996;10:526–30

32. Koval K, Sala DA, Kummer FJ, Zuckerman JD. Postoperative weightbearing after a fracture of the femoral neck or an intertrochanteric fracture. *J Bone Joint Surg* 1988;80:352–6

33. Barnes R, Brown JT, Garden RS, Nicoll EA. Subcapital fractures of the femur. A prospective review. *J Bone Joint Surg* 1976;58B:2–24

34. Schmidt AH, Swiontkowski MF. Femoral neck fractures. *Orthop Clin North Am* 2002:33:97–111

35. Cobb AG, Gibson PH. Screw fixation of subcapital fractures of the femur: A better method of treatment. *Injury* 1986;17:259–64

36. Garden RS. Malreduction and avascular necrosis in subcapital fractures of the femur. *J Bone Joint Surg* 1971;53B:183–97

37. Stromqvist B, Hansson LI, Nilsson LT, *et al.* Hook-pin fixation in femoral neck fractures: a two-year follow-up study of 300 cases. *Clin Orthop* 1987;218:58–62

38. Bentley G. Treatment of non-displaced fractures of the femoral neck. *Clin Orthop* 1980;152:93–101

39. Calder SJ, Anderson GH, Jagger C, *et al.* Unipolar or bipolar prosthesis for displaced intracapsular hip fractures in octogenarians. *J Bone Joint Surg* 1996;78B:391–4

40. Evans EM. The treatment of trochanteric fractures of the femur. *J Bone Joint Surg* 1949;31B:190–203

41. Koval KJ, Zuckerman JD. Hip fractures: II. Evaluation and treatment of intertrochanteric fractures. *J Am Acad Orthop Surg* 1994;2:150–6

42. Michelson JD, Myers A, Jinnah R, *et al.* Epidemiology of hip fractures among the elderly: risk factors for fracture type. *Clin Orthop* 1995;311:129–35

43. Kyle RF, Cabanela ME, Russell TA, *et al.* Fractures of the proximal part of the femur. Review. *Instr Course Lect* 1995;44:227–53

44. Tencer AF, Calhoun J, Miller BB. Stiffness of subtrochanteric fractures of the femur stabilized using a Richards interlocking intramedullary rod or Richards AMBI. *Orthop Biomech Lab Report*, no. 002. Memphis: Richards Medical Co., 1985

45. Tencer AF, Johnson KD, Johnston DWC, Gill K. A biomechanical comparison of various methods of stabilization of subtrochanteric fractures of the femur. *J Orthop Res* 1984;2:297–305

46. Allis OH. Fracture in the upper third of the femur exclusive of the neck. *Med News* 1891;59:585–9

47. Lauge-Hansen N. Fractures of the ankle. Analytic historic survey as basis of new experimental roentgenologic and clinical investigations. *Arch Surg* 1948;56:259–317

48. Lauge-Hansen N. Fractures of the ankle II. Combined experimental–surgical and

experimental roentgenologic investigation. *Arch Surg* 1950;60:957–85

49. Ramsey P, Hamilton W. Changes in tibiotalar area of contact caused by lateral talar shift. *J Bone Joint Surg* 1976;58A:356–7

50. Keene JS, Lange RH. Diagnostic dilemmas in foot and ankle injuries. *J Am Med Assoc* 1986;256:247–51

51. Beauchamp CG, Clay NR, Thexton PW. Displaced ankle fractures in patients over 50 years of age. *J Bone Joint Surg* 1983; 63B:329–32

52. Ali MS, McLaren AN, Routholamin E, O'Connor BT. Ankle fractures in the elderly: nonoperative or operative treatment. *J Orthop Trauma* 1987;1:275–80

53. Horak J, Nilsson BE. Epidemiology of fractures of the upper end of the humerus. *Clin Orthop Rel Res* 1975;112:250–3

54. Koval K, Gallagher MA, Marsicano JG, *et al.* Functional outcome after minimally displaced fracture of the proximal part of the humerus. *J Bone Joint Surg* 1997;79A: 203–7

55. Court-Brown CM, Garg A, McQueen MM. The translated two-part fracture of the proximal humerus: epidemiology and outcome in the older patient. *J Bone Joint Surg* 2001;83B:799–804

56. Bosch U, Skutek M, Fremerey RW, Tscherne H. Outcome after primary and secondary hemiarthroplasty in elderly patients with fractures of the proximal humerus. *J Shoulder Elbow Surg* 1998;7: 479–84

57. Goldman R, Koval KJ, Cuomo F, *et al.* Functional outcome after humeral head replacement for acute three- and four-part proximal humeral fractures. *J Shoulder Elbow Surg* 1995;4:81–6

58. Alffram P, Bauer G. Epidemiology of fractures of the forearm. *J Bone Joint Surg* 1962;44A:105–14

59. Fryckman G. Fractures of the distal radius including sequelae. *Acta Orthop Scand Suppl* 1967;180:1–153

60. Colles A. On the fracture of the carpal extremity of the radius. *Edin Med Surg J* 1814;10:182–6

61. Villar RN, Marsh D, Righton N, Greatorex RA. Three years after Colles' fracture: a prospective review. *J Bone Joint Surg* 1987;69B:635–8

62. Bhardwaj S, Holland JF. Chemotherapy of metastatic cancer in bone. *Clin Orthop Rel Res* 1982;169:34

63. Harrington KD. Impending pathological fractures from metastatic malignancy: evaluation and management. In *American Academy of Orthopaedic Surgeons Instructional Course Lectures*. New Orleans, 1986:357–381

64. Harrington KD, Sim FH, Enis JE, *et al.* Methylmethacrylate as an adjunct in internal fixation of pathological fractures. *J Bone Joint Surg* 1976;58A:1047–55

65. Ruchlin HS, Elkin EB, Allegrante JP. The economic impact of a multifactorial intervention to improve post-operatvie rehabilitation of hip fractures. *Arthritis Rheum* 2001;45:446–52

54 Polymyalgia rheumatica and temporal arteritis

T.S. Dharmarajan, MD, FACP, AGSF, *Shamim Ahmed,* MD, *and Barry Fomberstein,* MD, FACP, FACR

INTRODUCTION

Polymyalgia rheumatica (PMR) and temporal arteritis (TA) are two different but related entities belonging to the same spectrum of inflammatory disorders, characteristically presenting in older adults[1,2]. PMR, initially described by Bruce in 1888 as 'senile rheumatic gout', is a clinical syndrome of proximal muscle pain and stiffness and was given its current name in 1957 by Barber[3–5]. Co-morbid processes associated with aging make the diagnosis especially difficult, since there are no specific diagnostic laboratory tests. The syndrome often results in functional limitation and diminished quality of life. TA, also known as giant cell arteritis (GCA), typically presents with superficial headache, primarily affecting older individuals. Symptoms suggestive of TA were recorded by Ali Ibn Asa over a millennium ago[6]. In 1890 the entity was reported by Hutchinson, and in 1932 the term temporal arteritis was used by Horton[5,6]. The relationship of TA to PMR is unclear; the two entities may present together or in sequence[1,2]. Both disorders respond to corticosteroids and biopsy of the temporal artery may reveal evidence of arteritis in either syndrome[1,5]. The terms TA and GCA will be used synonymously for the rest of this discussion.

CRITERIA FOR DIAGNOSIS

PMR is characterized by pain and stiffness involving the neck, shoulders and/or pelvic girdle[1]. Commonly accepted criteria (Table 1) for diagnosis include:

(1) Age more than 50 years;

(2) Symptoms affecting at least two of the following locations: shoulders and arms, hips and thighs, neck and torso;

(3) Duration over 1 month;

(4) Elevated erythrocyte sedimentation rate (ESR), typically over 40 mm/h (but often much higher)[1,3,6].

Suddenness of onset is a feature, with the patient usually well prior to the appearance of symptoms. The presence of other specific disorders as a basis for such symptoms excludes the diagnosis of PMR[1].

TA, unlike PMR, is not primarily a musculoskeletal disorder but instead a form of systemic vasculitis. It typically affects people over 50 years of age, presents with new onset of localized headache, which may be severe, scalp tenderness overlying the temporal artery and a diminished temporal artery pulse[1,6,7]. An elevated ESR of 50 mm/h or greater accompanies an abnormal temporal artery biopsy[1,6,7]. The diagnosis of TA is suggested when three or

Table 1   Criteria for diagnosis of polymyalgia rheumatica and temporal arteritis

	Polymyalgia rheumatica	Temporal arteritis
Age	50 years or older	50 years or older
Symptoms	pain and morning stiffness in at least two of the following areas: shoulder girdle, pelvic girdle, neck and torso	new-onset localized headache, scalp tenderness, decreased or absent temporal artery pulse
Erythrocyte sedimentation rate	usually more than 40 mm/h	usually more than 50 mm/h
Duration	more than a month; sudden onset suggests diagnosis	more than a month
Biopsy	temporal artery biopsy may reveal vasculitis (not required for diagnosis)	multinucleated giant cells and evidence of vasculitis in temporal artery biopsy
Therapy	rapid response to low-dose (10–15 mg/day) corticosteroids	good response to higher-dose corticosteroids

more of the above criteria are present, even if temporal artery biopsy is negative[1,7].

Although cranial and ocular symptoms predominate in TA, musculoskeletal findings are also observed[8]. Up to 40–60% of cases of TA have evidence for coexisting PMR; conversely, 15–20% of those with PMR may have underlying GCA[1,9]. Other common arteries involved in GCA include the aorta and its proximal branches including the coronary, carotid, subclavian and ophthalmic arteries[2].

EPIDEMIOLOGY

The prevalence of PMR and TA vary with race and geographic area, but appear relatively common in the USA and Europe, particularly Scandinavian countries[1,2,6]. In the USA a higher prevalence has been reported in Minnesota, a state with a large population of Scandinavian origin[1,2,6]. The prevalence is lower in African-Americans, Latinos and Asians compared to non-Latino Whites[6]. The incidence of PMR increases with age, from approximately 20 per 100 000 per year in persons 50–59 years to 100 in persons aged 70–79 years[6]. The prevalence is approximately 600 cases per 100 000 persons[1,9]. More than two-thirds of all patients are women[1,6].

PMR may be even more prevalent than reported, as the entity is under-diagnosed[6]. TA, less common that PMR, has an incidence and prevalence of 17.8 and 200, respectively, per 100 000 persons over the age of 50 per year[1]. Even with specific clinical presentation and diagnostic tests for TA, this condition also appears under-recognized[6].

ETIOLOGY AND PATHOGENESIS

Symptoms of polymyalgia rheumatica are thought to be due to synovitis and proximal bursitis, characterized microscopically by T-cell and macrophage infiltration and vascular proliferation[1,2,10]. Even in the absence of vascular symptoms, T-lymphocyte infiltration of blood vessels may be found on biopsy[1]. Symptoms in TA are predominantly due to vasculitis of the affected artery. Multinucleated giant cells are the classic biopsy finding, serving as the basis for the alternative name, GCA. Degradation of elastic fibers is observed in the internal elastic lamina of large arteries[1,2,6].

Several causes have been suggested for both PMR and TA, but the exact etiology is unknown[1,2]. The association with age is also not clear[2]. Familial aggregations of cases and ethnic predisposition suggest a genetic basis[1,2,6]. Activated CD4+ T-helper lymphocytes have been implicated in the pathogenesis. HLA class II antigens probably influence the expression of these diseases, but the association is weaker than that for rheumatoid arthritis[1,11]. PMR and GCA have a significant association with HLA-DR4 alleles[1,11]. Levels of CD8+ T lymphocytes are often lower in patients or their asymptomatic family members[1]. It has also been suggested that PMR and GCA are autoimmune disorders triggered by infectious stimuli in susceptible persons[1]. An association between parvovirus B_{19} infection and GCA has been reported, as well as a higher prevalence of antibodies to adenovirus, respiratory syncytial virus and *Mycoplasma pneumoniae* in patients with PMR[1]. There is, however, no conclusive evidence to support the theory of viral etiology, nor is there a significant association between GCA and other autoimmune diseases, such as thyroid dysfunction[1,12].

CLINICAL FEATURES

Symptoms in PMR are most frequently sudden in onset, and may be accompanied by mild systemic manifestations, such as low-grade fever, anorexia, weight loss, malaise, fatigue and depression[2,6]. Less commonly, the onset may be more insidious, with symptoms present for weeks or months prior to diagnosis[6]. Musculoskeletal symptoms may be unilateral, involving one shoulder or hip, and progress to involve bilateral proximal muscles[2]. Stiffness is an especially prominent symptom. Morning stiffness and pain occur in the proximal muscles rather than in the joints, accentuated by movement of the affected area[2]. Pain from movement during sleep awakens the patient at night[2]. Severe disease interferes with mobility and may prevent simple motions such as transferring out of bed. The decrease in mobility is due to musculoskeletal pain rather than weakness *per se*, which is not a feature of PMR. In the advanced stages, muscle atrophy and contracture of the shoulder capsule may result in limitation of range of motion[2].

TA is a vasculitis having classic symptoms of severe headache and scalp tenderness, in association with a red, indurated temporal artery[1,2,6]. The temporal artery pulse may be weak or absent. Constitutional and skeletal manifestations are similar to those of PMR. Visual symptoms including diplopia, ptosis and sudden blindness are common in GCA[1,2,6]. Loss of vision may be partial or complete, transient or permanent, and requires prompt intervention[1,5]. Other common features are intermittent claudication of the jaw and/or extremities, cough and hoarseness of voice[1,2]. Angina, myocardial infarction and congestive heart failure may be due to coronary arteritis. Thoracic aortic aneurysms and dissection are also known to be late complications in GCA as well as other neurologic manifestations such as neuropathies, transient ischemic attacks or strokes[2]. Approximately 15% of patients with GCA may present with fever of unknown origin[2].

DIAGNOSIS

A variety of musculoskeletal problems including underlying degenerative joint disease, other inflammatory diseases and neurologic syndromes can obscure the diagnosis of PMR[1]. The most important diagnostic tool is a detailed history and physical examination, as the diagnoses of PMR and TA are largely based on clinical grounds. No diagnostic laboratory test is available for PMR, but temporal artery biopsy is considered standard for clinically suspected cases of GCA. The diagnosis of PMR should be considered in older patients with proximal muscle stiffness, pain and other criteria mentioned earlier, after exclusion of other possible entities, including occult or unsuspected neoplasm.

New-onset headache, transient or sudden loss of vision, unexplained fever and high erythrocyte sedimentation rate should raise the suspicion of TA in an older person; temporal artery biopsy is suggested in such

Table 2   Investigation of polymyalgia rheumatica (PMR) and temporal arteritis (TA)

Elevated erythrocyte sedimentation rate (usually more than 40 mm/h)
Normochromic normocytic anemia
Elevated C-reactive protein
Elevated alkaline phosphatase and transaminases
Normal serum creatine kinase
Negative antinuclear antibodies
Negative rheumatoid factor
Electromyography: unremarkable in PMR
Muscle biopsy: normal or non-specific atrophy in PMR
Temporal artery biopsy: evidence of arteritis in TA
Bone scan: non-specific increased uptake in affected areas in PMR

a situation[2]. Arterial disease occurs as 'skip lesions'; therefore segments of artery at least 1–2 cm long should be obtained to increase the diagnostic yield[1,7]. The biopsy may be negative in approximately 20–30% of cases. If there is high clinical suspicion for TA, the opposite side may be biopsied, or the patient may be treated despite a negative biopsy[5,7]. Temporal artery biopsy is relatively safe, with low morbidity, and is best performed prior to initiation of treatment[7]. However, biopsy specimens may still provide evidence for arteritis even after 2 weeks of corticosteroid therapy[7]. Temporal artery biopsy is also suggestive for arteritis in PMR in about a third of cases without obvious symptoms of vasculitis[6].

Other laboratory findings are common for both syndromes and are non-specific (Table 2). A mild to moderate normocytic, normochromic anemia is usually present in active disease[2,5,6]. Normal leukocyte counts and increased platelet counts are often observed. The ESR is a useful measure of disease activity or response to therapy. A markedly elevated ESR is characteristic for both PMR and GCA, and levels over 100 mm/h (Westergren method) are not uncommon[1,2,5]. It is worthwhile noting that a normal sedimentation rate in an untreated patient with high clinical suspicion does not exclude the diagnosis[10,13]. Serum

creatine kinase levels are normal. Antinuclear antibodies and rheumatoid factor are usually negative, while C-reactive protein and serum interleukin 6 levels have been found elevated[2]. Hepatic enzymes, particularly alkaline phosphatase, can be mildly abnormal in about a third of cases. Muscle biopsy in PMR is usually normal or may show non-specific atrophy; electromyographic studies are unremarkable[2,4].

In PMR, bone scans may demonstrate non-specific increased uptake in the shoulder and hip joints[5]. Color Doppler sonography of the temporal arteries reveals decreased blood flow velocity in patients with GCA, but has no role in PMR[14]. Another non-invasive technique is fluorodeoxyglucose positron emission tomography, which may suggest vasculitis in PMR and TA[15]. At present, expertise to perform this test is not widely available.

Ultrasound and magnetic resonance imaging (MRI) have been useful in demonstrating subacromial bursitis and subdeltoid bursitis as frequently found lesions in most patients with PMR. When complaints were present in the hands and feet, a tenosynovitis was demonstrated by MRI. Magnetic resonance angiography is helpful in demonstrating extra-cranial arteritis in TA[16].

Making a precise diagnosis is important, particularly in the case of TA, to avoid irreversible loss of vision. A recent study suggested that the most useful finding which predicted the likelihood of a positive temporal artery biopsy, was a normal ESR (value below 50 mm/h), which suggested that TA was unlikely[17]. Jaw claudication and diplopia substantially increased the probability of a positive biopsy. Beaded, prominent arteries were very likely to correlate with a diagnostic biopsy while synovitis did not favor the diagnosis of TA. A diagnosis was not suggested by any specific combination of features either[17]. Absence of a good response to steroids along with the presence of atypical features are indications to search for an alternate diagnosis[16].

Table 3 Differential diagnosis of polymyalgia rheumatica

Rheumatoid arthritis
Seronegative arthritis
Osteoarthritis (shoulders, spine and hips)
Polymyositis
Connective tissue disorders
Hypothyroidism
Endocarditis
Paraneoplastic syndromes

Table 4 Differential diagnosis of headache in temporal arteritis

Refraction errors
Ischemic cerebrovascular disease
Cervical spondylosis
Late-onset migraine
Drugs: nitrates
Intracranial mass lesions: primary or metastatic cancer, subdural hematoma
Psychological basis (depression)
Dental or temporomandibular joint-related

DIFFERENTIAL DIAGNOSIS

The initial presentation of rheumatoid arthritis in the elderly may mimic PMR. Symptoms in rheumatoid arthritis can be proximal and arise predominantly due to joint involvement[1,4]. The presence of subacromial and subdeltoid bursitis suggests PMR rather than rheumatoid arthritis[1]. Occasionally, in PMR, synovitis is present in the knees and wrists, and may raise the possibility of seronegative rheumatoid syndrome[1]. Osteoarthritis of the shoulder, spine and hips may also resemble the symptoms of PMR. Limited mobility in polymyositis is due to muscle weakness, whereas in PMR pain and stiffness are the predominant findings[1,4]. Bone pain is not a feature of PMR, and when present, suggests an alternative diagnosis[1]. Connective tissue diseases, hypothyroidism and cervical or lumbar degenerative diseases also enter the differential diagnosis (Table 3)[4]. Prominent musculoskeletal symptoms may be present in the course of bacterial endocarditis in up to a fourth of cases; the presence of leukocytosis and hematuria, along with altered ESR, suggests endocarditis[2,4]. Although some paraneoplastic syndromes may mimic PMR prior to diagnosis of the primary malignancy, the literature does not justify a search for underlying malignancy in patients with typical PMR[1,4]. However, multiple myeloma, leukemia, lymphoma, occult malignancy of the colon, prostate, and ovary may present with paraneoplastic syndromes resembling PMR[4]. Fibromyalgia is suggested by chronic fatigue, and diffuse pain in a setting of stress, depression, anxiety, insomnia and traumatic life situation. Normal laboratory tests are consistent with fibromyalgia[18].

TA or GCA shares a number of clinical and pathologic findings with Takayasu's arteritis, which affects almost exclusively females younger than 40 years[1,19]. However, ethnic background, localized scalp tenderness and shoulder stiffness are helpful in distinguishing GCA from Takayasu's arteritis[1]. Temporal arteries may be involved in other forms of vasculitis such as Wegener's granulomatosis, Churg–Strauss syndrome, sarcoidosis, lymphoma and amyloidosis[1]. Occasionally, refraction errors may cause new-onset headache in the elderly (Table 4), and progression of other common eye disorders, such as cataracts, glaucoma and macular degeneration may result in unilateral visual disturbances[1]. Osteoarthritis of the temporomandibular joint can also present with jaw pain[1]. Thus, a variety of presentations may create difficulties and delay in the diagnosis of TA.

TREATMENT

The mainstay of treatment for both PMR and TA is corticosteroids[1,2,6]. When TA presents with visual symptoms, prompt treatment with steroids is required to prevent possible loss of vision. The dramatic clinical response to steroids would also be suggestive of the diagnosis in both entities[1,4,5]. Within the first 12 h, symptoms begin to abate, and rapid relief of symptoms, usually within 24–48 h, is the characteristic response to steroid therapy in both PMR and TA[1,5].

For those who are not candidates for corticosteroids, in milder forms of PMR with no vascular symptoms and a negative temporal artery biopsy, an option is the use of nonsteroidal anti-inflammatory drugs (NSAIDs) for 2–4 weeks[1,2]. NSAIDs may adequately control musculoskeletal symptoms in a minority without affecting the ESR[1,2]. It should be emphasized that older persons are at high risk for developing NSAID-related complications in the presence of gastroesophageal diseases, renal insufficiency, hypertension and congestive heart failure[1]. We believe that low-dose steroids are more effective and perhaps safer than NSAIDs.

Since the manifestations and consequences of PMR and GCA differ, the dose of steroids required is different for each disorder[6]. The initial recommended dose of prednisone in PMR is 10–20 mg daily, and in GCA 40–60 mg daily in divided doses[1,2,4]. The laboratory responses follow clinical recovery; the ESR falls within 2 weeks and usually becomes normal in a month[1,6]. After resolution of symptoms and normalization of the ESR, the dose of prednisone can be reduced by 1–2.5 mg every 2–4 weeks[1]. More gradual tapering, such as 1 mg/month, is better tolerated when the dose is as low as 5–10 mg/day[1]. While the dose is being reduced, patients should be closely monitored for recurrence of symptoms or a rise in ESR[1,6]. Nevertheless, active arteritis may be present despite improving sedimentation rate[2]. Depending on the clinical response, the duration of steroid therapy may range from 2 months to more than 15 years[4]. From 15 to 70% of cases may still require corticosteroids at the end of 2 years, and syndromes may relapse in up to half the patients after discontinuation of therapy[4]. Of course, numerous adverse effects may result from the chronic use of steroids including osteoporosis, diabetes, hypertension, peptic ulcer disease, cataracts, insomnia, depression, anxiety and delirium[1,6].

Patients should be made aware of these possibilities, and routine monitoring should include inquiries or investigations to determine the presence of these possible untoward effects. Prophylaxis for osteoporosis with acceptable regimens is required for those on chronic steroid therapy. Age over 75 years, female gender, a cumulative prednisone dose over 2g, and initial dose of prednisone over 40 mg daily increased the risk of steroid-related complications. Use of alternate day steroids appears less effective in both TA and PMR[16]. Intravenous pulse therapy with methylprednisolone (1000 mg daily for 3 days) is an option when visual loss is imminent[16].

In an effort to reduce the dose and duration of steroid therapy, the use of methotrexate has been recommended. Opinions vary regarding the efficacy of methotrexate in both entities[1]. While some suggest it has steroid-sparing effects and helps preserve bone mineral density, others found no benefit in PMR without coexisting GCA[20,21]. Other disease-modifying agents, such as dapsone, hydroxychloroquine, penicillamine and cytotoxic drugs may be considered in patients unresponsive to steroids; these drugs have not been studied in a systematic fashion and their use is controversial[2,7].

SUMMARY

PMR and GCA are relatively common in the geriatric age group. They are closely related inflammatory disorders of unknown etiology, possibly attributable to an unidentified infectious pathogen in genetically susceptible persons. Clinical diagnosis can be suggested by typical symptoms relating to proximal muscle involvement or vasculitis. Both entities respond dramatically to steroid therapy, and the ESR is a useful marker of disease activity and treatment response. Despite severe consequences from vasculitis, overall life expectancy is normal. However, these diseases affect functional abilities and quality of life, and should be treated appropriately when suspected. Future research needs to focus on studies for the molecular basis of PMR and TA. Criteria for PMR needs to consider inclusion of ultrasound of the shoulders for bursitis and perhaps addition of C reactive protein. The precise role for methotrexate and other steroid sparing agents in these entities requires further elucidation[16].

References

1. Evans JM, Hunder GG. Polymyalgia rheumatica and giant cell arteritis. *Rheum Dis Clin North Am* 2000;26:493–515
2. Hunder GG. Giant cell arteritis and polymyalgia rheumatica. In Kelley WN, Ruddy S, Harris ED Jr, Sledge CB, eds. *Textbook of Rheumatology*, 5th edn. Philadelphia, PA: WB Saunders, 1997:1123–32
3. Bengtsson B-A. Polymyalgia rheumatica. In Klippel JH, Weyand CM, Wortmann RL, eds. *Primer on the Rheumatic Diseases*, 11th edn. Atlanta, GA: The Arthritis Foundation, 1997:305–6
4. Brooks RC, McGee SR. Diagnostic dilemmas in polymyalgia rheumatica. *Arch Intern Med* 1997;157:162–8
5. Dwolatzky T, Sonnenblick M, Nesher G. Giant cell arteritis and polymyalgia rheumatica: clues to early diagnosis. *Geriatrics* 1997;52:38–44
6. Goodwin JS. Progress in gerontology: polymyalgia rheumatica and temporal arteritis. *J Am Geriatr Soc* 1992;40:515–25
7. Lee AG, Brazis PW. Temporal arteritis: a clinical approach. *J Am Geriatr Soc* 1999;47:1364–70
8. Salvarani C, Hunder GG. Musculoskeletal manifestations in a population-based cohort of patients with giant cell arteritis. *Arthritis Rheum* 1999;42:1259–66
9. Sutej PG. Polymyalgia rheumatica. In Hazzard WR, Blass JP, Ettinger WH Jr, Halter JB, Ouslander JG, eds. *Principles of Geriatrics Medicine and Gerontology*, 4th edn. New York: McGraw-Hill, 1999:1121–4
10. Gonzalez-Gay MA, Rodriguez-Valverde V, Blanco R, *et al.* Polymyalgia rheumatica without significantly increased erythrocyte sedimentation rate. *Arch Intern Med* 1997;157:317–20
11. Guerne P, Salvi M, Seitz M, *et al.* Molecular analysis of HLA-DR polymorphism in polymyalgia rheumatica. *J Rheumatol* 1997; 24:671–6
12. Duhaut P, Bornet H, Pinede L, *et al.* Giant cell arteritis and thyroid dysfunction: multicentre case–control study. *Br Med J* 1999; 318:434–5
13. Brigden M. The erythrocyte sedimentation rate still a helpful test when used judiciously. *Postgrad Med* 1998;103:257–74
14. Lauwerys BR, Puttemans T, Houssiau FA, Devogelaer J. Color Doppler sonography of the temporal arteritis in giant cell arteritis and polymyalgia rheumatica. *J Rheumatol* 1997;24:1570–4
15. Blockmans D, Maes A, Stroobants S, *et al.* New arguments for a vasculitic nature of polymyalgia rheumatica using positron emission tomography. *Br J Rheumatol* 1999;38:444–7
16. Salvarani C, Cantini F, Boiardi L, Hunder GG. Polymyalgia rheumatica and giant cell arteritis. *N Eng J Med* 2002;347: 261–71
17. Smetana GW, Shmerling RH. Does this patient have temporal arteritis? *JAMA* 2002;287:92–101
18. Blumenthal DE. Tired, aching, ANA-positive: does your patient have lupus or fibromyalgia? *Cleveland Clin J Med* 2002; 69:143–52
19. Brack A, Martinez-Taboada V, Stanson A, *et al.* Disease pattern in cranial and large-vessel giant cell arteritis. *Arthritis Rheum* 1999;42:311–17
20. Ferraccioli G, Salaffi F, DeVita S, *et al.* Methotrexate in polymyalgia rheumatica: preliminary results of an open, randomized study. *J Rheumatol* 1996;23:624–8
21. Feinberg HL, Sherman JD, Schrepferman CG, *et al.* The use of methotrexate in polymyalgia rheumatica. *J Rheumatol* 1996;23: 1550–2

55 Vitamin B$_{12}$ deficiency

T.S. Dharmarajan, MD, FACP, AGSF, *G.U. Adiga*, MD,
Suresh Pitchumoni, MD, *and Edward P. Norkus*, PhD, FACN, ABNS

The relationship between vitamin B$_{12}$ and anemia has been recognized for years. Recent focus has expanded beyond the identification and treatment of megaloblastic anemia with attempts to understand subclinical B$_{12}$ deficiency states and the prevention of complications[1,2]. Newer tests and novel therapeutic approaches aid in this renewed interest.

Deficiency of vitamin B$_{12}$ (used synonymously in this chapter with the term cobalamin), either overt or covert, is amongst the most common nutritional disorders in older adults. It assumes significance in geriatric medicine for several reasons. First, the deficiency is common, with an estimated prevalence of 3–40%[3–5]. Second, it is increasingly recognized that tissue deficiency can coexist with serum B$_{12}$ levels that are borderline normal. Third, the recent implementation of folate fortification of foods to prevent birth defects has the potential to permit cobalamin deficiency to advance with complications that are unrecognized[6]. Fourth, the recognition that homocysteine is a marker for vascular disease and that cobalamin deficiency is one of several causes that increases homocysteine levels is another reason to screen for and treat B$_{12}$ deficiency in older subjects[7,8]. Fifth, failure to identify this deficiency has the potential to result in grave, sometimes irreversible, consequences.

The magnitude of the problem has been reported to be similar in nursing home and community elderly[9]. Our own data indicate that 17% of hospitalized elderly from nursing homes and 26% from the community have borderline or low B$_{12}$ status[5]. Further, patients from long-term care facilities are more likely to suffer from neuropsychiatric disturbances such as dementia, with cobalamin deficiency being one of several factors known to play a role[10].

CHEMISTRY

The cobalamin molecule is made up of a corrin nucleus with a central cobalt atom that is linked to a nucleotide. Different ligands are able to bind covalently with the cobalt atom to form the various cobalamin analogs. Of these, only methylcobalamin and adenosylcobalamin have physiological activity in humans. As both forms are labile, they are unsuitable for commercial preparations. Cyanocobalamin, with cyanide attached to the cobalt atom, is the stable commercial form available in the USA, while hydroxycobalamin is the preparation available in the UK and elsewhere. Cobalamin analogs, present in food or commercial preparations, must be converted to the physiologically active form in the body prior to utilization. Many cobalamin analogs are inactive in humans and some even possess anti-vitamin B$_{12}$ activity[11].

In humans, B$_{12}$ participates in two major enzymatic pathways. In the first, methylcobalamin is a coenzyme required for the conversion of homocysteine to methionine. This reaction is linked to the conversion of methyltetrahydrofolate to tetrahydrofolate (THF), which is essential for the synthesis of purine, pyrimidine and nucleic acids. Impairment of this reaction produces a deficiency of THF that results in elevated homocysteine levels with the accumulation of folate as methyltetrahydrofolate (methyl folate trap). B_{12} deficiency causes impaired DNA synthesis and hyperhomocysteinemia, the likely basis for some vascular and neurologic disorders.

The second enzymatic reaction uses adenosylcobalamin as coenzyme in the conversion of methylmalonyl coenzyme A (CoA) to succinyl CoA. This reaction has a role in fatty acid metabolism; deficiency of cobalamin can result in the accumulation of abnormal lipids in neuronal membranes that may contribute to neurological dysfunction. When this reaction is impaired, methylmalonyl CoA accumulates with subsequent conversion to methylmalonic acid (MMA). Thus, B_{12} deficiency results in elevation of both MMA and homocysteine[12].

SOURCES AND REQUIREMENTS

The ultimate source for dietary cobalamin is microbial synthesis. Fruits and vegetables lack B_{12} unless contaminated by microorganisms. Foods rich in vitamin B_{12} include organ meat such as liver, kidney and heart. Moderate amounts of the vitamin are present in dairy products, some seafood, muscle meats and egg yolk[11]. Normal colonic bacteria synthesize sufficient B_{12}; however, this is not bioavailable, as B_{12} absorption occurs predominantly in the distal small intestine[13].

The recommended dietary allowance (RDA) for vitamin B_{12} is 2.4 µg/day[14]. The average American diet with 5–30 µg of cobalamin far exceeds the RDA. Since food-cobalamin malabsorption is the most common cause of deficiency and the elderly suffer from multiple conditions that can affect the complex absorption pathway for B_{12}, adequate dietary intake alone does not ensure normal cobalamin status in the elderly. As vegetable sources lack B_{12}, strict vegetarians (vegans) are at risk for deficiency unless they consume supplements[13].

ABSORPTION, STORAGE AND EXCRETION

Cobalamin in food is protein bound and must undergo a series of elaborate digestive steps prior to absorption. Initially, cobalamin is released from polypeptide linkages by gastric acid and pepsin in the stomach. Free cobalamin binds with salivary R-protein, due to its high binding affinity, rather than to intrinsic factor (IF)[11]. In the duodenum, alkaline pH and pancreatic trypsin degrade the R-protein, to release free cobalamin which then binds to IF. This cobalamin–IF complex is resistant to further proteolytic digestion and is carried down to the ileum. In the terminal ileum, the cobalamin–IF complex binds to specific receptors in the brush border in the presence of ionic calcium and is internalized. Once inside the enterocyte, cobalamin is released from IF and attaches to transcobalamin-II (TC-II), a carrier protein, and is released into portal venous blood[12]. When B_{12} is consumed in large quantities, small amounts are absorbed by passive diffusion throughout the length of the small intestine without requirement for IF[11]. This minor pathway assumes significance when considering oral therapy, especially in the absence of IF.

TC-II is the major carrier and delivery protein for B_{12}. TC-II-bound cobalamin (holo- transcobalamin II) is taken up by the liver, bone marrow and other cells by a receptor-mediated uptake in the presence of ionic calcium. The significance of TC-II in vitamin B_{12} utilization is best exemplified in congenital TC-II deficiency, which manifests with florid features of cobalamin deficiency. Vitamin B_{12} is also bound to TC-I and TC-III, collectively referred to as haptocorrins. Both forms mainly serve a storage function[11].

The liver contains about 2–5 mg of vitamin B$_{12}$ which represents 50–90% of the body's stored cobalamin. A small amount of the vitamin undergoes enterohepatic circulation with nearly complete reabsorption. A fully functioning enterohepatic circulation is essential for vitamin B$_{12}$ economy, particularly for vegetarians. When large doses of B$_{12}$ are administered, the excess vitamin is excreted in the urine.

PATHOGENESIS

Vitamin B$_{12}$ is ultimately required for DNA synthesis and a constant supply is required by all dividing cells. Deficiency effects are seen in rapidly dividing hematopoietic cells and in the gastrointestinal epithelium. The pathogenesis of neurologic involvement is poorly understood. Postulated mechanisms include homocysteine toxicity[15], incorporation of abnormal neuronal lipids[12] and defective methylation of basic myelin proteins[7]. Pathologically the involved nerves become demyelinated followed by axonal degeneration, resulting in eventual neuronal death.

CAUSES OF DEFICIENCY

Since the absorption and utilization of cobalamin involves several unique interdependent pathways, conditions that affect any step predispose to deficiency. Food-cobalamin malabsorption is the most common basis, accounting for up to 50% of cases[3,16,17]. Pernicious anemia (PA), once considered a common etiology of deficiency, contributes to a much smaller proportion. Nevertheless, the cause of cobalamin deficiency remains unclear in many individuals. While diet-induced B$_{12}$ deficiency is rare, it should be considered in vegetarians or vegans and whenever malnutrition is suspected.

Food-cobalamin malabsorption is the inability to absorb food-bound cobalamin, while the absorption of free cobalamin remains intact. Since cobalamin in food is protein bound, the first step is the release of vitamin in the presence of acid. Conditions predisposing to food-cobalamin malabsorption include atropic gastritis, *Helicobacter pylori* infection and achlorhydria, irrespective of the cause. Food-cobalamin malabsorption is more common in Blacks and Latin Americans than in Caucasians, although cobalamin deficiency itself is more common in Caucasians[17]. Up to half the elderly may have hypochlorhydria and so may not effectively cleave protein-bound cobalamin[18]. An association between *H. pylori* infection and B$_{12}$ deficiency has been observed with correction of B$_{12}$ status after treatment of *H. pylori* infection alone[17,19].

PA causes B$_{12}$ deficiency due to the lack of IF following the antibody-mediated destruction of parietal cells. PA is a cause of up to 17% of all cases of B$_{12}$ deficiency[16]. In addition, about 2% of older adults may have undiagnosed PA[3]. In contrast to food-cobalamin malabsorption, PA involves the inability to absorb both free and protein-bound B$_{12}$.

Small intestinal bacterial overgrowth (SIBO) is an important, often unrecognized cause of malnutrition in older adults[20]. These individuals typically suffer from conditions predisposing to SIBO such as achlorhydria, decreased intestinal motility, previous intestinal surgery and the use of acid-lowering agents. In these cases, B$_{12}$ deficiency is secondary to the consumption of the vitamin by bacterial overgrowth.

Several medications, widely used in the geriatric population, may contribute to the development of cobalamin deficiency (Table 1). Aminoglycoside antibiotics, metformin, para-aminosalicylic acid and anticonvulsants cause intestinal B$_{12}$ malabsorption. Nitrous oxide anesthesia can irreversibly inactivate the vitamin by an oxidative process and may even precipitate an acute myelopathy in patients with true or borderline deficiency[21]. It has also been suggested that high intakes of vitamin C can interfere with B$_{12}$ metabolism by converting the vitamin

Table 1 Etiology of cobalamin deficiency in older adults*

Mechanism	Cause
Dietary deficiency	strict vegetarianism (vegans)
	chronic malnutrition
Food-cobalamin malabsorption	hypochlorhydria
	achlorohydria
	atropic gastritis
Microbial consumption	small intestinal bacterial overgrowth
Other defective absorption	pernicious anemia
	Helicobacter pylori gastritis
	Crohn's disease
	gastric/intestinal resections
	chronic pancreatitis
	other causes of malabsorption
Insufficient stores	advanced liver disease
Defective utilization	congenital transcobalamin-II deficiency
Medications	
malabsorption	acid-lowering agents
	antibiotics
	metformin
	phenytoin
	colchicine
	para-aminosalicylic acid
	cholestyramine
inactivation	vitamin C
	nitrous oxide anesthesia

*The list is for illustration only. Any cause of deficiency may be applicable to the elderly

into an inactive form and by destroying IF. Long-term proton pump inhibitors and other acid-lowering agents have the potential to cause food-cobalamin malabsorption by causing diminished acid peptic activity or by predisposing to SIBO[22,23]. Oral contraceptives, though associated with falsely low B_{12} levels, are not believed to be associated with true deficiency[24,25].

Other causes of cobalamin deficiency include Crohn's disease, gastric and/or intestinal resection, HIV infection, chronic pancreatitis and advanced liver disease. Crohn's disease is common in older adults, with one in six patients presenting for the first time after age 60. Here, the risk of B_{12} deficiency is proportional to the extent (length) of terminal ileal involvement. Advanced liver disease predisposes to deficiency, due to decreased vitamin stores. HIV infection, though underrecognized in the elderly, may become a significant problem in the future[26].

CLINICAL FEATURES

Clinical features of B_{12} deficiency vary widely. Manifestations range from nonspecific lethargy or weakness to obvious hematologic and/or neuropsychiatric features. Development of cobalamin deficiency has been described by Herbert[4] to occur in four stages. Stages 1 and 2 represent biochemical deficiency in the presence of normal serum vitamin B_{12} levels, while stages 3 and 4 represent a more definite deficiency with metabolic and/or clinical features. The correlation of clinical features with blood B_{12} levels is poor, and hematologic and neurologic findings may occur concurrently, in sequence, or independently of each other (Table 2).

The typical laboratory abnormality is a macrocytic anemia with or without thrombocytopenia and leukopenia. Hypersegmentation of neutrophils may be evident on a blood smear. Ineffective erythropoiesis in the

Table 2 Features of cobalamin deficiency

	Manifestations
Neurologic	
cerebral	dementia, depression, psychosis, cerebrovascular disease
spinal cord	subacute combined degeneration, gait abnormalities
peripheral nerve	sensory and motor neuropathy, mononeuropathy
autonomic	urinary and fecal incontinence, impotence
Hematologic	anemia, leukopenia, thrombocytopenia, hypersegmented neutrophils, macro-ovalocytosis
Bone marrow	hypercellular marrow, nuclear–cytoplasmic asynchrony, increased myeloid/erythroid ratio
Biochemical	low serum B$_{12}$ levels, elevated serum MMA, normal or elevated serum homocysteine, normal or elevated serum bilirubin and/or LDH
Miscellaneous	anorexia, lassitude, apathy, diarrhea, glossitis

MMA, methylmalonic acid; LDH, lactate dehydrogenase

marrow with intramedullary destruction of red blood cells results in elevated lactate dehydrogenase and bilirubin levels. Neurologic abnormalities differ widely, based on varying involvement of the peripheral nerves, spinal cord and/or cerebrum. The classic manifestation is subacute combined degeneration of the spinal cord resulting in ataxia, loss of vibration and position senses, weakness, brisk tendon reflexes, extensor plantars and incontinence. Romberg's sign may be present. Symptoms from neuropathy are more pronounced in the lower rather than the upper extremities. Cerebral involvement results in neuropsychiatric disturbances ranging from irritability and apathy to delirium, psychosis and dementia. As symptoms and signs from deficiency may be amenable to timely therapy, prompt evaluation is warranted. Long-standing neurologic disease may or may not respond to treatment. The effect of deficiency on the rapidly proliferating gastrointestinal epithelium may manifest as anorexia, oral ulcers, weight loss, diarrhea and malabsorption.

ASSOCIATIONS

Cobalamin deficiency has been associated with Alzheimer's disease and other dementias[7,15]. A strong association has also been observed between elevated homocysteine

and the risk of dementia including Alzheimer's disease[27]. Low B$_{12}$ levels have been noted in the serum and cerebrospinal fluid of patients with Alzheimer's disease, with improved cognitive function following B$_{12}$ therapy. Multiple sclerosis is another neurologic disorder associated with B$_{12}$ deficiency[28]. In these conditions, the precise relationship between deficiency and disease has not been elucidated. Since B$_{12}$ is essential for DNA synthesis, concern has been raised about genomic stability and mutations in those with deficiency[29]. An increased frequency of breast cancer has also been suggested with the deficiency state[30].

LABORATORY DIAGNOSIS

As measurement of serum vitamin B$_{12}$ level is essential for the diagnosis, it should be the initial test. However, the serum B$_{12}$ assay does not accurately depict tissue cobalamin status, particularly when the serum values fall in the borderline to low-normal range[31]. Levels below 100 pg/ml clearly suggest a deficiency state, while values of more than 400 pg/ml usually confirm normal status[32,33]. Levels between 100 and 400 pg/ml discriminate poorly between states of deficiency and normalcy. When serum levels fall in this borderline range, additional tests are better

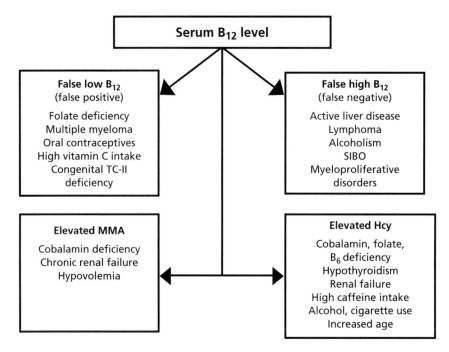

Figure 1 Laboratory diagnosis of vitamin B_{12} deficiency and possible misinterpretation
TC-II, transcobalamin-II; SIBO, small intestinal bacterial overgrowth; MMA, methylmalonic acid; Hcy, homocysteine

equipped to identify subclinical or tissue deficiency.

Serum MMA is a measure of tissue B_{12} activity and it is fairly specific[34,35]. Serum homocysteine is another sensitive indicator, but lacks the specificity of MMA[32,36]. Holo-TC-II measurements may prove to be the earliest indicator of deficiency[11], as low levels are observed even in stages I and II of deficiency. The test is not widely available at present. Elevation of both MMA and homocysteine occur in chronic renal failure, with other conditions shown in Figure 1.

The deoxyuridine suppression test (dUST) and the Schilling test are cumbersome for routine use. dUST, based on abnormal DNA metabolism in bone marrow cells, helps differentiate between cobalamin and folate deficiency, but it involves the use of radioisotope material and bone marrow aspiration[31]. The Schilling test involves measurement of urinary B_{12} after oral administration of radio-labeled vitamin. It is performed in three stages: without IF, with IF and after a course of antibiotics. Absorption improves with IF in PA, while antibiotic therapy improves absorption in SIBO. In small intestinal disease all three stages are abnormal, and in food-cobalamin malabsorption, all stages are normal[37].

SCREENING

Though not mandatory, routine screening for B_{12} deficiency appears to be reasonable considering the magnitude of the problem, the irreversibility of the consequences when left untreated and the short window of opportunity for effective treatment once diagnosed. While suggestions range from screening every individual to treating everyone, a rational approach may be to initiate screening at age 50[3,32,33,35]. Individuals with conditions that predispose them to deficiency (Table 1) may be offered screening at the first opportunity, irrespective of age. The frequency of screening and the further use of laboratory tests should be guided by results from the initial screening. Individuals with B_{12} levels in

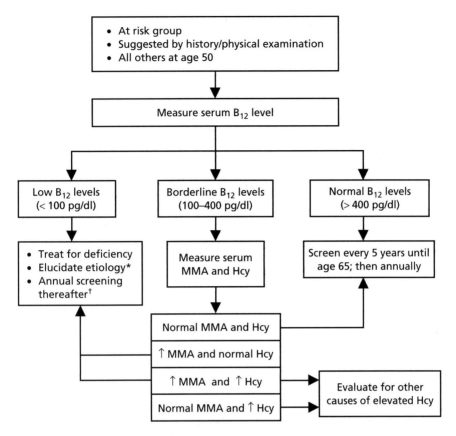

Figure 2 Screening for vitamin B$_{12}$ deficiency: a suggested approach
MMA, methylmalonic acid; Hcy, homocysteine. *Example: tests for pernicious anemia, small intestinal bacterial overgrowth, HIV disease, etc. †Not required if maintenance parenteral B$_{12}$ given by health-care provider

the normal range may be screened at 5-year intervals until age 65, and yearly thereafter. For individuals with borderline levels, additional tests may be utilized to define their cobalamin status (Figure 2).

PROPHYLAXIS AND TREATMENT

Since food-cobalamin malabsorption is widely prevalent, prophylaxis in the form of nutritional supplements may be recommended for elderly patients[1,38,39]. In view of this, the National Academy of Sciences' Institute of Medicine recommends that adults over 51 years obtain most of their recommended intake in the form of fortified foods or supplements containing B$_{12}$[14]. Commercial supplements vary in their B$_{12}$ content.

Although there are no recommendations for a precise prophylactic dose, $\geq 25\,\mu g$ daily should be adequate[40]. Prophylaxis assumes further relevance since the Food and Drug Administration (FDA) has regulated the fortification of cereals with folic acid in the USA since 1998.

When identified, deficiency is corrected with adequate replacement of cobalamin to replenish body stores. Traditionally, treatment has been via intramuscular administration of the vitamin in doses from 100 to 1000 μg/day for 3–7 days, followed by maintenance injections every 1–3 months for life (Table 3). The utility of oral cobalamin has been successfully demonstrated in several studies[40–42]. While small amounts are adequate in food-cobalamin malabsorption and

Table 3 Maintenance treatment options for cobalamin deficiency

Route	Dose	Comments
Intramuscular	100–1000 µg (every 1–3 months)	expense related to need for administration by health-care personnel suitable for any etiology of deficiency discomfort related to injection
Oral	500–2000 mg (daily)	easy to administer compliance an issue if cognitively impaired not suitable for patients with extensive intestinal resection
Sublingual	2000 µg (daily)	easy to administer insufficient long-term data compliance is an issue
Intranasal	500 µg (weekly)	easy to administer not be used with nasal mucosal disease insufficient long-term data

for vegetarians, larger amounts are required in PA. Here, oral B_{12} in amounts of 500–2000 µg/day are needed, as only minute amounts are absorbed in the absence of IF[1]. When oral maintenance therapy is provided, periodic B_{12} levels should be measured to ensure compliance. Oral preparations have varying bioavailability, are not well regulated by the FDA and are ineffective in patients with extensive intestinal resection.

Vitamin B_{12} is also available as an intranasal gel (administered weekly) and as a sublingual preparation (administered daily). Both formulations offer distinct advantages to special populations[43]. The intranasal gel is useful for administration by a caregiver to a homebound and cognitively impaired individual. However, this route is contraindicated for individuals with concomitant nasal mucosal disease.

References

1. Carmel R. Current concepts in cobalamin deficiency. *Ann Rev Med* 2000;51:357–75
2. Dharmarajan TS, Narayanan SL, Poduval RD. Life threatening vitamin B_{12} deficiency: will timely screening make a difference? *World J Gastroenterol* 2000;6:456–57
3. Carmel R. Cobalamin, the stomach and aging. *Am J Clin Nutr* 1997;66:750–9
4. Herbert V. Vitamin B_{12} – an overview. In Herbert V, ed. *Vitamin B_{12} Deficiency*. London: Royal Society of Medicine Press, 1999:1–8
5. Dharmarajan TS, Ugalino JT, Kanagala M, *et al*. Vitamin B_{12} status in hospitalized elderly from nursing homes and the community. *J Am Med Dir Assoc* 2000;1:21–4
6. Rothenberg SP. Increasing the dietary intake of folate: pros and cons. *Semin Hematol* 1999;36:65–74
7. Bottiglieri T. Folate, vitamin B_{12} and neuropsychiatric disorders. *Nutr Rev* 1996;54:382–90
8. Sarkar PK, Lambert LA. Etiology and treatment of hyper homocysteinaemia causing ischaemic stroke. *Int J Clin Pract* 2001;55:262–8
9. Smith RL. Evaluation of vitamin B_{12} and folate status in the nursing home. *J Am Med Dir Assoc* 2001;2:230–8
10. Dharmarajan TS, Koshy A, Sipalay M, Norkus EP. The need to screen: a case in point. In Herbert V, ed. *Vitamin B_{12}*

Deficiency. Round Table no. 66. London: The Royal Society of Medicine Press, 1999:9–14

11. Herbert V, Das KC. Folic acid and vitamin B$_{12}$. In Shils ME, Olson JA, Shike M, eds. *Modern Nutrition in Health and Disease*, 8th edn. Philadelphia: Lea & Febiger, 1994:402–25

12. Fairbanks VF, Klee GG. Biochemical aspect of hematology. In Burtis CA, Ashwood ER, eds. *Tietz Textbook of Clinical Chemistry*, 3rd edn. Philadelphia: WB Saunders, 1999:1642–710

13. Herbert V. Vitamin B-12: plant sources, requirements and assay. *Am J Clin Nutr* 1988;48:852–8

14. Christina HO, Kauwell GPA, Bailey LB. Practitioners' guide to meeting the vitamin B$_{12}$ recommended dietary allowance for people aged 51 years and older. *J Am Dietetic Assoc* 1999;99:725–7

15. Wang HX, Wahlin A, Basun H, *et al.* Vitamin B$_{12}$ and folate in relation to the development of Alzheimer's disease. *Neurology* 2001;56:1188–94

16. Andres E, Goichot B, Schlienger JL. Food cobalamin malabsorption: a usual cause of vitamin B$_{12}$ deficiency. *Arch Intern Med* 2000;160:2061

17. Carmel R, Aurangzeb I, Qian D. Associations of food cobalamin malabsorption with ethnic origin, age, *Helicobacter pylori* infection and serum markers of gastritis. *Am J Gastroenterol* 2001;96:63–70

18. Pitchumoni S, Dharmarajan TS. Vitamin B$_{12}$, the gastrointestinal system and aging. *Pract Gastroenterol* 2001;25:27–40

19. Kaptan K, Beyan C, Ural AU, *et al. Helicobacter pylori* – is it a novel causative agent in vitamin B$_{12}$ deficiency? *Arch Intern Med* 2000;60:1349–53

20. Lewis SJ, Potts LF, Malhotra R, Mountford R. Small bowel bacterial overgrowth in subjects living in residential care homes. *Age Aging* 1999;28:181–5

21. Flippo TS, Holder WD Jr. Neurologic degeneration associated with nitrous oxide anesthesia in patients with vitamin B$_{12}$ deficiency. *Arch Surg* 1993;128:1391–5

22. Richter JE. Should patients receiving long term gastric acid inhibition therapy be evaluated for vitamin B$_{12}$ deficiency? *Cleve Clin J Med* 2000;67:785, 787

23. Kapadia C. Cobalamin (vitamin B$_{12}$) deficiency: is it a problem for our aging population and is the problem compounded by drugs that inhibit gastric acid secretion? *J Clin Gastroenterol* 2000; 30:4–6

24. Gardyn J, Mittelman M, Zlotnik J, *et al.* Oral contraceptives can cause falsely low vitamin B$_{12}$ levels. *Acta Haematol* 2000; 104:22–4

25. Carmel R, Howard JM, Green R, *et al.* Hormone replacement therapy and cobalamin status in elderly women. *Am J Clin Nutr* 1996;64:856–9

26. Paltiel O, Falutz H, Veilleux M, *et al.* Clinical correlates of subnormal vitamin B$_{12}$ levels in patients infected with the human immunodeficiency virus. *Am J Hematol* 1995;49:318–22

27. Seshadri S, Beiser A, Selhub J, *et al.* Plasma homocysteine as a risk factor for dementia and Alzheimer's disease. *N Engl J Med* 2002;346:476–83

28. Wynn M, Wynn A. The danger of B$_{12}$ deficiency in the elderly. *Nutr Health* 1998;12: 215–26

29. Fenech M. The role of folic acid and vitamin B$_{12}$ in genomic stability of human cells. *Mutat Res* 2001;475:57–67

30. Choi SW. Vitamin B$_{12}$ deficiency: a new risk factor for breast cancer? *Nutr Rev* 1999;57: 250–3

31. Zittoun J, Zittoun R. Modern clinical testing strategies in cobalamin and folate deficiency. *Semin Hematol* 1999;36: 35–46

32. Snow CF. Laboratory diagnosis of vitamin B$_{12}$ and folate deficiency. *Arch Intern Med* 1999;159:1289–98

33. Dharmarajan MD, Norkus EP. Approaches to vitamin B$_{12}$ deficiency. Early treatment may prevent devastating complications. *Post Grad Med* 2001;110:99–105

34. Elin RJ, Winter WE. Methylmalonic acid. A test whose time has come? *Arch Pathol Lab Med* 2001;125:824–7

35. Stabler SP. Screening of older population for cobalamin (vitamin B$_{12}$) deficiency. *J Am Geriatr Soc* 1995;43:1290–7

36. Wickramasinghe SN. The wide spectrum and unresolved issues of megaloblastic anemia. *Semin Hematol* 1999;36:3–18

37. Babior BM, Bunn FH. Megaloblastic anemias. In Fauci AS, Braunwald E, Isselbacher KJ, *et al.*, eds. *Harrison's Principles of Internal Medicine*. New York: McGraw Hill, 1998:653–9

38. De Jong N, Marijke JM, Paw CA, *et al.* Nutrient dense foods and exercise in frail elderly: effects on B vitamins, homocysteine, methylmalonic acid and neuropsychological functioning. *Am J Clin Nutr* 2001;73:338–46

39. Tice JA, Ross E, Coxson PG, *et al.* Cost effectiveness of vitamin therapy to lower plasma homocysteine levels for the prevention of coronary heart disease. Effect of grain fortification and beyond. *J Am Med Assoc* 2001;286:936–43

40. Seal EC, Metz J, Flicker L, Melny J. A randomized, double-blind, placebo-controlled study of oral vitamin B_{12} supplementation in older patients with subnormal or borderline serum vitamin B_{12} concentrations. *J Am Geriatr Soc* 2002;50: 146–51

41. Kuzminski AM, Del Giacco EJ, Allen RH, *et al.* Effective treatment of cobalamin deficiency with oral cobalamin. *Blood* 1998;92:1191–8

42. O'Dowd P. B_{12} supplementation: must be parenteral. *Med Health Rhode Island* 2000;83:252–3

43. Slot WB, Merkus FWHM, Van Deventer SJH, Tytgat GNJ. Normalization of plasma vitamin B_{12} concentration by intranasal hydroxycobalamin in vitamin B_{12} deficient patients. *Gastroenterology* 1997;113:430–3

56 Cutaneous infections in older adults

Jeffrey M. Weinberg, MD, Noah S. Scheinfeld, MD, and Robert A. Norman, DO, MPH

The treatment of bacterial skin and skin structure infections in the elderly is an issue of growing importance. There has been an alarming increase in the incidence of Gram-positive infections, including resistant bacteria such as methicillin-resistant *Staphylococcus aureus* (MRSA) and drug-resistant pneumococci. While vancomycin has been considered the drug of last defense against Gram-positive multidrug-resistant bacteria, the late 1980s saw a rise in vancomycin-resistant bacteria, including vancomycin-resistant enterococci (VRE). More recently, strains of vancomycin-intermediate resistant *Staphylococcus aureus* (VISA) have been isolated[1]. Gram-positive bacteria, such as *Staphylococcus aureus* and *Streptococcus pyogenes*, are often the cause of skin and skin structure infections, ranging from mild pyodermas to complicated infections including post-surgical wound infections, severe carbunculosis and erysipelas. With treatment options limited, it has become critical to identify antibiotics with novel mechanisms of activity. Several new drugs have emerged as possible therapeutic alternatives, including linezolid and quinupristin/dalfopristin.

HERPES ZOSTER

Herpes zoster is caused by reactivation in adults of the varicella-zoster virus (VZV) that causes chicken pox in children. It is primarily a disease of older adults. After acute varicella infection, VZV becomes latent in the dorsal root ganglia. An unknown triggering mechanism, possibly caused by declining or impaired cell-mediated immunity, results in a reactivation of VZV. Infection involves the ganglia and satellite cells of the affected region. In immunocompetent persons, herpes zoster is usually confined to a single dermatome. Cutaneous or visceral dissemination of herpes zoster in immunocompetent individuals is rare.

Herpes zoster is also associated with a characteristic pain syndrome. The infected, inflamed and damaged nerve is the source of the acute and chronic pain of herpes zoster. Pain associated with zoster can be divided into the following three types[2]. Prodromal pain is a sharp stabbing pain that occurs before the onset of rash. Depending on the affected dermatome, prodromal pain may be misdiagnosed as myocardial infarction, appendicitis, cholecystitis or renal colic. Acute pain is often classified as lasting throughout the course of the vesicular eruption. Chronic pain, also known as post-herpes zoster pain or postherpetic neuralgia (PHN), can last from months to years after the disappearance of the herpes zoster lesion. PHN will be described in detail as a complication of herpes zoster later in this chapter.

Antiviral therapy

Antiviral therapy is aimed at decreasing viral replication, thereby lessening nerve damage or inflammation, and reducing the duration and severity of long-term pain syndromes. The benefits of antiviral therapy in reducing the extent and duration of pain have been seen primarily in patients older than 50 years of age, reflecting the age-related association of long-term pain[2].

Regardless of age, early antiviral therapy should be considered for any patient who has prodromal pain and early moderate or severe pain, and should be instituted in patients with known or suspected states of immune system compromise. To be effective, antiviral therapy must be instituted early, usually within 72 h of the onset of the rash. Antiviral therapy may be of benefit after 72 h in patients who are at high risk of PHN, in whom there is evidence of viral replication. After 72 h, antiviral therapy should be strongly encouraged for any immunocompromised patient who still has vesicles or an increasing number of vesicles[2].

For many years, acyclovir was the gold standard of antiviral therapy for the treatment of patients with herpes zoster. Therapy with acyclovir should be instituted within 72 h of onset of the rash at 800 mg five times a day for 7 days. In herpes zoster patients with HIV infection, therapy should be continued until new lesions stop forming, and those that have formed crust over. Failure to maintain an adequate antiviral regimen in this population may lead to a clinical entity known as verrucous zoster. These wart-like lesions continue to display ongoing viral replication and are very difficult to treat once they have been allowed to develop[2]. VZV is less acyclovir-sensitive than herpes simplex virus (HSV), and therefore higher doses are needed to reach the IC_{90} for patients with VZV. It is particularly important that elderly patients receive the full herpes zoster dose of acyclovir, because they are at the highest risk of chronic pain. Although the proper dose of acyclovir for the treatment of patients with VZV is four times greater than the dose for the treatment of patients with HSV, serum levels are only double.

Acyclovir remains one of the safest antimicrobial agents. It is preferentially taken up by infected cells and requires activation by viral enzymes to be active. Once phosphorylated into its active moiety, acyclovir has 100 times the affinity for viral DNA polymerase than for cellular DNA polymerases. Maintenance of adequate hydration is needed because the drug is excreted via the kidneys[2]. Analysis of pooled data from various placebo-controlled trials shows the significant impact of acyclovir on the severity, duration and relative risk of long-term pain[3].

Famciclovir is the oral form of the antiviral agent penciclovir. It is rapidly absorbed and efficiently converted in virally infected cells through phosphorylation to its active metabolite, penciclovir-triphosphate. Penciclovir-triphosphate competitively inhibits viral DNA polymerase, thereby halting DNA synthesis and viral replication[4].

Valacyclovir is the L-valine ester of acyclovir. It is converted *in vivo* to acyclovir and the naturally occurring amino acid valine. Valacyclovir provides three to five times the oral bioavailability of acyclovir compared with the unesterased compound. This results in acyclovir exposures similar to those seen with intravenous acyclovir[2].

Analgesics for herpes zoster

Concomitant use of pain medications is required for optimal management of patients at risk for PHN. Prompt analgesic control of pain may shorten the duration of the zoster-associated pain. The pain in herpes zoster stems from damage to the nerve and not to the epidermis. A theoretically attractive approach that would prevent long-term pain would be to maximize pain relief initially, controlling pain with opioid sedation, particularly in elderly patients. Once the pain has been brought under control, trials of stepped-down pain control can be instituted[2].

The burning and itching commonly felt as a result of the herpes zoster rash itself responds to some extent to proper skin care, which includes topical lotions such as colloidal oatmeal and topical soaks.

Postherpetic neuralgia

Spontaneous pain, pain provoked by trivial stimuli and altered sensation accompany herpes zoster, and may continue long after its characteristic rash has healed, a condition known as PHN[5]. It may develop after a pain-free interval.

Nearly all patients have pain in association with acute herpes zoster, and 10–70% have PHN[6–9]. The severity and duration of pain are age-related, but it is not related to the degree of immunocompetence[3]. The risk of PHN and the intractability of pain increases with age. Few children have PHN, whereas 27, 47 and 73% of untreated adults over 55, 60 and 70 years of age, respectively, develop PHN[7,10,11]. The duration of chronic pain is greatest in patients with prodromal pain, in those older than 60 years and in those with severe or very severe pain during the first 3 days of the rash[2]. The risk of PHN is increased in patients with ophthalmic zoster and may be higher in women than in men[6,7,12–14]. The incidence among HIV-positive patients is difficult to determine, because such patients have high rates of recurrent and chronic zoster[5].

Treatment of established postherpetic neuralgia

The pain associated with acute zoster and PHN is neuropathic and results from injury of the peripheral nerves and altered central nervous system processing. The excessive peripheral activity is thought to lead to hyperexcitability of the dorsal horn, resulting in exaggerated central nervous responses to all input. These changes require a combined therapeutic approach. It is important to introduce and modify interventions sequentially and to discard those that are ineffective or poorly tolerated. Elderly patients are at greatest risk of drug interactions, and the quality of life must be considered in designing a treatment plan for an older patient.

As initial therapy, topical lidocaine–prilocaine cream or 5% lidocaine gel may be utilized[5]. The efficacy of this treatment can be determined in a day or two. A double-blind, controlled trial of topical lidocaine demonstrated a clear short-term benefit[15]. Aspirin and other mild analgesic drugs are commonly used in patients with PHN, but their value is limited; ibuprofen is ineffective[16]. Topical formulations of aspirin with ether, indomethacin with ether, lidocaine, and lidocaine with prilocaine have all been reported to be useful in uncontrolled trials[17–20]. Intravenous/local injections of anesthetic drugs such as lidocaine, procaine and mepivacaine are reported to offer transient benefit[21–24]. Topical capsaicin is not recommended, even though it is the only drug approved by the Food and Drug Administration (FDA) for the treatment of PHN, because the burning elicited during its application is intolerable for up to one-third of patients, and it makes blinded studies impossible[5].

As the second step, a trial of non-narcotic analgesic drugs may be indicated, but is usually ineffective. Narcotics, depending upon the risks of sedation and dependence, may be tried, but if relief is incomplete, they should be withdrawn.

The third and the most important step involves the addition of a tricyclic antidepressant drug. Because of their ability to block the reuptake of norepinephrine and serotonin, these drugs may relieve pain by increasing the inhibition of spinal neurons involved in pain perception.

Adverse reactions to tricyclics include confusion, urinary retention, postural hypotension and arrhythmias, which limit their usefulness in older patients. Patients should be advised that there may be a delay of several weeks in achieving their maximal benefit and the appearance of side-effects from the tricyclics is seen much sooner than their benefit is seen[5]. If only partial relief is achieved with tricyclics, an anticonvulsant drug can be added. Anticonvulsant drugs can reduce the lancinating component of neuropathic pain[25]. Phenytoin or valproate sodium have been reported to reduce shooting pain[26]. Carbamazepine has been shown to reduce lancinating pain, but is ineffective for continuous pain[27].

Non-pharmacologic, non-invasive and non-traditional therapies, such as transcutaneous electrical nerve stimulation, ethyl chloride spray, 'counterirritation', hypnosis, biofeedback and other cognitive and behavioral techniques, complement the traditional medical treatment of PHN and may provide partial to complete relief of pain[5].

Prevention of postherpetic neuralgia

Five controlled trials have evaluated the use of corticosteroids to reduce the inflammatory features of zoster and prevent the injury that follows (Table 1)[11,28–31]. In these studies, the benefit of corticosteroids for PHN appeared variable.

Although nerve blocks are effective for the immediate, short-term relief of acute zoster pain[32], well-designed, controlled trials of their efficacy in preventing PHN neuralgia have not been performed.

Combination therapy

Combination therapy with a corticosteroid and an antiviral drug in patients with zoster has been evaluated in two trials. In both trials there was a definite benefit in reducing acute pain in patients receiving prednisolone plus acyclovir versus those receiving acyclovir alone or placebo. However, there was no difference in PHN at 6 months among the three groups[31,33].

Other therapies

Antagonists to N-methyl-D-aspartate receptors may lessen neuropathic pain by altering abnormal central nervous system processing. The available antagonists of these receptors, such as ketamine and dextromethorphan, reduce neuropathic pain but have many adverse effects[34].

The best way to prevent PHN may be to prevent zoster itself. The live Oka-strain vaccine prevents varicella. As humoral and cellular responses to VZV wane with age, vaccination may reinvigorate these responses. Immunization of both adults who are immune to VZV and those who are not immune has yielded promising increases in humoral and cytotoxic cellular immune responses, as compared with age-related baseline levels[5,35,36].

Cutaneous reactions following herpes zoster infections

Many cutaneous reactions are known to develop within resolved varicella-zoster lesions. These include granuloma annulare, sarcoidal granulomas, tuberculoid granulomas, lymphoma, pseudolymphoma, granulomatous vasculitis and Kaposi's sarcoma[37]. The interval between the varicella-zoster infecton and any of the above is relatively short (average 6 months; range 2 weeks to 4 years)[37].

ONYCHOMYCOSIS

Onychomycosis is found frequently in older adults, and in more males than females[38]. Onychomycosis, or tinea unguium, is caused by dermatophytes in the majority of cases, but can also be caused by *Candida* and non-dermatophyte molds[39]. There are four

Table 1 Placebo-controlled trials of oral corticosteroids for the prevention of postherpetic neuralgia. From reference 5

| Trial | Corticosteroid treatment | Comparative treatment | No. of patients | Average age or range (years) | Duration of rash at entry | Definition of pain | Efficacy | | Effect on PHN at last visit |
							Reduced early pain	Reduced pain at 1 month	
Eaglstein et al.[28]	triamcinolone 16 mg three times a day tapered over a period of 21 days	placebo	35	21–91	'early'	persisting > 2 months	yes	yes (in patients > 60 years)	yes at 3 years
Keczkes and Basheer[29]	prednisone 40 mg/day tapered over a period of 28 days	carbamazepine	40	67	2–8 days	persisting > 2 months	—	yes	yes at 1 year
Clemmensen and Andersen[11]	prednisone 40 mg/day tapered over a period of 21 days	corticotropin or placebo	60	56	< 7 days	persisting > 6 weeks	yes	no	no at 4 months
Esmann et al.[30]	prednisolone 40 mg/day tapered over a period of 21 days	placebo	78	72	< 96 h	zoster-associated	yes	no	no at 26 weeks
Whitley et al.[31]	prednisone 60 mg/day tapered over a period of 21 days	acyclovir or placebo	208	62	< 72 h	zoster-associated	yes	yes	no at 6 months

PHN, postherpetic neuralgia

types of onychomycosis: distal subungual onychomycosis, proximal subungual onychomycosis, white superficial onychomycosis and candidal onychomycosis. Distal subungual onychomycosis is the most common type of onychomycosis. A whitish-brown discoloration begins at the free edge or the lateral nail fold, invades the distal nail bed and travels proximally. Subungual hyperkeratosis may lead to separation of the nail plate from the nail bed, thus providing a conducive environment for secondary bacterial infections. Proximal subungual onychomycosis, the least common variant, presents as a whitish-brown area on the proximal part of the nail plate that eventually enlarges to affect the entire nail. White superficial onychomycosis, an infection in which the toenails, not the fingernails, are affected, produces a friable, sharply delineated, white nail. Candidal onychomycosis, seen in patients with chronic mucocutaneous candidiasis, affects both fingernails and toenails. The nail bed and nail plate both thicken. The surface of the nail turns a brownish-yellow and becomes furrowed. Paronychia often develops concurrently.

Before initiation of therapy, it is important to document the presence of fungi utilizing one or more diagnostic techniques, including KOH preparation, fungal culture and nail plate biopsy with periodic acid–Schiff stain. Proper diagnosis is necessary because other disorders can mimic onychomycosis, including psoriasis, irritant dermatitis and trauma.

Laboratory monitoring, including liver function tests, should be performed at baseline and at variable intervals (at 4 and 8 weeks for itraconazole, at 6 weeks for terbinafine, for 3-month courses) on patients taking either medication for over 1 month[39]. Recently, ciclopirox lacquer, a topical agent, has been approved for the treatment of onychomycosis. This agent may be useful in patients who are not candidates for the other therapies, but it has significantly lower efficacy than the oral medications[39].

ADVANCES IN ANTIBACTERIAL THERAPY

Linezolid (Zyvox)

This is an oxazolidinone antibiotic, shown to be effective for nosocomial and community-acquired pneumonias, vancomycin-resistant *Enterococcus faecium* (VREF) infections and skin infections due to certain staphylococcus or streptococcus species[40]. The oxazolidinones are a novel class of antibiotics first discovered in 1987[41]. They are the first new antibiotics to have been discovered in the past 35 years.

Currently linezolid is FDA approved for the treatment of various Gram-positive infections, including both nosocomial and community-acquired pneumonias, complicated and uncomplicated skin and skin structure infections and vancomycin-resistant *Enterococcus* infections.

The recommended dosage of linezolid depends on the severity of the skin or soft tissue infection. The recommended dosage for uncomplicated infections is 400 mg every 12 h for 10–14 days. For complicated infections, 600 mg twice daily either via intravenous infusion or orally is recommended. Because the absolute bioavailability after oral dosing is nearly 100%, no dosage changes are needed when switching from intravenous to oral therapy[42].

Quinupristin/dalfopristin (Synercid, 30 : 70 ratio)

This is a combination of two semisynthetic pristinamycin derivatives and is the first parenteral streptogramin antibacterial agent. Both quinupristin and dalfopristin have antibacterial capability individually, but demonstrate synergistic activity when used in combination. Much of the clinical experience with this antibiotic is derived from five comparative trials and an FDA-sanctioned emergency-use program for patients without alternative therapies.

FDA indications for quinupristin/dalfopristin are serious infections associated with VREF bacteremia and complicated skin and skin structure infections caused by methicillin-sensitive *Staphylococcus aureus* or *Streptococcus pyogenes*. VREF infections are difficult to treat and few therapeutic options are currently available. These pathogens are resistant to most β-lactam and aminoglycoside antibiotics. For complicated skin or skin structure infections, the recommended dose is 7.5 mg/kg intavenously twice daily for at least 7 days. The drug can be administered up to three times daily for bacteremic patients. Dose adjustment to 5 mg/kg is recommended for patients with hepatic insufficiency. No dose adjustment is needed for older or renally impaired patients.

CONCLUSION

The diagnosis and management of diseases of the skin are significant issues in the elderly population. With advances in these areas, we have new tools to combat these diseases and limit morbidity. It is important for clinicians to aggressively monitor and treat these diseases in the elderly, because of the potential for immunosuppression in this population. Further advances in therapy and the potential for the development of vaccines will aid in the therapy of these diseases.

References

1. Centers for Disease Control. Reduced susceptibility of *Staphylococcus aureus* to Vancomycin-Japan 1996. *Morbid Mortal Weekly Rep* 1997;46:624–6
2. Beutner KR. Clinical management of herpes zoster in the elderly patient. *Compr Ther* 1996;22:183–6
3. Soong SJ, Whitley R. A comprehensive analysis of the effect of acyclovir versus placebo on herpes zoster pain. Presented at the *35th Interscience Conference on Antimicrobial Agents and Chemotherapy*, San Francisco, CA, 17–20 September 1995
4. Tyring SK. Efficacy of famciclovir in the treatment of herpes zoster. *Semin Dermatol* 1996;15:27–31
5. Kost RG, Straus SE. Postherpetic neuralgia – pathogenesis, treatment, and prevention. *N Engl J Med* 1996;335:32–42
6. Ragozzino MW, Mellon LJ, Kurland LT, *et al.* Population-based study of herpes zoster and its sequelae. *Medicine (Baltimore)* 1982;61: 310–16
7. De Moragas JM, Kierland RR. The outcome of patients with herpes zoster. *Arch Dermatol* 1957;75:193–6
8. Epstein E. Treatment of zoster and post-zoster neuralgia by the intralesional infection of triamcinolone: a computer analysis of 199 cases. *Int J Dermatol* 1976;15: 762–9
9. Balfour HH. Varicella zoster virus infections in immunocompromised hosts: a review of the natural history and management. *Am J Med* 1998;85:68–73
10. Rogers RS, Tindall JP. Geriatric herpes zoster. *J Am Geriatr Soc* 1971;19:495–504
11. Clemmensen OJ, Andersen KE. ACTH versus prednisone and placebo in herpes zoster treatment. *Clin Exp Dermatol* 1984; 9:557–63
12. Hope-Simpson RE. Postherpetic neuralgia. *JR Coll Gen Pract* 1975;25:571–5
13. Cobo LM, Foulks GN, Liesegang T, *et al.* Oral acyclovir in the treatment of acute herpes zoster ophthalmicus. *Ophthalmology* 1986;93:763–70
14. Harding SP, Lipton JR, Wells JC. Natural history of herpes zoster ophthalmicus: predictors of postherpetic neuralgia and ocular involvement. *Br J Ophthalmol* 1987;71: 353–8
15. Rowbotham MC, Davies PS, Fields HL. Topical lidocaine gel relieves post herpetic neuralgia. *Ann Neurol* 1995;37: 246–53
16. Max MB, Schafer SC, Culnane M, *et al.* Association of pain relief with drug side effects in post herpetic neuralgia: a single-dose study of clonidine, codeine, ibuprofen, and placebo. *Clin Pharmacol Ther* 1988;43:363–71

17. Rowbotham MC, Fields HL. Topical lidocaine reduces pain in postherpetic neuralgia. Pain 1989;38:297–301

18. De Benedittis G, Besana F, Lorenzetti A. A new topical treatment for acute herpetic neuralgia and post-herpetic neuralgia: the aspirin/diethyl ether mixture. An open-label study plus a double blind controlled clinical trial. Pain 1992;48: 383–90

19. Milligan KA, Atkinson RE, Schofield PA. Lignocaine–prilocaine cream in post herpetic neuralgia. Br Med J 1989; 298:253

20. Slow PJ, Glynn CJ, Minor B. EMLA cream in the treatment of post-herpetic neuralgia: efficacy and pharmacokinetic profile. Pain 1989;39:301–5

21. Watson CP, Evans RJ, Watt VR, et al. Post-herpetic neuralgia: 208 cases. Pain 1988; 35:289–97

22. Dan K, Higa K, Noda B. Nerve-block for herpetic pain. In Fields HL, Dubner R, Cervero F, eds. Proceedings of the Fourth World Congress on Pain, Seattle, vol 9 of Advances in Pain Research and Therapy. New York: Raven Press,1985:831–8

23. Colding A. The effect of regional sympathetic blocks in the treatment of herpes zoster: a survey of 300 cases. Acta Anaesth Scand 1969;13:133–41

24. Fine PG. Nerve blocks, herpes zoster and postherpetic neuralgia. In Watson CPN, ed. Herpes Zoster and Postherpetic Neuralgia. Pain Research and Clinical Management, vol 8. Amsterdam: Elsevier Science, 1993:173–83

25. Swerdlow M. Anticonvulsant drugs and chronic pain. Clin Neuropharmacol 1984; 7:51–82

26. Swerdlow M. The treatment of 'shooting' pain. Postgrad Med J 1980;56:159–61

27. Killian JM, Fromm GH. Carbamazepine in the treatment of neuralgia: use of side effect. Arch Neurol 1968;9:129–36

28. Eaglstein WH, Katz R, Brown JA. The effects of early corticosteroid therapy on the skin eruption and pain of herpes zoster. J Am Med Assoc 1970;211:1681–3

29. Keczkes K, Basheer AM. Do corticosteroids prevent post-herpetic neuralgia? Br J Dermatol 1980;102:551–5

30. Esmann V, Geil JP, Kroon S, et al. Prednisolone does not prevent post-herpetic neuralgia. Lancet 1987;2:126–9

31. Whitley RJ, Weiss H, Gnann J, et al. The efficacy of steroid and acyclovir therapy of herpes zoster in the elderly. J Invest Med 1995;43(Suppl 2):252A (abstr)

32. Portenoy RK, Duma C, Foley KM. Acute herpetic and post-herpetic neuralgia: clinical review and current management. Ann Neurol 1986;20:651–64

33. Wood MJ, Johnson RW, McKendrick MW, et al. A randomized trial of acyclovir for 7 days or 21 days with and without prednisolone for treatment of acute herpes zoster. N Engl J Med 1994;330: 896–900

34. Eide PK, Jorum E, Stubhaug A, et al. Relief of post herpetic neuralgia with the N-methyl-D-aspartic acid receptor antagonist ketamine: a double-blind, cross over comparison with morphine and placebo. Pain 1994;58:347–54

35. Levin MJ, Murray M, Rotbart HA. Immune response of elderly individuals to a live attenuated varicella vaccine. J Infect Dis 1992;166:253–9

36. Hayward A, Villanueba E, Cosyns M, et al. Varicella-zoster virus (VZV)-specific cytotoxicity after immunization of non-immune adults with Oka Strain attenuated VZV vaccine. J Infect Dis 1992;166: 260–4

37. Gibney MD, Nahass GT, Leonardi CL. Cutaneous reactions following herpes zoster infections: report of three cases and a review of the literature. Br J Dermatol 1996;134:504–9

38. Gupta AK. Onychomycosis in the elderly. Drugs Aging 2000;16:397–407

39. Weinberg JM. Fungal diseases of the skin. In Demiss DJ, ed. Conn's Current Therapy 2002, 54th edn. Philadelphia: WB Saunders, 2002:827–9

40. Zyvox [package insert]. Kalamazoo, MI; Pharmacia & Upjohn, 2000

41. Slee AM, Wuonola MA, McRipley RJ, *et al.* Oxazolidinones, a new class of synthetic antibacterial agents: *in vitro* and *in vivo* activities of DuP 105 and DuP 721. *Antimicrob Agents Chemother* 1987;31: 1791–7

42. Swaney SM, Aoki H, Ganoza MC, *et al.* The oxazolidinone linezolid inhibits initiation of protein synthesis in bacteria. *Antimicrob Agents Chemother* 1998;42:3251–5

57 Hormone replacement therapy

T.S. Dharmarajan, MD, FACP, AGSF, and Seema Sami Rizvi, MD

INTRODUCTION

Despite numerous studies, systematic reviews and meta-analyses, definitive clinical practice guidelines for hormone replacement therapy (HRT) continue to be unavailable. HRT is a complex subject with areas of uncertainties and inconsistent information. Data from completed trials and ongoing studies continually appear, with new information influencing decisions on hormone therapy. The decision to begin HRT is individualized based on risks and benefits – often a difficult choice for both patient and health-care provider. For definitive answers, many women seek the advice of a primary care provider; questions often follow regarding indications for HRT, duration of therapy, risks, benefits and side-effects. In this chapter, the term HRT is used for both estrogen and progesterone therapy, while estrogen replacement therapy (ERT) is used for estrogen alone.

MENOPAUSE

Currently, one application where HRT appears to be approved is for manifestations of menopause[1]. Menopause is defined as permanent cessation of menstruation due to loss of ovarian function. The mean age of natural menopause is 51 years (range 45–55) for women in the USA; smokers attain menopause about 1.5 years earlier compared to non-smokers[2]. In the USA, women spend

Table 1 Signs and symptoms of menopause

Menstrual
Irregular menses
Hot flushes
Dyspareunia
Pruritus
Vaginal dryness

Psychological
Anxiety
Insomnia
Mood swings
Depression

about a third of their life in the post-menopausal period.

In women of reproductive age, the primary source of estrogen is the ovary; the predominant form of estrogen is estradiol. At menopause, there is a progressive loss of ovarian oocytes, resulting in a decline in the secretion of estradiol, with estrone becoming the predominant estrogen. The gradual decline of estrogen and progesterone reduces the negative feed-back inhibition of the hypothalamic–pituitary axis and causes an increase in follicle stimulating hormone (FSH) and luteinizing hormone (LH)[3]. The signs and symptoms of menopause are listed in Table 1.

There are two estrogen receptors, alpha (α) and beta (β). Each person has heterogeneity of receptor type specific to the individual, explaining the differing response of women

Table 2 Hormone replacement therapy: risks versus benefits

Benefits
Menopausal symptoms
Osteoporosis

Uncertain benefit
Colorectal cancer
Cognitive function

Risks
Endometrial cancer
Breast cancer
Cardiovascular disease
Venous thromboembolism
Gall bladder disease

to estrogen deprivation and replacement. α-Receptors are present in the breast and endometrium. β-Receptors are present in the bone, brain and vascular tissues.

HORMONE REPLACEMENT THERAPY

Risks and benefits

The risks and benefits of HRT are not fully defined and remain controversial. On the application of HRT, several trials have been completed and many are still underway, with some results likely to be available in only a few years. While every woman may consider HRT, not every one is a candidate. All guidelines recommend risk–benefit assessment and individualization of therapy. Prior to initiating HRT, a woman should undergo gynecologic and breast examinations, a PAP smear and a mammogram. A broad perspective on risks and benefits is outlined in Table 2.

Menopausal symptoms

As women undergo menopause due to estrogen deficiency, they develop genitourinary atrophy, leading to sexual and urinary dysfunction including vaginal dryness, dyspareunia, frequency and urgency. There is a high

concentration of estrogen receptors in the vulva, vagina, urethra and trigone of the bladder. About 40–60% of women experience hot flushes during menopause. Hot flushes may be present for years in the perimenopausal period, or can be life-long in a minority of women. The Heart and Estrogen/Progestin Replacement Study (HERS) demonstrated that HRT has a positive or negative effect on quality of life, depending on the presence or absence of symptoms. Women with hot flushes given HRT showed improvement in depressive symptoms and mental health, while interestingly, those without flushing had greater decline in physical function and energy level. Randomized clinical trials suggest that estrogen therapy is highly effective in controlling vasomotor and genitourinary symptoms during menopause[4].

Cardiovascular prevention

The leading cause of death in American women is coronary heart disease. Observational studies in postmenopausal women provide data on the role of HRT for primary and secondary prevention of cardiovascular disease. Data from select randomized trials are provided in Table 3.

Primary prevention

Studies in the past have suggested that HRT decreases the risk of coronary artery disease (CAD) by nearly 50%[5]. This reduction is unlikely to result in substantial absolute benefit and is not enough to support its use. Recently, in the Women's Health Initiative (WHI) the estrogen plus progestin arm was abruptly discontinued (after 5.2 years) on the grounds that there was a higher absolute risk for CAD; the results indicate that estrogen plus progestin should neither be initiated nor continued for the primary prevention of CAD[6]. At present, primary prevention of CAD should not be considered an indication for initiating HRT.

Table 3 Select randomized trials of hormone replacement therapy (HRT) for cardiovascular disease

---

Heart and Estrogen/Progestin Replacement Study (HERS)
2763 women, with intact uterus and documented CAD
Women were randomly assigned to estrogen/progestin or placebo
Randomized clinical trial, secondary prevention
Mean duration: 4.1 years
Result: No benefit with HRT for secondary prevention
     Higher incidence of deep vein thrombosis and pulmonary embolism

Estrogen Replacement and Atherosclerosis Trial (ERA)
309 women with angiographically documented CAD
Secondary prevention study
Mean duration: 3.2 years
Result: No benefit with either estrogen or combined therapy for women with CAD

Nurses' Health Study
59 337 women, 2489 patients with CAD
Prospective, observational study (biennial questionnaire)
Duration: 20 years
Result: The risk of major coronary events seemed to increase among short-term hormone users, but
     decreased with long-term use

Women's Health Initiative (WHI)
27 500 women at usual risk for CAD, but without CAD, 16 608 on estrogen + progestin
Primary prevention study
Estrogen plus progestin arm terminated (2002), estrogen arm being continued
Mean duration: estrogen + progestin arm 5.2 years, entire study 8.5 years
Result: Increase in absolute excess risk for CAD; all-cause mortality not affected.
     Results of estrogen arm pending (2005?)

CAD, coronary artery disease

Secondary prevention

The HERS data do not support the use of HRT in women with pre-existing heart disease[7]. The study failed to demonstrate a net beneficial effect of estrogen on overall CAD after an average follow-up of 4.1 years[8]. In women with pre-existing heart disease, studies have shown an increased risk of recurrent CAD with HRT used for a short period of time, whereas there appeared to be a decreased risk of coronary events in those who had used HRT for longer periods. HRT when added to anti-ischemic medications did not reduce the prevalence of angina in postmenopausal women with a history of unstable angina[9]. Recently, the American Heart Association has opposed the use of HRT for secondary prevention in post-menopausal women[10].

Lipid profile and menopause

In perimenopausal women CAD is rare, although CAD is more age dependent in women then in men[11]. There is a significant change in postmenopausal lipoproteins, with an increase in low-density lipoprotein (LDL)-cholesterol, apolipoprotein B and total cholesterol. The lipid alterations result in an increase in the risk of CAD. Modest elevations occur with triglyceride and lipoprotein(a) (Lp(a)). High-density lipoprotein (HDL) levels remain unchanged or decline only slightly after menopause.

Role of HRT

Estrogens increase the level of HDL-cholesterol and triglycerides and decrease LDL-cholesterol, Lp(a) and homocysteine

Table 4 Candidates for hormone replacement therapy in osteoporosis. Based on recommendations of the National Osteoporosis Foundation (reference 17)

Women with T score on BMD below −1.5 with the following risk factors:

(1) Family history of osteoporosis
(2) Smoking
(3) Low body weight

Women with T score on BMD below −2.0 in the absence of risk factors
Women over 70 years of age with multiple risk factors: treat even without BMD testing

BMD, bone mineral density
Note: Recommendations for treatment must be weighed against risks and use of alternatives

levels. No effect or a decrease is noted for total cholesterol. The best predictor for CAD risk in women appears to be HDL-cholesterol rather than LDL-cholesterol for secondary prevention of CAD. The 4S and CARE studies suggest that aggressive lipid-lowering therapy has a greater impact in women than in men[12,13]. Significant variability in HDL-cholesterol levels occur, perhaps influenced by genetic factors. Postmenopausal women with CAD with certain genotypes have an augmented response of HDL-cholesterol to HRT. The HERS data suggested that lowering lipids alone does not achieve greater risk reduction of CAD.

Osteoporosis

Osteoporosis may be postmenopausal, age-related or secondary to other causes. Estrogen deficiency is a primary cause of osteoporosis; estrogen replacement inhibits bone resorption, increases bone density and reduces the risk of fracture. The unresolved issue is whether estrogen causes additional gain in bone mass after the bone-remodeling transient has been closed[14]; 'transient' is the time taken for bone changes from a higher to a lower turnover state, with a gain in bone mass. The Postmenopausal Estrogen/Progestin Interventions (PEPI) study showed that after discontinuation of HRT there appeared to be no accelerated bone loss or decline in bone mineral density (BMD)[15]. A meta-analysis of randomized controlled trials suggested that

ERT significantly reduces the incidence of non-vertebral fractures, if ERT is initiated before age 60 years compared to after age 60. To prevent fractures, HRT should ideally begin within 5 years of menopause[16]. The WHI study also demonstrated a risk reduction from osteoporosis-related hip fractures after 5 years of estrogen and progestin[6]. If HRT is initiated after age 60, the benefit may be attenuated. On the other hand, if HRT is postponed until after age 60, we can reduce the overall cost and risk associated with prolonged therapy. HRT is recommended as standard therapy for both prevention and treatment of osteoporosis, with guidelines provided by the National Osteoporosis Foundation (Table 4)[17]. However, it is recommended that the risk for cardiac events, strokes and breast cancer be weighed against the benefits from reduction in fractures following treatment for osteoporosis[6].

Cancer

Breast

One of the most common reasons for patients to discontinue HRT is the fear of breast cancer. Meta-analysis studies suggest that with HRT continued for more than 5 years there is an increased (30%) risk of breast cancer[18]. The WHI data was also consistent with an absolute increase in breast cancer[6]. When compared to non-users, those on HRT have smaller breast tumors with favorable histology[19]. Prospective studies have shown that an increase in serum estradiol levels may increase the risk of breast cancer[19]. The Multiple Outcomes of Raloxifene Evaluation Trial (MORE) data revealed that in postmenopausal women estradiol level could be a sensitive assay for those at risk of breast cancer and identifies those who may benefit from selective estrogen receptor modulators (SERMs) such as raloxifene[19]. When counseling women about risks and benefits of HRT the risk of breast cancer should be discussed. Women should not be advised to stop progestin and continue estrogen just to lower the risk of breast cancer[20]. The average woman has a risk of developing breast cancer at some stage during her life time; the risk increases to 14% overall and by 30–35% after 5 years of HRT[18,21]. The data stresses the need for regular breast examinations and mammograms while on HRT.

Endometrium

Endometrial cancer has an incidence of 1 in 1000 per year in postmenopausal women[22]. Long-term use of unopposed estrogen increases the risk of endometrial cancer, while addition of progesterone to estrogen eliminates this risk. Therefore, women with an intact uterus should be given estrogen and progesterone together to prevent endometrial hyperplasia. Women who have had a hysterectomy should not have concerns regarding endometrial cancer and are not candidates for progesterone. They are to be given estrogen alone.

Colon and rectum

Analysis of epidemiological data found a reduction in colon and rectal cancers by nearly 20% in women who had ever used HRT, compared with never users, regardless of duration of HRT[23]. However, the study could not confidently demonstrate that HRT decreases the risk of colon cancer. The

WHI study demonstrated an absolute, small reduction in risk for colorectal cancer following use of estrogen and progestin for 5 years[6].

Venous thromboembolism

A meta-analysis revealed that postmenopausal estrogen replacement increases the risk of venous thromboembolism, highest in the first year of use[24,25]. The HERS trial demonstrated an increased risk for both deep vein thrombosis (DVT) and pulmonary embolism two- to four-fold in postmenopausal women with preexisting heart disease given HRT. Preliminary data from the WHI also confirms an increased risk for DVT[6].

Cognition

Long-term benefits to the brain have been attributed to estrogen, including a reduction in plaque formation in Alzheimer's disease[26]. However, the existing data do not confirm a benefit for estrogen in women with preexisting Alzheimer's disease of improved cognitive function, not did it slow the progression of disease. For primary prevention, in the area of cognition, the role of estrogen is still under study in the WHI and the Preventing Postmenopausal Memory Loss in Alzheimer's with Replacement Estrogen study.

Stroke

Observational studies suggest that HRT should not be prescribed for the secondary prevention of cerebrovascular disease[27]. Data on HRT for primary prevention of cerebrovascular disease in the WHI study suggest a higher absolute risk of strokes after 5 years of therapy[6].

Urinary incontinence

HRT is not recommended for the treatment of urinary incontinence[28]. The HERS data

Table 5 Side-effects of estrogen therapy

Withdrawal bleeding
Nausea and bloating
Headache
Elevation in blood pressure
Breast tenderness
Breakthrough bleeding in 80–90% of patients
Venous thromboembolism

Table 6 Contraindications to estrogen therapy

Absolute
Coronary artery disease
Endometrial cancer
Estrogen-responsive breast cancer
Active thromboembolic disease
Abnormal vaginal bleeding

Relative
Gallbladder disease
Chronic liver disease
Endometriosis
Prior thromboembolic disease

Table 7 Non-adherence to hormone replacement therapy (HRT). From references 6, 31–33

Use and reluctance to use HRT
HRT is commonly prescribed, but remains underused by the patient
Only 10–30% of those prescribed HRT take it on a regular basis
50% discontinue use within the first year

Causes of non-adherence
Fear of breast and endometrial cancer
Breakthrough and cyclic bleeding (most common cause)
Fear of thromboembolism
Inadequate counseling and communication by health provider
Side-effects, including weight gain
Lack of understanding of the effects of estrogen deficiency
Fear of cardiovascular disease from recent data

Table 8 North American Menopausal Society recommendations to help long-term compliance. From reference 36

Explain the risks and benefits clearly
Involve the individual in decision-making
Discuss women's preferences
Provide educational material
Schedule follow-up visits

suggested that daily oral HRT given to postmenopausal women in fact caused worsening of symptoms related to urinary incontinence. Transvaginal estrogen appears to be more effective then oral estrogen for treatment of incontinence.

SELECTIVE ESTROGEN RECEPTOR MODULATORS

Although ERT/HRT have benefits, some women may choose not to accept therapy, because of side-effects. Therefore, there is a growing interest in SERMs, which have both estrogen agonist and antagonist properties. SERMs differ from estrogens in that the latter act as estrogen agonists in all tissues. SERMS are non-steroidal compounds and do not lead to estrogen-dependent risks or side-effects. Examples of SERMs include tamoxifen, clomiphene and raloxifene. The MORE trial performed in over 7700 osteoporotic women, mean age 67 years, had a placebo group and a raloxifene group (60 mg or 120 mg/day) treated for 4 years. Those on raloxifene demonstrated a decrease in total and LDL-cholesterol levels. There was no increased risk of breast and endometrial cancer. Raloxifene suppressed bone turnover, and improved BMD. The MORE study demonstrated a 50% reduction in vertebral fractures[29]. Measurement of estradiol level by sensitive assay in postmenopausal women identifies those at high risk of breast cancer who may most benefit from the use of raloxifene[19]. Raloxifene given for 4 years significantly reduced the risk of cardiovascular events in the cohort of women with increased

Table 9 Estrogen–progesterone preparations. From references 1, 2, 6, 33 and 35

Oral estrogen preparations
Conjugated equine estrogen (Premarin®) 0.3, 0.625, 0.9, 1.25, 2.5 mg
Micronized estradiol (Estrace®) 0.5, 1.0, 2.0 mg
Estrified estrogen (Estratab®) 0.3, 0.625, 2.5 mg

Combination preparations (estrogen and progesterone)
Premphase®
  conjugated estrogen 0.625 mg and medroxyprogesterone 5 mg
Prempro®
  conjugated estrogen 0.625 mg and medroxyprogesterone 2.5 mg or 5.0 mg

Vaginal preparations
Conjugated estrogen cream (Premarin) 0.625 mg/g
Micronized estradiol (Estrace) 0.01% or 0.1 mg/g

Transdermal estradiol preparations
Climara®, Estraderm®, Alora®

Women with an intact uterus
Cyclic combined
  estrogen days 1–25
  progesterone days 16–25
Continuous combined
  estrogen + progesterone daily

Women without a uterus
Continuous estrogen daily

Note: while the above preparations are available options, recent data suggest weighing the risks, benefits and alternatives in each case. In particular, combination estrogen/progestin therapy has been associated with side-effects over time

cardiovascular risk, but did not significantly affect the overall cardiovascular risk in women[30].

HORMONE REPLACEMENT THERAPY/ESTROGEN REPLACEMENT THERAPY: SIDE-EFFECTS, CONTRAINDICATIONS, COMPLIANCE, RECOMMENDATIONS AND REGIMENS

Information is provided in easy-to-read format in Tables 5, 6, 7 and 8[31–36]. The material is intended only for general guidance. The health provider should decide in conjunction with each individual candidate what is best for that person. A discussion on risks, benefits and alternatives is indicated in each and every case. Hormone replacement may be offered in several forms, including oral, vaginal and transdermal routes. Vaginal estradiol in low doses is safe and effective for relief of localized symptoms. It is particularly preferred for urogenital symptoms related to atrophic vaginitis as compared to systemic estrogen therapy. As hepatic metabolism is bypassed with vaginal estrogen, an enhanced vaginal tissue response with fewer systemic side-effects may result. Continuous combined regimen (conjugated equine estrogens and medroxyprogesterone acetate) is the most widely prescribed HRT, and causes less regular bleeding than the cyclic form of therapy. Postmenopausal women generally dislike cyclic regimens because of resumption of menses. A list of preparations is provided in Table 9.

SUPPLEMENTARY THERAPIES

Alternative therapies are generally on the increase in women. Many herbal remedies have been promoted to help manage menopausal symptoms, but most lack scientific proof of efficacy, and are not regulated by the Food and Drug Administration. Phytoestrogens are weaker estrogens, as they bind poorly to estrogen receptors compared to estradiol. Many plants contain estrogen activity. Isoflavones are a major class of phytoestrogens; a major dietary source of isoflavone is soy. Osteoporosis-related fractures appear to be less frequent in Asian women because they ingest large quantities of phytoestrogens in their diet. There is fair evidence that soy decreases vasomotor symptoms, which explains why hot flushes are less common in Japanese women. Asians consume many times more isoflavones in the diet then people in the West[37].

HORMONE REPLACEMENT THERAPY: WHERE DO WE GO FROM HERE?

The American College of Obstetricians and Gynecologists[38], the US Preventive Services Task Force (USPSTF)[39], the American Heart Association/American College of Cardiology[40], American College of Preventive Medicine[41], and the North American Menopause Society[36,42] provide recommendations on various aspects of HRT, which may be reviewed. Most organizations do not fully address the issue of HRT, stating that more research is required. While the public is awaiting a clear direction, the early termination of one arm of the WHI study surprised many; the USPSTF is presently attempting to formulate a guidance[43]. Many women will stop or have stopped taking HRT, and the decisions may not be correct in all cases[43]. A meta-analysis of several studies of fair or good quality (from the years 1966 to 2000) was consistent with recent randomized trials in that there was no benefit in the secondary or primary prevention of cardiovascular disease; on this basis, no consideration for cardiovascular disease prevention is to be recommended while discussing HRT use with women[44].

Where do we go from here? With the lack of favorable evidence from trials we should discourage its use for the prevention and treatment of at least some diseases and its use should be for shorter rather than longer periods[45]. It is also conceivable that modified dosing or refined products in the future may have differing effects and benefits for vascular disease, cognition, osteoporosis, incontinence, overall well being and quality of life[45]. Low dose HRT may be as effective as standard dose HRT, with fewer side-effects[46]. Small studies have demonstrated benefits in depression[46]. Genetic testing may reveal a rational manner to use HRT in the future by predicting proneness to fracture, cardiovascular disease, thrombosis and breast cancer[46].

Overall, the value of HRT appears to be diminishing. While the danger to an individual woman is small, over years the results indicate more harm than good[47]. HRT is unquestionably effective for menopausal symptoms. The small benefit in reduction of osteoporosis-related fractures appears outweighed by the increase in risk of heart attacks, strokes, thrombo-embolism, and cancer. For women who stop taking estrogen for osteoporosis, alternatives such as raloxifene or bisphosphonates should be offered. The emerging trend is in the direction of questionable long-term use and a search for alternatives[47].

In summary, HRT should be customized to each and every individual. While there is no consensus, it is even more important that adequate explanations of the risks, benefits and alternatives to HRT be offered by the health care provider. In the next few years, more data should be available, including results from the WHI estrogen-only trial.

References

1. Kenny AM. Hormone replacement therapy. In Cobbs EL, Duthie EH, Murphy JB, eds. *Geriatrics Review Syllabus: a Core Curriculum in Geriatric Medicine*, 5th edn. Malden, MA: Blackwell Publishing for the American Geriatrics Society; 2002:345–50

2. Noblett KL, Ostergard DR. Gynecologic Disorders. In Hazzard WR, Blass JP, Ettinger, WH Jr, Halter JB, Ouslander JG, eds. *Principles of Geriatric Medicine and Gerontology*, 4th edn. New York: McGraw Hill, 1999:797–807

3. Belchetz PE. Hormonal treatment of postmenopausal women. *N Engl J Med* 1994; 330:1062–71

4. Hlatky MA, Boothroyd D, Vittinghoff E, *et al.* Quality-of-life and depressive symptoms in postmenopausal women after receiving hormone therapy. Results from the Heart and Estrogen/Progestin Replacement Study (HERS) trial. *J Am Med Assoc* 2002;287:591–7

5. Stampfer MJ, Colditz GA. Estrogen replacement therapy and coronary heart disease: a quantitative assessment of the epidemiologic evidence. *Prev Med* 1991;20:47–63

6. Writing Group for the Women's Health Initiative Investigators. Rossouw JE, Anderson GL, Prentice RL, *et al.* Risks and benefits of estrogen plus progestin in healthy postmenopausal women: principal results from the Women's Health Initiative randomized controlled trial. *J Am Med Assoc* 2002;288:321–33

7. Hulley S, Grady D, Bush T, *et al.* Randomized trial of estrogen plus progestin for secondary prevention of coronary heart disease in postmenopausal women. *J Am Med Assoc* 1998;280:605–13

8. Grodstein F, Manson JE, Stampfer MJ. Post menopausal hormone use and secondary prevention of coronary events in the Nurses' Health Study. *Ann Intern Med* 2001; 35:1–8

9. Schulman SP, Thiemann DR, Ouyang P, *et al.* Effects of acute hormone therapy on recurrent ischemia in postmenopausal women with unstable angina. *J Am Coll Cardiol* 2002;39:231–7

10. Mosca L, Collins P, Herrington DM, *et al.* Hormone replacement therapy and cardiovascular disease: a statement for health care professionals from the American Heart Association. *Circulation* 2001;104:499–503

11. Bonithon-Kopp C, Scarabin PY, Darne B, *et al.* Menopause-related changes in lipoproteins and some other cardiovascular risk factors. *Int J Epidemiol* 1990;19:42–8

12. Grodes D, Tonglet R. Scandinavian simvastatin study (4s). *Lancet* 1994;344:1768

13. Lewis SJ, Sacks FM, Mitchell JS, *et al.* Effect of pravastatin on cardiovascular events in women after myocardial infarction: the Choleseterol and Recurrent Events (CARE) trial. *J Am Coll Cardiol* 1998;32:140–6

14. Greendale GA, Espeland M, Slone S, *et al.* Bone mass response to discontinuation of long term hormone replacement therapy. Results from Postmenopausal Estrogen/Progestin Interventions (PEPI) Safety follow-up study. *Arch Intern Med* 2002; 162:665–72

15. Torgerson DJ, Bell-Syer SEM. Hormone replacement therapy and prevention of nonvertebral fractures; a meta-analysis of randomized trials. *J Am Med Assoc* 2001; 285:2891–7

16. Cauley JA, Zmuda JM, Ensrud KE, *et al.* Timing of estrogen replacement therapy for optimal osteoporosis prevention. *J Clin Endocrinol Metab* 2001;86:5700–5

17. National Osteoporosis Foundation. *Physician's Guide to Prevention and Treatment of Osteoporosis*. Washington, DC: NOF, 1998

18. Nanda K, Bastian LA, Schulz K. Hormone replacement therapy and the risk of death from breast cancer: a systemic review. *Am J Obstet Gynecol* 2002;186:325–34

19. Cummings SR, Duong TU, Kenyon E, *et al.* Serum estradiol level and risk of breast cancer during treatment with raloxifene. *J Am Med Assoc* 2002;287:216–20

20. Schairer C, Lubin J, Troisi R, *et al.* Menopausal estrogen and estrogen–progestin replacement therapy and breast cancer risk. *J Am Med Assoc* 2000;283:485–91

21. Gapstur SM, Morrow M, Sellers TA. Hormone replacement therapy and risk of breast cancer with a favorable histology: results of the Iowa Women's Health Study. *J Am Med Assoc* 1999;281:2091–7

22. Speroff L. Menopause and hormone replacement therapy. *Clin Geriatr Med* 1993;9:33–55

23. Grodstein F, Newcomb PA, Stampfer MJ. An incentive to start hormone replacement: the effect of postmenopausal hormone replacement therapy on the risk of colorectal cancer. *J Am Geriatr Soc* 2002;50:768–70

24. Miller J, Benjamin KS, Chan MS, Nelson HD. Postmenopausal estrogen replacement and risk for venous thromboembolism: a systemic review and meta-analysis for the U.S Preventive Task Force. *Ann Intern Med* 2002;136:680–90

25. Grady D, Wenger NK, Herrington D, *et al.* Postmenopausal hormone therapy increases risk for venous thromboembolic disease. The Heart and Estrogen/Progestin Replacement Study. *Ann Intern Med* 2000;132:689–96

26. Mulnard RA, Cotman CW, Kawas C, *et al.* Estrogen replacement therapy for treatment of mild to moderate Alzheimer's disease: a randomized controlled trial. Alzheimer's Disease Cooperative Study. *J Am Med Assoc* 2000;283:1007–15

27. Viscoli CM, Brass LM, Kernan WN, *et al.* A clinical trial of estrogen-replacement therapy after ischemic stroke. *N Engl J Med* 2001;345:1243–9

28. Grady D, Brown JS, Vittinghoff E. Postmenopausal hormones and incontinence: The Heart and Estrogen/Progestin Replacement Study. *Obstet Gynecol* 2001;97:116–20

29. Johnston CC Jr, Bjarnason NH, Cohen FJ, *et al.* Long term effects of raloxifene on bone mineral density, bone turnover, and serum lipid levels in early postmenopausal women: three-year data from 2 double-blind, randomized, placebo-controlled trials. *Arch Intern Med* 2000;160:3444–50

30. Barrett-Connor E, Grady D, Sashegyi A, *et al.* Raloxifene and cardiovascular events in osteoporotic postmenopausal women: four-year results from the MORE (Multiple Outcomes of Raloxifene Evaluation) randomized trial. *J Am Med Assoc* 2002;287:847–57

31. Ettinger B, Pressman A, Silver P. Effect of age on reason for initiation and discontinuation of hormone replacement therapy. *Menopause* 1999;6:282–9

32. Valleur JL, Wysocki S. Selection of oral contraceptives or hormone replacement therapy: patient communication and counseling issues. *Am J Obstet Gynecol* 2001;185:S57–64

33. Ansbacher R. The pharmacokinetics and efficacy of different estrogens are not equivalent. *Am J Obstet Gynecol* 2001;184:255–63

34. Notelovitz M, Funk S, Nanavati N. Estradiol absorption from vaginal tablets in postmenopausal women. *Am Coll Obstet Gynecol* 2002;99:556–62

35. Cutson TM, Mueleman E. Managing menopause. *Am Fam Physician* 2000;61:1391–406

36. North American Menopause Society. Achieving long term continuance of menopausal ERT/HRT: consensus opinion of The North American Society. *Menopause* 1998;5:69–76

37. Albertzaal P, Panisini F, Bottazzi M, *et al.* Dietary soy supplementation and phytoestrogen levels. *Obstet Gynecol* 1999;91:6–11

38. American College of Obstetricians and Gynecologists. *Hormone Replacement Therapy*. ACOG educational bulletin 247. Washington, DC: ACOG, 1998

39. U. S. Preventive Services Task Force. *Guide to Clinical Preventive Services*, 2nd edn. Baltimore: Williams & Wilkins, 1996

40. Mosca L, Grundy SM, Judelson D, *et al.* Guide to preventive cardiology for women:

AHA/ACC Scientific Statement Consensus Panel statement. *Circulation* 1999;99: 2480–4

41. Nawaz H, Katz DL. American College of Preventive Medicine practice policy statement: perimenopausal and postmenopausal hormone replacement therapy. *Am J Prev Med* 1999;17:250–4

42. North American Menopause Society. A decision tree for the use of estrogen replacement therapy or hormone replacement therapy in postmenopausal women: consensus opinion of the North American Menopause Society. *Menopause* 2000;7:76–86

43. Kaine C. Postmenopausal hormone replacement therapy: how could we have been so wrong? *Ann Intern Med* 2002; 137:290

44. Humphrey LL, Chan BKS, Sox HC. Postmenopausal hormone replacement therapy and the primary prevention of cardiovascular disease. *Ann Intern Med* 2002;137:273-84

45. Gupta G, Aronow WS. Hormone replacement therapy. An analysis of efficacy based on evidence. *Geriatrics* 2002;57:18–24

46. Thacker HL. The case for hormone replacement: new studies that should inform the debate. *Cleveland Clin J Med* 2002;69:670–8

47. *The New York Times* Editorial. Hormone therapy woes. 2002; July 11

58 HIV and aging

Robert A. Norman, DO, MPH

OVERVIEW

Over 10% of all new AIDS cases in the USA occur in people over the age of 50[1]. New AIDS cases in the past several years rose faster in middle age and older people than in people under 40[2]. Although many of these AIDS cases are the result of HIV infection at a younger age, several are due to becoming infected after age 50. Because very few persons over the age of 50 at risk for HIV routinely get tested, it is difficult to determine rates of HIV infection among older adults[3]. Older adults are often first diagnosed with HIV at a late stage of infection, when they seek treatment for an HIV-related illness. HIV cases among older people may be under-reported because HIV symptoms and infections may coincide with other diseases associated with aging and therefore be overlooked. Fatigue, weight loss and other early HIV symptoms may be dismissed as a normal part of aging. AIDS-related dementia is often misdiagnosed as Alzheimer's disease[4].

Many characteristics of HIV are specific for older persons. The elderly with AIDS get sick and die sooner than younger persons, due to late diagnosis of the disease as well as co-infection with other diseases that may speed the progression of AIDS[5]. In addition, new drugs for HIV treatment may interact with medications the older person is taking to treat pre-existing chronic conditions.

A common stereotype is that – 'older people don't have sex or use drugs'. Few HIV-prevention efforts are aimed at people over 50, and most educational advertising campaigns rarely show older adults, selecting them as an invisible at-risk population[6]. Older adults, therefore, are generally less knowledgeable about HIV/AIDS than younger individuals and less aware of how to protect themselves against infection. This lack of awareness is especially true for older injecting drug users, who comprise over 16% of AIDS cases over age 50.

DEMOGRAPHICS/EPIDEMIOLOGY

Men who have sex with men form the largest group of AIDS cases among adults over 50. Older gay men tend to be invisible and ignored both in the gay community and in prevention. Among the HIV risk factors for older gay men are internalized homophobia, denial of risk, alcohol and other substance use, and anonymous sexual encounters[7].

Although AIDS has afflicted persons of all ages, only recently has attention been devoted to AIDS in older persons. To examine the epidemiology of AIDS in persons aged ≥ 50 years in the USA, cases reported to the Centers for Disease Control were analyzed. From 1981 to 1989 the number of AIDS patients reported annually in persons ≥ 50 years old increased from 13 to 3562. Through December 1989, 11 984 cases had been reported, which represented 10% of all cases. Male homosexual contact accounted for most cases in persons aged 50–69.

However, blood transfusion became a more common means of exposure with increasing age, accounting for 28% of cases in persons aged 60–69 and 64% of cases in individuals aged ≥ 70. The proportion of women increased from 6.1% in persons with AIDS aged 50–59 to 28.7% of those aged ≥ 70. Older women are at higher risk for HIV infection during intercourse, contributed by normal aging changes such as a decrease in vaginal lubrication and thinning vaginal walls[8].

The proportion of AIDS diagnoses made in the same month as death increased from 16% in persons aged 50–59 to 37% in those aged ≥ 80, which suggested either more rapid progression of disease or increasing delay in diagnosis. As the incidence in older persons continues to increase, clinicians caring for older patients must become more familiar with AIDS[9].

PREVENTION BARRIERS

Few Americans over age 50 who are at risk for HIV infection either use condoms or get tested for HIV. In a national survey, at-risk people over 50 were one-sixth as likely to use condoms and one-fifth as likely to have been tested for HIV than at-risk people in their 20s[3]. Factors that influence condom use in older persons are not clear. Doctors and nurses often do not consider HIV to be a risk for their older patients. A study of doctors in Texas found that most doctors rarely or never asked patients older than 50 years questions about HIV/AIDS or discussed risk factor reduction. Doctors were much less likely to ask patients over age 50 about HIV risk factors (40%) than they were to ask patients under 30 (6.8%)[10].

LONG-TERM CARE

Many older people live in assisted living communities, where there is still great stigma attached to HIV/AIDS, often associated with homosexuality and/or substance abuse.

Management may be resistant to providing HIV/AIDS educational materials or presentations in their facilities.

KNOWLEDGE, ATTITUDES AND BEHAVIOR

Cultural and generational issues need to be considered in crafting HIV prevention efforts. Older persons may not be comfortable disclosing their sexual behaviors or drug use to others. This can make it difficult to find older adults who attend support groups[11]. Also, older adults may not view condom use as important or necessary. This is especially true in postmenopausal women, who need not worry about pregnancy protection.

Older adults may have fewer surviving friends and a smaller social network to provide support and care. Also, they are more likely to be caregivers themselves, as about one-third of AIDS patients are dependent on an older parent for financial, physical or emotional support[12].

SERVICE MODELS

Unfortunately, few prevention programs exist that target adults over 50. Most programs for older adults offer support for HIV-positive persons, or target clinicians and caregivers of older adults. Promising prevention programs incorporate generational concerns, target high-risk groups such as older gay men and older women (especially recent widows), and involve older adults in their design and as peer educators.

The Senior HIV Intervention Project (SHIP) in Florida's Dade, Broward and Palm Beach Counties trains older peer educators to present educational and safer sex seminars at retirement communities. Trained AIDS educators meet with health-care professionals and aging services workers to help them understand the risk posed to seniors by HIV[13].

In six regional senior centers in Chicago, a program used peer-led 'study circles' to increase HIV awareness and knowledge. Participants viewed a video, 'The Forgotten Tenth', and did their own research as to how HIV affected their lives physically, politically and economically. They then shared their knowledge at the next meetings. After the program, many participants became AIDS educators[14].

An HIV education program for older adults was conducted at meal sites in Florida. Based on the Health Belief Model, the program included facts and statistics on older persons and HIV, condom use instruction, HIV testing information and case studies of older persons with AIDS. After the session, participants reported a significant increase in knowledge about AIDS and perceived susceptibility to HIV[15].

Older adults need support and education to ensure that their lives over 50 are as rewarding and safe as before 50. A comprehensive HIV prevention strategy uses many elements to protect as many people at risk for HIV as possible. Adults over 50 are an especially important group to target with prevention messages, both for their own risk behaviors and for their role as leaders and teachers of younger generations.

CASE STUDIES

Women in midlife and older represent over 25% of all women with AIDS and 4% of all reported AIDS cases in the USA. Overall safer sex practices among older women who reported sexual risk behaviors were minimal. Between 90 and 100% had not used condoms in the previous 6 months. Moreover, almost 90% of the women who reported a risk behavior did not perceive themselves to be at risk[16].

In New York City, to assess the extent of HIV infection among elderly patients, serum samples were retrieved from patients 60 years or older without a history of HIV infection, but who died during a 1-year period at an institution. Serum samples were tested for the presence of HIV antibodies and the charts of all those found to be infected with HIV were reviewed. The results showed 13 (5.05%) of 257 serum samples were HIV-antibody positive. Six (6.5%) of 92 men and seven (8.9%) of 78 women between the ages of 60 and 79 years were infected with HIV, with more women having HIV infection. The death of none of the 13 patients with HIV infection was attributable to HIV infection. The researchers concluded that elderly patients from certain high HIV seroprevalence communities might be at significant risk of HIV infection. The impact of this unrecognized infection on health requires further evaluation. HIV prevention and education programs should include the elderly, and studies of HIV seroprevalence in this population should be supported[17].

An estimated 8–10 million people worldwide are infected with HIV, the virus causing AIDS; a large proportion live in developing countries. A review of the recent literature by de Bruyn[18] revealed that the impact of HIV/AIDS is particularly great on women in developing countries for four reasons:

(1) Stereotypes related to HIV/AIDS have meant that women are either blamed for their spread or not recognized as potential patients with the disease. The consequences can include delayed diagnosis and treatment, stigmatization, loss of income and violations of human rights;

(2) Women are at increased risk of exposure to HIV infection for reasons related indirectly and directly to their gender;

(3) The psychologic and social burdens are greater for women than men in a similar situation. These may include problems related to pregnancy and motherhood, rejection as marital partners, loss of security and income (if they or their partners

are seropositive) and greater demands to cope with the effects of the epidemic, both as lay persons and as professionals;

(4) Women's frequently low socioeconomic status and lack of power make it difficult for them to undertake prevention measures.

de Bruyn stated that 'prevention programs targeting sex workers have begun and need to be continued. More programs are needed for women in general, including older women, men, traditional health practitioners and opinion leaders, incorporating seropositive women wherever possible. In addition, HIV/AIDS-related research involving women must be increased as well as their access to adequate health services and income-earning opportunities'[18].

Gordon and Thompson described the epidemiology of HIV infection diagnosed in persons aged 60 years and older at a large urban county hospital[19]. Retrospective chart reviews were performed on patients aged 60 years and older, diagnosed with HIV infection, among 6493 patients identified with positive enzyme immunoassay HIV tests. The results showed a total of 32 HIV-infected elderly patients, including 27 men and five women, with a mean age of 64.8 years (range 60–83 years). HIV testing of 47% (15/32) patients was performed after a diagnosis of opportunistic infection. Among 24 elderly patients who presented with signs or symptoms of HIV infection, testing for HIV was often delayed (median 3.1 months). Eleven patients underwent workups to rule out a malignancy, and three were initially diagnosed with organic brain syndrome. Ten of the 32 patients (31%) had a history of syphilis.

Gordon and Thompson concluded that the majority of HIV-infected patients 60 years or older acquired their infection through sexual intercourse or intravenous drug use. The diagnosis of HIV infection in the elderly was usually not considered by clinicians until late in the course of infection, despite a high prevalence of prior sexually transmitted diseases (STDs). Their data indicated that clinicians who take care of elderly patients should take a complete sexual history and offer sexual education. HIV testing and counseling should be considered for all individuals with a history of recent STDs or reporting behaviors placing them at risk for HIV infection[19].

Lieberman[20] prepared an epidemiologic perspective on HIV and concluded as follows. The elderly population is increasing as baby boomers are beginning to approach retirement. People 65 years of age or older already constitute approximately one-eighth of the population of the USA; this proportion is expected to double in the next 50 years. Older Americans have their own population-specific health challenges, such as Alzheimer's disease, osteoporosis, adult-onset diabetes, prostate cancer, menopause and hypertension. HIV infection and AIDS are seldom discussed within this community. Prevention, counseling, testing and education efforts are not being directed their way. In addition, few practitioners are experts in both HIV and health problems associated with aging, resulting in misdiagnosis, especially in the early stages when AIDS symptoms such as fatigue, weight loss, night sweats and diminished appetite are dismissed as part of the aging process.

Very few HIV-related social support services have been aimed at the needs of the elderly, perhaps because older Americans are not suspected of being sexually active or are assumed to be in a monogamous, heterosexual relationship. Older Americans are not suspected of drug use. Nevertheless, many are sexually active, often demonstrating risky sexual behavior, such as dispensing with the use of condoms; and the isolation that frequently accompanies old age can lead to alcoholism and injectable drug use. Primary and secondary prevention of HIV/AIDS in older Americans, the cost of these efforts and organizations that gear their efforts toward reaching and educating older Americans regarding their risks are reviewed by Lieberman[20].

Many Americans mistakenly believe that older adults are not at risk for HIV/AIDS. Older people do not perceive themselves to be at risk for HIV infection, either, according to a study by Wooten-Bielski[21]. In reality, approximately 10% of AIDS cases are among people older than 50. Many health care providers lack an awareness of the risk of HIV/AIDS in the elderly population and, as a result, many older people with these conditions are misdiagnosed with other ailments. Major manifestations of HIV/AIDS in elderly adults include *Pneumocystis carinii* pneumonia, herpes zoster, tuberculosis, cytomegalovirus, oral thrush, *Mycobacterium avium* complex and HIV dementia. Elderly HIV-positive women have special health concerns, such as cervical cancer[21].

PREVENTION AND EDUCATION

There has been a striking lack of interest in people over 50 in HIV prevention efforts. Prevention programs are needed specifically for older adults. Mainstream advertising campaigns need to incorporate images and issues concerning persons over 50 and encourage at-risk older adults to be routinely tested for HIV. More research on sexual and drug using behavior of older adults is needed, as well as research on disease progression and treatments, including recruiting HIV-positive older persons for clinical trials.

Clinicians and service providers for older adults, including caregivers and nursing home staff, need to be educated on HIV risk behaviors and symptoms of HIV infection pertinent to older adults. Clinicians need to conduct thorough risk assessments for sex and drug use in patients over 50, and challenge any assumptions that older people do not engage in these activities or will not discuss them.

As Laura Engle wrote, 'We often hear how the face of AIDS is changing, with people of color, women, children, and heterosexuals now making up a greater proportion of the HIV community. What we seldom hear is that the face is also aging. People are living longer with the virus than ever before, and if new medications live up to even a fraction of their promise, the HIV-positive baby boomers will continue to swell the older AIDS population as well as demand services that meet their needs'[22].

References

1. Centers for Disease Control and Prevention. *HIV/AIDS Surveillance Report.* 1997;8:15
2. Genke J. HIV, AIDS, and older adults the invisible 10%. *Care Manag J* 2000;2: 196–205
3. Stall R, Catania J. AIDS risk behaviors among late middle-aged and elderly Americans. The National AIDS Behavioral Surveys. *Arch Intern Med* 1994;154:57–63
4. Whipple B, Scura KW. The overlooked epidemic: HIV in older adults. *Am J Nurs* 1996;96:22–8
5. Skiest DJ, Rubinstien E, Carley N, et al. The importance of comorbidity in HIV-infected patients over 55: a retrospective case–control study. *Am J Med* 1996;101: 605–11
6. Feldman MD. Sex, AIDS, and the elderly. *Arch Intern Med* 1994;154:19–20
7. Grossman AH. At risk, infected, and invisible: older gay men and HIV/AIDS. *J Assoc Nurs AIDS Care* 1995;6:13–19
8. Catania JA, Turner H, Kegeles SM, et al. Older Americans and AIDS: transmission risks and primary prevention research needs. *Gerontologist* 1989;29:373–81
9. Ship JA, Wolff A, Selik RM. Epidemiology of acquired immune deficiency syndrome in persons aged 50 years or older. *J Acquired Immune Defic Syndromes* 1991;4:84–8

10. Skiest DJ, Keiser P. Human immunodeficiency virus infection in patients older than 50 years. A survey of primary care physicians' beliefs, practices, and knowledge. *Arch Fam Med* 1997;6:289–94

11. Nokes K, ed. *HIV/AIDS and the Older Adult*. Washington DC: Taylor & Francis, 1996

12. Ory MG, Zablotsky D. Notes for the future: research, prevention, care, public policy. In Riley MW, Ory MG, Zablotsky D, eds. *AIDS in an Aging Society*. New York: Springer Publishing, 1989

13. Senior HIV Intervention Project (SHIP). Contact: Lisa Agate (954) 467-4774

14. Dill D, Huston W. AIDS education for older adults. Healthpro UIC. 1996; Fall: 18–19. Contact: Rita Strombeck, HealthCare Education Associates (760) 323-4032

15. Rose MA. Effect of an AIDS education program for older adults. *J Commun Health Nurs* 1996;13:141–8

16. Binson D, Pollack L, Catania JA. AIDS-related risk behaviors and safer sex practices of women in midlife and older in the United States: 1990 to 1992. *Health Care Women Int* 1997;18:343–54

17. el-Sadr W, Gettler J. Unrecognized human immunodeficiency virus infection in the elderly. *Arch Intern Med* 1995;155: 184–6

18. de Bruyn M. Women and AIDS in developing countries. *Soc Sci Med* 1992;34: 249–62

19. Gordon SM, Thompson S. The changing epidemiology of human immunodeficiency virus infection in older persons. *J Am Geriatr Soc* 1995;43:7–9

20. Lieberman RJ. HIV in older Americans: an epidemiologic perspective. State University of New York (SUNY) Health Science Center at Brooklyn, USA. *Midwifery Womens Health* 2000;45:176–82

21. Wooten-Bielski K. HIV and AIDS in older adults. *Geriatr Nurs* 1999;20: 268–72

22. Engle L. Old Aids. *Body Positive* 1998;xi:1

USEFUL CONTACTS

Center for AIDS Prevention Studies at the University of California San Franciso
Collaborative HIV Prevention Research in Minority Communities
74 New Montgomery St, Suite 600
San Francisco, CA 94105
(415) 597-9162
(415) 597-9213 Fax
BMarin@psg.ucsf.edu

National Library of Medicine
(Internet search)

NY HIV Over 50 Task Force
Brookdale Center on Aging
Hunter College
425 E 25th Street
New York, NY 10010
(212) 481-7594

American Association of Retired Persons (AARP)
Social Outreach and Support (SOS)
601 E Street, NW
Washington, DC 20049
(202) 434-2260

National Association on HIV Over Fifty (NAHOF)
Midwest AIDS Training & Education Center
(Source of HIV and Aging Issues Bibliography)
University of Illinois
808 S. Wood Street m/c 779
Chicago, IL 60612
(312) 996-1426

American Association of Retired Persons. (1997) HIV/AIDS: It Could Happen to Me (Video Kit). Washington, DC: AARP.

HealthCare Education Associates.
The Forgotten Tenth (Video)
1729 E. Palm Canyon Drive, Suite A
Palm Springs, CA 92264

Index